Eberhard Teuscher
Medicinal Spices

Medicinal Spices

A Handbook of Culinary Herbs, Spices, Spice Mixtures and Their Essential Oils

Eberhard Teuscher, Triebes, Germany

With contributions from
Ulrike Bauermann, Bergholz-Rehbrücke, Germany
Monika Werner, Montjoi, France

Translated from German by
Josef A. Brinckmann, Sebastopol, USA
Michael P. Lindenmaier, Eugene, USA

With a foreword by
James A. Duke, Fulton, USA

173 full color illustrations
36 black-and-white illustrations
498 chemical structures

medpharm
Scientific Publishers Stuttgart

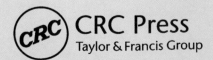
CRC Press
Taylor & Francis Group

Addresses of the Authors:

Prof. Dr. Eberhard Teuscher
Goethestr. 9
D-07950 Triebes, Germany

Ulrike Bauermann
Institut für Getreideverarbeitung
Arthur-Scheunert-Allee 40-41
D-14558 Bergholz-Rehbrücke, Germany

Monika Werner
Place de la Fontaine
F-11330 Montjoi, France

Translators:

Josef A. Brinckmann
Sebastopol, California USA

Michael P. Lindenmaier
Eugene, Oregon USA

Title of original German edition:
Gewürzdrogen. Ein Handbuch der Gewürze, Gewürzkräuter, Gewürzmischungen und ihrer Ätherischen Öle
© 2003 Wissenschaftliche Verlagsgesellschaft mbH, Birkenwaldstrasse 44, 70191 Stuttgart, Germany
All rights reserved

Translated from the German by Josef A. Brinckmann and Michael P. Lindenmaier

Bibliographic information published by Die Deutsche Bibliothek
Die Deutsche Bibliothek lists this publication in the Deutsche Nationalbibliografie; Detailed bibliographic data is available in the Internet at http://dnb.ddb.de.

Cataloguing-in-Publication Data available from the Library of Congress

Sole distribution for North America granted to CRC Press, Taylor and Francis Group, LLC, 6000 Broken Sound Parkway, NW, Suite 300, Boca Raton, FL 33487, USA

ISBN 3-88763-103-X medpharm Scientific Publishers, Stuttgart
ISBN 0-8493-1962-5 CRC Press, Boca Raton, London, New York, Washington, D.C.

Printed in Germany
Composition, Printing and Binding: Stürtz GmbH, Würzburg
Cover Design: Atelier Schäfer, Esslingen

Foreword

Most of us are aware that herbs and spices can work magic on drab entrees, converting them into exciting culinary experiences. But few of us realize that these aromatic plants are also among the most important antiinflammatory, antioxidant (hence antiaging) and immune-boosting foods that we have, with the power to improve and even extend our lives.

It is with genuine pleasure and anticipation that I welcome a new translation by medpharm Scientific Publishers. Covering some 300 plant species with nearly 100 monographs, Eberhard Teuscher and translators Josef A. Brinckmann and Michael P. Lindenmaier dish us up a well-formatted overview of the herbs and spices. **Medicinal Spices** not only covers their culinary and medicinal potential, but also provides information on cultivation, production, constituents, organoleptic characteristics and biological activities, warning us where potential toxicity lurks.

This great translation tells us why, when and where to usc herbs and spices. Equally importantly, the authors reveal **how** to utilize them to convert dull dishes into tasty, satisfying experiences that are at the same time health-boosters, enhancing and possibly even extending our lives when they are combined with good dietary, exercise and stress-management regimes.

Having read their account of a European shrub, the juniper, and one of the most important of American spices, the vanilla, I can say that the reader is in for a treat.

James A. Duke
Ethnobotanist
Fulton, Maryland, USA

Preface to the English Edition

For good reason, there exists a popular German folk saying: *The seasoning makes the roast*. Besides visual appearance, odor and taste play the most important role in terms of acceptance and wholesomeness of foods. Nutritious food products are often rejected by people if they are not enjoyable. Therefore, we zest the foods. Spices do not only add to the enjoyment of foods and increase the love of life, they can also be beneficial to human health if they are used appropriately within a reasonable dosage range.

Hundreds of books on culinary herbs and spices as well as spice mixtures are currently on the market. This indicates that the ancient art of seasoning is still popular and continues to gain momentum.

The aim of this book is to present the scientific and medical aspects of culinary herbs and spices, and among others to work up our knowledge of botany, cultivation of spice plants and the production of culinary herbs and spices, their chemistry, and the analysis of their constituents, physiological effects as well as their toxicology and medicinal application. In order to fascinate the reader about the fine art of seasoning, this book also includes information about the cultivation of culinary herbs in the garden or on the balcony, their commercial forms as well as their storage and use in cooking. The use of spices can be a special event particularly if the fragrances of exotic foods are captured at home. In order to give the reader the possibility to appreciate the value of culinary herbs and spices, in many of the monographs simple recipes for experimenting and aroma testing are included. An attempt has been made to choose those types of dishes, which only include one type or just a few culinary herbs and spices in order to demonstrate the typical flavor of an herb or spice. Try yourself!

The book is divided into 2 parts, a general section and the specific monographs. The general section provides an overview of facts about herbs and spices that can be generalized; it also should contribute to a better understanding of the specific monographs. The monograph section describes the most important culinary herbs and spices. Many monographs are followed by short supplementary paragraphs describing herbs and spices, which are only used rarely or not at all in Central Europe. Since thousands of plants are used as spices, the list is, of course, not exhaustive. Evaluated were scientific papers that were found through literature research of periodicals relevant for this particular field, from the author's own file of references and from Hager's Handbook of Pharmaceutical Practice (4th edition, 5th edition and subsequent volumes), as well as from references of the last 5 annual volumes of Chemical Abstracts, internet literature, specialty literature and cook books (→ Index of books and monographs used as general references at the back of this book) and the secondary literature cited in the aforementioned publications. Not all of the publications cited were read by the author in their original form. Sometimes facts were taken from abstracts or review papers. Hence, the page numbers are not always noted. The literature list is structured in such a way that the reader can access it in order to solidify his/her knowledge and possibly conduct one's own investigations. The book also tries to verify relevant findings. A complete verification was of course not possible since the literature list would have become far too large. The individual herbs and spices were investigated quite differently by various international research groups. An internet search for soybean generated about 35,000 hits for literature citations; for garlic, there

were about 1,300 citations. For a few other herbs and spices, relevant literature citations were not available; the selection and "omission" criteria were difficult for the author, particularly for the well-researched spices (e.g. garlic, paprika, pepper, and soy bean).

This book is intended primarily for pharmacists, physicians, biologists, and interested students and laypersons, but also for food scientists who are interested in the chemical and pharmacological-toxicological aspects of culinary herbs and spices.

The color illustrations should familiarize the reader with the appearance of herbs and spices and their plant sources. Pictures of comminuted herbs and spices were not included since they are only of minor importance for the consumer. Line drawings of microscopic images are only shown if the powder shows conspicuous features or if they are significant for trade and as a component of spice mixtures. Only relevant microscopic features are shown; atypical powder components, e.g. parenchymatic, sclerenchymatic and vascular tissue, starch, etc., are mentioned in the text. Chemical structures are only shown for selected substances that contribute to the odor, taste or color, or in some cases to the therapeutic and toxicological effects. The more important structures of chemicals, which are typical for a specific culinary herb or spice, are reproduced in the individual monographs. Chemical structures of common essential oil components are compiled in chapter 2.2, mostly without indicating their steric structures; individual components can be found using the subject index. From compounds with unequivocal rational names chemical structural formulae (chemical structure diagrams) are not drawn.

I am especially grateful to Prof. M. Wichtl, Mödling (Austria), who inspired me to write this book, and I also would like to thank Dr. K.G. Brauer, Medpharm Scientific Publishers, Stuttgart (Germany), for accepting me as an author. I am also thankful to the staff of Medpharm Scientific Publishers, particularly Dr. E. Scholz, for his cooperative effort preparing the design of the book.

Many thanks also go to Mrs. U. Bauermann, Potsdam-Rehbrücke (Germany) and Mrs. M. Werner, Montjoi (France), for their contributions and support. My thanks also go out to all of my colleagues who placed their photos at my disposal for illustration of the book.

Constructive discussions and valuable advice from many colleagues helped the author to write this book, above all agronomist Dipl. Ing. P. Achermann, Basel (Switzerland), Dr. M. Börnchen, Drensteinfurt (Germany), Dr. Ch. Rotta, Stuttgart (Germany), apothecary Mr. K.H. Schnitter, Oberwolfach (Germany), Mrs. I. Schönfelder and Prof. P. Schönfelder, Regensburg (Germany), Mrs. A. Teige, Gera (Germany), Dipl. pharm. S. Tiemann and Dr. D. Tiemann, Dassow (Germany), as well as Mrs. Dr. W. Wichtl and Prof. M. Wichtl (Austria); I would like to express my gratitude to all of them. For providing the specimens of dried culinary herbs and spices, I would like to thank the companies Caesar and Loretz GmbH, Hilden (Germany), Gera Gewürze GmbH, Gera (Germany), Hamburger Gewürzmühle GmbH, Hamburg (Germany), and especially the firm SUNDAVital OHG, Wolfach (Germany).

I am also very grateful to my wife, Dr. G. Teuscher, in her tireless effort to proofread the German manuscript and galley proof. I express my gratitude to Josef A. Brinckmann, Sebastopol (California, USA) and Michael P. Lindenmaier, Eugene (Oregon, USA), translators and specialists, for the translation of the sometimes very difficult texts and for good cooperation with the author.

Due the diversity of the presented data, and the inherent possibilities for errors, I am grateful for any critical suggestions and advice on the content and layout of the book.

Triebes, Thuringia, Germany, Winter 2005
Eberhard Teuscher

Table of Contents

List of Abbreviations

AB-DDR   Pharmacopoeia of the former German Democratic Republic, final valid edition 1989
ADI   Acceptable daily intake

BAnz   Bundesanzeiger (German Federal Gazette), edited by the German Federal Minister of Justice
Bcq   Becquerel, the unit for measuring of the activity of radioactive substances
BfArM   Bundesinstitut für Arzneimittel und Medizinprodukte (German Federal Institute for Drugs and Medical Devices)
BGBl   Bundesgesetzblatt (German Federal Law Gazette), edited by the German Federal Minister of Justice
BHP   British Herbal Pharmacopoeia, BHP 83, 2nd edition 1983, BHP 90, 3rd edition 1990

cfu   Colony forming units
ChinP IX   Chinese Pharmacopoeia, IX edition 1988

Da   Dalton, atomic mass unit
DAB   Deutsches Arzneibuch (German Pharmacopoeia) 2001
DAB 6   Deutsches Arzneibuch (German Pharmacopoeia), 6th edition, 1926
DAC   Deutscher Arzneimittel-Codex (German Drug Codex) 2001
DAC 86   Deutscher Arzneimittel-Codex (German Drug Codex) 1986
DAD   Diode array detector
DIN   Deutsches Institut für Normung (German Institute for Standardization), Berlin

EB6   Ergänzungsbuch zum Deutschen Arzneibuch (Supplement Volume to German Pharmacopoeia), 6th edition 1941
EC$_{50}$ The average active concentration that can cause a defined effect in 50% of the test animals
ELISA   Enzyme linked immunosorbent assay, immunological method for determination of content
ESCOP   European Scientific Cooperative on Phytotherapy, Exeter, GB

FDA   Food and Drug Administration, regulatory authority for foods and drugs in the USA
FID   Flame ionization detector
FTIR   Fourier-transformation infrared spectroscopy detection

GC   Gas chromatography
GLC   Gas liquid chromatography
GUS   Russian Federation, comprises a large part of the former Soviet Union
Gy   Gray, a unit for the absorbed dose of ionizing radiation (replaces "Rad")

HAB   Homöopathisches Arzneibuch (German Homoeopathic Pharmacopoeia) 2001
HDL   High density lipoproteins
HPLC   High performance liquid chromatography

IFN   Interferon
i.p.   Intraperitoneal, in the abdominal area
i.v.   Intravenous, in the veins
IRMS   Isotope ratio mass spectrometry
ISO   International Organization for Standardization, Geneva

kDa   Kilodalton, → Da

LC   Liquid chromatography
LD$_{50}$ Lethal dose, the dose at which 50% of the test animals will die
LDL   Low density lipoproteins
LPS   Lipopolysaccharides, cell wall components of gram-negative bacteria

MEKC   Micellar electrokinetic chromatography
MIC   Minimum inhibitory concentration of a compound that stops the growth of microorganisms
MS   Mass spectrometry

ÖAB   Österreichisches Arzneibuch (Austrian Pharmacopoeia) 2001

p.o.   Peroral, through the mouth
PF X   Pharmacopée Française (French Pharmacopoeia), 10th edition 1988
Ph Eur   Pharmacopoea Europaea (European Pharmacopoeia), 4th edition 2002
Ph Helv   Pharmacopoea Helvetica (Swiss Pharmacopoeia) 2001; Ph Helv V, 1933 edition; Ph Helv VI, 1972 edition; Ph Helv VII, 1987 edition

RP-HPLC   Reversed phase HPLC

s. c.   Subcutaneous, under the skin
SDS-PAGE   Sodium-dodecyl-sulphate-polyacrylamide gel electrophoresis
SFC   Supercritical fluid extraction chromatography
SFE   Supercritical fluid extraction

TLC   Thin-layer chromatography
TMS   Tetramethylsilane
TPA   12-Tetradecanoyl-phorbol-13-acetate (cocarcinogenic active substance)

VLDL   Very low-density lipoproteins

General Part

1 Spices, Herbs, Seasoning Ingredients

Spices are biogenetic substances of complex nature that serve as food ingredients, providing taste and odor. They are also used in the commercial production of such food ingredients. Thus spices are not only fresh, dried or otherwise preserved plants or plant parts that are intended for seasoning, but also compounds that are obtained from plants, e.g. essential oils or oleoresins. In the industrial food sector, individual seasoning ingredients are defined differently. In this sector the definitions are rendered as those stipulated in the Guidelines of the German Food Compendium (LBM) [Ü40].

Herbs and spices are plant parts, which due to their natural constituents content are intended for use as food ingredients for providing taste and odor. Spices are flowers, fruits, buds, seeds, barks, roots, rhizomes, bulbs or parts thereof, usually in dried form. Herbs are fresh or dried leaves, flowers, shoots or parts thereof. So for example caraway, clove, and cinnamon are spices while lemon balm, marjoram, and borage are herbs. The same plant can produce either spices, e.g. dill fruits, or an aromatic herb, e.g. dill tops.

Spice mixtures are blends that are composed exclusively of spices, e.g. → Curry powder, → Gingerbread spice, → Herbes de Provence.

Seasoning blends or spice preparations are mixtures of one or more spices with other ingredients that provide and/or affect taste, as well as with technologically necessary substances. They contain minimum 60% spices. Spice aromas are also used, e.g. onion-pepper-spice preparations. Spice preparations are intended for sale to product manufacturers, e.g. spice preparation for making pork sausage.

Spice aromas are products that are obtained from spices with suitable extraction solvents and contain only these extracts and/or natural flavoring substances.

Seasoning salts are mixtures of table salt with one or more spices and/or seasoning blends/spice preparations that are also used as seasonings. They contain minimum 15% spices (except for garlic) and more than 40% table salt, e.g. celery-, chicken-, cutlet-, garlic-, and onion-spice salt.

Spice aroma preparations are spice preparations, in which the spices are partly or completely replaced by spice aromas, e.g. spice aroma preparations for roast chicken.

Aromatic salts are seasoning salts, in which the spices are partly or completely replaced by spice aromas, e.g. vegetable seasoning salt.

Seasonings are liquid, paste-like or dry products, which are used to impact the taste and/or odor of soups, meat broths and other foods. They are manufactured by hydrolysis of protein-rich substances, e.g. soy sauce and soup spice.

Seasoning mixes are solid or liquid products, which are composed mainly of flavor enhancers, table salt, and the usual types of sugars or other carriers; additionally they may contain seasonings, as well as yeasts, vegetables, mushrooms, spices, aromatic herbs and/or extracts thereof, e.g. spaghetti seasoning mix. Powdered seasoning mixes can be added to foods with a seasoning shaker. Seasoning pastes have a pasty consistency.

Seasoning sauces are flowable or paste-like preparations with distinctively spicy taste made of crushed and/or liquid ingredients, e.g. Worcestershire sauce and pepper sauce [Ü40].

Other frequently used terms include:

Spice additives include all commercially produced products that indeed have a flavor impact on food, but are not classified within the named product groups according to the above-cited guidelines. Ingredients belonging to this category include, among others, bouillon cubes, organic acids (e.g. acetic acid), cooking salt, flavor enhancers (e.g. glutamate), essential oils, sweeteners and foods, being suited as seasonings (e.g. tomato purée, sugar, fruit syrup).

Collectively, spices and spice-containing products and condiments can be combined under the term **flavoring substance** [Ü30].

Spice concentrates (spice extracts) are obtained by extraction of spices and spice mixtures, with the use of carriers, e.g. starch, salt, glucose or lactose, dried or concentrated, aqueous, ethanolic or microencapsulated liquid, pasty or powdery seasonings with a precisely defined spicing strength. They are traded in sealed airtight containers, practically sterile, and good to measure [Ü92, Ü98].

Instant seasonings are industrially produced spice preparations that are mostly cube-shaped and contain admixtures, e.g. offered in the flavor types curry or sweet herbs [Ü92].

Spice granulates are made by granulating powdered spices or powdered spice mixtures with or without the addition of salt or glutamate. They are easily measured for food preparation [Ü92].

Essences are concentrated preparations of flavor compounds of natural or synthetic origin that are not intended for direct consumption [Ü98]. Natural essences are made from natural products such as fruit, fruit parts, spices or the essential oils obtained from them, e.g. lemon essence. They serve as flavorings of bakery goods, refreshing beverages, confectionaries, margarine, noodles, and desserts, e.g. pudding or ice cream, of effervescent powder, chewing gum, potable spirits and liqueurs [Ü92, Ü98].

2 Quality-indicating constituents of spices

2.1 Spectrum of constituents and content ratios

The spectrum of plant constituents, i.e. the compounds present and their content ratios, is mostly dependent on genetics. Plants belonging to the same species often have a number of genetically different chemical races with characteristic constituent profiles. For example, thyme, *Thymus vulgaris* L., has chemical races with e.g. thymol, carvacrol, *p*-cymene, linalool or α-terpineol as the dominant components of the essential oil obtained from the herb. For the cultivation of medicinal plants, chemical races with a specific constituent profile are selected. Thus, thyme must contain at least 0.5% steam-distillable phenols (thymol and carvacrol), calculated with reference to the dried herb [Ph Eur]; races with *p*-cymene, linalool or α-terpineol as the dominant essential oil components are excluded from cultivation. For growing culinary herbs and spice plants, cultivars with distinct sensory qualities are selected; hence, variations of the constituent profile are also limited to a narrow range.

The spectrum of constituents is also dependant on the plant parts. The essential oil from the bark of the Ceylon cinnamon tree, for example, contains mostly cinnamic aldehyde while the main component of the essential oil from the leaves is usually eugenol, or in some races safrole; in the essential oil of the root bark, camphor is the predominant constituent.

The stage of development of the plant influences its spectrum of constituents in a similar way. For example, caraway fruits show an increase of the carvone content of the essential oil during ripening, while at the same time, the limonene content decreases.

Environmental factors can also modify the spectrum of plant constituents within a certain range. A number of modifying environmental factors should be considered: Type and intensity of light exposure, temperature, air circulation, amount of precip-

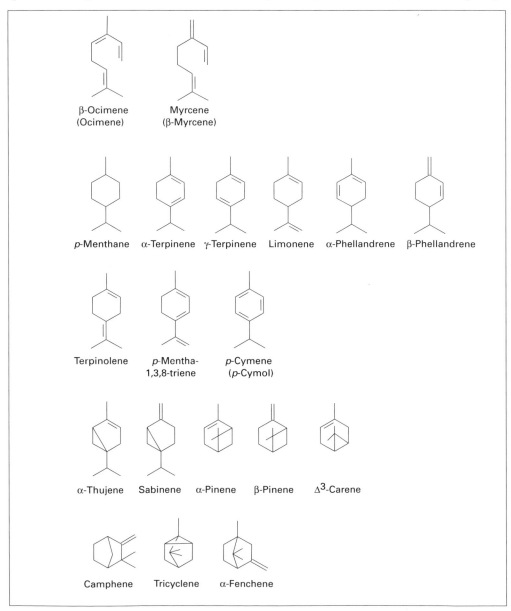

Fig. 1 Monoterpene hydrocarbons as essential oil components

itation, physical as well as chemical soil conditions and stress factors (for example, infection with certain microorganisms can lead to an increased content of toxic plant constituents, known as phytoalexins). Other factors which significantly influence the qualitative and quantitative composition of the constituents of herbs and spices are growing techniques (time of planting and harvest, plant care, use of fertilizers, etc.), degree of maturity and weather at the time of harvest, method of harvest, temporal succession of cuts, type of post-harvest processing (fermentation, drying, transport, comminution), as well as possible sterilization and/or disinfestation treatment, type of packaging, as well as duration of and conditions of storage. Therefore, standards for spice crops (DIN- and ISO-Standards, Austrian and Swiss Food Codex) are in effect, which regulate the concentration range for certain constituent groups, for example essential oils, and also require upper and lower limits for important components of constituent groups.

The following sections deal with the different constituent groups mostly responsible for odor, taste and color of culinary herbs and spices.

2.2 Essential oils

Essential oils (also designated as volatile oils) are mixtures of lipophilic, volatile and mostly liquid constituents, which are produced by plants and deposited by them in their special storage structures. These oils can be separated with physical methods from the plants, and they also carry their characteristic odor. In the spice trade, they are sometimes called "spice oils".

Essential oils are produced in the cytoplasm by the plant's secretory cells and stored in these cells (the cell turns into an oil cell) or are transported into intercellular lumina (forming oil cavities or oil ducts in the tissue). Secretory cells along the surface deposit their oils beneath a membranaceous lamina, the cuticula (forming glandular trichomes, glandular scales and papillae). In the storage structures, the essential oil deposits are enclosed by specialized membranes, which consist of highly polymerized esters of hydroxylated fatty acids that are further linked by peroxide groups (cork, cutin). Due to their very low gas permeability, they reduce volatilization of the essential oils as well as their reaction with atmospheric oxygen. As a result, essential oils remain unchanged for longer periods of time in uncomminuted herbs and spices when compared to spice powders, whose protective tissue structures have been destroyed. In a few plants, particularly in herbaceous ones, which store the essential oil in thin-walled leaves (e.g. parsley and dill), this protection is less effective. Plants with glandular trichomes are less prone to loss of essential oils from drying. Only a small amount of essential oil is lost from oil cells or oil cavities that are situated deep within the tissue, for example in umbelliferous fruits such as anise, caraway, and fennel. In a number of plants,

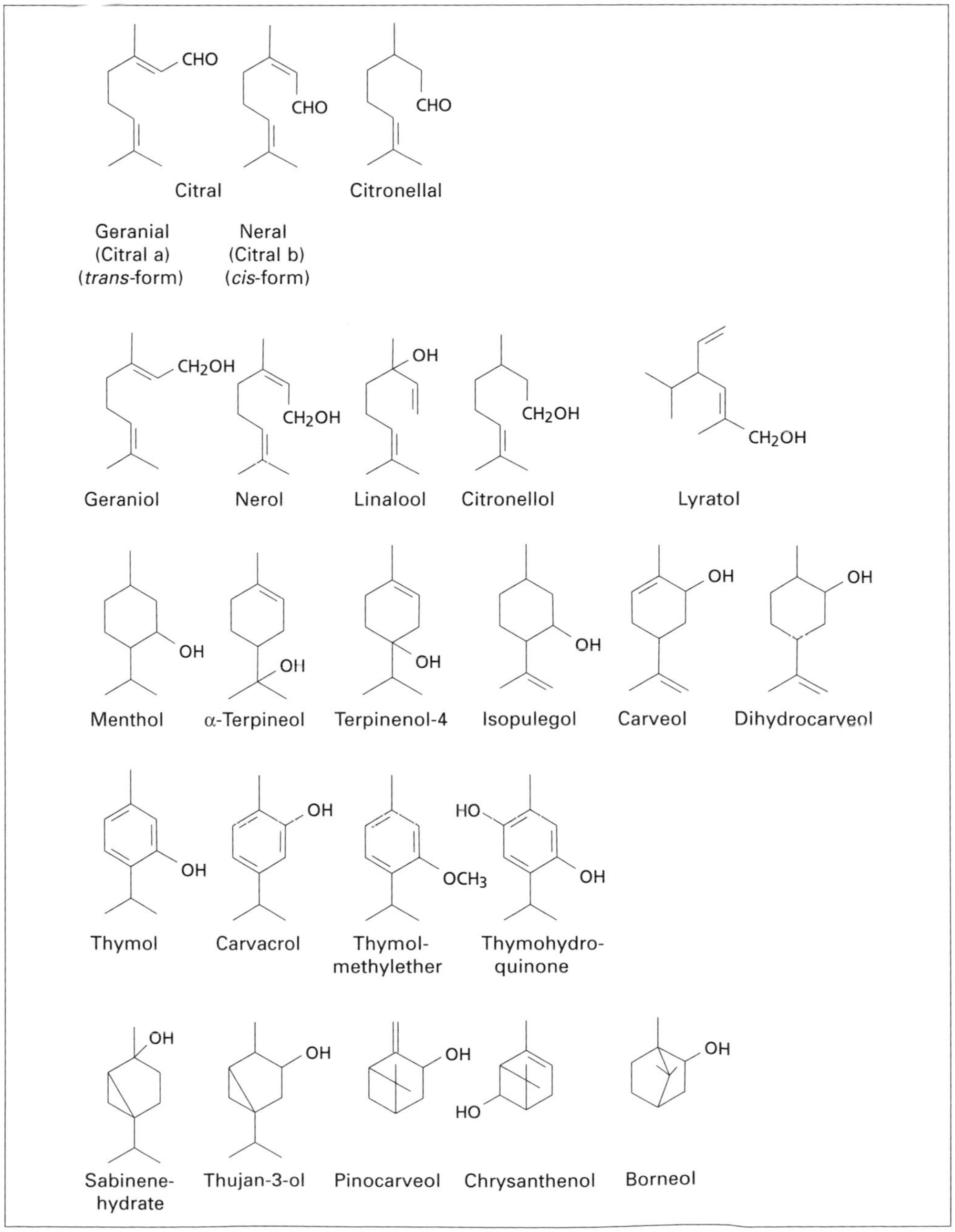

Fig. 2 Monoterpene aldehydes and -alcohols as essential oil components

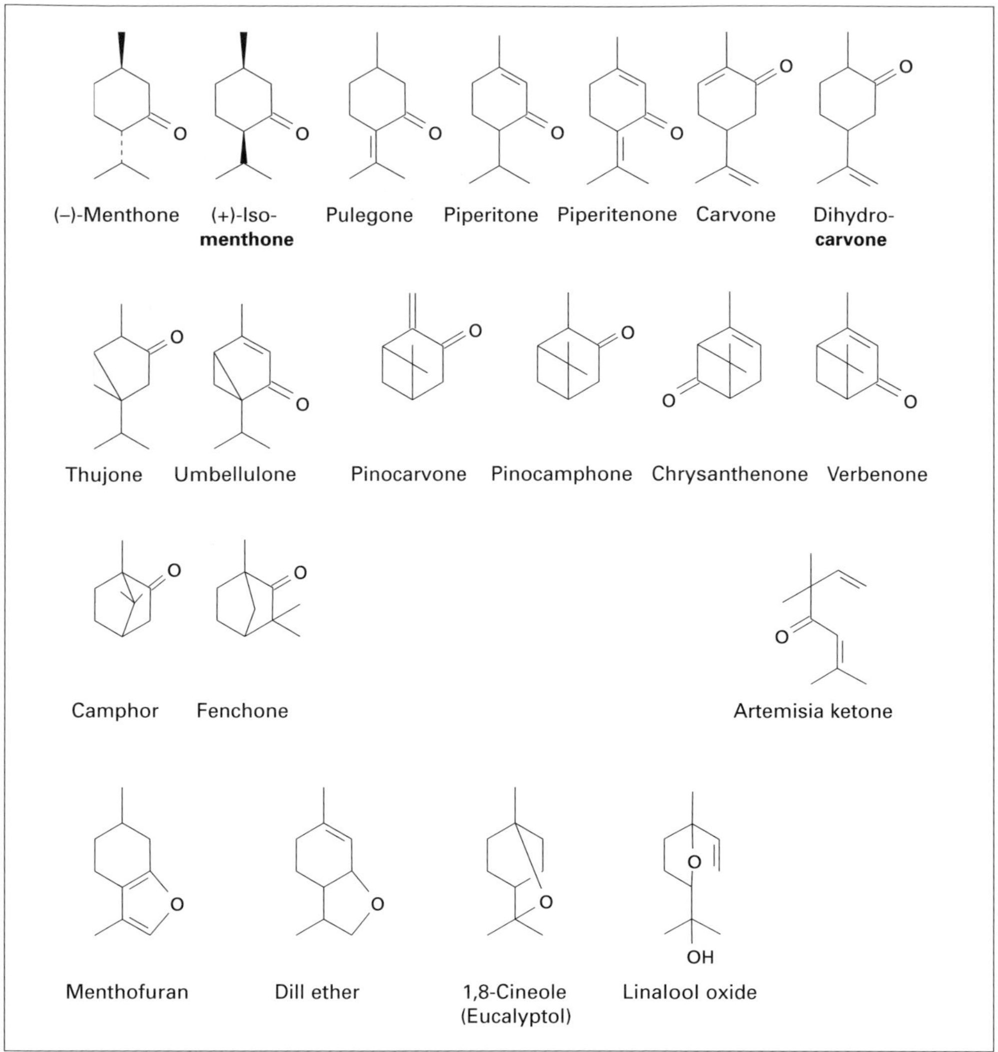
(–)-Menthone
(+)-Isomenthone
Pulegone
Piperitone
Piperitenone
Carvone
Dihydrocarvone
Thujone
Umbellulone
Pinocarvone
Pinocamphone
Chrysanthenone
Verbenone
Camphor
Fenchone
Artemisia ketone
Menthofuran
Dill ether
1,8-Cineole (Eucalyptol)
Linalool oxide

Fig. 3 Monoterpene ketones and -epoxides as essential oil components

glycosides of alcoholic and phenolic essential oil components have also been detected. In peppermint for example, 5% of the menthol can occur as menthol glucoside. The cleavage of these glycosides after the plant dies off is possibly related to the often-observed increase in the absolute essential oil content during the drying process.

The industrial production of essential oils is mostly carried out with steam distillation and more rarely with fractionating extraction using supercritical CO_2. The food industry often uses oleoresins (→ Chapter 9.4), containing mainly essential oils obtained by extraction with lipophilic solvents, rather than the essential oils themselves.

Up to this date, more than 3,000 chemical compounds have been isolated from essential oils. Most of these constituents are acyclic or cyclic monoterpene hydrocarbons (Fig. 1), monoterpene aldehydes (Fig. 2), monoterpene ketones (Fig. 3), monoterpene epoxides (Fig. 3), sesquiterpene hydrocarbons (Fig. 4), sesquiterpene alcohols (Fig. 5), sesquiterpene ketones (Fig. 6) and sesquiterpene epoxides (Fig. 6). Polyfunctional terpenes also occur. Often, also present are phenylpropane derivatives (Fig. 7) or their breakdown products, e.g. hydroxy- or methoxyderivatives of benzaldehyde (Fig. 8) or benzyl alcohol. Some of the alcohol and phenolic components are esterified with carboxylic acids, often with acetic acid (Fig. 9). Even though these esters only occur in small amounts, they are often determining the odor. Unbranched aliphatic hydrocarbons and their oxygenated derivatives (particularly aldehydes or ketones but also alcohols, epoxides, esters of carboxylic acids, rarely compounds with polyine character) can also be components of essential oils. Volatile sulfur- and/or nitrogen-containing compounds, such as alliaceous- and mustard oils (see below) are often attributed to the essential oils.

The composition of the essential oils in plants is very complex. Modern analytical methods now allow for the identification and quantification of over 100 components in an essential oil of a plant. For example in lavender oil, over 250 components have been detected. Of these compounds, only a few usually influence the odor of a culinary herb or spice. Other constituents, often occurring as the main components, have little or no significance in contributing to the odor.

How much an odorous component of an essential oil is contributing to the odor of a culinary herb depends on its vapor pressure at room- or body temperature, or, in other words, on its concentration in the gas phase that reaches our sensory organs. Head-space-chromatography, an analytical method that determines the concentration of individual essential oil components in the air space above the herb sample, nevertheless does not allow for a conclusive determination of the expected odor qualities. Not only the type and concentrations of the volatile constituents that reach our olfactory sense cells determine the odor impression but also the odor-threshold of individual components. For example, the threshold concentration for the odor perception of limonene is 0.01 mg/l (aqueous solution), of linalool 0.006 mg, of β-ionone 0.000007 mg and of 2-isobutyl-3-methoxypyrazine (odor component of fresh paprika) only 0.000002 mg.

As a result, odorous qualities of culinary herbs and spices cannot be deduced from the spectrum of constituents alone. Sensory evaluations are irreplaceable (see Chapter 3). One such method, among others, known as the so-called sniff-GC, allows following up a gas-chromatographic separation of essential oil olfactory components. In the course of separation, parts of the separated, gaseous constituents are diverted to a special valve where a technician can access an odor sample for establishing an aromagram. In this way, it can be ascertained which constituents contribute to the odor of the essential oil. Through AEDA (aroma extract dilution analysis), FD (flavor dilution)-factors can be established, which indicates at what lowest dilution the isolated odorous component can still produce an odor sensation. These FD factors allow for a distinction of the different components to their significance for the typical odor of an essential oil. This facilitates the work of the flavorist, whose job it is to "recreate" natural odors from combinations of isolated natural- or nature-identical odorous substances [23, 74, Ü30].

2.3 Pungent constituents

2.3.1 Alliaceous oils

Alliaceous oils are mixtures of lipophilic, liquid, volatile, strongly odorous, sulfur-containing compounds, which trigger the sensation "pungent" upon contact with the buccal cavity. In terms of their physicochemical characteristics, they are similar to essential oils but they are not present in the intact plant. They are mostly alk(en)yl-alkane/alkene thiosulfinates, dialk(en)yl-monosulfides and dialk(en)yloligosulfides. They constitute the pungent- and aroma constituents of alliaceous species (Alliaceae) that serve as culinary herbs, e.g. chives, garlic, leek, onion, ramsons, shallot, and Welsh onion.

The components of the alliaceous oils develop from non-volatile constituents, the alliins. Alliins are S-alk(en)yl-L-cysteine-sulfoxides (Fig. 10). The S-atom is mostly substituted with methyl-, ethyl-, propyl-, allyl- and prop-1-enyl groups (see Figs. → Garlic, → Leek, and → Onion). They occur in dormant plant parts partially as γ-glutamyl conjugates, from which they are released by peptidases. The alliins are ac-

companied by alliinase (EC 4.4.14), an enzyme being a C-S-lyase, which is separated spatially in intact plants from the alliins. Upon tissue injury, the alliinase comes into contact with the alliins, and in the first instance the characteristic pungent smelling alk(en)ylsulfenic acids are formed (Fig. 10). They undergo a number of spontaneous concurrent reactions; usually they are transformed to dimers, the alk(en)yl-alkane/alkenethiosulfinates, by dehydration.

These compounds are chemically esters of alkane- or alkene-thiosulfenic acids or dialkyl-disulfide-mono-S-oxides and represent the flavor compounds of raw alliaceous plants. They can disproportionate, particularly during heating (e.g. boiling, frying, or steam distillation), to dialk(en)yldisulfides and dialk(en)ylthiosulfonates or to dialk(en)yldisulfides, dialk(en)ylmonosulfides and SO$_2$, respectively. From the dialk(en)yldisulfides, dialk(en)yltrisulfides

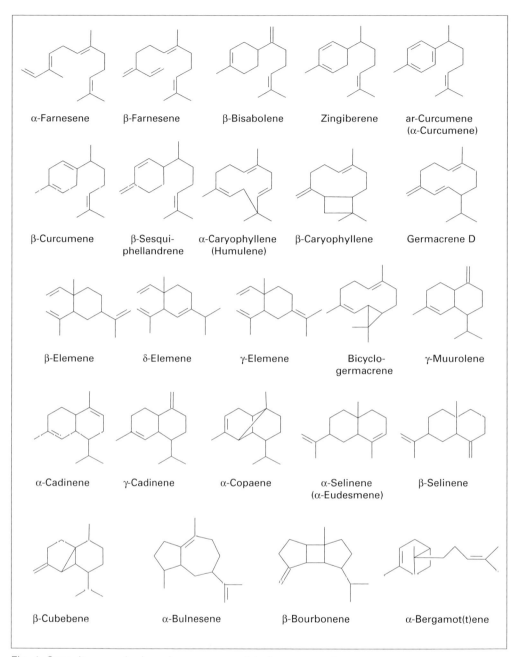

Fig. 4 Sesquiterpene hydrocarbons as essential oil components

α-Farnesene   β-Farnesene   β-Bisabolene   Zingiberene   ar-Curcumene (α-Curcumene)

β-Curcumene   β-Sesqui-phellandrene   α-Caryophyllene (Humulene)   β-Caryophyllene   Germacrene D

β-Elemene   δ-Elemene   γ-Elemene   Bicyclo-germacrene   γ-Muurolene

α-Cadinene   γ-Cadinene   α-Copaene   α-Selinene (α-Eudesmene)   β-Selinene

β-Cubebene   α-Bulnesene   β-Bourbonene   α-Bergamot(t)ene

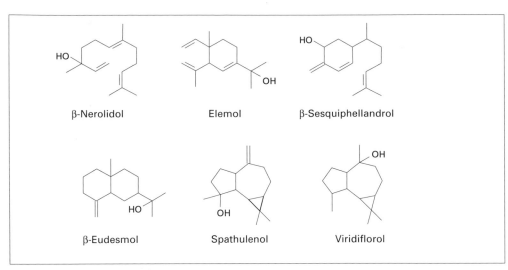

Fig. 5 Sesquiterpene alcohols as essential oil components

β-Nerolidol Elemol β-Sesquiphellandrol

β-Eudesmol Spathulenol Viridiflorol

are formed, or, with advanced reaction, dialk(en)ylpolysulfides and dialk(en)yl-monosulfides, respectively. 3 molecules of alk(en)yl-alkane/alkene thiosulfinates can transform into 2 molecules of the odorless dialk(en)yl-tri-thia-alkane-monoxide (α-sulfinyldisulfide); in garlic, they are known as ajoenes and in the onion, as cepaenes. Cyclic compounds are also formed, e.g. vinyldithiins and zwiebelanes.

According to this reaction scheme, allyl-sulfenic acid develops from alliin or its storage form γ-glutamyl-alliin (Fig. 11) respectively, which are often present in Allium-species; allylsulfenic acid then dimerizes to allicin (allyl-prop-2-enthiosulfinate). Allicin can be transformed to diallyldisulfide and diallylsulfide, and it can also be broken down to allylsulfenic acid and thioacrolein. 2 molecules of thioacrolein form 2-vinyl-[4H]-1,3-dithiin (besides 3-vinyl-[4H]-1,2-dithiin). The ratio of the secondary breakdown products is influenced by the pH value of the milieu, among other factors. Alliins with alkenyl residues, such as alliin, can be transformed into cyclo-derivatives, e.g. cycloalliin, by addition of the amino group to the double bond. Deviating from the above mentioned reaction scheme, prop-1-enyl-sulfenic acid formed from S-prop-1-enyl-L-cysteine sulfoxide is partially converted to thiopropanal-S-oxide (lacrimator principle of → Onion), which is reduced to thiopropanal and hydrolyzed to propionaldehyde, H_2SO_4 + H_2S or cyclisised to compounds with complicated ring systems [6].

2.3.2 Mustard oils

Mustard oils are mixtures of lipophilic sulfur- and nitrogen-containing compounds triggering the sensation "pungent" when absorbed in the mouth. They are usually volatile, then pungent smelling compounds. All of them have conjunctiva-, skin- and mucosa irritant effects. The components of mustard oil are mostly volatile alkyl-, alkenyl-, ω-methylthioalkyl-, benzyl- or phenylethylisothiocyanates as well as the non-volatile p-hydroxybenzyliso-

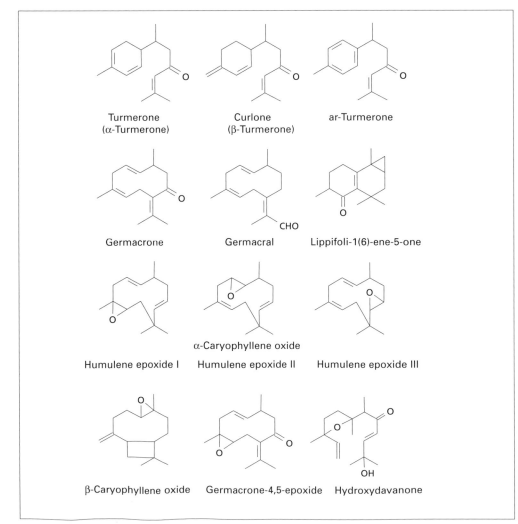

Turmerone (α-Turmerone) Curlone (β-Turmerone) ar-Turmerone

Germacrone Germacral Lippifoli-1(6)-ene-5-one

Humulene epoxide I α-Caryophyllene oxide Humulene epoxide III
  Humulene epoxide II

β-Caryophyllene oxide Germacrone-4,5-epoxide Hydroxydavanone

Fig. 6 Sesquiterpene ketones and -epoxides as essential oil components

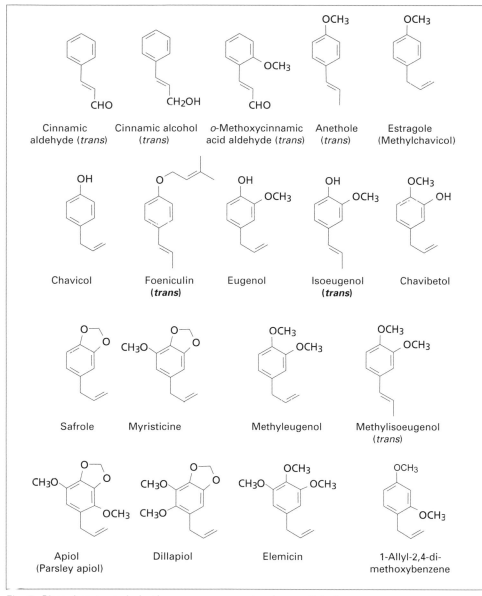

Cinnamic aldehyde (*trans*)   Cinnamic alcohol (*trans*)   *o*-Methoxycinnamic acid aldehyde (*trans*)   Anethole (*trans*)   Estragole (Methylchavicol)

Chavicol   Foeniculin (**trans**)   Eugenol   Isoeugenol (**trans**)   Chavibetol

Safrole   Myristicine   Methyleugenol   Methylisoeugenol (*trans*)

Apiol (Parsley apiol)   Dillapiol   Elemicin   1-Allyl-2,4-di-methoxybenzene

Fig. 7 Phenylpropane derivatives as components of essential oils

thiocyanate or the non-volatile ω-methyl-sulfinylalkyl- and ω-methylsulfonylalkyl-isothiocyanates (Fig. 12, see also → Capers and → Horseradish). The mustard oils have similar physico-chemical characteristics as the essential oils, but they do not occur in the intact plant. They represent the pungent principle of spices obtained from cruciferous plants (Brassicaceae), e.g. black mustard, garden cress, horseradish, Sarepta mustard, scurvy grass, watercress, and white mustard.

The components of the mustard oils arise from non-volatile constituents, the glucosi-nolates ("mustard oil glycosides", C-substituted *S*-(β-D-glucopyranosyl)-methane-thiohydroximic-*O*-sulfates, Fig. 12). Glu-cosinolates are formed in many plants from different botanical families; they are stored in the vacuoles. Upon destruction of the cell, they come into contact with the enzyme myrosinase (β-thioglucoside-glu-cohydrolase, EC 3.2.3.1), which is located in the so-called myrosine-cells. It catalyzes upon contact with the glucosinolates the cleavage off of the sugar moieties. The re-sulting C-substituted methanethiohydrox-imic acid-*O*-sulfates transform, in a neu-

tral environment around pH 7, to the *N*-substituted isothiocyanates upon elimination of the sulfate moieties. Under certain conditions, nitriles are formed, and in some other plants also S-alkylated thio-cyanates. Under natural conditions, mixtures of isothiocyanates and nitriles are predominantly formed.

2.3.3 Gingerols

Gingerols are non-volatile derivatives of phenylethyl-n-alkyl-ketones (phenylalka-nones), which produce the sensation "pungent"; of particular importance are especially [6]-gingerol, [8]-gingerol and [10]-gingerol ([n] = number of C-atoms of the fatty acids participating in the biosynthesis; with the cleavage of the retroaldols, aldehydes with corresponding chain lengths are formed, see chemical structures, → Ginger). Gingerols are accompanied by methylgingerols (methylation at the asymmetrical C-atom or the phenolic OH-group), among others, and the very pungent shogaols (5-desoxy-4,5-dehydro-gingerols, particularly [6]-, [8]- and [10]-shogaols (→ Ginger), which form from the gingerols by dehydration during storage and drying, including methylshogaols and gingerdiols (3-desoxo-3,5-dihydroxy-gin-gerols). They represent the pungent principle in plants from the family Zingi-beraceae, for example ginger and galangal.

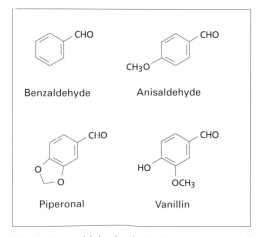

Benzaldehyde   Anisaldehyde

Piperonal   Vanillin

Fig. 8 Benzaldehyde derivatives as essential oil components

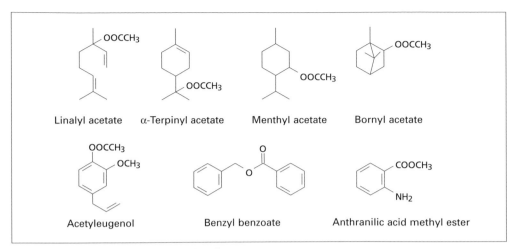

Fig. 9   Ester components of essential oils

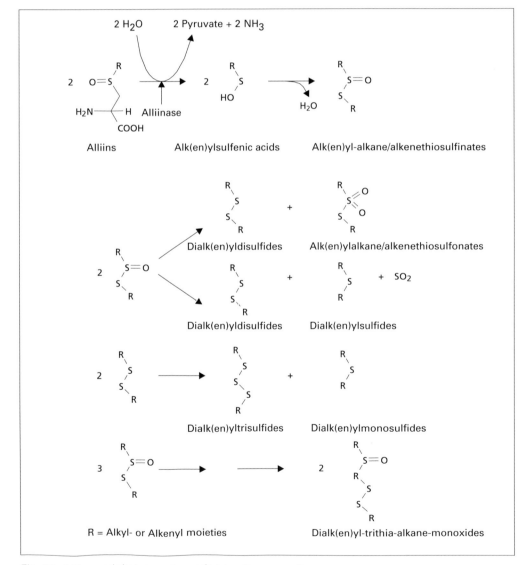

Fig. 10   Alliins and their transformation to alliaceous oils

2.3.4 Carboxylic acid amides

Carboxylic acid amides, responsible for the sensation "pungent" include the capsaicinoids and amides of Piper-species. Capsaicinoids (chemical structures, → Paprika) are amides of saturated or monounsaturated C_8- to C_{13}-fatty acids or -methyl fatty acids with vanillylamine (4-hydroxy-3-methoxy-benzylamine), respectively. Up to this point, 15 capsaicinoids have been detected. The main components of the capsaicinoid mixture in paprika and chilies are capsaicin (acid component: 8-methyl-non-6(Z)-enoic acid), dihydrocapsaicin (acid components: 8-methyl-nonoic acid) and nordihydrocapsaicin (acid component: 7-methyloctanoic acid). Other acid components include, among others, n-octanoic acid (octylvanillylamide), n-decanoic acid (decylvanillyl amide), 9-methyl-dec-6(E)-enoic acid and 8-methyl-dec-6(E)-enoic acid.

The acid amides of Piper-species (chemical structures, → Black pepper) are composed of alkaryl acids, such as chavicinic acid, piperettine, piperic- as well as trimethoxycinnamic acid, and amines, such as piperidine, Δ^5-piperidine-2-one or isobutylamine. The main components are piperine (*all-trans*), piperyline (trichostachine), piperolein A, piperolein B, piperanine (4,5-dihydropiperine), pipercide, guineensine and piperlongumine.

2.3.5 Protoanemonine

Protoanemonine is a lactone of 4-hydroxy-penta-2,4-dienoic acid (Fig. 13). This liquid, easily volatilized, pungent smelling compound is a strong skin- and mucous membrane irritant, producing the sensation "pungent". It is relatively unstable and dimerizes easily to the crystalline anemonine with weak skin-irritant effects. Protoanemonine develops in injured plant tissue that contains ranunculin, via enzyme catalysis by non-hydrolytic splitting off of the glucose moiety. Ranunculin occurs in numerous species of the crowfoot family (Ranunculaceae). Protoanemonine is the pungent principle of the flower buds from marsh marigold (*Caltha palustris* L.), used as a caper substitute [Ü99, → Capers].

2.4 Bitter principles

Bitter principles are bitter tasting plant constituents, which, aside of the reflectory increase in the production of gastrointestinal secretions triggered by the bitter taste, have no other pharmacological effects within this range of application. There are numerous other strongly bitter plant constituents, which, due to their strong pharmacological effects however, are not counted among the bitter principles (e.g. strychnine).

The bitter compounds are structurally very diverse. According to the so-called AH-B-hypothesis (which is also valid for the taste sensation "sweet"), bitter compounds require a proton-donator (AH-group, e.g. **OH, CHCO, CHOCOCH₃, CHCOOCH₃**) and a proton-acceptor (B-group, e.g. **COOCH₃, C=C-O-, OCOCH₃**), with a distance of 1 to 1.5 Å to each other (in sweet tasting constituents 2.5 to 4 Å) [49].

Due to the chemical heterogeneity of bitter tasting constituents, the bitter tasting culinary herbs and spices can only be evaluated with sensoric examination, e.g. by determining the bitter value. The bitter value of a culinary herb or spice is defined as the reciprocal value of that most diluted extract concentration, which still has a perceptible bitter taste. In order to compensate for individual sensitivity to taste, a standard substance is used, for example quinine hydrochloride whose bitter value has been normalized to 200,000 (meaning that a test solution with 1 g in 200,000 ml water still has a bitter taste).

The bitter constituents of culinary herbs and spices are mostly monoterpenes (see for example the bitter constituents of → Bitter fennel, → Olives, and → Saffron), sesquiterpene lactones (e.g. bitter constituents of many Artemisia-species such as mugwort, southernwood, wormwood, see chemical structures → Mugwort), diterpenes (e.g. bitter principle of rosemary and sage, see chemical structures → Sage), triterpenes (e.g. limonoids in the

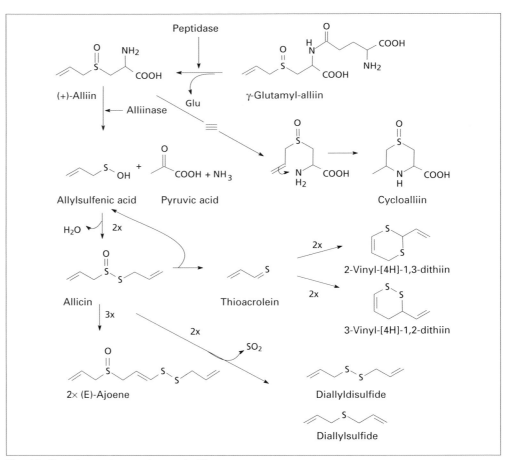

Fig. 11 Transformation products of alliin

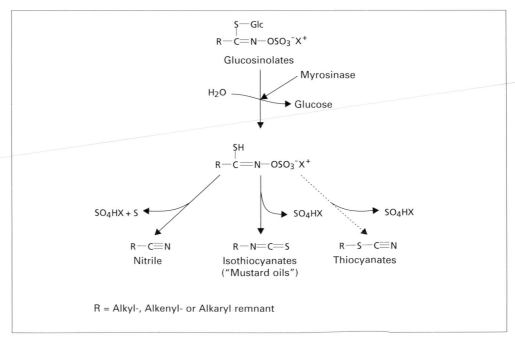

Fig. 12 Glucosinolates and their transformation to mustard oils

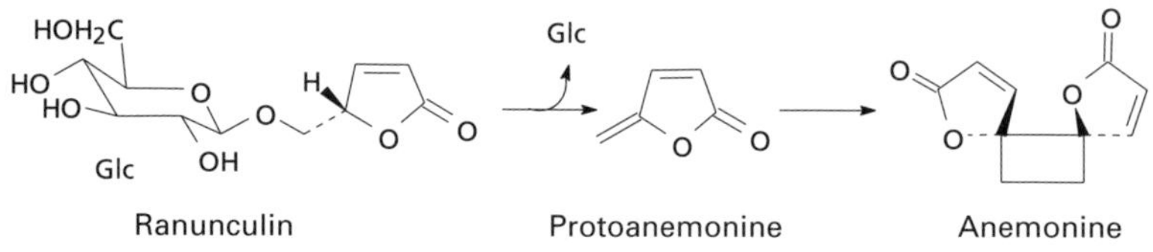

Fig. 13 Ranunculin and its transformation to Protoanemonine

seeds of citrus fruits, → Citrus species), acylphloroglucinols (e.g. bitter acids of hops, chemical structures, → Hops), flavonone glycosides (e.g. bitter constituents in the pulp of many citrus fruits, such as bitter orange and citron, chemical structures → Citrus species), lignans (e.g. bitter principle of nutmeg) or saponins (bitter princi-ple of soybean, see chemical structures → Soybean).

2.5 Coloring matters

An important coloring matter of culinary herbs and spices is chlorophyll. Addition-ally the anthocyans, flavonoids, betacyans, and carotenoids also play a significant role. Particularly relevant are the strong coloring carotenoids capsanthin and capsorubin from → Paprika, crocin from → Saffron, and bixin from → Annatto, as well as phenylpropane derivatives, such as curcumin from → Turmeric. These coloring matters are light sensitive and partially broken down during heating, for example, from the heat generated during grinding. A few pigments of culinary herbs and spices, for example the polymerization products of the orthodiphenols of black pepper, develop only later during fermentation.

3 Sensory effects of culinary herbs and spices

3.1 The role of odor, taste and appearance of foods

Our experiences in odor and taste sensations allow us to decide whether materials, looking edible, are indeed possibly suitable for consumption. If the food item has an agreeable odor and taste, the positive sensations trigger conditioned and unconditioned reflex stimuli and thus prepare the digestion by stimulating secretion of the salivary glands, the glands of the stomach, of the pancreas and of the intestine as well as by influencing the composition of the secretions depending on the type of food ingested. Odor and taste sensations also exercise an influence on our emotional well being since the odor and taste sense cells are connected to the limbic system. Our digestive tract is also "wired" to the brain. This is exemplified by the fact that toxic compounds can activate those areas in the brain (metencephalon), which trigger vomiting. Possibly, there are also "positive" signals transmitted from the gastrointestinal tract to the brain, indicating "good food" and thus influencing our emotional life in a positive way.

In most cases, but not always (!), foods with an appealing odor and taste are beneficial. The exceptions to this rule had to be learnt by mankind from experience by observing victims of poisonings. It is empirical knowledge that informs us not to consume the agreeable smelling and tasting death cap mushroom, or the mucilaginous sweetish tasting belladonna fruits. Often, we also learn that foods, which have a disagreeable taste at first, will be food items liked by us later on. One such example is beer, which tastes bitter due to hop bitter acids and their breakdown products that are formed during the fermentation process. People who have not yet learned to appreciate its taste, for example children, reject it; for many adults, however, it is an enjoyable drink. The bitter taste, originally an "invention" of plants to signalize the occurrence of poisonous substances to predators (in the case of hops used by an "impostor"), is easily found out by us to be an "empty threat". Another example is the consumption of certain cheese varieties; some of these specialty products smell like decomposing foods and indicate contamination with bacteria, but to many, they are desirable food items.

Humans have tried to use odor and taste as a mood enhancer since ancient times, for example by adding spices to foods. We are not really aware of the fact that the psychological as well as the direct systemic effects of odorous- and taste substances also have a positive effect on physical human health.

The subjective evaluation of odor and taste of foods, that means to determine if the foods have an agreeable smell and taste to us or not, is partially genetically based but to a large extent, it is acquired empirically. Such food preferences can already be influenced for example by substances we came in contact with because of the eating habits of our mothers during pregnancy or nursing. American studies have shown that infants born by mothers who drank carrot juice in the last trimester of pregnancy also prefer carrot juice. The taste of baby food also influences our later food preferences considerably. For example, it could be shown that people, who received vanillin in their baby food, developed considerably different food preferences compared to the individuals who were fed a vanillin-free diet [26].

Changes of odor and taste perception and -appreciation are likely due to psychological and physiological factors. The memories associated with odor or taste significantly influence how we esteem foods. Thereby, negative experiences have a greater impact than positive ones. The physiological shape of the body also influences how we valuate odor, for example, it makes a difference if the sensory impression took place before or after hard work. A number of illnesses, e.g. Diabetes mellitus and migraine attacks, as well medications and smoking can also influence the way we perceive and valuate odor and taste. Later in life, the sensitivity to odor and taste is diminished. That is why older people often prefer more strongly seasoned foods. Smokers too apparently have a reduced sense of smell and taste.

Aromachology examines and utilizes the relationship of odor perception and psychological as well as physiological processes, for example with regard to perception of certain odors and how they relate to feelings and emotions such as relaxation, elation, sensuality, and well-being or how they can reduce stress and anxiety and influence behavior, such as shopping habits, or also how they influence physical parameters, for example, brain waves, blood pressure, diameter of peripheral blood vessels, pulse rate, skin potentials, mydriasis as well as ability, such as capacity of learning and memory [39].

The reflex and direct systemic effects of odor substances are used in **aromatherapy** for the treatment of disturbances of well-being and illnesses [Ü105].

Besides odor and taste, the appearance of foods, but also the ambience where the meal is presented, also influences appetite and thus the whole digestive process. Hence, we are using many culinary herbs and spices not only to enhance taste but also to make food visually more appealing. Culinary herbs and spices are used for garnishing (decorative- or visually appealing herbs such as parsley and sesame) and as coloring ingredients (e.g. paprika, saffron, and turmeric). Even though the addition of nitrites to meats is perceived as a potential health hazard (possible formation of carcinogenic nitrosamines), we often prefer the "mouth-watering" nitrite-containing, red sausage products over the unappetizing gray ones.

While the color of a food is easily defined, the definition of a taste is more complex since only a few culinary herbs and spices can be described with the 4 basic taste sensations. Describing an odor is nearly impossible. Attempts to reduce odor impressions to 6 "basic odors" (spicy, smoky, resinous, fruity, flowery, fetid) have not been generally accepted. Comparative descriptions (odor: lemon-like) are usually better understood but their application is limited. Hence, the general terms used in literature (including this book) to describe odors (odor: aromatic?) are of little value.

Odor and taste also play a large role for the efficacy of many herbs used in phytotherapy. Unfortunately, the phytopharmaceutical industry often completely neglects this fact. Dry extracts from essential oil containing herbs, or extracts of such herbs that have been strongly concentrated by evaporation and thus are free of essential oils are often produced (e.g. from caraway, fennel, hops, and lemon balm) since patients usually prefer solid dosage forms. Dry extracts obtained from bitter herbs (e.g. from condurango bark, gentian root) are incorporated into coated tablets or sugar coated pills (dragées) in order to hide the bitter taste and not to discourage the patient from taking the product even though the bitter taste is crucial for its efficacy. Moreover, for the extraction of essential oil containing herbs, solvents with a low or no alcohol content are used. They only dissolve a small amount of the essential oil. They are produced to guarantee the miscibility with aqueous solutions, e.g. with sugar syrup, or to assure that the alcohol content is limited to 30% so that the

product can be used not only for adults but also in pediatric medicine (e.g. thyme fluid extract).

3.2 Physiology of olfaction

For the sensory perception of foods, olfaction probably plays the most crucial role. Before we taste a food item, we consciously or unconsciously examine its odor (olfactory impression). Also during eating, we obtain olfactory impressions in addition to taste sensations (gustatory impressions). The odorous components reach the olfactory sense cells during chewing via the nose-throat connection (retronasal impression, gustatory odor perception). If the olfactory senses are impaired, for example due to a virus infection of the nasal mucous membranes, foods will taste insipid despite a normally functioning taste perception. The entire odor and taste impression (in addition to trigeminal sensations, see below) is designated as flavor [55].

Odor components reach the "odor receptors", the **olfactory sense cells,** through the nostrils or while eating, also through the pharyngonasal connection (choana). These cells originate from neuronal tissue of the telencephalon. Up to 30 million of them exist in the **olfactory epithelium** of humans. This type of tissue can be found primarily in the **olfactory region** (Regio olfactoria), which covers an area of about 2.5 cm² each, located on the upper right and upper left sides of the turbinate bone (Concha nasalis). In addition, the nose and throat regions also contain neuronal projections from other nerves (Nervus trigeminus, N. glossopharyngeus, N. vagus), which are also able to detect odors but have a much higher sensitivity threshold than the olfactory sense cells. The olfactory sense cells are associated with supporting and basal cells (Fig. 14). The ducts of the Bowman's glands lead also to the olfactory epithelium. Bowman's glands in addition to the supporting cells produce a secretion covering the olfactory epithelium. The olfactory sense cells have a relatively short life span. About every 10 days, they are regenerated from the basal cells. The

heads of the olfactory sense cells are exposed towards the mucous membranes, bearing 5 to 10 olfactory cilia, which constitute the sensitive part of the bipolar neurons.

A volatile substance that can be detected with the olfactory senses must be a lipophilic one but also somewhat water-soluble, and its molecular weight should not exceed 300 Da. The odorous substances first dissolve in the mucus, which covers the olfactory epithelium and are carried to the olfactory sense cells by **odorant-binding-proteins** (OBPs). There, they react with the **olfactory receptor proteins**, which are located in the membranes of the ciliae of the olfactory sense cells. The contact of the odorous substance with its "corresponding" receptor protein leads to a three-dimensional structure change of that protein and as a result, a reaction cascade is triggered, resulting in a change of ion permeability of the olfactory sense cell membrane and thus to a change of its electrical potential.

The occurrence of about 1,000 different olfactory proteins in the olfactory epithelium is assumed. Each olfactory sense cell probably only produces one type of olfactory receptor protein. Since considerably more than 1,000 odorous constituents can be differentiated by humans, it is assumed that there are overlapping reactions of odorous constituents with different receptor proteins. This "accord" of odor impressions probably determines the odor sensation of a specific constituent. The multitude of detectable, odorous substances does not allow for a clear distinction of odor qualities, as is possible for the 4 basic taste qualities.

The changes in the electrical potential of olfactory sense cells after contact with the "corresponding" odorous substance are transmitted through their axons, traversing about 100 perforations of the ethmoid (located in the middle of the base of skull) to reach the **olfactory bulb** (Bulbus olfactorius). There, the signals are redirected from about 1,000 glomeruli (Glomeruli olfactorii) to the so-called mitral cells. It is likely that each glomerulus only receives signals from the axons of olfactory sense cells with one specific receptor-type. About 30,000 of such specific olfactory sense cells, recognizing one substance only, occur in our nasal mucosa. A network of the mitral cells interlaced with other nerve cells (granular cells, periglomerular cells), modulates the received signals, which are then transmitted by the olfactory nerve to the **olfactory cortex**. After the signals have been redirected by other nerve cells, they reach also the hippocampus and the autonomous nuclei of the hypothalamus. This connection with the limbic system, from which feelings, desires and emotions originate, explains the strongly emotional component of odor impressions. As a result, the respiratory center is also activated by the myelencephalon (Medulla oblongata), among other brain regions, including influences on endocrine functions and the immune system through the thalamus and hypothalamus.

In order to identify the odor of an essential oil that often contains over 100 components and therefore interacts with over a 100 different olfactory sense cell types, e.g. originating from lemon balm, we only require the odor sensations of a few substances known as lead substances, in the case of lemon balm oil, particularly the odor of citral.

The sense of odor is subject to **adaptation**, meaning that a constant odor can no longer be detected after a few seconds. Only a short interruption of the odor exposure, allows the detection of a specific odor to return for a few seconds.

The ability to detect a wide spectrum of odors is genetically based. Some humans are not able to detect certain odors, for example of hydrocyanic acid. The inability of an individual to detect a specific odor is called **anosmia** (olfactory anesthesia). If the threshold for odor sensitivity is very high, **hyposmia** is present. Illnesses, chemical or thermal influences can also temporarily or permanently damage the sense of smell.

With regard to the effects of volatile substances, the **vomeronasal organ** (VNO) located on both sides of the anterior nasal septum is of particular importance. If this organ comes into contact with specific

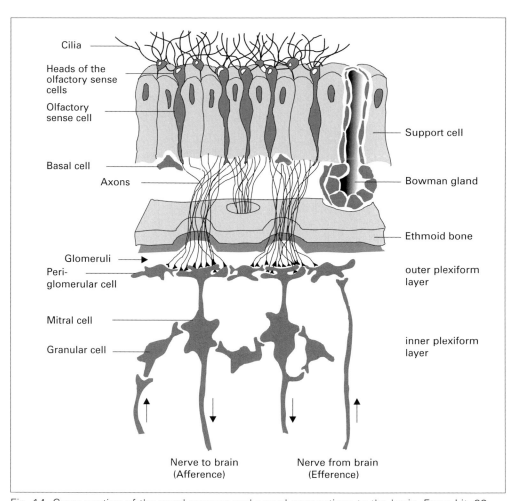

Fig. 14 Cross section of the nasal mucosa and neural connections to the brain. From Lit. 29

volatile substances, the so-called vomerophenines, a number of physiological reactions take place without an odor impression, e.g. release of gonadotropic hormones. Emotional patterns can also be influenced by such substances. The vomeronasal organ plays an essential role, clearly not only in animals but also in humans, for communication between individuals of the same species [1, 7, 28, 29, 37, 69, Ü36].

3.3 Physiology of taste

The sense of taste is clearly less differentiated than that of olfaction. We are able to detect 4 different qualities of taste, sweet, sour, bitter, and salty, with our taste buds located almost entirely on the surface of the tongue. Furthermore, there are the so-

called Umami-receptors (umami is Japanese and means delicious). These receptors are stimulated by the presence of salts of L-glutamic acid (glutamates), inosine-5′-monophosphate and guanosin-5′-monophosphate. These substances have a synergistic effect and are also known as flavor potentiators (Umami substances). Umami-receptors mediate the typical taste of meat broth. The postulation that a few oligopeptides, particularly with an L-glutaminyl component, also have Umami-taste, could not be confirmed [2, 5, 55, 68, 86, 94]. The food we eat mostly generates mixed taste sensations, for example the sweet-sour-bitter taste of a grapefruit.

In contrast to earlier opinions, the entire area of the tongue generates taste sensations for all taste qualities, but there are slight differences in the intensity of the

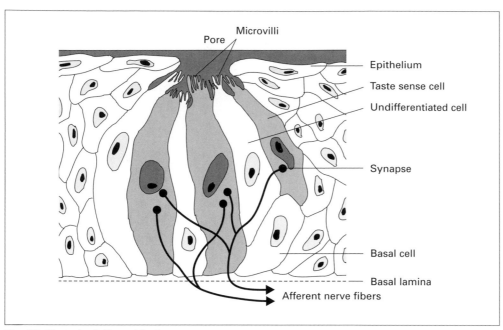

Fig. 15 Taste bud. From Lit. 1

perception of the different taste qualities between the different surface areas [21, Ü36].

The detectors of taste impressions are the **taste sense cells** (gustatory sense cells, Fig. 15). They have cilia (taste hairs, microvilli), in analogy to the olfactory sense cells, facing the exposed surface of the tongue. Similar to the olfactory sense cells, they also have a limited life span of about 10 days. In combination with indifferent cells and basal cells, they occur mostly in groups of 40 to 60 on the surface of the tongue, forming the 50 to 70 μm wide, pitted groups, known as **taste buds.** Between the

taste buds are glands, which cover the taste buds with secretions. The so-called circumvallate papillae at the base of the tongue contain up to 200 taste buds. The smaller fungiform- or foliate-papillae at the lateral and anterior part of the tongue only contain a few taste buds.

The taste sense cells also experience a change in their electrical potential if they come into contact with a corresponding taste substance. This change of the potential is transmitted via the afferent fibers to brain nerves (Nervus facialis, N. lingualis, N. glossopharyngeus). The potentials transmitted by these nerve fibers are redi-

rected to other dendrites near the myelencephalon (Medulla oblongata) and finally reach the cerebral cortex via the thalamus. Similar to the olfactory sense cells, the taste sense cells also undergo **adaptation** after extended exposure to a constant concentration of a solution of a taste substance. Only after a considerable change in its concentration, the taste sensation can be detected again.

The ability of taste sense cells can also be influenced by environmental factors, for example by nicotine or caffeine, as well as by age of a human being in a similar way as the olfactory sense cells. Newborns can only detect the taste quality "sweet". All other taste sensations develop later. During old age, the amount of active taste buds decreases (8,000 to 12,000 in newborns, 4,000 to 6,000 in adults, and 2,000 to 3,000 in old age).

The condition of increased sensitivity threshold to taste sensations is called **hypogeusia**. The total absence of taste sensations is called **ageusia.**

The sensations of pungent, burning, cooling and warming are not detected by taste sense cells. They are part of the **trigeminal sensations** (somato-sensoric impressions) and are triggered by the stimulation of fibers from the Nervus trigeminus, which is also responsible for the innervation of the facial area, including nose and mouth [Ü36]. The astringent sensation is mostly caused by suppression of the taste detection due to the formation of a protein/tannin membrane precipitate over the taste sense cells.

4. Pharmacology of culinary herbs and spices

4.1 Assessment of experimental-pharmacological studies

For investigating the action of culinary herbs and spices, pharmacological studies are of particular interest wherein extracts, essential oils or isolated constituents are orally administered (peroral, p.o.).

Studies in which extracts or solutions of constituents of culinary herbs and spices are applied in a way that bypasses the digestive system (parenteral), e.g. by injection into the veins (intravenous, i.v.) or in the peritoneum (abdominal cavity, intraperitoneal, i.p.), have only significance in very few cases. Often it remains unclear as to whether the observed effect would also occur following oral use. Many substances that show efficacy with parenteral administration are changed if they move through the digestive tract, either in the stomach by the gastric acid or in the intestine by the body's enzymes or enzymes of the intestinal flora, or they cannot pass through the intestinal wall, thus not entering into the bloodstream, respectively. Should they enter into the blood, nevertheless, they can, before reaching their target organs, be altered in their passage through the liver into physiologically inactive products. Therefore, the effects observed in studies with parenterally administered substances do not always occur with peroral application. There can also be an absence of effects with parenteral application, however that would occur with peroral application, because the aroma effect and/or the direct action on the digestive organs do not occur.

Drawing conclusions on the action of culinary herbs and spices in humans based on animal studies, even if the herb materials were administered orally, is also not possible without reservations. Reflex actions in humans caused by color, odor and taste, are not expected to occur in animal tests in the same manner. Not only because the drug or extracts are often administered in animals by gavage (that means without any contact with oral or nasal mucosa), but also due to potentially divergent reaction behavior of the animals. With regard to the pharmacokinetics and pharmacodynamics, there are often significant differences between humans and animals.

Results from studies with isolated organs in vitro can only be meaningful in those cases where spice materials come into direct contact with the isolated organs (such as preparations of stomach and intestines).

Drawing conclusions from cell cultures studies is also problematic. In these test systems, the cells are exposed directly to the test substances without protection from absorption barriers and biotransformation mechanisms. The assertion that a substance has antitumor action because it is lethal against isolated tumor cells is quite questionable. The substance is usually injurious to the viability of all cells due to its cytotoxicity. Like tests with isolated enzymes, studies with cell cultures can at most contribute to the clarification of the mechanism of action of reactions obtained with other methods. Such tests are considered only in exceptional cases in this book.

In vitro studies of the antimicrobial effects of extracts or isolated substances from culinary herbs and spices permit conclusions to be made on their action in the intestine, if one takes into consideration the concentrations, which can occur after the application of the spices as a seasoning agent after the meal in the digestive tract.

Studies of the chemical reactivity, particularly the antioxidative activity, of constituents of culinary herbs and spices are also of interest. These substances can act as radical scavengers, among other actions, contributing to the prevention of formation of carcinogenic compounds in foods or in the gastrointestinal tract.

Generalizations of the results of a test with a specific culinary herb or spice on culinary herbs and spices in general are not valid. Although culinary herbs and spices have many common actions, e.g. their digestion promoting and appetite stimulating action, in addition they also have specific effects. Due to the multitude of chemical races of a plant species and due to the variability of the constituent spectrum of a race under the influence of environmental conditions, generalizations about the actions that were attained with a one specific herbal drug, when applied to all races and origins of a species, are likewise often not possible. As an example, the anthelmintic action of tansy is probably dependent on its thujone content, so low thujone or thujone-free races are not likely to have this action.

It is unclear as to whether effects other than the appetite stimulant and digestive promoting action that are observed in pharmacological experiments, often with high doses of culinary herbs or spices, likewise corresponds to effects that would occur with the small amounts used for seasoning in daily life. However the results appear in a somewhat favorable light, if one also considers that the concentrations of toxic substances used in studies to demonstrate protective effects of culinary herbs or spices are levels that we are not exposed to in daily life.

Culinary herbs and spices are certainly only one "voice" in the "concert" that brings about positive effects from our food. But what would an orchestra be without the first violin?

4.2 Appetite stimulant and digestive promoting action

The main activity of culinary herbs and spices is in the stimulation of the secretion of enzyme-rich secretions of the salivary glands, gastric glands, the pancreas and intestine as well as in an intensified excretion of biliary juice and thereby a promotion of digestion [21, 64, 67].

This digestive aid effect probably occurs in three ways:

- By way of an "appetizing" appearance of the food, through pleasant olfactory sensations and bitter, salty, sour and/or "umami" taste impressions or the perception of pungency (cephalic phase),
- through irritation of the gastric mucosa (gastric phase),
- through irritation of the intestinal mucosa (intestinal phase).

Active substances of culinary herbs and spices in the cephalic phase are mainly aromatic smelling essential oils, pungent compounds as well as bitter substances, salt and substances that stimulate the umami-receptors. In the gastric- and intestinal-phases particularly active substances are the essential oils and pungent compounds. That the secretion-promoting action of culinary herbs and spices can also be independent of odor and taste perception has been demonstrated in animal tests. The gastric acid secretion of pentobarbitone-anesthetized rats was also increased when aqueous spice extracts were brought directly into the stomach, in the following declining order of activity intensity: paprika, fennel, ajowan, cardamom, black pepper, cumin, or coriander [87]. Some authors postulate that bitter substances also have secretomotor action when they bypass the mouth (?). An increased metabolic rate effect has also been observed with a range of culinary herbs and spices, for example with paprika and mustard [35].

4.3 Antimicrobial action

All herbs and spices with essential oils and isolated essential oils are more or less strongly antimicrobial in action. The components of the essential oils are integrated in the cell membranes of the microorganisms due to their lipophilic nature and inhibit, among others, the membrane-bound electron flow of the oxidative phosphorylation and therewith energy metabolism. High concentrations in essential oils also lead to lysis of the cell membranes and to denaturation of the cytoplasmic proteins. The disinfectant effect of many essential oils or their components is comparable to, or often significantly surpasses, that of phenol. So for instance the so-called phenol coefficient, that is rendered as the measure of the bactericidal activity for a specific test bacterium in relation to phenol (phenol = 1), for the essential oil of lavender it amounts to 1.6, for that of fennel fruit to 13.0 and for that of thyme to 13.2. For selected components of essential oils, e.g. for menthol the phenol coefficient is calculated at 0.9, for cinnamic aldehyde 3.0, for camphor 6.2, for eugenol 8.6, and for thymol at 20. Mustard oils and alliaceous oils also have good antibiotic action. 1 mg allylmustard oil/100 g in a food can inhibit the growth of yeasts and molds. The growth of lower fungi is also suppressed by the essential oil present in the gas phase. Some culinary herbs and spices, e.g. garlic, thyme and turmeric, also inhibit the growth and urease formation of *Helicobacter pylori* [e.g. Lit. 12, 47, 48, 60, 81, 96, Ü98].

4.4 Carminative action

The carminative action (flatulence relieving effect) of spices is attributable primarily to three factors.

Culinary herbs and spices **stimulate the secretion of the digestive glands**. By increasing the acid production in the stomach, disinfection of chyme is improved and by stimulating the secretion of enzymes through the digestive organs as well as by the enhanced excretion of biliary juice,

rapid decomposition of food is guaranteed. For this reason faulty fermentation is constrained (see Chapter 4.2).

Culinary herbs and spices with essential oils have **spasmolytic action**. The low-molecular, lipophilic components of essential oils are reversibly integrated in the membranes of the smooth muscle cells of the upper orifice of the stomach (cardia) and of the intestines, impairing the permeability of ionic channels and therewith inhibiting the contractibility of these organs. Accumulations of air in the stomach are thus prevented and intestinal spasms resolved. The spasmolytic action of culinary herbs and spices and of their isolated essential oils in vitro in intestinal preparations has been documented repeatedly. The introduction of diluted emulsions of essential oils into the human large bowel has also resolved spasms. However, in most cases, concentrations were used that will not be attained with the normal use of spices (see for example → Anise, → Fennel, → Caraway).

Culinary herbs and spices have **antimicrobial action**. Therefore they can inhibit the reproduction of pathogenic bacteria and thereby prevent the formation of gases and toxic metabolic products in the intestine [22, 71, see Chapter 4.3].

Culinary herbs and spices with good carminative action include, among others, anise, caraway, cinnamon bark, fennel, marjoram, peppermint, star anise, and summer savory.

4.5 Antioxidative, radical scavenging action

Culinary herbs and spices contain, like most other plant products, a multitude of constituents, which are able to exhibit antioxidative activity, by scavenging radicals, reactive oxygen species (particularly the extremely aggressive hydroxyl- and superoxide- radicals), reactive nitrogen species (including, among others, NO, NO_2), hypochlorite radicals or fatty acid radicals, among others [Ü83].

These reactive compounds originate with the exposure of food to oxygen and with metabolic processes in the organism, among others. Our body has at its disposal a range of defensive measures that serve to eliminate these aggressive substances. If these physiological mechanisms of inactivation are overcharged, then these substances can attack lipids, proteins as well as DNA and in this way, damage cell membranes, enzymes and genetic material. Particularly high concentrations of superoxide radicals occur in the area of inflammatory processes, because macrophages as well as neutrophilic- and eosinophilic leukocytes use these radicals in the course of immune defense, e.g. for the destruction of bacteria. Many age-related diseases, e.g. cardiac circulatory diseases, arthritis, various forms of tumors and Alzheimer's disease are possibly initiated by these radicals [101].

Antioxidants transfer the hydrogen of their phenolic-OH-groups to the oxygen radicals or form stable products with fatty acid radicals and therewith interrupt the radical chain reaction. In this process they are themselves consumed.

Good radical scavengers include mainly *o*-dihydroxybenzene derivatives such as flavonoids, isoflavonoids, caffeic acid derivatives (e.g. rosmarinic acid, caffeoylquinic acids), anthocyans, *o*-dihydroxycoumarins, lignans, and aromatic *o*-dihydroxyditerpenes, as well as alliaceous oils, mono- and diterpene aldehydes, benzoic- and cinnamic-acid derivatives (vanillin, cinnamic aldehyde), hop bitter acids, tocopherols, carotenoids, ascorbic acid, capsaicin, curcumin, oleuropein, phthalides), and monophenols, which can form relatively stable semiquinones (e.g. eugenol). Culinary herbs and spices with good antioxidative properties include, among others, clove, ginger, mace, marjoram, nutmeg, onions, oregano, paprika, pepper, rosemary, sage, summer savory, thyme, and turmeric.

The antioxidative and radical scavenging activity of spices, that is for the most part still retained after cooking, can be demonstrated in vitro quite well. Thus many spices can inhibit the formation of carcinogenic compounds, e.g. nitrosamines, in foods and subsequently in the stomach and in this way block tumor genesis. Radical

scavenging substances of culinary herbs and spices are also partially absorbed and enter into the bloodstream. In these cases the oxidation of LDL (low density lipoprotein, deposits in its oxidized form cholesterol in the blood vessels) is blocked and thereby so is the formation of arteriosclerotic plaques. Moreover they also retard lipid peroxidation and thereby protect cell membranes from oxidative changes. Thus it could be shown in mice that the concentrations of phospholipid peroxides in blood plasma and in the erythrocytes were reduced after supplementation with turmeric rhizome extracts (curcumin!), rosemary leaves (aromatic *o*-dihydroxyditerpene derivatives!), and paprika fruits (capsaicin!) [3]. The activities of radical inactivating enzymes (glutathione reductase, superoxide dismutase) can be increased in humans by consumption of parsley with food [61]. It is also accepted that herbs with alliaceous oils have an antioxidative systemic action and therewith an antiarteriosclerotic effect (→ Garlic).

Because foods also contain radical scavengers, it is likely that only those culinary herbs and spices, which are ingested in relatively large amounts, are contributing significantly to the protective effect (e.g. chives, garlic, olives, onions) [e.g. 11, 24, 25, 32, 34, 43, 63, 65, 66, 75, 76, 82, 91, 101, Ü30]. Spices also play a large role as radical scavengers for food preservation (→ Chapter 7).

4.6 Anticarcinogenic and antitumor action

A range of studies point to tumor genesis inhibition, therefore an anticarcinogenic action of culinary herbs and spices. This effect is probably contingent upon, among others:

- Prevention of the formation and activation of carcinogens, e.g. of nitrosamines, which can develop in the food or in the gastrointestinal tract [54, 75],
- the antioxidative, radical scavenging action, which protects the DNA from oxidative assaults (see above),
- effects on liver metabolism, particularly inhibiting the induction of cytochromes

(cytochrome P450 and cytochrome P448), e.g. by isothiocyanates, which cause the metabolic activation of carcinogens in the liver [17, 30],

- activation of enzymes, that leads to the detoxification of carcinogens, e.g. of glutathione-S-transferase, or of UDP-glucuronosyltransferase [4, 31, 50, 99, 100],
- inhibition of enzymes involved in carcinogenesis, e.g. of protein kinase C, tyrosine kinase and topoisomerase II [92],
- inhibition of the activation of tumor-triggering viruses, e.g. of the Epstein-Barr-Virus [57, 58, 89],
- prevention of the reaction of carcinogens with the DNA [9, 80],
- suppression of the activation of oncogens [10].

A few culinary herbs and spices can also contribute to the prevention of carcinogenesis in the stomach by providing protection against *Helicobacter pylori* infections. Whether this chemoprevention is actually of relevance for the small amounts of spices used in daily life remains to be studied.

The tumor growth inhibiting action of culinary herbs and spices is supposed to be based on, among other things, the induction of apoptosis (self-destruction) of tumor cells and/or on the inhibition of neoangiogenesis (formation of a tumor-associated blood vessel system). With estrogen-dependent tumor cells, it is conceivable that the estrogens that are necessary for their growth are displaced in this process by phytoestrogens that do not promote their growth [46, 92].

Anticarcinogenic and antitumor actions are assumed particularly for herbs and spices (or their isolated constituents) that contain essential oils (nutmeg, parsley, rosemary), alliaceous oils (asafetida, garlic, onions), mustard oils (garden cress, watercress), curcuminoids (turmeric), as well as for saffron and soybeans.

4.7 Hepatoprotective action

The liver protective action of culinary herbs and spices is likely attributable to their radical scavenging activity as well as to the stimulation of the increase of the content of soluble SH-compounds and of the activity of glutathione-S-transferase in the liver, in this way protecting cellular components, e.g. DNA, from fatal reactions with radicals and promoting the conjugation of hepatotoxic substances with SH-compounds and thereby their detoxification. For an example, it could be shown that the age-related decline of the antioxidative status of rat hepatic tissue can be improved with the administration of thyme oil [95]. Hepatoprotective action is accepted for, among others, black cumin, celery, nutmeg, pepper, and soybean.

4.8 Antihypercholesterolemic and antiarteriosclerotic action

Antihypercholesterolemic and antiarteriosclerotic action have been demonstrated, for example for citrus flavonoids, coriander, fenugreek seeds, garlic, ginger, mustard, nutmeg, olives, onions, Oswego tea, saffron, sesame, and soybean, among others. The anticholesterolemic action is probably attributable to the stimulation of the biliary excretion by the spices, which leads to an enhanced elimination of sterane derivatives from the body. The radical scavenging effect of many culinary herbs and spices, particularly of the alliaceous oils, which inhibit the oxidation of LDL and in doing so prevent the formation of arteriosclerotic plaque (see Chapter 4.5), can in addition to the anticholesterolemic action be jointly responsible for the antiarteriosclerotic action.

4.9 Estrogenic and gestagenic action

A number of spices have been found to contain phytoestrogens and phytoprogestins, which bind to the estrogen receptors (e.g. hops, soybean, thyme, turmeric) or the progestin receptors (e.g. clove, cumin, fennel, nutmeg, oregano, thyme, and turmeric). The substances bind to estrogen receptors but antagonize, due to their weak estrogenic activity with the body's own estrogens, being in this way potentially anticarcinogenic substances for hormone-dependent tumors of the breast and of the endometrium. The substances that bind to the progestin receptors are partly progestin antagonists, in that they inhibit, for example progesterone-induced formation of alkaline phosphatase [98].

Estrogenic actions have been demonstrated for, among others, anethole-containing culinary herbs and spices, e.g. anise and fennel, as well as for cumin, hops, and lovage root. How the action of saffron on the uterus and the anti-fertility effect of rue and of juniper take place remains unclear. A few herbs and spices are also used for the alleviation of symptoms of dysmenorrhea. Their effects, if any at all, are probably due the content of phytoestrogens and spasmolytic components (cinnamon bark, cumin, European pennyroyal, rosemary, rue, sage, and vanilla).

4.10 Other actions

Culinary herbs and spices with essential oils, particularly anise, fennel, star anise, and thyme, have bronchospasmolytic and secretolytic action for treating bronchial catarrhs, if the vapors of their essential oils enter the bronchi via direct inhalation (cough -teas, -drops, -rubs and -baths) or by percutaneous application (cough -rubs and -baths). With oral application, a large portion of the essential oil components are altered by oxidation and are secreted through the urinary tract in conjugated form without having reached the bronchi. Antiulcerogenic action has been shown for clove, garlic, ginger, paprika, tansy, and also for fenugreek. It is possible that this action takes place through the elimination of *Helicobacter pylori* or, in the case of fenugreek, by protection of the mucosa of the stomach by the mucilage.

Blood sugar lowering activity has been observed for fenugreek and tamarind (by the mucilage causing a delay in sugar absorption?), bay leaves, cumin, olives, onions, and Sarepta mustard.

Juniper, lovage, and parsley, among others, have diuretic action, which may essentially be due to the flavonoid content. Urinary antiseptic action has been postulated for herbs and spices that contain mustard oils, particularly garden cress, garden nasturtium, and horseradish.

In animal tests, antiphlogistic and analgesic actions have been demonstrated for black cumin, capers, celery, cinnamon, clove, ginger, hops, juniper, lemongrass, onions, and tansy. This can likely be attributed to the radical scavenging action and to the action of their lipophilic components to inhibit cyclooxygenase, lipoxygenase or protein kinase activity. Through injury of C-fibers, the capsaicinoids of paprika have analgesic action. Onions have antasthmatic activity (lipoxygenase-inhibition?).

Thrombocyte aggregation is reduced, probably by inhibition of the formation of thromboxane A_2, through clove oil, garlic, nutmeg, olives, and onions. Garlic and onions contribute to increasing the fibrinolytic activity of the blood.

Antidiarrheal action has been observed for nutmeg. The oleuropein from olives has antihypertonic action. Sage has shown an antiperspirant effect. The volatile components of hops, lavender, lemon balm, and rosemary, among others, are supposed to have sedative action. Nutmeg has shown a psychotomimetic effect at high doses.

The virostatic action of many Lamiaceae plants, e.g. of peppermint, rosemary, and sage, is caused mainly by the rosmarinic acid. Because rosmarinic acid is probably not absorbed with oral administration, these herbs display this action only with topical application. Immunostimulation is supposed to be caused by black cumin oil, garlic, and tamarind fruits, among others.

A range of culinary herbs and spices have shown anthelmintic action, e.g. herb materials that contain alliaceous oils such as asafetida and garlic, or essential oil containing herbs such as basil, cinnamon, or tansy, among others. Insecticidal and insect repellant action has been demonstrated for mugwort, bay, clove, and pepper, among others.

5 Medicinal use of herbs and spices

In higher doses, not typical for their employment as spices, individual culinary herbs and spices have a range of specific effects in addition to their appetizing and digestive promoting actions.

Herbs and spices are used prophylactically and therapeutically as **stomachic** remedies. Particularly used for these purposes are those herbs with essential oils (Aromatica), with essential oils and bitter substances (Aromatica amara), as well as essential oils and/or pungent compounds (Aromatica acria), e.g. angelica, caraway, cardamom, cinnamon bark, clove, coriander, fennel, ginger, lemon balm, nutmeg, orange peel, peppermint, spearmint, and wormwood. The appetizing action of spices can also be employed when a low-sodium diet is indicated, e.g. in cases of hypertension, in order to make foods more palatable. In cases of flatulence and meteorism, these herbs or their essential oils, preferably caraway and fennel, are used as **carminatives**. Stomachic and carminative herbs are taken about 30 to 60 minutes before eating in the form of tea infusions, tinctures, essential oils, powdered crude herbs or as finished medicinal products.

Due to their content of essential oils with secretolytic and secretomotor actions, many herbs and spices are also used as **expectorants**, e.g. anise, fennel, star anise and thyme. They are used in the form of tea infusions (drunk slowly, warm and well sweetened) or of essential oils (per inhalation, percutaneous, less beneficial perorally).

Some herbs and spices, e.g. juniper berries, lovage root, and parsley root, are used as **diuretics** in the form of infusions, e.g. for irrigation therapy in cases of urinary tract infections. Garden nasturtium and horseradish, among others, are used as **urinary antiseptics**.

Hops and lemon balm serve as **sedatives.**

Due to the radical scavenging action of alliaceous oils, which inhibit LDL oxidation by blocking the uptake of LDL into macrophages that are responsible for atherosclerotic plaque formation, herbs and spices that are capable of forming alliaceous oils are used as **antiatherosclerotic remedies**, e.g. garlic, onion, and ramsons. Herbs and spices with alliaceous oils, e.g. asafetida and garlic, or with thujone, e.g. tansy, are used in folk medicine as **anthelmintic**.

The essential oils of a few herbs and spices, e.g. of basil, clove, juniper, lavender, and rosemary, herbs and spices that contain mustard oils (black mustard, Sarepta mustard, white mustard) or capsaicinoids, e.g. paprika, are used topically, usually in the form of alcoholic solutions or ointments, as **agents for skin irritant therapy** for rheumatic, neuralgic and arthritic complaints as well as for muscle pains.

6 Toxicology of culinary herbs and spices

6.1 Acute toxic effects

Based on existing data, there is no acute or chronic toxicity with the use of culinary herbs and spices by healthy individuals at normal doses. This is evidenced by the use of today's commonly used herbs and spices over the past millennia. Potential risks are discussed in chapters 6.2 and 6.3.

In cases of certain gastric illnesses, e.g. gastritis or stomach ulcers, the consumption of spices that trigger a sensation of "pungent" such as garden cress, garlic, horseradish, paprika, pepper, Sarepta-, white- and black mustard as well as other herbs and spices, such as turmeric, which strongly increase the production of gastric juice, may aggravate those ailments. In cases of kidney diseases, the inflammatory processes can be worsened by the intake of high doses of spices that contain essential oils, mustard oil or capsaicinoids. Herbs and spices should only be used sparingly during pregnancy; some of them, e.g. black cumin, caraway, parsley fruit, pepper, and saffron, are suspected to induce abortion at high doses. In cases of spice overdoses, even healthy individuals can experience toxic symptoms, for example photodermatosis from the use of angelica, citrus fruits, lovage, parsley, and rue, as well as psychotomimetic effects and general symptoms of intoxication from high doses of nutmeg; atypical, partially serious cases of poisonings have also been reported with overdoses of cinnamon bark, saffron, sage, sweet woodruff, and tansy.

6.2 Allergic reactions

As it is the case with many other substances, a number of herb and spice components are able to start allergic inflammations. These allergies belong to the Type I and Type IV. Allergic reactions of the Type II and III are not relevant for herbs and spices.

Type I allergic reactions (anaphylactic or immediate-type hypersensitivity) are caused by sensitization to certain proteins occurring in plants. This sensitization leads to the production of IgE-type antibodies, which are bound to mast cells or basophilic granulocytes. Upon subsequent contact with the allergy-causing antigens (allergens), these cells release inflammatory mediators, for example histamine. The observed reactions, which can start after seconds or minutes, differ depending on the location where they occur. Contact with allergenic dust leads to conjunctivitis, rhinitis, and asthma attacks, among other reactions. Upon intake of allergens present in foods, swelling of the lips, tongue and throat may occur, as well as gastrointestinal symptoms, skin reactions (urticaria), respiratory symptoms (asthma) and cardiovascular effects. The sensitization and allergic reactions are triggered by the contact of the allergen with the mucous membrane. Negative environmental factors are facilitating the occurrence of these allergies [45].

Allergens responsible for Type I allergies are mostly proteins with a relatively small molecular mass (10 to 70 kDa); most always, they are destroyed during the cooking process (only rarely, for example in celery, its allergenic constituents are heat stable). Well known is the birch pollen allergen Bet v 1 (155 amino acid residues, over 20 isoallergens). Another allergen is profilin (124 to 153 amino acid residues, numerous isoallergens) occurring in most of the eukaryotes. Such allergens are mostly found on the surface of pollen grains. Hence, pollen grains have a considerable sensitization potential. 50 to 93% of the individuals who are allergic to birch pollen also suffer from allergies against many foods and spices. For culinary herbs and spices, the birch-mugwort allergy plays a particular role. Individuals with this allergy show allergic reactions towards birch and mugwort pollen as well as towards spices from umbelliferous plants (Apiaceae), for example towards anise, celery, carrots, cumin, coriander, dill, fennel, and parsley. In these cases, cross reactions occur, which means that sensitization by birch- and mugwort surface proteins is leading to allergic reactions even after contact with other plants that contain the same or structurally similar allergens [40, 79, 88, 93].

Contact allergies (delayed type, Type IV reactions) are also frequently observed. In these cases, human proteins react with chemically very reactive plant constituents, known as haptens. The reaction product, an allergen, then sensitizes T-lymphocytes that form specific antibodies to recognize the hapten. These T-cells release lymphokines upon repeated contact with the hapten, and subsequent immunological chain events trigger skin reactions, most often eczema. The outbreak of the symptoms is delayed and usually manifest within 12 to 96 hours. Culinary herbs and spices with contact allergenic activity and moderate to high sensitization potential include bay leaf, cinnamon, garlic, hops, tansy, and vanilla, among others [Ü39].

Such haptens include the sesquiterpenes with α-methylene-γ-lactone group or β-unsubstituted cyclo-pentanone ring. They alkylate nucleophilic groups of proteins, in particular SH-groups, according to a

Michael-Addition type mechanism and thus convert them into complete antigens. This type of allergy only manifests upon skin contact with the allergen, not with peroral intake. Such sesquiterpene lactones occur especially in the glandular trichomes of the aster family (Asteraceae), for example mugwort and tansy, but also in the laurel family (Lauraceae), such as bay leaf. 00Other haptens include, among others, alkylphenols (e.g. occurring in pink pepper) [Ü100].

6.3 Cancerogenic and hepatotoxic effects

Estragole (methylchavicol, → Fennel), safrole (→ Sassafras) and pulegone (→ European pennyroyal) showed hepatocarcinogenic and/or hepatotoxic effects in animal tests at high doses. Since culinary herbs and spices are used sparingly and only contain small amounts of estragole (a few basil varieties, fennel, French tarragon, chervil), safrole (particularly in sassafras, in small amounts also in caraway, ginger, nutmeg, pepper, and star anise) or pulegone (buchu leaf, European pennyroyal, and few other races of mint species), any danger to human health is unlikely.

Administration of high coumarin doses led to serious liver damage in a number of animal species (for example in rats, mice, and rabbits). The toxic effects in these animals are due to the biotransformation of coumarin to coumarin-3,4-epoxide, which can react with proteins and/or DNA. In humans however, coumarin is mainly transformed into the non-hepatotoxic 7-hydroxycoumarin (umbelliferone). Coumarin-3,4-epoxide, occurring as a metabolic by-product, is detoxified in the liver with glutathione by formation of N-acetyl-S-(3-coumarinyl) cysteine. Only with the intake of very high coumarin doses (→ Sweet woodruff, tonka beans) that exceed the detoxification capacity of the liver, hepatotoxic effects occur. However, they are not to be expected if the herbs are used at normal doses. To avoid possible risks, the use of both of the above-mentioned two herbs is limited by applicable food laws (see also → Sweet woodruff, food law regulations) [53].

Due to its content of hepatotoxic and hepatocarcinogenic pyrrolizidine alkaloids, a few authors caution against the use of → Borage. Its use as a medicinal plant is not recommended. It is assumed that high doses of → Black cumin also have hepatotoxic effects.

In a few animal tests, → Paprika or → Pepper facilitated the development of tumors.

7 Culinary herbs and spices as preservatives

Culinary herbs and spices are not only used to improve the odor, taste and appearance of foods but they also can extend their shelf-life, especially by inhibiting fat spoilage due to radical scavenging and antioxidative properties and to a lesser extent due to their antimicrobial activity.

Fats, which contain unsaturated fatty acids, e.g. linoleic- or linolenic acid, are easily subjected to autoxidation reactions. This process is facilitated by the presence of heavy metal traces, chlorophyll, hemoglobin or riboflavin and accelerated by light, water and high temperatures. The higher the number of double bonds in the molecule, the quicker the autoxidation reaction takes place. Autoxidation is a very complicated and not yet fully understood process which is initiated by activated oxygen molecules that are formed by light and enzymatic processes. Thereby, hydroperoxides are formed, which are split into aldehydes and alkoxy radicals, among other reaction products. Short chain fatty acid residues are converted into ketones. The ketones and aldehydes thus formed can spoil fats due to their disagreeable odor and taste as well as by their irritant effects (aldehyde- or ketone rancidity). A concomitant process is the polymerization of fatty acid radicals, which leads to resinification of fats [Ü99].

Many culinary herbs and spices are able to inhibit autoxidation processes due to the radical scavengers they contain (→ Chap 4.5). Particularly effective are lamiaceous culinary herbs due the content of aromatic o-dihydroxyditerpenes and caffeic acid derivatives. Their effects are comparable to butylhydroxyanisol, which is used as a synthetic food preservative. The food preserving effects can be quantified using the so-called antioxidant-factor. It represents the ratio of a product's shelf-life with and without spices added. For example for pork lard with sage, the ratio is 14.1 (meaning that the shelf-life is increased by a factor of 14.1) or for rosemary 17.6, for minced pork with both aforementioned spices 5.3 and for mayonnaise 2.4 to 2.2. Allspice, cinnamon, clove, ginger, nutmeg, and turmeric have shown good preservative effects particularly in oil/water emulsions. Oxidation-sensitive coloring matters, e.g. carotenoids, which are subjected to a similar oxidation as fats due to the presence of numerous double bonds, can also be stabilized by the aforementioned spices [Ü30]. Black pepper showed good effect in fat preservation during the smoking and curing of sausages [56, 73, Ü30]. Particularly sage, but also juniper berries, oregano, and thyme were able to retard the spoilage of rapeseed oil; the same is true for rosemary and thyme in pork lard [36, 83]. The development of carcinogenic heterocyclic amines in meat was suppressed by → Garlic [85].

Due to their antimicrobial effects (→ Chap 4.3), culinary herbs and spices can retard food spoilage caused by microorganisms, for example in meat products. A significant delay in spoilage was achieved with clove (0.5 g/kg), mace (1 g/kg), and cinnamon (0.2 g/kg). Particularly effective were the essential oils of cinnamon, clove, coriander, garlic, ginger, mace, pepper, and thyme [Ü30]. The antimicrobial effect is in some cases contributing to the growth inhibition of mycotoxicogenic fungi, or their mycotoxin production (→ Cumin). Since spices themselves often contain mycotoxins, this effect cannot be generalized.

The food preserving and antimicrobial effects of culinary herbs and spices can of course only be used to a limited extent since the required concentrations for the preservation of foods in most cases lead to undesired changes in the taste of the product. Extracts, whose essential oils have been removed, however, can be used in relatively high concentrations.

8 Spice plants: Breeding, cultivation and harvest

8.1 Breeding

The breeding of spice plants is oriented towards producing:

- Favorable sensory properties,
- high content of flavor-substances, e.g. essential oils,
- increased yield (crop) performance,
- improvement of certainty of the yield, e.g. resistance against drought, frost, insects and plant diseases,
- attainment of yield stability, i.e. preservation of the favorable properties of the plant that were acquired from breeding and also of its progeny,
- improvement of harvest certainty, e.g. simultaneous maturity of fruits, inhibition of fruit opening to prevent seeds from falling out, firmer fruit set or high standing ability for the facilitation of mowing,
- improvement of growth characteristics, e.g. ability to produce large leaves and higher leaf proportion for leaf drugs, higher yield of root for root drugs [8].

Compared to the breeding of other economic crops, the breeding of spice crops is still in its infancy. Only those plants with a very high market demand, e.g. caraway, marjoram, and peppermint, have been subjected to intensive breeding programs. The methods used are the same as those used for the breeding of other economic crops. The primary method is selective breeding and, less often, combination breeding and mutation breeding. Biotechnological methods will certainly play a large role in the future breeding of spice plants [8, 15].

8.2 Cultivation

The wild collection of spice plants plays almost no role in Central Europe in contrast to the wild collection of medicinal plants. At the most, just a few herbs are obtained by wild collection for home use, e.g. angelica, juniper berries, mugwort, ramsons, salad burnet, watercress, and wild thyme.

In cultivation, yield and quality of spice plants are strongly influenced by quality and quantity of light, temperature, water- and nutrient-supply; but it should also be taken into consideration that each plant has very specific demands. Light already plays a role in the germination of the seeds. Some seeds germinate only in the dark (dark germinators), e.g. anise, garlic, lavender, and lovage, some others only in the light (light germinators), e.g. angelica and caraway. The quantity of light influences the yield of foliage. For many plants, the light cycle determines whether a plant will bloom or not. Short-day-plants bloom only when the duration of daily light exposure falls below a certain level and long-day-plants bloom only when the duration of daily light exposure exceeds a specific time. On the other hand, blooming is often a prerequisite for the formation of a certain spectrum of flavor substances and of course for development of fruits. The same is true for a specific optimum temperature. Each plant species also poses its own requirements for water-, mineral- and nutrient supply. These factors not only influence the yield of biomass, but also the spectrum of flavor constituents and their concentrations.

For cultivation, only recognized, varietally pure seeding material should be used. That is not only important with regard to

yield performance, but also to the desired sensory properties, due to the existence of different chemical races of one plant species. Data on the properties of individual varieties can be found in the database of descriptive variety lists of the German Bundessortenamt [Ü14, Ü15, Ü16].

In industrial cultivation, sowing takes place facilitated by mechanical inter-row cultivation almost always as drill sowing, accomplished today usually with precision drill planters, which are fitted with, for example, perforated seed plates, belt feeders or bucket wheels. In some cases transplanting into the open field occurs after planting in advance in a hotbed or in the greenhouse. Vegetative propagation is also frequently done, carried out using tubers, bulbs, cuttings or also by stock division. Planting in small areas is done by hand, and in large areas with mechanical planters (flexible disc transplanters, snap picker arm, etc.) [Ü21].

Certainly in the future, propagation by way of cell cultures will also become important. This allows a vegetative mass propagation of genetically uniform plant materials, because any cell of a culture that originated from a plant can, under suitable conditions, be regenerated to grow the plant again. Because of the relatively high costs, this method is used only in cases where it provides big advantages, e.g. where seeds are not easily accessible or germinate poorly, or where it is necessary to attain a great uniformity of plant material. If one uses apical cones, being free of viruses also in infected plant, to start cell cultures, virus-free clones are obtained.

Many spice plants are self-incompatible by toxic metabolites excreted into the soil that can kill themselves. 4 to 5 years should elapse before planting them again in the same location (e.g. umbellifer and mint family plants).

Spice plants, which can be cultivated outdoors in Central Europe with good yields include, among others (life span in parenthesis: 1 = annual, 2 = biennial, St = perennial): angelica (St), basil (1), black mustard (1), borage (1), caraway (2, also 1), celery (St), chervil (1), chive (St), clary sage (St), coriander (1), dill (1), fennel (1), fenugreek (1), garden cress (1), garden nasturtium (St), garlic (St), hops (St), horseradish (St), hyssop (St), lavender (St), lemon balm (St), lovage (St), marjoram (1 or 2), mints (St), mountain savory (St), mugwort (St), onion species (St), oregano (St), Oswego tea (St), parsley (2, in the 2nd year only useable for leaf harvest in the spring, then flowering and fruiting), peppermint (St), leek (St), rue (St), safflower (1), sage (St), Sarepta mustard (1), southernwood (St), summer savory (1), sweet cicely (St), tarragon (St), thyme (St), watercress (1), white mustard (1).

Controlled cultivation in Central Europe for the most part eliminates quality defects, such as those that often occur with imported materials, especially from developing countries, e.g. impurities, quite uncontrollable pesticide residues, high levels of microbiological contamination, high heavy metals content, and mycotoxins, especially with imports from countries with a humid warm climate.

Integrated plant protection consists of the prevention of pest infestation of plants, e.g. by use of healthy seed- and planting-stock, selecting suitable cultivation sites as well as by suitable crop rotation, intensive crop maintenance, adequate fertilization, breeding resistant strains and eradication of intermediate (bridging) hosts, but also in the treatment of diseased or insect-infested plants with crop protection chemicals.

As far as possible, the use of crop protection chemicals in the cultivation of spice plants is to be avoided. The soil should also be free of residues from previous chemical treatments. It is however important to keep in mind that crop protection chemicals are still used in the cultivation of spice plants. Contamination with these chemicals is also possible by way of drift from spraying in neighboring fields.

Insecticides, acaricides, molluscicides and rodenticides are used for the control of insects, mites, snails and rodents. Herbicides serve to limit weed infestation of the fields. Weeds interfere with not only the growth of spice plants, but also cause contamination of the botanical raw materials. Herbicides are usually used before sowing or before the shoots emerge. If the use of an herbicide on a fully developed plant stand must be carried out, a preharvest interval, from application of the herbicide up until harvest of the plants, must be adhered to. Fungicides are directed against plant infestation by microbial fungi. The preparations used for plant protection are mostly organic compounds of very many substance classes, which for the most part are also toxic for humans.

8.3 Harvest

Not only is the quality of the spice plants of decisive importance for the quality of the spices produced, but also the harvest date, proper harvesting technique and the type of post-harvest treatments. Although plant-specific harvesting standards are applied to each spice plant, there are some generalizations that can be made.

Herbs, that are to be dried, are collected at the start of the blooming period, at which time the concentration of active principles is the highest. The leaves of dill, mugwort, peppermint, and sage are harvested, however, before the blooming period. Basil, lemon balm, summer savory and tarragon are harvested when the plant buds. Leaves, which are to be used fresh, e.g. of borage, chervil, cutting celery, dill, fennel, leek, lemon balm, mints, parsley, sage, and summer savory, can be picked at any time.

Subterranean organs are to be harvested during the dormant period of the plants, that means preferably in the late autumn (October, November), but if there are unfavorable weather conditions in the autumn they can be harvested also in the spring (February, March). During the vegetation period, the content of flavor components of subterranean organs is low.

Seeds and **fruits** are harvested just prior to reaching maturity, the content of active principles in unripe fruits is in many cases low, and with mature fruits there is the risk that the fruits may drop off before or during the harvest. In some cases, however, the unripe fruits are also harvested (e.g. vanilla and pepper).

Flowers, leaves and herbs, that are to be dried, should not be harvested during or shortly after rainy periods, but always after 1 to 2 rain-free days, because water-soluble active principles are leached out by the rain or they can be degraded by post mortem reactions during an extended drying process due to the high moisture content of plants after rainfalls. The most favorable harvest time is in the late morning, if the dew has evaporated. Plants with essential oil should be harvested if possible under overcast skies. Solar radiation lowers the content of volatile substances.

The harvest of herbs is done by hand on small farming operations (e.g. with a knife, hand sickle or scythe), and for industrial scale cultivation they are machine harvested by mowing with special swathes, cutter-loaders, green forage harvesters or loader combines, e.g. for peppermint, for the harvest of fruits or seeds with combine harvesters, e.g. fennel, for the harvest of roots, if the above ground parts of the plants do not die off, after removal of the herb with a flail chopper, the roots are lifted with oscillating share-, vibrating screen- or chain-uprooters, e.g. for horseradish. Some plant parts must also be harvested by hand, e.g. clove, saffron, and vanilla. The heavy-duty separator, air separator and sheller installations are used for cleaning of the fresh or dried crop and for root drugs washing installations are used [Ü21].

8.4 Herbs in the garden or anywhere else

Because most herbs are best used when fresh, home growing is highly recommended. You can raise spice plants on your own but they can also be purchased at nurseries, building centers or supermarkets and often grown at home in the same container, or also after planting them into pots, balcony boxes or in the garden. Bay and rosemary can be planted in a sufficiently large pot. They must over-winter indoors.

What can be grown in Western and Central Europe is described in Chapter 8.1.

For **propagation,** seeds are sown either in pots, cultivating trays, seed pans or frames or directly in the field. The propagation vessels should contain fine crumbly, light soil (fine compost + vermiculite or perlite 1:1). After planting, the containers should be covered with glass discs or plastic film (for dark germinators also with newspaper). The covering is removed after germination. Seeds of light germinators should only be pressed on, but not covered with soil. The temperature in the night should not drop below 18 °C. If the seedlings grow too close together, they are thinned out by clipping some of them with scissors (if pulled out the neighboring plants can be uprooted). As soon as the plants have developed two foliage leaves over the cotyledons, they are pricked out. For that purpose, one to three plantlets are removed together, preferably using a spatula, with as much of the adhering soil as possible (in order to accomplish this, it is helpful to moisten the soil somewhat in advance) and then transplanted into small pots filled with compost. One can also sow the seeds directly into Jiffy pots, paper pots or soil blocks (recommended especially for plants with taproots, e.g. caraway or parsley). In these cases the plants are not pricked out, but rather after germination all of the seedlings are removed except for the strongest. If the plantlets are strong enough, they are hardened, by placing the pots in the garden during the daytime. After about three to four weeks, weather permitting, they are transplanted in the open field. Plants that do not produce seeds, e.g. French tarragon and some mints, are planted in the summer from cuttings. All lignescent herbs such as hyssop, lavender, rosemary, sage, thyme, and winter savory are also easily propagated in this way. The cuttings are rooted in a warm location, if necessary after their base is dipped into rooting powder; then, a few of them are planted in a pot covered with a plastic bag that has ventilation holes. They are transplanted in the following spring. Another possibility for the propagation of herbaceous perennial plants, e.g. of lemon balm, oregano, peppermint or thyme, is by division of the unearthed plant cushion.

Plants that are largely cold resistant, e.g. caraway, dill, and chives, are sown in March to April in the open field, cold-sensitive plants only after the last night frosts in May, and frost germinators (angelica, ramsons, sweet cicely) in the autumn. After the emergence of seedlings they are thinned out by cutting.

Perennials and annual plants should be planted as neighbors, which make caring for them easier. Highly rampant plants (e.g. mints or lemon balm) are planted in tubular containers with open bottoms dug in the soil. Otherwise their rapid spreading is hardly controllable.

Annual plants, from which the fresh herb will be used (e.g. chervil, dill), should be sown several times annually, in intervals of about 1 month.

If one does not have a garden and would also like to have fresh herbs available in the winter, they can be grown in **herb pots** or **herb trays**. They can, if sufficiently large enough (Ø minimum 30 cm), hold several spice plants, e.g. basil, chives, dill, oregano, parsley, rosemary, and sage. Also an ensemble of small pots (Ø 10 to 12 cm) with only one plant species has proven to be useful. In summer they are placed outdoors, in the autumn they are brought into a warm (13 to 18 °C), light room, e.g. in a light corridor, on the steps of the staircase inside the house, in a paned veranda or in the winter garden, rotated every couple of days so that they do not become "one sided." Naturally such pots provide for only a modest yield, but they are decorative and their spice plants are well suited as an addition to salads or as a garnish of cold plates, among others. The pots must contain loose soil (coarse sand + loamy soil + peat in equal parts, enriched with slow-release fertilizer) and have good drainage holes. They should be kept on the terrace and on the balcony on flower saucers so that no unsightly stains are produced. In the spring they should be repotted. Annual plants (basil, dill, parsley) are then also replaced by new ones, and the perennial plants that have grown too large are divided.

An **herb tower** is also suitable for the balcony or terrace. For this purpose, mesh wire (about 1 × 1.5 m, mesh size about 5 to 7 cm) is rolled together and connected to a cylinder with its loose wire ends. The cylinder is placed on a large flower saucer. The inside is lined with waterproof material, e.g. plastic film, and then filled with soil. Finally, using the wire meshes as frames, the plastic lining is perforated in specific intervals with a sharp knife. The cuttings of the spice plants are placed in these perforations on a slight angle: the smaller, upright plants are planted in the upper part, the fast growing and moisture-loving ones in the lower part [Ü95].

If constructing an **herb bed**, it should be situated as close to the house as possible and be quickly accessible, for example through the terrace. Because one may perhaps desire to grow herbs more extensively later, one should allow for expansion possibilities. Many spice herbs prefer sun (e.g. anise, basil, caraway, clary sage, coriander, dill, fennel, garden nasturtium, hyssop, marjoram, oregano, Oswego tea, rosemary, rue, sage, southernwood, summer savory, tarragon, and thyme), but others also thrive quite well in half-shade (e.g. angelica, arugula, chervil, chives, horseradish, lemon balm, lovage, mints, parsley, sweet cicely, and sweet woodruff). Decorative plants, e.g. hyssop, lemon thyme, marjoram, oregano, Oswego tea, and sage, can also be integrated into a stone garden.

The soil should be permeable. If not, one can construct a right-angled or round raised bed, which can be filled up with suitable soil (e.g. mixture of coarse-grained sand, loam and humus). Making an herb spiral or an herb mound (see below) also takes care of this problem. The raised bed should be constructed only so wide that one can reach the plants in the center of the bed. Other types of herb beds should also be accessible up to the center (about

1.2 to 1.5 m wide, near separation walls or house walls 0.9 m). Paths are put in, that are as easy to care for as possible, e.g. from bricks, paving stones or natural slabs (also installed as stepping stones).

If the herb bed is large, the smaller spice plants should be put on the outside, if possible, on the side that is aligned with the most solar radiation, e.g. basil, marjoram, parsley, and thyme, followed by the medium height plants, e.g. borage, dill, tarragon, and sage, and completely in the center of the bed the tall plants such as angelica, fennel, and lovage. One can certainly also grow caraway, celery, garlic, horseradish, leek, and onions, but they are also commercially available in good quality [Ü33].

In order to prevent plant diseases and insect infestations, annual and biennial plant varieties and location should be changed annually or after two years, respectively. Insecticides should not be applied to culinary herbs which are used as seasonings. Even with adherence to a preharvest waiting period, it is not certain whether the plants will actually be free of insecticide residues when used. The use of non-toxic snail bait (e.g. ferric phosphate) is harmless; otherwise, snails need to be removed manually. Aphids can be sprayed off with a strong water-jet. Individual branches infested with insects or fungi are to be immediately removed and destroyed (best burned up, not composted!). One should not touch dripping wet plants. Fungal spores could be transferred via water drops [Ü1, Ü47, Ü64, Ü67].

An **herb spiral** makes it possible to grow spice plants in a tight space. It should be laid out in the warmest and sunniest spot in the garden. The diameter can be up to about 3 m. To construct, dig out a flat pit and fill it with a thick layer of gravel. Then build an ascending, spiral-shaped wall with large stones stacked as close to one another as possible, which reach the center with 1 1/2 revolutions. A pile of stones is heaped in the center, which serve to store heat. Then it is filled with garden earth. Moreover, starting at the outside with loamy garden earth and compost in a ratio of 1:1, followed by loamy garden earth and compost in a ratio of 3:1 and finally a mixture of sand, garden earth and compost in a ratio of 1:1:1. The center of the spiral should be situated about 50 cm above the ground. According to the moisture requirements and the size of the plants, they are planted in an approximate order (from the exterior to the interior of the spiral) of mint, borage, parsley, chervil, chives, mugwort, lovage, rosemary, dill, tarragon, sage, summer savory, hyssop, fennel, coriander, and caraway [Ü33, Ü71].

Enclosed by round wood, an **herb mound** is built by piling first a layer of brushwood, reversed sod bricks, half-ripe compost and then garden earth. Concerning the reachability of the plants, the herb mound should not be more than 1.5 m wide [Ü71].

Herb gardens serve as a useful adornment that pleases the eyes and the nose and they can also be a nice little place to relax. There are no limits placed on the design of your fantasy. There are however good books, in which one can find suggestions for the design of herb gardens [Ü17, Ü18, Ü33, Ü47, Ü64, Ü67].

9 Processing of spice plants

9.1 Preservation

Fresh culinary herbs should be put with their petioles in water (like a bunch of flowers) immediately after harvest even if they will be used within 24 h. If they are not used on the same day, they can be stored for a few days in the refrigerator, in sealed plastic bags with a few drops of water.

Comminuted fresh herbs can also be frozen with water in the ice-tray and kept for a few weeks in the freezer compartment. These "spice-cubes" can be stored in the freezer in a freezer bag for up to one year. Culinary herbs that have been flash frozen (e.g. basil, chervil, cutting celery, dill, fennel, lemon balm, lovage, marjoram, mint, parsley, and tarragon) keep their full flavor even after months of storage, and can be used until the next harvest. Before freezing, the herbs should be briefly washed, spot dried and then chopped. By applying manual pressure, as much air as possible should be removed from the freezer bag before flash freezing. The herbs can also be frozen whole and cut to size immediately before use. Deep frozen culinary herbs are also encountered in commerce. Since they are mostly packed in cartons, they dry out quickly due to the sublimation of water.

Another method of preservation is salt curing. With this method, the fresh herbs (e.g. basil, chives, garlic, marjoram, oregano, rosemary, summer savory, and thyme) are comminuted and alternately covered with layers of table salt (one part of salt for 5 parts of herb) in a container with a cork-glass- or plastic closure. The herbs can be used to season sauces and casserole dishes [Ü1, Ü55, Ü67].

Usually, herbs and spices are preserved by drying. During the drying process when the plant parts die off, the cell membrane and the endomembrane system are destroyed. The enzymes which previously have been spatially separated from the substrate are now able to chemically alter the constituents. Spontaneous reactions also lead to the breakdown of constituents and to the discoloration of the herbal material. Microorganisms contained in the plants or on their surface can negatively influence the dried herb, for example by the formation of bacterial- and mycotoxins. If the water content remains under 10 to 12%, the enzymatic processes and bacterial growth are interrupted. Due to these reasons, the drying process must occur as quickly as possible immediately after harvest. Excessive drying not only leads to discoloration but also to fragmenting of herbal materials and particularly in spice plants with essential oils, to losses of active constituents. In a few leaf herbs, which store their essential oil in oil cells or secretory canals (e.g. parsley, dill), the essential oils are almost completely lost in the course of drying. In the herbal industry, a solution of table salt, cane sugar and flavor enhancers is sprayed on fresh herbs, such as basil, chervil, dill, lovage, and parsley, to protect volatile flavor components from evaporation before they are dried.

Post-mortem processes are sometimes desirable. In these cases, they are facilitated by the delay in drying. Examples are the fermentation of vanilla pods in order to release the vanillin from the glycoside vanilloside and the fermentation of unripe peppercorns to obtain black polymers from orthodiphenolic constituents.

For natural drying of herbs, as it is practiced only on small cropping areas, the culinary herbs or spice plants are layered about 2 to 5 cm thick onto a cloth or paper (not printed!), if possible on racks or trays in a drying chamber, spread out separated by plant species. The plants should not be turned over to accelerate dehydration, particularly when drying herbs which fragment easily. Exposure to sunlight is to be avoided. The drying process is finished when the leaves make a brittle sound, the stalks break easily and the seeds and fruits are also hard in the interior. On an industrial scale, the drying is carried out at elevated temperature in commercial dryers (batch-, shelf-, conveyor band-, dumping floor-, belt-, rotary drum- or spray dryers). The optimal drying temperature for leaves, herbs and seeds is 38 to 42 °C (caution when drying in attics since the temperature there can be considerably higher!) and for roots, which should preferably be peeled and cut, 50 to 60 °C [33, 38, Ü21].

For the production of dried culinary herbs, the plants are sometimes cut into smaller pieces before drying with field choppers or forage cutters. Subsequent separation of the leaf- and stem fragments using an air separator produces a quality known in German as "Blattkrüll" (curly cut leaves). Leaves and flowers can be separated from stalks by so-called "rubbing" process, that means stripping them off from the stems by hand. Only roots, rhizomes as well as tubers are washed and split, and sometimes also peeled.

Freeze drying is also used for drying herbs and spices. With this method, the herb materials are flash frozen at –18 °C and then dehydrated under vacuum by water sublimation. Freeze dried spices are especially used in the food industry but they can also be found in family size packages in retail commerce. They have a good flavor since the essential oil is almost completely retained. Freeze dried spices also have a good water absorption capacity and regain their natural color when reconstituted with water; however, they then attain a spongy consistency [Ü30].

A more advanced method is vacuum-microwave-drying. This process does not generate any essential oil losses and produces an attractive dried herb product with good water absorption capacity [97].

For domestic use, the herbs are cut with garden scissors and dried in bunches, while hung upside down in a warm, well-ventilated area. Only plants that are visibly soiled need to be shortly (!) washed with cold (!) tap water, and then immediately spot dried, for example with a paper towel. During wet weather, culinary herbs can be dried in an electric baking oven with temperature control at about 40 °C. Thereby, the oven door should always be kept open slightly. Drying in the microwave oven is also possible. With this method, the plants are layered between paper towels suitable for microwaving. During this drying process at a low setting for 1 minute, a cup of water is placed in the microwave [Ü67]. After drying, the leaves are stripped from the stems. For → Bouquet garni, whole and dried twigs, which have not been rubbed, are used. Cool storage in sealed airtight containers is recommended (see below).

For obtaining fruits, e.g. anise, coriander, cumin or fennel, the entire infructescences are harvested and dried, to avoid loss of the fruits dropping off, in large paper bags, on paper towels or linen, in a warm place. In order to eliminate insect infestation, some fruits, e.g. coriander, should be wrapped in gauze and immersed briefly into boiling water before drying.

The dried herbs are mostly comminuted in order to take up less space in transport. Comminution leads to considerable losses, particularly in herbs with essential oils, and decomposition of flavor constituents due to oxidative processes, (see below).

Another suitable method of preservation for herbs is the immersion in liquids (see below) such as vinegar (→ Herb vinegars), oil (→ Herb oils) and salt brine (→ Olives). Storage containers should be labeled with the month and year of harvest, date of purchase, and if prepared the date of preparation.

9.2 Disinfestation and sterilization

Disinfestation, i.e. elimination of storage pests and their eggs can be carried out with exposure to vapors of methylbromide, hydrogen phosphide or hydrogen cyanide. Due to the risk of toxic residues, decontamination with pressurized CO_2 (at about 40 bars, Carvex-process) or super cooled air (–100 °C) is most suitable [72, Ü30].

In a few food industry applications, the use of sterilized, i.e. microorganism-free spices, is recommended, especially for seasoning of raw sausages, prosciutto, preserves, ice cream, yogurt, fresh cheese and mayonnaise. Sterilized spices are of particular importance for use in diets for immunosuppressed patients, for example after transplantations.

There are no suitable sterilization methods for the elimination of bacteria, bacteria spores, yeast, fungi and fungi spores, however, that are legal (!) in the German speaking countries. Due to the heat sensitivity of the flavor constituents, heat sterilization is not recommended for most herbs and spices. Other known methods, such as treatment with ozone, carbon dioxide, and high frequency, also lead to undesirable losses of organoleptic properties and to only an unsatisfactory reduction of the microbial count. Due to the not clarified, toxicological risks of the breakdown products arising during sterilization with gamma-, X-, or electron radiation (possible formation of radicals and reaction products?) or with ethylene oxide (chemical reaction of the plant constituents), these methods are, in contrast to many other European countries, not approved in Germany, Austria and Switzerland. For reducing microbial counts, the Bactosafe-process is recommended; therein, herb batches are shortly (up to 2 minutes) exposed to superheated steam (3 bar) [41, Ü83].

In order to reduce microbial counts in seasoned foods, the food industry and particularly the meat sector, has started to use more and more oleoresins, essences, and essential oils due to the resulting reduction of the microbial count during manufacturing.

9.3 Comminution

Only a few culinary herbs and spices reach commerce in whole form (e.g. allspice, bay leaves, cinnamon, clove, mustard seeds, nutmeg, and pepper) mostly however, they are ground, which makes them easier to use for the consumer. Disadvantageous are the partial losses of essential oil and coloring matters during grinding and the limited shelf life of spice powders. Due to the destruction of the oil cavities, the essential oil easily dissipates and the large surface area and the small paths of diffusion facilitate contact of the constituents with atmospheric oxygen, which are therefore easily oxidized.

On an industrial scale, the preferred grinding methods are rod- and roller mills but also cross-beater-, hammer-disk-, tooth-plate- and rigid-hammer-mills, among others. Loss of essential oils during the milling process can be reduced with the application of additives, such as cane sugar, or the use of coating techniques. Most optimal are grinding techniques with coolants such as dry ice, liquid CO_2 or liquid nitrogen. During cooled processes, the loss of essential oil is small and the mechanical grinding process is more effective (the hardness of the ground material is higher, which is partially due to the hardening of fats) [Ü30].

For household use, the herbs should be cut with a sharp (!) knife or scissors. Dried spices are ground immediately before use in a spice mill. Nutmeg is comminuted in a special nutmeg grater or nutmeg mill (see Chapter 13.1).

9.4 Extraction, steam-distillation

The use of spice extracts and essential oils has a number of advantages, including the near sterility of the product, its easy standardization as well as only minor transport and storage costs. Since these types of products are more difficult to measure out, they are often mixed with inert carriers (ethanol, vinegar, fatty oil) or spray dried with protective substances (e.g. tragacanth, gummi arabicum, soy flour + maltodextrin, cyclodextrin) [Ü30].

Most often used are **oleoresins**; these extracts of culinary herbs or spices are manufactured with lightly volatile organic solvents. The extraction of the comminuted spices is mostly carried out at normal pressure by maceration, percolation or digestion. Suitable solvents include methanol, ethanol, acetone, hexane or dichloromethane, among others. Upon distilling of the solvents, which is mostly carried out under vacuum, a small amount of the flavor components is lost. A two-step process is applied to first obtain the essential oil by steam distillation, and subsequently, the non-volatile flavor substances are extracted. Both fractions are then combined. However, this process causes thermal changes of the essential oil components and reduces the amount of their water-soluble components.

The mostly liquid or pasty oleoresins obtained after evaporation of the solvent often have a better odor profile than the essential oils produced by steam distillation. However, they also contain non-volatile lipophilic constituents, for example high molecular paraffin-type hydrocarbons, fatty oils, ester waxes, triterpenes, and pungent compounds [Ü30].

A less destructive but relatively expensive extraction method is supercritical CO_2 fluid extraction (SFE). The dissolving power of supercritical CO_2 increases at constant temperature with higher density. With gradual pressure changes, a step-by-step extraction of the constituents is possible (starting with essential oils, followed by fatty oils and waxes) [27, 52, 77, 78, Ü30].

Essential oils (spice oils) are mostly obtained by steam distillation. Usually fresh plants are brought to a boil in water or exposed to water vapor. In the condensate, the essential oil mostly floating on top, not miscible with water, is easily separated from the water phase (hydrolate). Obtaining the essential oil by steam distillation is the most economical method of production. However, the odor qualities are often changed with this process, mostly in a negative way. Esters are partially hydrolyzed, unstable compounds are thermally broken down, water-soluble volatile components remain completely or partially in the aqueous phase of the steam distillate and the ratio of the more volatile monoterpenes to the less volatile sesquiterpenes changes at the cost of the latter. For example, the odor-determining cis-sabinene hydrate of marjoram is mostly transformed during steam distillation into terpinenol-4, α-terpinene, and limonene. Even though the changes of the constituent profile are not as extreme as in the case of marjoram, the analytical data with regard to the composition of essential oil, that is obtained by steam distillation, does not exactly match the ratios found in the starting plant material.

Differences in the content of main components of essential oils or oleoresins depending on the different types of extraction of the same herb material are exemplified in the case of cardamom oil; product obtained by steam distillation contained, among other constituents, 35.5% α-terpinyl acetate and 31.2% 1,8-cineole; product obtained by hexane extraction contained 57.3% α-terpinyl acetate and 16.6% 1,8-cineole; celery oil obtained by steam distillation contained among others, 50.5% limonene and 23.6% phthalides, with supercritical CO_2 33.4% and 40.6% respectively [77, Ü30].

A more protective but more expensive method of extraction is fractionating extraction of the essential oils with supercritical CO_2 (see above).

In rare cases, the oils are obtained by mechanical methods, e.g. in the case of citrus fruits the oil is expressed from the peel by machine, by centrifuging after mechanically rupturing the oil cavities of the peel or by separating the top layer during the production of citrus juices by homogenization of unpeeled fruits.

10 Contamination of culinary herbs and spices

Culinary herbs and spices can be contaminated with microorganisms, their toxic metabolites, heavy metals, pesticides, herbicides, fertilizers, radioactive substances, environmental poisons, alive or dead insects, sand, soil, dust and foreign plant matter, among other contaminants.

The microbial count of untreated herbs and spices is usually very high (not seldom up to 10^4 to 10^5 cfu/g, in some cases up to 10^8/g). The contaminating **microorganisms** are especially aerobic spore and mold forming germs, which mostly originate from soil. In producing countries with low hygienic standards, the microbial contamination takes place during the harvest and drying processes, for example due to contact with fecal matter, particularly of animals. During the time of harvest and processing in tropical countries, the microorganisms in spices multiply quickly regardless of the content of antimicrobial constituents in the spices; this is due to the high temperature and humidity and leads to the formation of toxic metabolites, particularly mycotoxins. Endogenous microorganisms that live inside the plant also contribute to microbial contamination and the formation of toxic metabolites. Despite high microbial counts, the risks of human infection are low with the use of culinary herbs and spices. In about 90% of the cases where spices are used, the microorganisms are destroyed by the cooking process. In other cases (for example with seasoning of hamburger eaten raw, and with spices used after cooking), our body with its natural defenses against infections is almost always able to eliminate these microorganisms through the disinfecting effects of the stomach acid and the non-specific immune defenses of the gastrointestinal system. Most critical is the use of highly contaminated herbs and spices in the food industry. On raw materials, the microbes multiply quickly and lead to food spoilage, or, with massive growth, the bacterial toxins formed in the substrate can cause food poisoning [41, 51, 84, Ü30, Ü69].

The most important toxic metabolites of microorganisms are **mycotoxins**. It is assumed that about 30 to 40% of all mold fungi species are able to produce mycotoxins. Of particular importance are aflatoxins, zearalenones, ochratoxins, cytochalasans and trichothecenes. Many mycotoxins are relatively heat resistant and remain intact during cooking, baking or extract production. When taken in high doses, they lead to acute symptoms in humans and some of them also cause liver damage and tumors in chronic consumption. Aflatoxins can for example lead to the so-called aflatoxicosis, usually with extreme symptoms of hepatitis. Ochratoxins cause kidney damage. Particularly spices (e.g. chilies, nutmeg, paprika, and pepper) imported from tropical countries, frequently showed relatively high levels of aflatoxins. Acutely toxic concentrations of mycotoxins are not likely to be reached even with the intake of spices, which contain high levels of mycotoxins. However, the risks of cancerogenic effects in chronic consumption should not be underestimated [Ü100, Ü30].

Little is known about the concentrations of **heavy metals** (e.g., lead, mercury, copper, arsenic) occurring in spices. **Nitrates** that are formed in the plant in relatively high concentrations due to the copious application of nitrogen fertilizers, are mostly deposited in the aerial part of some of the spice plants. Upon reduction in the stomach, they can contribute to the formation of carcinogenic nitrosamines. The amount of heavy metals and nitrates ingested through culinary herbs and spices, however, is extremely low when compared to the amounts ingested through other plant-based foods [59].

Even though **pesticides** (antiviral substances, bactericides, fungicides, acaricides, nematicides, rodenticides) are only used very carefully in herb and spice farming, it should be assumed that residues of these agents can occur in culinary herbs and spices. Little is known about the use of such agents in tropical countries, but it may also be that health risks from their use in these countries are rarely encountered [Ü30].

Considerable amounts of **radionuclides** were released by nuclear testing and by the accident at the Chernobyl nuclear power plant. The radioactive contamination of spices, however, is relatively small [Ü30].

Contamination with fragments of large insects, aphids, mites, animal hair, parts of bird feathers, insect excrement, rodent droppings, sand and soil are called **filth** in the spice trade. They are found particularly in culinary herbs and spices with hairy plant parts (e.g. sage and rosemary) or rough surfaces (e.g. clove) [Ü30].

11 Storage and shelf life of culinary herbs and spices

During the **storage of dried culinary herbs and spices**, the quality can decrease. Volatile constituents, e.g. essential oils, evaporate. Spontaneous or enzymatically catalyzed chemical reactions, particularly oxidation-, hydrolysis- or polymerization processes lead to losses of active constituents. Pigments are also broken down. Herbs and spices discolor or turn brown. Decomposition products with disagreeable odor and taste form. Microorganisms can lead to the accumulation of toxic bacterial- or mycotoxins in herbs and spices. Insect infestation can render herbs and spices worthless. Volatile substances from the environment can be absorbed.

Therefore, a number of measures must be taken to inhibit or delay some of the mentioned processes.

- The herbs must be dried well (water content below 12%, for onions below 10%), otherwise, there is a risk of mold growth and undesirable enzymatic reactions, as well as spontaneous ignition.
- The herbs should be stored in uncomminuted form. Destruction of the cellular matrix, particularly the tearing of secretory vessels, as well as the increase in surface area, facilitate the loss of volatile substances and the penetration of oxygen, and thus cause oxidative changes.
- The storage temperature should not exceed 20 °C. The herbs should under no circumstances be stored in the attic, as this was traditionally practiced, but in a dry basement. The most optimal storage temperature is at or below 5 °C. High temperatures accelerate decomposition processes and evaporation of volatile substances. The storage temperature should be kept as constant as possible, since the effect of warm air on cold botanical raw materials leads to the formation of condensation water (transpiration, for example during transport on ships). For large-scale storage, the herbs are therefore stored most optimally in air-conditioned facilities.
- Exposure to light is to be avoided. Light contributes to the formation of radicals and facilitates oxidative changes.
- Herbs and spices with volatile constituents should be stored in gas-tight containers. Polyethylene and polypropylene bags are not suitable for storage; lipophilic materials indeed retain moisture, but volatile, lipophilic constituents such as components of essential oils are adsorbed and do permeate the plastic material, even though this process is slow. Storage bags made of polyamides retain volatile compounds much more effectively, but they can release bitter tasting monomers from the plastic material. For retail commerce, when only limited storage is required, parchment paper or cellophane bags can be used. For the extended storage of small amounts, for example for household use, polyethylene-lined aluminum foil, brown glass- or porcelain containers as well as tin or aluminum boxes are most suitable. Even herbs with non-volatile flavor substances should be stored in airtight containers. In this way, water adsorption and insect infestation can be avoided. The effect of atmospheric oxygen is also diminished.
- Herbs and spices which are not stored in airtight containers must be kept in dry storage facilities. The relative humidity should not exceed 60%. They should not be stored together with other strongly odorous substances or other herbs and spices. The stored herbal material will absorb the odor of these substances.
- The storage of dried herbs in bags is not recommended. During stacking of bags, the herbs experience a high degree of fragmentation, particularly in leaf- and (aerial) herb materials. Hard containers are preferred for storage.
- Herbal materials that are prone to insect infestation must be decontaminated in a suitable manner to remove all living insects including their eggs; they also must be protected from renewed infestation.
- Storage containers for herbs and spices should always be completely emptied and cleaned before they are filled with the next lot. Residual microorganisms and insect infested remains, in the case of fatty and essential oils, the radicals formed can accelerate spoilage.
- Fresh ginger, garlic and onions are stored in baskets or clay pots permeable to air, otherwise they become moldy.

For household use, the following rules continue to be valid: Do not store your spices above the stove (heat!) and do not sprinkle the spices directly from the spice jar or the spice mill onto the boiling or heated dish. Water vapors will enter the container and lead to aroma losses, clumping of its contents as well as mold growth.

Even with careful storage, the **shelf life of culinary herbs and spices** is limited. Particularly relevant are flavor changes or losses as well as discoloration. The shelf life depends on the type of active constituents and decreases with higher degree of comminution. Essential oils and uncomminuted herbs and spices containing essential and/or fatty oils should not be stored for longer than 3 years after harvest, chilies, dill tops, and paprika not longer than 2 years.

Long-term **storage of ground spices** is not recommended. This is especially true for spice powders with characteristic odor qualities. Disruption of the tissue, in particular of the oil vessels, and the increased surface area of the ground material, leads quickly to the evaporation of volatile constituents, to oxidation reactions due to increased contact with atmospheric oxygen and adsorption of foreign aroma substances. The microbial count is mostly higher in spice powders compared to whole spices. The short-term storage of spice powders can occur under the same condition as whole spices (see above).

The **storage of essential oils and oleoresins** should occur in a cool, dry location, protected from light and if possible in containers with minimal headspace or under inert gas. Essential oils, particularly if they contain a high amount of unsaturated hydrocarbons, only have a very short shelf life. Exposure to oxygen as well as heat, moisture and light lead to oxidative changes of the components. Reaction products with disagreeable odor and strongly skin- and mucous membrane irritating effects form, e.g., aldehydes or peroxides, and through polymerization resin-like substances occur. Since the decomposed constituents are catalysts, the containers need to be emptied completely and washed thoroughly before a new essential oil batch is filled in. Oils from different shipments should not be mixed. Very sensitive essential- or fatty oils, e.g. caraway oil, citronella oil, lavender oil, and lemon oil, should not be stored longer than 1 year. If necessary, preservatives can be added.

12 Analysis of culinary herbs and spices

12.1 Tests for identity

The determination of identity serves to exclude misidentification and adulteration. Such tests are carried out based on the description of a culinary herb or spice and specific identity tests.

Uncomminuted culinary herbs and spices and powdered spices first undergo a preliminary sensory examination of their appearance, sometimes with a magnifying glass, as well as of their odor and taste. If whole culinary herbs and spices cannot be fully identified with this procedure, microscopic examination of a tissue cross-section should be carried out. Color reactions with herbs or extracts thereof can supplement this examination. If powdered herbs or spices are purchased in large amounts, a microscopic examination is absolutely necessary. A comparison of the pictures of the microscopically observed tissue features of an herb or spice to be identified and of those of the components of the powder with the pictures of an unequivocally identified herb or spice and with descriptions, microphotographs and line drawings, as found in standardized specifications and literature sources, can be of great help [for overviews with illustrations see 13, 16, 20, Ü25, Ü35, Ü48, Ü49, Ü94, Ü106, DAC, DAC 86]. In order to assist the reader in the identification, this book contains photos of herbs and spices and short descriptions of whole spices, and in some cases, of their anatomical structures. Only the monographs of herbs and spices that are often traded in powdered form include a description of powder components, and if present, typical reproductions of powders in the form of line drawings.

Despite great progress in analytical technology and especially due to the considerable variability in the spectrum of constituents of herbs and spices, sensory examination is still the fastest and most reliable way to determine from which plant the raw material originated. Preliminary indications of the chemical race that an herb or spice belongs to can be deduced from its odor and taste.

Another identification method is to make visible selected odor- and taste constituents as well as pigments with chemical reagents or physical methods after chromatographic separation. The separation methods of choice are usually TLC (= thin-layer chromatography) [see review in Lit. Ü101, Ü102], HPLC (= high performance liquid chromatography) [see review in Lit. Ü62] or GC (= gas chromatography) [review in Lit. Ü110]. With the help of these methods, information on the chemical race of the herbal material can simultaneously be obtained. If the analysis of odor- and taste constituents as well as the pigments is not sufficient for the identification of the herbal material, or they can only be ascertained with difficulties, other characteristic constituents, the so-called marker compounds are utilized for identification. Since the R_f values or retention times, respectively, are strongly influenced by experimental conditions, the chromatographic parameters of the herbal constituents are compared with chromatographically pure compounds (reference substances) or herbal reference materials [18, 42, Ü99].

Spices without cellular structure, for example essential oils, are also first examined for their appearance, odor and taste, as well as with chromatographic methods. Also used are physico-chemical parameters, such as solubility, relative density, UV- and visible light absorption, refractive index, optical rotation, melting point, boiling point and freezing point. Another method for the identification of essential oils is infrared spectroscopy (IRS), near infrared (NIRS) and medium infrared red spectroscopy (MIRS). Based on the IR spectra, a great number of adulterants can be detected. The determination of the stable isotope ratio ($^{13}C : {}^{12}C$ or $^2H : {}^1H$) in specific positions of the molecule can reveal information about the way the material was produced, for example, if vanillin was obtained naturally or semi-synthetically. Hyphenated methods are also frequently applied, e.g. GC/MS (gas chromatography/mass spectroscopy), IRMS (SIRA, isotope ratio mass spectroscopy) as well as GC-IRMS, HPLC/MS and HPLC/DAD [62, Ü36].

12.2 Tests for purity

For purity testing, the sensory examination is also of primary importance. Many of the **visible impurities**, known as filth (see Chapter 10), as well as foreign plant parts, can be detected with a magnifying glass. To evaluate the extent of the impurities in herbal materials with cellular structure, plant parts, which do not conform to the standards or official descriptions, for example pieces of stems, parts of other plants, mineral components and foreign matter, are all separated out. By weighing the impurities, it is determined if the amount of foreign material is below the official maximum allowable limit, usually below 2%. The amount of filth can also be recognized by suspending the herbal material in chloroform or aqueous organic solvents. In the first case, the heavy filth (e.g. sand, insect feces) sinks to the bottom, in the second case, it floats on the surface (light filth, insect fragments, animal hairs and dander).

Untypical smelling and/or tasting impurities can be recognized by evaluating odor and taste. These impurities can be caused by oxidative changes of fat components (rancidity) or volatile oils (e.g. oxidation products of unsaturated terpenes), as well as by mold (moldy odor) and adsorbed volatile constituents.

The **ash content**, particularly of acid-insoluble ash, indicates whether the material contains impurities, such as soil and sand, beyond the extent that is technically unavoidable or has been adulterated with mineral components. In pharmacy, the test for ash content or content of acid-insoluble ash is carried out according to the European Pharmacopoeia [Ph Eur, 2.4.16 or 2.8.1, respectively]. The allowable limits are defined in the herbal drug monographs. In the food industry, it can be carried out based on DIN 10 223 or ISO 930 specifications. In the revised rules for spices and other seasoning ingredients published in the German Federal Gazette (BAnz 183a, Sept 30, 1998), limits for many culinary herbs and spices have been issued, which normally should not be exceeded [Ü36].

The **water content** of dried culinary herbs or spices should not exceed 12%, in order to inhibit spoilage, for example due to mold and microbial growth as well as enzymatic reactions. In pharmacy, the assay for water content is carried out volumetrically with steam distillation of toluol according to the European Pharmacopoeia [Ph Eur, 2.2.13] or with the loss-on-drying method [Ph Eur 2.2.32]. In the food industry, this test can be carried out according to the DIN 10229 or ISO 939 specifications (for mustard seeds and saffron, the oven-drying method in DIN 10221-2). For the determination of the water content by the loss-on-dry value, a correction is necessary to account for the essential oil content [Ü36].

Purity testing also includes the evaluation of **microbial and mold fungi contamination** [overview in Lit. Ü7]. Usually, the total microbial count lies between 10^3 and 10^8 cfu per gram of herbal material. The microbi-

al count is about proportional to the surface area of the herbal material, and is therefore especially high in leaf-, flower- and aerial herb raw materials. These microbes usually involve aerobic spore-forming germs, yeast, mold spores and coliforms, which are not harmful to humans. Pathogenic bacteria occur only very rarely. With regard to microbiological quality, the European Pharmacopoeia has different specifications depending on the dosage form of a pharmaceutical product (see Chap. 14.2.1). In the spice trade, there are approximate values and limits for culinary herbs and spices which are intended for direct use by the consumer or are added, in the form tested, to food products without microbial reduction treatment (see Chap. 14.1.2).

From the group of **bacterial- and mycotoxins**, today only aflatoxins are assayed quantitatively. This test can be carried out with two-dimensional TLC and UV detection, with ELISA-assays or with immuno-affinity chromatography combined with HPLC and fluorescence detectors [Ü30, Ü36]. There are different maximum allowable limits for the food- (see Chap. 14.1.2) and pharmaceutical industry (see Chap. 14.2.1); nevertheless, both industry sectors limit the content of aflatoxins in a similar way.

Testing for heavy metals, e.g. cadmium, lead, nickel, and mercury ions, is also required. The level of these contaminants is usually determined with atomic-absorption-spectroscopy (AAS) [Ü30, Ü36]. Maximum allowable limits for herbal drugs are in effect (see Chap. 14.2.3), and for culinary herbs and spices recommended values have been established (see Chap. 14.1.4).

Pesticide residues are also analyzed. Due to the chemical diversity of pesticides, presently about 500 different chemical compounds are used globally, their analysis is very difficult. The analytical work is facilitated if the origin of the herbs or spices and agricultural practices are known. Particularly risky is the collection of herbs for household use, which are growing along roadsides and fields. Imported spices from developing countries

can also contain high levels of pesticides. Allowable limits of 34 of the most important pesticides in pharmaceutical products have been issued by the European Pharmacopoeia (see Chap. 14.2.2), and, for the food sector, they are determined by the German regulation for the maximum allowable limits of pesticides (see Chap. 14.1.3).

Disinfestants and sterilization agents or their reaction products, for example with plant constituents, can lead to impurities if no residue-free methods for disinfestation treatment are used.

Radioactive isotopes, for example from nuclear reactor accidents and nuclear testing, can also be present in biological material. Therefore, culinary herbs and spices should be examined for γ-radiation. EU regulations limit such contamination to 600 Bcq/kg, calculated with reference to the fresh herb.

Methods for the **purity testing of essential oils** include:
- Determination of the above mentioned physico-chemical parameters for identity tests, such as relative density, refractive index, optical rotation, freezing point, distillation range, as well as residue on evaporation and solubility in ethanol.
- Evaluation of the chromatographic profile with the aforementioned methods, especially GC or HPLC.
- Chemical parameters, for example content of esters, free alcohols and ketones.
- Testing for defined impurities such as water, foreign esters, fatty oils, resinified essential oils, ethanol-insoluble and water-soluble fractions, halide-containing components, e.g. chlorinated hydrocarbons, heavy metals and peroxide levels above the maximum allowable limits [Ü99].

12.3 Quantitative evaluation of odor-, taste- and coloring substances

Qualitative and quantitative variations in the spectrum of odor- and taste substances as well as coloring matters of culinary herbs and spices, and possible changes of their chemical structure during processing, lead to strong fluctuations in the content of quality-indicating constituents.

If the odor- and taste constituents can be analyzed with a reasonable effort, the standards and specifications, and in the spice trade also the purchaser, demand a minimal content of one or more odor- and taste-determining constituents. Quantitative tests are carried out with physicochemical and/or chemical assays. Since conventional methods are often used, only relative and not absolute values are obtained, which means that the contents required by the standards or specifications must be determined with the method specified.

The most important evaluation of aroma constituents is the determination of the essential oil content. This technique always involves a volumetric determination using steam distillation in a reflux-condenser (Neo-Clevenger apparatus) after the distillate has been captured in a graduated cylinder containing a measured amount of xylol (to prevent the essential oil, whose density is higher than that of water, from sinking to the bottom). In pharmacy, this analysis is carried out according to the European Pharmacopoeia [Ph Eur, 2.8.12]. In the spice industry, this analysis can be carried out according to the DIN 10 228 and ISO 6571 specifications or AOAC method 30.020-30.027. These are convention methods that only produce comparable results under standardized conditions.

In order to determine the quantitative proportion of individual components of the total weight (or volume) of essential oils, the following methods are mainly used:

- Gas chromatography (GC), for culinary herbs and spices Headspace-Gas chromatography (HSGC, analysis of volatile constituents in the gas phase above the herb sample) is also carried out, particularly with the use of microcapillaries (HRGC, High Resolution GC), combined with mass spectroscopy (GC/MS) and detection of ions of selected mass/charge ratio fragments as well as Fourier-Transformation-Infrared-Spectroscopy,

- High Performance Liquid Chromatography (HPLC),
- ^{13}C-NMR-spectroscopic multicomponent analysis.

These methods allow for identification and quantification of almost all components, often more than 100, in one sample of essential oil.

If results of an essential oil analysis are used for determining the essential oil composition of the culinary herb or spice from which the oil was originally obtained from, the type of production method has to be considered. The analysis of essential oils obtained by steam distillation often does not appropriately reflect the composition of the essential oil as it occurs in the culinary herb or spice. During steam distillation, the heat sensitive constituents are broken down to form artifacts, water-soluble constituents remain in the water phase and esters are partially hydrolyzed. If essential oils are obtained with organic solvent or supercritical CO_2 extraction, the content ratios of the constituents change due to solubility differences of the individual components. Even the analytical procedure itself can produce additional artifacts due to thermal stress.

The quantitative determination of an individual constituent or a group of constituents is not sufficient to evaluate the quality of culinary herbs and spices. Most often, the "ensemble" of all odor- and taste constituents as well as coloring matters determines their quality. Therefore, quantitative measurements of constituents do not allow judgment on the sensory properties of herbs and spices.

12.4 Sensory evaluation

For culinary herbs and spices, the sensory evaluation is of crucial importance. Above all other things, it determines if the spice is accepted by the consumer. Such testing is necessary for purchasing, product development and quality assurance [review in Lit. Ü72].

Appearance, odor, taste, aftertaste and mouth feel are examined.

Laboratory methods include, among others:

- Duplicate differential testing according to DIN 10 954 and ISO 5495.
- Threshold value testing according to DIN 10 961, Part 1: Examination of a test series with increasing odor- and taste intensity.
- Triangle testing according to DIN 10 951 and ISO 4120: Comparison of 3 samples of which 2 are identical.
- Duo-trio-method: Comparison of two samples, 1 of which is identical with the standard, performed by 2 analysts.

Quality-evaluating methods include:

- Basic description according to DIN 10 964: Verbal, value-neutral description of properties.
- Sensory profile determination according to ISO 6564: Description of successively perceived sensory impressions. For example initial odor (top note, head), main odor (body, bouquet, base note), after-taste (finish) or initial-, main- and after taste, respectively.
- Sensory analysis ranking according to DIN 10 963 and ISO 8587: Arrangement of test samples of one taste type in a series of increasing taste intensities.
- Sensory analysis with a quantitative response scale according to DIN 10 952, part I, ISO 8587 and ISO 4121: Quality evaluation based on point scale, for example following ASMW-VW 1149.

The test individuals (analysts) must be selected based on their aptitude and training in sensory evaluation. For hedonic examinations, training is not necessary. The group of analysts involved in the testing form a panel, which is led by a team leader [70, Ü36].

For **odor evaluation**, a certain amount of the spice sample to be tested is placed into a sealable container. After storage at a defined temperature for a specific amount of time, the odor is evaluated after opening the container. By varying the temperature, an odor profile is established (sniffing method) [Ü30].

A **taste evaluation** is possible with analysis of a dilution profile. A direct taste evaluation of spices is not possible due to the high concentrations of aroma compounds.

Therefore, taste-neutral diluents in powder or paste form are used, for example lactose and quark as well as gels obtained from starch, gelatin, tragacanth, or carob bean flour. Suspended in water, the spice particles would settle quickly; extracts would not reflect the taste accurately due to different solubility parameters of the aroma components [Ü30].

The easiest method for **essential oil testing** consists of moistening a strip of filter paper with essential oil to repeatedly obtain an odor impression during evaporation. Due to this evaporative "fractionation", odor deviations are more easily detected [Ü38]. The European Pharmacopoeia [Ph Eur 2.2.8] describes the sensory examination as follows: "Mix 3 drops essential oil with 5 ml ethanol, add 10 g saccharose powder and shake. The odor and taste must be similar to that of the plant or parts thereof, from which the essential oil originated."

Furthermore, attempts are made to make the sensory evaluation more objective through the use of new sensory analytical equipment, known as sniff-detectors (electronic nose machines) [19, Ü30].

These examinations are only supportive tools for the evaluation of spices that are used to season specific foods. Additionally, testing under reality conditions is necessary, including taste evaluations of the seasoned foods. Therefore, most manufacturers of seasonings and spice mixtures have in-house test kitchens.

13 Use of herbs and spices in the kitchen

13.1 Aromatic herbs and spices

The directions for use, as to which spice one should add in what amount in order to season a food, can only be given quite hypothetically. Seasoning, in the truest sense of the word, is all a matter of taste. Our directions only serve as advice, in order to stimulate experimentation and thereby come across the individual preferences of your family and dinner guests. With seasoning, some amount of boldness is needed and the saying "learning by doing" also applies here. In any case, one should avoid overseasoning, especially when trying out an unknown spice. The spice must bring out the typical taste of the food, and it should not mask it. A cautious approach and the adding of seasoning according to taste are precautions against overseasoning.

Fresh herbs are excellent supplements to salads. Especially well suited for salads are basil, chervil, chives, dill, oregano, or thyme. These, as well as parsley, also provide an outstanding taste and give good appearance to soups (e.g. potato soup), sauces, stews and omelets. Fresh herbs, e.g. basil, chervil, chives, coriander, dill, hyssop, lemon balm, lemongrass, marjoram, parsley, peppermint, rosemary, tarragon, and thyme are also well suited for the preparation of non-alcoholic herb drinks [Ü57].

If fresh herbs are visibly soiled, they should be washed before use and then any adhering water should be removed (clean kitchen towel, paper towels, salad spinner). Cutting of herbs should be done only immediately before use. If immediate use is not possible, cover the cut herbs with foil. Cutting should not be carried out on a wooden cutting board (wood soaks up the juice of herbs and it is difficult to clean).

Many herbs are best when cut with a scissors or with a sharp (!) knife, e.g. chives and all herbs with large leaves. When cutting a large amount, an herb mill is also suitable. Herbs should only be cut in the blender if they are going to be worked in with other ingredients into a stuffing.

Most herbs are added to cooked dishes only at the end of the cooking process. Some herbs, however, need the cooking process to develop their full aroma, e.g. bay leaf, marjoram, oregano, rosemary, sage, tarragon, and thyme. They are added to the pot about 15 minutes before the end of the cooking time. Basil should be added after cooking, otherwise it becomes bitter. The same goes for horseradish. For seasoning of salads, the herbs should be placed in the salad dressing or vinegar about 10 minutes before use. For grilled dishes it is recommended to put aromatic herbs in oil.

Dried culinary herbs and spices should be ground, but as shortly as possible, before their use. By grinding, a better release of their odor- and taste substances is achieved. Spice mills are suited for comminuting, preferably ceramic mills. For frequently used herbs and spices it is beneficial to use a specific mill. This is especially the case for fatty spices, e.g. cardamom, because the grist leaves a residue in the mill and the flavor of the next grist is masked by it. For comminuting nutmeg, a nutmeg grater or preferably a nutmeg mill is used, and a peppermill for pepper, allspice or black cumin. Cardamom (after removing of the pericarp), coriander fruit, caraway, fennel, and juniper berries can be crushed in a mortar.

Culinary herbs with hard stems and/or leathery leaves are added to foods in their whole form, e.g. bay leaf, rosemary or thyme. Whole allspice, caraway, cinnamon, clove, coriander, juniper, or pepper, must also be cooked with the food, because their essential oil is only slowly released. These spices are removed before serving the meal. In the case of marjoram, mugwort, rosemary, summer savory, and thyme a whole branch should be used or better yet bundled in gauze for → Bouquet garni. For pieces of cinnamon bark or for small or coarsely-cut spices, a stainless steel spice ball or a large tea ball is used. In this case the food during cooking should be stirred frequently or the position of the spice ball should be changed. If pieces of meat are to be grilled or fried, they are rubbed with the spice (e.g. with garlic or rosemary). Saffron and tamarind pulp must be soaked before use. Some spices develop their full aroma only after careful roasting (e.g. sesame).

For dishes requiring a long cooking time, the seasoning agents are first added just before (killing of microorganisms!) the end of the cooking time in order to prevent the escape of volatile substances during long times of cooking. Moreover, with longer cooking exposure, undesired changes in taste can occur through chemical reactions (e.g. to a bitter taste). In particular, allspice, coriander, mace, marjoram, and nutmeg are heat-labile. In the food industry, spice extracts are often used, added after cooking; in such way chemical reactions occur to a lesser extent. Preparing dishes with cooking time of under 20 minutes, one can add spices in whole form at the start of cooking (e.g. allspice, bay leaves, pepper corns, and summer savory). For the seasoning of cold dishes, the spice is added 20 to 30 minutes before eating. Some spices, such as, for example, pepper or paprika, are also on hand at the table to further season the finished dish.

Spice mixtures (→ see chapter at the back of this book) are almost always necessary for the optimization of the taste of meals. These can be prepared at home from coarsely-cut or powdered spices or they can be purchased at the store. It is best to purchase coarsely-cut mixtures and, just before using them, grind them in a spice mill.

Other seasoning ingredients, e.g. seasoning blends, spice aromas, seasoning salts, spice aroma preparations, aromatic salts, seasonings, seasoning sauces (→ Chapter 1) or essential oils (→ Chapter 13.2), can be used likewise. For foods that will be heated, → Herb cubes, herb mixtures embedded in vegetable fat together with table salt, are particularly suitable. They are added to unsalted dishes shortly before the end of the cooking process and stirred in after they liquefy [Ü30, Ü92].

13.2 Essential oils

Monika Werner, Munich

Seducingly aromatic is the odor of culinary herbs and spices, but especially sophisticated, and yet still easy, is seasoning with essential oils. They give foods that special something. Whether used as a substitute for fresh herbs or as an accentuating spice: They are the dot that tops the "i" and are always handy.

We have a distinct memory of odor: Haven't you ever experienced the pleasant smell of cinnamon and vanilla suddenly transporting you back to your childhood – A vivid recollection of grandmother's baked apples and warm living room? On these grounds, the seasoning of foods is the coronation of culinary art: Because fragrances leave an impression and can exert a downright magical power on us. Yet the use of a variety of herbs and spices also serves good health. Aromas alone get the digestive juices flowing. They stimulate the production of salivary enzymes and gastric juices. Thereby foods are more easily digested.

Precisely because of their combined sensuality and healing power, herbs and spices have firmly established themselves in the kitchen. Yet what is one to do, if one has neither an herb garden nor the opportunity to buy fresh herbs and spices? In these cases, reaching into a special aroma- and spice- bag-of-tricks will help: Experience the versatility of essential oils. In no way are essential oils in the kitchen thought of as a complete substitute for fresh herbs, spices or citrus fruits. But rather they can be a supplement and enrichment to your cuisine. They expand your seasoning spectrum in simple and uncomplicated ways. Pepper oil, for example, gives a dish the typical taste of pepper – but without the pungency, and then not everyone likes it hot. Many children and also some adults dislike fresh or dried herbs in their food. Through discreet seasoning with essential oils, however, you do not have to give up enjoying their taste and their pleasant, often health-promoting effect. Moreover, essential oils are superbly suited to accentuate the characteristic taste of a food, without overpowering it. So, for example, oil of bay and carrot seed oil can accentuate the fine characteristic taste of carrots.

Sophisticated and surprising taste combinations are possible to make easily and quickly. A pinch of pepper- and citrus oil gives whipping-cream with fresh strawberries that special something.

Essential oils bring variety into your cooking: They can spontaneously give an Indian or Mediterranean flavor to a vegetable, completely according to your desire or at your whim. And besides, seasoning with essential oils involves absolutely no witchcraft. If you observe certain rules, you will then experience lots of fun and pleasure.

And there is another advantage: You are freed from much of the preparation work. In the meantime, the variety of essential oils offered today has become immense. You can find small bottles of fragrant oils at fairs and in souvenir shops, often at an astoundingly affordable price. For the **purchase of essential oils** one should make certain to only buy them in places where competent consultation is provided, for example in natural foods stores. Also make certain that the following information is found on the bottle label or in the price list:

- 100% pure essential oil
- English and Latin plant names
- Declaration of the plant part from which the oil was obtained (e.g. cinnamon bark, cinnamon leaf)
- Filling quantity in ml or g
- Country of origin
- Method of production (steam distillation, extraction, expression)
- With extraction: Declaration of the extraction solvent; is the oil tested for solvent residues?
- Quality designations, for example: Produced from controlled biological (organic) cultivation, from controlled wild collection, from conventional cultivation (thus from plants treated with pesticides)
- Lot number.

Be watchful since essential oils are offered in translucent bottles. Essential oils that are very light-, air- and temperature sensitive must be stored in light-impermeable glasses. Small bottles of brown, blue or milky-white glass are suitable. You should also consider such types of storage for your essential oils and spice oil mixtures – thus, stored essential oils retain their quality over many years. One exception is lemon oil obtained by expression. It has a shelf-life of only about one year.

Essential oils are highly concentrated, liquid and fat-soluble substances. Hence, there are a **few rules for the use of essential oils** that must always be observed, in order that the seasoning achieves the desired effect.

One drop too many can already spoil everything. Be cautious initially with your dosing – adding more seasoning afterwards is always possible. Never drop the undiluted essential oils directly on your foods, but rather first onto a spoon. It can happen that, instead of one drop, several drops come out at the same time. In this case, rinse the spoon off and start over.

- With very intense aromas – for example cinnamon bark – just a tinge is sometimes sufficient. In this case, put only 1 drop of the essential oil on a coffee spoon, let it afterwards drop off again. You can flavor the dessert with the oil that has remained adhering to the spoon.

- If you want particularly fine and discreet seasoning, you must then remember that the essential oil is volatile. For this purpose, I mainly add the essential oil or the spice oil mixture to warm soups and sauces just before serving.
- In order for the aroma of essential oils to fully develop and to penetrate the entire dish, **emulsifiers** are necessary.

In these cases, the following rule also applies: Pure, undiluted essential oils are dispensed drop by drop into an emulsifier. Substances suitable for emulsification, dissolving or distribution include: Egg yolk, all edible oils, butter, cream, crème fraîche, sour cream, yogurt, mayonnaise, mustard, vinegar, alcohol, honey, maple syrup, cane sugar, raw cane sugar, and salt.

With homemade **spice oil mixtures** you can please not only yourself, but also your cooking-enthusiast friends. I have spice oil mixtures all the time on hand because they are practical to dose.

The preparation of spice oils is simple, if you observe the following rules:

- For the mixing of spice oils, use only qualitatively, high-quality edible fatty oils (e.g. olive-, sunflower-, peanut-, sesame oil) and 100% pure essential oils.
- Add 1 drop of essential oil per 10 ml of fatty oil.
- It is best to allow the mixtures to set for 2 to 4 weeks, in doing so the essential oils and the fatty oil can bind well with one another and the full aroma can also develop.
- Use small 50 ml brown bottles.
- First pour the base oil into the bottles, then the essential oil and then blend them together well. Do not forget to label your spice oil mixes.
- Take to heart the rule: Less is often more!

Important: Spice oil mixes are used by the teaspoon to the tablespoon – according to the desired spicing intensity.

Here are a few examples:

Basil spice oil (e.g. for improving the taste of tomato dishes)
5 drops basil oil per
50 ml olive oil

Provençal spice oil
1 drop thyme oil
3 drops oregano oil
2 drops rosemary oil
1 drop lavender oil
1 drop sage oil
50 ml olive oil, cold pressed

Italian spice oil
4 drops mandarin red oil
2 drops rosemary oil
1 drop thyme oil
50 ml olive oil, cold pressed

Indian spice oil
1 drop black pepper oil
2 drops cinnamon bark oil
1 drop oil of bay
2 drops coriander oil
2 drops ginger oil
3 drops cumin oil
1 drop cardamom oil
50 ml sesame oil

Recipes

With these spice oils in your kitchen, you can give a simple vegetable casserole or a soup the most distinct taste options. Here are some examples:

Carrot-potato-pot
Ingredients for 4 persons:
500 g carrots
500 g potatoes
2 tablespoons soft butter
40 g shallots
2 drops carrot seed oil
2 tablespoons "Indian" spice oil mix
1 bunch fresh cilantro (can be substituted for parsley)
Salt

Wash and peel the carrots and potatoes, and cut into slices. Heat about 1 tablespoon of butter in a cast iron pot. The carrots with the finely chopped shallots are dropped in and stirred constantly for about 5 minutes. Then the potatoes are added and lightly salted. Cover the pot and cook on a low flame for about another 10 minutes. Preheat the oven to 200º. The carrot seed oil and the "Indian" spice oil mix should be stirred well with the remaining butter and then mixed in with the vegetables. Grease a casserole dish with butter and spread out the vegetables in it. Strew the finely chopped parsley over it and bake lightly in the oven for 15 minutes.

Rosemary cream
Ingredients for 4 persons:
400 g crème double
50 g sugar
2 drops rosemary oil
2 tablespoons of your favorite dessert wine
1 twig of fresh rosemary

Whisk the crème double, sugar, rosemary oil and dessert wine in a bowl until foamy. Fill the cream into glasses and garnish with the rosemary twig.

Antipasti with zucchini

Ingredients for 4 persons:
500 g small zucchini
2 to 4 tomatoes (about 300 g)
2 tablespoons butter
2 tablespoons olive oil, cold pressed
Salt
1 clove of garlic
2 drops oregano oil
5 drops pepper oil
1 teaspoon aceto balsamico (balsamic vinegar, can be substituted with red wine vinegar)

Wash the zucchini, dry off and cut off the stem- and flower appendages. Cut the zucchini lengthwise into quarters in about 5 cm long pieces. Pour boiling water over the tomatoes, skin them and cut small, and at the same time remove the stems and the cores. Heat the butter and 1 tablespoon of olive oil in the pan. Then brown the small pieces of zucchini in it. Add the tomatoes and salt. Peel the clove of garlic and squeeze it in. Cook the zucchini on a low flame for about 10 minutes until al dente. Then put it on a flat plate and let it cool down. Mix the remaining olive oil with the oregano oil and pepper oil. Drizzle the oil and vinegar over the zucchini pieces. Mix all carefully, and season it with salt according to your taste preference. It is suitable to serve with a fresh white bread and a cool, rich rosé.

Tomato-orange-soup

Ingredients for 4 persons:
1 onion
1 small clove of garlic
1 kg tomatoes
2 tablespoons olive oil
2 tablespoons butter
2 slices of toasted bread
1/8 liter orange juice
1 teaspoonful honey
2 drops mandarin oil
2 drops ginger oil
1 drop black pepper oil
Salt

Peel the onion and chop finely. Peel the clove of garlic. Wash the tomatoes and quarter them, at the same time remove the stem appendages. Heat the olive oil with half of the butter. Add the onion and squeeze the clove of garlic through the garlic press. Blanch both on low heat until glassy. Add the tomatoes and cook everything together, covered, for about 15 minutes on a low flame, until the tomatoes become soft. Meanwhile cut the toasted bread into cubes. Heat the remaining butter in a pan. Roast the bread cubes in the pan until golden brown on both sides and put it aside. Purée the soup with a hand-held blender. Then pass it through a fine mesh sieve. Pour on the orange juice. Boil the soup again one time and then keep warm. Mix the honey and the essential oil and stir into the soup with a whisker. Season the soup with salt to taste. Serve on preheated plates and garnish with the bread cubes.

Literature [Ü34, Ü52, Ü104].

14 Food- and drug regulations for the trade of spices

Ulrike Bauermann, Bergholz-Rehbrücke

In Germany, the legal basis for all commercial activities involving culinary herbs and spices is the **Foodstuffs and Commodities Act (LMBG).** All universally valid statutory provisions that food product sellers must follow are set forth therein, as well as generally accepted test methods for the testing of food products, e.g. for the determination of dry weight, total ash and acid-insoluble ash. A legal basis does not exist for spice producers, for example in the requirements that are specified for microbiological purity or for the content of specific constituents and the corresponding analytical methods.

Herbs and spices or spice mixtures that are sold in the pharmacy for medicinal purposes must comply with the drug regulations. If the individually, or as components of spice mixtures, traded herbs and spices are monographed in the **European Pharmacopoeia** (Ph Eur), the **German Pharmacopoeia** (DAB) or in other official compendia, e.g. in the **German Drug Codex** (DAC), they must comply with the standards of these monographs.

14.1 Quality standards for spices

Because no statutory provisions exist for certain foods, nor for spices, with regard to their hygienic-microbiological quality or allowable limits for content of undesired contaminants, such as for example heavy metals content, and because the commercial trade lacks references of what to go by for official food inspection monitoring, other institutions thus compiled and published reference- and maximum values, e.g. the German Society for Hygiene and Microbiology (DGHM) or the (former)

German Federal Institute for Health Protection of Consumers and Veterinary Medicine (BgVV); BgVV was dissolved in 2002, now absorbed into the Federal Agency for Consumer Protection and Food Safety (BVL) and the Federal Institute for Risk Assessment (BfR). These values, determined by the requirements of Good Manufacturing Practice (GMP), are adapted to the current state of science and technology. Thus, they are not codified, but rather they represent up-to-date findings, standards and possibilities of food technology that are consistently readjusted. These rules have no statutory but administrative, informing character. If the maximum values are exceeded, "...all persons in charge of food quality, including the producer as well as the supervisory party, are required to investigate the sources of the contamination and to take corrective action if possible. Additionally, according to circumstances, it should be examined critically as to whether further measures are to be activated, such as for example a recall from the market" (German Federal Health Gazette: Bundesgesundhbl. 37, p. 204, 1995).

The basic quality-determining criteria for spices include:

- Chemical-physical parameters
- Microbiological parameters/toxins
- Pesticide residues load
- Heavy metal residues load
- Sensory science.

14.1.1 Chemical and physical parameters

First and foremost, this concerns the following parameters:

- Essential oil content   DIN 10228

- Water content   DIN 10229
- Total ash content/Sand content
  (acid-insoluble ash)   DIN 10223
- Foreign matter   —

Up until recently the Federal Republic of Germany did not have available standardized methods for determination of any of these parameters. Of the existing national standards only a few are relevant for the German producer in the herb and spice sector. Since May 1993, a working committee established through the German Institute for Standardization (DIN) has worked on the codification and revision of test methods. Methods available since December 1995 include DIN 10228 "Analysis of spices and condiments – Determination of essential oil content", since 1996 DIN 10223 "Analysis of spices and condiments – Determination of total ash and acid-insoluble ash" and since August 2000 DIN 10229 "Analysis of spices and condiments - Determination of moisture content – Entrainment method". At the time being, other draft standards are being discussed and will be confirmed through interlaboratory testing.

With the codification of these analytical methods, the comparability of test results can be assured. Minimum- and maximum content levels will not (!) be specified. Such standards are agreed upon contractually between the buyer and the seller. For orientation, the existing standards of the German Institute for Standardization (DIN), the International Organization for Standardization (ISO), the AOAC methods (official methods of the Association Of Analytical Communities International) or the ASTA specifications (American Spice Trade Association), among others, can be accessed.

For international standards in the spice trade (ISO Standards), there is quite an extensive work of 68 standards available at this time. Among these are three standards of terms, definitions, and nomenclature, two standards for sampling plans and sample preparation, 21 testing standards and 42 product specifications. Included in these specifications, e.g. for dried marjoram, basil or peppermint, are minimum essential oil content values and maximum levels for the content of, e.g. moisture, ash and extraneous matter presented as reference values (!). The standards are revised on a rotational basis and adapted to the current level.

The current listing of existing national and international standards, as well as the standards themselves, can be obtained from Beuth-Verlag GmbH, Burggrafenstraße 6, D-10787 Berlin, Germany.

In the September 1998 edition of the German Federal Gazette (BAnz), the so-called guidelines for spices and other seasoning ingredients were published. These guidelines also contain, in addition to definitions and general quality criteria, reference levels for acid-insoluble ash (sand) in individual spices.

14.1.2 Microbiological parameters/ toxins

No legal basis exists yet concerning limits for the microbiological load of spices. Therefore, to this end, **reference- and maximum levels** (Table 1) were developed by the Food-Microbiology and Food-Hygiene Committee of the German Society for Hygiene and Microbiology (DGHM). The applicable test methods are published in §35 LMBG (L 00.00-20/21).

Materials with bacterial counts below or the same as the reference levels are always saleable.

Findings of a transgression of the reference level, on occasion of a legal official food inspection monitoring, result in a suggestion or an instruction to prevent such occurrences or the taking of follow-up samples, respectively, or in an unscheduled process control. With a transgression of

the maximum levels, the requisite food law measures are taken under adherence of the commensurability of the remedial action.

Mycotoxins are secondary metabolites of mold fungi. Aflatoxins, ochratoxins, fumonisins, and patulins are among the main group of mycotoxins that occur in foods. Cancerogenic activity has been shown for aflatoxins. Therefore, in the Federal Republic of Germany the maximum aflatoxin content has been legally established in the **Maximum Allowable Limits of Mycotoxins in Foods Regulation (MHmV)** of June 2, 1999 (German Federal Law Gazette (BGBl, Part I, p. 2243, June 11, 1999):

- Aflatoxin B_1 < 2 µg/kg
- Sum of aflatoxins
  B_1, B_2, G_1, and G_2 < 4 µg/kg

A regulation for the maximum content of ochratoxins is at a preliminary stage of discussion.

14.1.3 Pesticide residue load

The use of pesticides in the cultivation of herbs and spices is allowed, unless their application will violate the requirements of compliance issued in the permit, the pesticide application regulation and the regulation for the maximum levels of residues.

Concerning the allowance and application of pesticides, a plant protection products list is published annually by the German Federal Biological Research Centre for Agriculture and Forestry (BBA). The approvals are limited in time; a conclusion is later published in the German Federal Gazette (BAnz).

The maximum pesticide residues content has been legally established in the **Maximum Allowable Limits of Residues Regulation (RHmV)** of October 21, 1999 (German Federal Law Gazette (BGBl Part I, p. 2083-2144, November 5, 1999).

Here it must be pointed out that the new pesticide law took effect already in July 1998. Hitherto, in Germany, distribution licenses for pesticides were available, i.e. the pesticides were also allowed to be used for non-specific, permitted fields of application, considering the above-mentioned conditions and regulations. With the new regulated indication approvals, the use of a pesticide is still only allowed for the field of application that is designated with the license or permit. Pesticides that were licensed prior to July 1998 were allowed to be traded and used up until June 30, 2001, according to the regulations of the hitherto legal provisions. Up until February 1, 1999, license holders had to apply for further application of these agents to the German Federal Biological Research Centre.

14.1.4 Heavy metal residue load

No legal framework exists for the content of heavy metal residues. The **Reference Values for Contaminants in Foods** were published in the German Federal Health Gazette (Bundesgesundhbl. 40, No. 5, p. 182, 1997) (Table 2). The values speci-

Table 1 Reference- and maximum values for spices that are intended for the end consumer (§6 LMBG) or are added to the food in the tested form and subjected to bacterial reduction processes. Data shown in colony forming units per gram (cfu/g)

Microorganism	Reference value	Maximum value
Salmonella	—	ND in 25 g
Staphylococcus aureus	1.0×10^2	1.0×10^3
Bacillus cereus	1.0×10^4	1.0×10^5
Escherichia coli	1.0×10^4	—
Sulfite-reducing clostridia	1.0×10^4	1.0×10^5
Mold fungi	1.0×10^5	1.0×10^6

fied for spice plants are also applied to culinary herbs.

The sampling of the spices can be carried out according to DIN 10220 or ISO 948.

14.2 Quality standards for herbs and spices in the pharmacy

At the present time in Germany, the official, legally binding pharmacopoeias are the **European Pharmacopoeia** (Ph Eur), the **German Pharmacopoeia** (DAB) and the **German Homoeopathic Pharmacopoeia** (HAB).

The pharmacopoeias are compilations of recognized pharmaceutical rules for the

- Quality
- Testing
- Storage
- Dispensing
- Designation

of pharmaceuticals and of the ingredients that are used to manufacture them. Pharmaceuticals are not allowed to be manufactured and may not be brought into commerce for dispensing to consumers unless they comply with these rules.

In the general sections of the pharmacopoeias, all universally valid test methods that must be used are described and the requirements for packaging materials and containers are stated in detail.

The specific sections of the pharmacopoeias contain the monographs of materials, arranged in alphabetical order that may possibly be used in the preparation of

Table 2 Reference values for heavy metals in foods

Heavy metal	Reference value (mg/kg fresh produce) according to BGBl	Converted to dry weight reference value (mg/kg). Drying ratio 1:5
Lead	2.0	10.0
Cadmium	0.1	0.5
Mercury	0.05	0.25

drug products. In these monographs, sensory (e.g. color, odor, taste) and chemical-physical quality parameters (e.g. foreign matter, water content) are described as well as test methods specific to the corresponding material (e.g. identity tests, determination of content).

Beyond the requirements of the specific monographs of the pharmacopoeias, additional quality requirements, among other requirements, apply to medicinal substances with regard to

- Microbiological purity
- Maximum allowable limits of pesticide residues and aflatoxins.

14.2.1 Microbiological parameters/ toxins

For these, the requirements of the European Pharmacopoeia are in effect [Ph Eur, 5.1.4.9]. Accordingly, the microbiological purity of the starting materials should be of the type that will allow for the purity requirements of the finished product to be

adhered to. Categories 3a, 4a and 4b are of particular relevance. The prescribed upper limits are summarized in tables (Table 3).

For the maximum levels of mycotoxins, the regulation about their prohibition, the **Use of Substances Contaminated with Aflatoxins in the Manufacture of Drug Products** (AVV) of July 19, 2000 (German Federal Law Gazette (BGBl Part I, No. 33, p. 1081, July 25, 2000), applies to medicinal plants. The maximum levels correspond to the same statutory rules as for foods (Chapter 14.1.2).

14.2.2 Pesticide residue load

The application of pesticides in the cultivation of medicinal plants is regulated in similar ways to the cultivation of culinary herbs and spices. Since 1996 there have been a few regulations concerning the maximum allowable levels of pesticide residues for medicinal plants. The European Pharmacopoeia contains a listing of the respective, officially required upper

Table 3 European Pharmacopoeia Categories 3a, 4a and 4b for microbiological purity

Category 3a	Category 4a	Category 4b
Preparations for oral and rectal administration	Herbal medicinal products to which boiling water is added before use	Other herbal medicinal products
Per gram or milliliter: – Maximum 10^3 aerobic bacteria – Maximum 10^2 fungi – *E. coli* and Salmonellae absent	Per gram or milliliter: – Maximum 10^7 aerobic bacteria – Maximum 10^5 fungi – Maximum 10^2 *E. coli* – Salmonellae absent	Per gram or milliliter: – Maximum 10^5 aerobic bacteria – Maximum 10^4 fungi – Maximum 10^3 enterobacteria – *E. coli* and Salmonellae absent

limits for the 34 substances or substance groups that are used in plant protection. Moreover, the specified Maximum Allowable Limits of Residues Regulation (RHmV) for the food sector is also in effect for herbal drugs.

14.2.3 Heavy metal residue load

For maximum levels of heavy metals in botanical raw materials that are used in medicinal products, the **Recommendations of the former German Federal Ministry of Health (BMG)** on heavy metal loads exist (Heavy Metal Contaminants of Drugs-Recommendation, October 17, 1991, Table 4, unpublished).

These values fall below the reference values in effect for spices. If a heavy metal determination is required in a particular monograph, the herbal drug must always comply with the prescribed upper limit tests of the European Pharmacopoeia [Ph Eur, 2.4.8.]. The type and amount of sampling of crude drugs has to be carried out according to the official method of the German Pharmacopoeia, DAB 2.8.N6, and powdering of the material for analytical purposes according to DAB 2.8.N7.

Table 4 BMG-Recommendations for maximum levels of heavy metals in herbal drugs

Heavy metal	Reference value (mg/kg dry weight)
Lead	5.0
Cadmium	0.2
Mercury	0.1

15 General part literature

[1] Altner H., Boeckh J., in: Schmidt R.F., Thews G. (Hrsg.): Physiologie des Menschen, Springer-Verlag Berlin, Heidelberg, New York 1993, p. 320–328 (1993)

[2] André H.A. et al., Z. Lebensm. Unters. Forsch. A 205:125–130 (1997)

[3] Asai A. et al., Biosc. Biotechnol. Biochem. 63(12): 2118–2122 (1999)

[4] Badary O.A. et al., Eur. J. Cancer. Prev. 8(5):435–440 (1999)

[5] Bellisle F., Neurosci. Biobehav. Rev. 23(3):423–428 (1999)

[6] Block E., Angew. Chem. 104:1158–1203 (1992)

[7] Buchbauer G., Selos S., Dtsch. Apoth. Ztg. 137(42):3719–3736 (1997)

[8] Buschbeck E., Drogenreport 10(18): 74–79 (1997)

[9] Cai Y.N. et al., Carcinogenesis 18(1): 215–222 (1997)

[10] Chuang S. et al., Food Chem. Toxicol. 38(11):991–995 (2000)

[11] Cuppett S.L., Hall C.A. 3rd, Adv Food Nutr. Res. 42:245–271 (1998)

[12] De M et al., Phytother. Res. 13(7): 616–618 (1999)

[13] Deutschmann F. et al., Drogenanalyse I: Morphologie und Anatomie, Gustav Fischer Verlag, Stuttgart, New York (1981)

[14] Dewilde A., et al., J. Photochem. Photobiol. B - Biology 36(1):23–29 (1996)

[15] Diekmann W., Drogenreport 10(18): 80–85 (1997)

[16] Eschrich W., Pulver-Atlas der Drogen, 6. Aufl., Fischer-Verlag Stuttgart 1997

[17] Fiala E.S. et al., Annu. Rev. Nutr. 5:295–321 (1985)

[18] Formacék, V., Kubeczka K H , Essential Oil Analysis by Capillary Gas Chromatography and Carbon-13-NMR Spectroscopy, John Wiley & Sons, Chicester, New York, Brisbane, Toronto, Singapore 1982

[19] Franz Ch., Auer M., Drogenreport 4(6): 31–37 (1999)

[20] Gassner G., Deutschmann B., Mikroskopische Untersuchung pflanzlicher Lebensmittel, 5. Aufl., Fischer Verlag, Stuttgart 1989

[21] Glatzel, H., Ernährungsschau 12(10): 295–301 (1965)

[22] Gordonoff T., Rödel S. , Hippokrates 31: 335–338 (1960)

[23] Grosch W., Trends Food Sci. Technol. 4:68–73 (1993)

[24] Haenen GRMM, Bast A., in: Nitric Oxide, Pt. C (Series: Methods in Enzymology, 1999, 301:490-503 (1999)

[25] Hall III C.A., Cuppett S.L., Antioxid Methodol 1997:141–172 (1997)

[26] Haller R. et al. Chem. Senses 24(4): 465–467 (1999)

[27] Hamburger M., Drogenreport 10(17): 66–70 (1997)

[28] Hatt H., Forum Aromather. Aromapflege 10:7–17 (1996)

[29] Hatt H., Forum Aromather. Aromapflege 16:5–13, (1999)

[30] Hecht S.S. et al., Cancer Epidemiol. Biomarkers Prev 4(8):877–884 (1995)

[31] Hecht S.S. et al., Cancer Epidemiol. Biomarkers Prev 8(10):907–913 (1999)

[32] Heilmann J. et al., Planta Med. 61(5): 435–438 (1995)

[33] Heindl A., Drogenreport 12(21):45–53 (1999)

[34] Helen A. et al., Vet. Hum. Toxicol. 41(5):316–319 (1999)

[35] Henry C.J., Emery B., Hum. Nutr. Clin. Nutr. 40(2):165–168 (1986)

[36] Herrmann K., Z. Lebensm. Unters. Forsch. 116:224–228 (1961)

[37] Hose S., Dtsch. Apoth. Ztg. 131(37): 1925–1927(1991)

[38] Jaquet H., Herba Germanica 2(2): 124–132 (1994)

[39] Jellinek J.S., dragoco report: 5–31 und 83–93 (1995)

[40] Jensen-Jarolim E. et al., Clin. Exp. Allergy 27(11):1299–1306 (1997)

[41] Kabelitz L., Z. Phytother. 17(1, Supplement):9–16 (1996)

[42] Kabelitz L., Herba Germanica 2(2): 95–114 (1994)

[43] Kamal-Eldin A. et al., in: Spec. Publ. R. Soc. Chem. 1996, 181 (Natural Antioxidants and Food Quality in Atherosclerosis and Cancer Prevention), p. 230–235, (1996)

[44] Kelkar S.M., Kaklij G.S., Phytomedicine 3(4):353–359 (1997)

[45] Keller R., Immunologie und Immunpathologie, Thieme Verlag Stuttgart, New York 1994

[46] Khar A. et al., FEBS Lett. 445(1): 165–168 (1999)

[47] Knobloch K. et al., J. Essential Oil Res. 1:119–128 (1989)

[48] Knobloch K. et al., Planta Med 52:556 (1986)

[49] Kubota T.I., Kubo I., Nature 223:97–9 (1969)

[50] Kumari M.V.R., Cancer Lett. 60:291–294 (1991)

[51] Küpper C., Ernährungsumschau 43: 249–252 (1996)

[52] Lack E., Seidlitz H., in: Process Technol. Proc. 12 (High Pressure Chemical Engineering): 253–258 (1996)

[53] Lake B.G., Food Chem. Toxicol. 37: 423–453 (1999)

[54] Martinez A. et al., J. Agric Food Chem. 46(2):585–589 (1998)

[55] Matheis G., dragoco Bericht für die Geschmacksstoffe verarbeitende Industrie 39:50–65, (1994)

[56] Milivojevic J., Tehnol Mesa 37(1):32–34 (1996)

[57] Murakami A. et al., J. Agric. Food Chem. 48(5):1518–1523 (2000)

[58] Murakami A. et al., Biosci. Biotechnol. Biochem. 64(1):9–16 (2000)

[59] Namiki K. et al., J. Agric. Food Chem. 32:948–952 (1984)

[60] Nielsen P.V., Rios R., Int. J. Food Microbiol. 60(2/3):219–229 (2000)

[61] Nielsen S.E. et al., Br. J. Nutr. 81(6): 447–455 (1999)

[62] Nürnberg E., Surmann P. (Hrsg.), Hagers Handbuch der pharmazeutischen Praxis, Bd. 2, Methoden, Springer-Verlag, Berlin, Heidelberg; New York 1991

[63] Oya T. et al., Biosc. Biotechnol. Biochem. 61(2):263–266 (1997)

[64] Platel K., Srinivasan K., Int. J. Food Sci. Nutr. 47(1):55–59 (1996)

[65] Paya M., et al., Biochem. Pharmacol. 48(3):445–451 (1994)

[66] Pérez-Garcia F. et al., 45th Ann. Congr. Soc. Med. Plant Res. (Abstracts) (1997)

[67] Platel K., Srinivasan K., Nahrung 44(1): 42–46 (2000)

[68] Reilly C.E., J. Neurol. 247(5):402–403, (2000)

[69] Restrepo D., Brand J.G., dragoco report 122–127 (1992)

[70] Schiede S., Drogenreport 4(5):12–17 (1991)

[71] Schilcher H., Therapiewoche 36: 1100–1112 (1986)

[72] Schneider E., Kutscher V., Drogenreport 10(16): 37–40 (1997)

[73] Shahidi F. et al., J. Food Lipids 2(3): 145–153 (1995)

[74] Sheen L.Y. et al., J. Agric. Food Chem. 39:939–943 (1991)

[75] Shenoy N.R., Choughuley R., J. Agric. Food Chem. 37:721–725 (1989)

[76] Shobana S., Naidu K.A., Prostaglandins Leukot. Essent. Fatty Acids 62(2): 107–110 (2000

[77] Simandi B. et al., Solvent Extraction in the Process Industries, II, Proceedings of ISEC '93, Logsdail DH, Slater MJ (Eds) (1993)

[78] Simandi B. et al., J. Agric. Food Chem. 47(4):1635–1640 (1999

[79] Stäger J. et al., Allergy 46:475–478 (1991)

[80] Suaeyun R. et al., Carcinogensis 18(5): 949–955 (1997)

[81] Tabak M. et al., J. Appl. Bacteriol. 80(6): 667–672 (1996)

[82] Tagashira M. et al., Biosc. Biotechn. Biochem. 59:740–742 (1995)

[83] Ternes W. et al., in: Oils-Fats-Lipids 1995, Proc. World Congr. Int. Soc. Fat. Res., 21st 1995 2:347-348 (1996)

[84] Teuscher E., Lindequist U., Dtsch. Apoth. Ztg. 132(42):2231–2238 (1992)

[85] Tsai Sh.J. et al., Mutagenesis 11(3): 235–240 (1996)

[86] Van Eijk T., dragoco Bericht für Geschmacksstoffe verarbeitenden Industrien 32:3–17 (1987)

[87] Vasudevan K. et al., Indian J. Gastroenterol. 19(2):53–56 (2000)

[88] Vieths S., in: Felix D'Mello J.P. (Ed.) Handbook of Plant and Fungal Toxicants I CRC Press inc., p. 157 (1997)

[89] Vimala S. et al., Br. J. Cancer 80(1/2): 110–116 (1999)

[90] Wagner H., Forum Aromather. Aromapflege 16:14–19 (1999)

[91] Wang H. et al., J. Nat. Prod. 62(2): 294–296 (1999)

[92] Wiseman H., Bioact. Components Food 24:795–800 (1996)

[93] Wüthrich B., Hofer T., Dtsch. Med. Wschr. 109:981–986 (1984)

[94] Yamaguchi S., Ninomiya K., J. Nutr. 130(4S Suppl):921–6S (2000)

[95] Youdim K.A., Deans S.G., Mech. Ageing Dev. 109(3):163–175 (1999)

[96] Yousef R.T., Tawil G.G., Pharmazie 35:698–701 (1980)

[97] Yousif A.N. et al., J. Agric. Food Chem. 47(11):4777–4781 (1999)

[98] Zava D.T. et al., Proc. Soc. Exp. Biol. Med. 217(3):369–378 (1998)

[99] Zheng G.Q. et al., Planta Med. 58(4): 338–341 (1992)

[100] Zheng G.Q., Kenney P.M., Lam L.K.T., J. Agric. Food Chem. 40(1):107 (1992)

[101] Zittermann A., Dtsch. Apoth. Ztg. 134(32): 2991 (1994)

Literature references identified by Ü can be found in the general listing of books and monographs at the back of this book.

Monographs

of Spice Plants

and Culinary Herbs

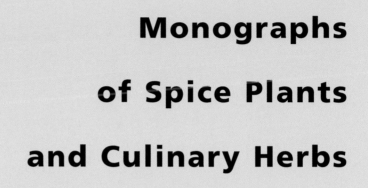

Ajowan

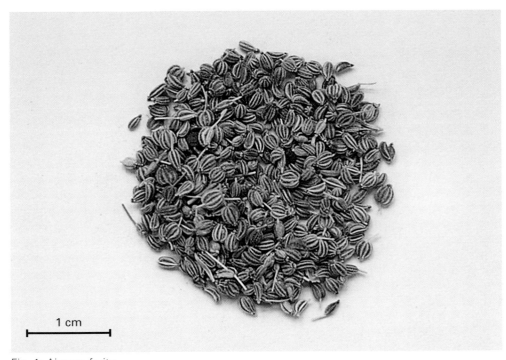

1 cm

Fig. 1: Ajowan fruits

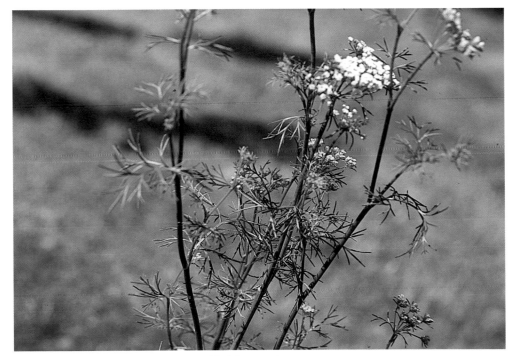

Fig. 2: Ajowan (*Trachyspermum ammi* (L.) SPRAGUE)

Plant source: *Trachyspermum ammi* (L.) SPRAGUE.

Synonyms: *Carum copticum* (L.) BENTH. et HOOK. f. ex C.B. CLARKE, *Carum ajowan* BAILL., *Trachyspermum copticum* (L.) LINK.

Family: Umbelliferous plants (Apiaceae, synonym Umbelliferae).

Common names: Engl.: ajowan, ajowain, omum, omum plant, bishop's weed (this name is also used for *Ammi majus* L.), white cumin, Ethiopian caraway, in Indian cookbooks incorrectly called lovage (*Levisticum officinale* W.D.J. KOCH); Fr.: ammi de l'Inde; Ger.: Ajowan, Ajowain, Adjowan, Ajowainkümmel, Ajowankümmel, Kretischer Kümmel, Ägyptischer Ammei, Schnabelsame.

Description: An up to 1.5 m high annual with a glabrous stem and multiple pinnate leaves having filiform lobes; the inflorescences are composed of umbels with 5 to 15 rays, and the radial quinate flowers have a white corolla, 5 stamina, and an inferior bilocular ovary with two styles. The fruit is a double achene (cremocarp), consisting of 2 mericarps mostly remaining attached to each other [Ü60].

Native origin: Probably native to India, only known in cultivation.

Main cultivation areas: India, Pakistan, Egypt, Ethiopia, Afghanistan, Yemen, Iran, Russian Federation, Indonesia, and China.

Main exporting countries: India.

Cultivation: Ajowan is cultivated only in tropical and subtropical regions, prefers sunny locations and well-drained soil, and is very tolerant of dry heat.

Culinary herb

Commercial forms: Ajowan seed: dried fruits; commercial varieties include Desi Ajowain (large), Nadiad Ajowain (small), ajowan essential oil, and ajowan oleoresin.

Production: The fruits are harvested shortly before ripening, then dried.

Forms used: Fresh or dried fruits, ajowan essential oil, and ajowan oleoresin.

Storage: The ripe, dried fruits can be stored for a long time, protected from light and moisture in well-sealed metal- or glass containers.

Description: The **whole fruits** are ovate, similar to parsley fruits but somewhat smaller; depending on the commercial variety (see above), 1 to 4 mm long and up to 1 mm wide, reddish to dark brown with 5 light-colored ribs. The texture is rather rough due to the presence of numerous dull papillae, which easily rub off; the achenes are only partially separated into their mesocarps (Fig. 1) [11].

The **powdered fruits** are yellowish-brown, microscopic examination shows conspicuous papillary protuberances of the epicarp of varying sizes (maximum 50 μm long, Fig. 3) and tissue fragments with polygonal, irregularly thickened cells, striated cuticula, orange-brown remains of the oil ducts as well as the layers of collenchyma cells and of stone cells of the mesocarp; the endosperm contains oil deposits, tiny aleuron grains and very small oxalate microrosette crystals [16, Ü48, Ü60].

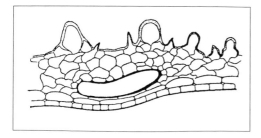

Fig. 3: Ajowan. Cross section of the fruit wall with secretory duct and papillary protuberances. From [16]

Odor: Thyme-like upon crushing the fruits, **Taste:** Pungent and burning.

History: The drug reached Central Europe in 1549; attempts to cultivate it there failed due to unsuitable climate conditions [Ü92].

Constituents and Analysis

Constituents

- Essential oil: 2 to 5% (in high performance strains for thymol production, up to 10%); the main components vary depending on chemotype:
  Thymol (24 to 37%, some authors isolated up to 60%), *p*-cymene (20 to 23%, in part as a distillation artifact?), γ-terpinene (15 to 20%), carvacrol (2 to 4%) as well as α-pinene [3, 4, 5, 9, 10, 14, 16]; carvone (about 46%), limonene (about 38%), dillapiol (about 9%) [6]; carvacrol (about 69%); additionally, α-phellandrene (about 11%), α-terpinene (about 10%) and α-pinene (about 6%) [7].
- Fatty oil: 25 to 32%.

Tests for Identity: Organoleptic, macroscopic and microscopic examinations as well as TLC or GC analyses [16, Ü102].

Quantitative assay: The content of essential oil can be determined volumetrically with steam distillation and xylol in the graduated tube, according to Ph Eur.

Adulterations, Misidentifications and Impurities are possible with → Cumin (*Cuminum cyminum* L.) or the fruits of bishop's weed (*Ammi majus* L.). The fruits of both species lack the characteristic papillae.

Actions and Uses

Actions: It is assumed that, due to the aromatic-pungent taste of the drug, it stimulates salivation, gastric juice secretion, bile excretion and intestinal motility. An increase in gastric juice secretion has been demonstrated experimentally [15]. Preparations of the drug have a blood pressure lowering effect. The active principle is presumed to be thymol, which acts as a calcium channel blocker [1]. Extracts of the drug inhibit thrombocyte aggregation [13]. The essential oil has good antimicrobial activity [2, 12].

Toxicology: Based on existing data, there is no acute or chronic toxicity with the regular use of this drug as a spice. For the toxicology of higher doses of thymol → Thyme.

Culinary use: In India, ajowan is a very frequently used spice. It serves, particularly, as a flavor-enhancing ingredient of pungent dishes such as ompadi, boondi, nambin and sov, as a spice component in Indian flat breads and spicy baked breads (naan, pakora, paratha, ser) as well as of legume dishes (dal, puree of mung beans). In Ethiopia, ajowan is used similarly as a spice in bread (alicha wet), but also as a component of alcoholic beverages.

In the European kitchen, ajowan is utilized as a spice component in dishes made from legumes, root vegetables, meat-, vegetable- and rice dishes (e.g. pilaf, an oriental rice dish) as well as spice of pickles. Ajowan can also serve as an ingredient in marinades for fish and for spicing of baked goods or crackers [8, Ü2, Ü51, Ü55, Ü73, Ü92, Ü93].

Combines well with cumin or garlic.

As a component of spice mixes and preparations: → Curry powder, → Chat masala, → Sarawak spice mix.

Other uses: Thymol is obtained from the essential oil through freezing out. The fruits are used as pig feed or in the form of oil cakes as fish feed in fish breeding operations.

Cultivation: Allspice has minimal soil requirements, but it thrives especially well in calcareous, loamy, water permeable, deep soil at temperatures around 25 °C and annual rainfall of 1000 to 2000 mm, with the occurrence of a dry season. These conditions are best fulfilled in the Caribbean Islands or neighboring mainland. Allspice is propagated through seeds, which first are germinated damp and shaded in baskets or plastic bags. After one year, when the plants are about 30 cm tall, they are transplanted. The majority of male trees are removed after the first flowering. In order to eliminate the risk of a very high number of male plants, the practice of increasing the proportion of female trees by grafting has taken hold. After about 8 years the first harvest is possible. After 15 years the peak harvest is attained. The trees are productive for over 100 years [Ü89].

Culinary herb

Commercial forms: Allspice or pimento: unripe dried fruits, whole, shredded or ground, essential oil of allspice (obtained from the leaves), allspice oleoresin.

Production: The fully-grown, but still green fruits are harvested at about 4 months after the tree flowers, in Jamaica from August to September. The infructescences or the fruit-bearing twigs are cut off from the cultivated trees, and also from wild growing trees. Then they are sun dried, sometimes after 2 to 5 days fermentation in heaps or in sacks, in larger operations also in drying ovens or in band driers at 70 to 75 °C. Afterwards, the stalks are rubbed off from the fruits [8, Ü55, Ü89, Ü92].

Forms used: Unripe dried, whole, crushed or ground fruits.

Storage: The whole fruits should be stored in a cool place, in tightly sealed glass- or porcelain containers, protected from light and moisture. Whole allspice can be stored for a very long time without aroma loss; in

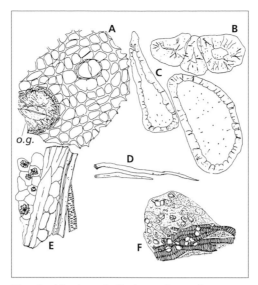

Fig. 3: Allspice. **A** Surface view of exocarp fragment, o.g. translucent oil reservoir, **B** and **C** Stone cells of the mesocarp, **D** Trichomes of the epidermis, **E** Side view of fragments from the mesocarp **F** Vascular bundles with spiral vessels, oxalate prisms and crystal clusters. From Ü48.

comminuted form, it loses its aroma quickly.

Description. Whole fruit (Fig. 1): Globose to ovoid or indistinctly quadrangular, red to gray-brown fruits, without peduncle, diameter 4 to 8 mm, finely warty rough on the outside, with a circular depression at the pointed end, crowned by a small 4-toothed rim of the calyx and the remains of the style, with the stalk's stigma at the base, each of the two locules containing one dark-violet, plano-convex, indistinctly spiral-twisted seed; fruit-wall about 0.5 mm thick, brittle, covered by a microcellular cuticula with stomata and a few scattered, short hairs that are strongly thickened [Ü29, Ü60].

Powdered fruit: The chloral hydrate preparation of the reddish-brown powder shows the fragments of the exocarp with stomata and the translucent parenchyma with brown cell walls, in which large, schizogenous, globular secretory spaces are embedded; also present are single or aggregated groups of colorless stone cells

from the mesocarp, short, unicellular, strongly thickened hairs of the epidermis, fragments of the mesocarp which, in longitudinal view, show parenchyma cells with oxalate druses, and sclerenchyma fibers and pitted vessels, vascular bundles with spiral vessels and oxalate prisms, as well as oxalate crystal clusters (Fig. 3), pigmented cells of the testa and yellow clumps of pigment. Suspensions of the powder in water show numerous single or aggregated, up to 12 μm wide, starch grains [Ü48, Ü60].

Odor and **Taste:** Reminiscent of clove, nutmeg, pepper and cinnamon (hence the names "Allspice" and "Quatre-épice"), weakly anesthetizing upon chewing.

History: The original inhabitants of Central America used allspice not only as a seasoning (e.g. as a flavoring in chocolate) but also as an ingredient, among other components, for the embalming of their dead. In the 16th century, allspice was brought to Europe by the Spaniards. When the English conquered Jamaica in 1655, they already encountered extensive allspice plantations. From Jamaica, allspice was shipped in large amounts to England. The seafarers of the 17th century used allspice for its food preserving properties to conserve meat and fish supplies [8, Ü55, Ü68, Ü89, Ü97].

Constituents and Analysis

DIN and ISO Standards: ISO 973 (Pimento (Allspice), whole or ground).

Constituents

- Essential oil: In the dried fruits 2 to 5%, the main components significantly depend on the origin, and include eugenol (65 to 87% in Jamaican, 8 to 15% in Mexican material), methyleugenol (eugenol methyl ether, 3 to 13% in Jamaican, 48 to 68% in Mexican material), myrcene (less than 1% in Jamaican, up to 18% in Mexican material), β-caryophyllene (3 to 6%), as well as 1,8-cineole (1 to 15%), α-terpineol (0.2 to 1.8%), α- and β-phellandrene, among others [3, 6–8, 10, 16]. The hydroxy-constituents also occur partially as glucosides [5].

The composition of the essential oil from the leaves and the fruits is very similar. In both cases, eugenol, methyleugenol and β-caryophyllene dominate [8, 11].

- Tannins: Galloyl glucosides including, among others, α-terpineol-8-*O*-β-D-(6-*O*-galloyl)glucopyranoside, and catechin derivatives [5, 13].
- Flavonoids [17].
- Starch: 3% [8].
- Fatty oil: 6 to 8% [Ü92].

Tests for Identity: Based on morphological and anatomical characteristics, TLC [8, 15] or GC of the essential oil [3].

Quantitative assay: The content of essential oil is determined volumetrically with steam distillation using a graduated tube with xylol [analogously to the essential oil assay for clove in the Ph Eur]; eugenol levels in the essential oil are measured with HPLC [14].

Adulterations, Misidentifications and Impurities are possible with crown allspice (see below) whose fruits are up to 1 cm long and 0.5 cm wide, bearing the remains of the 5-partite calyx, or with tabasco allspice (see below) whose ash-gray fruits have little aroma [Ü60]. Sometimes allspice is illegally adulterated with iron oxide-containing red ocher (ruddle) to improve appearance (iron detection assay!) [8].

Actions and Uses

Actions: On the basis of its aromatic taste, allspice has appetizing and digestion promoting effects.

Allspice may also possess all of the same activities that have been observed for → Clove and eugenol, but to a lesser degree because its eugenol content is lower.

Extracts of allspice show, similar to many other spice herbs, good radical scavenging properties [2, 9], which in part can be attributed to the galloyl glucosides [15]. Allspice extracts have good antimicrobial, especially fungistatic action and in refrigerated ready-to-eat foods are able to inhibit the growth of psychrotrophic bacteria, e.g. *Listeria monocytogenes* [4, 12].

Toxicology: Based on existing data, there is no acute or chronic toxicity with the use of allspice as a seasoning at usual doses. The sensitization potential of allspice due to the eugenol content is likely lower than that of → Clove. There are no case reports.

Culinary use: Allspice is especially popular in Finland and Sweden, among others, as a fish spice, especially for herring, and to season the meat dish kalops. In England, it is an indispensable component of plum pudding. In the USA, allspice is used mainly to season desserts, soufflés, pickles, fruit conserves and ketchup. The national drink of Jamaica is Jamaica dram (Pimento dram), which is made from rum and allspice. In Central European cooking, perhaps unjustly, it has lost its former importance. In Germany, the bulk of imported allspice is used in the food industry for the production of meat- and fish conserves [Ü68, Ü89].

Allspice is used whole or ground. Powdered allspice should always be prepared fresh, e.g. using a pepper mill or a mortar. Whole allspice granules can be cooked with the food or added 1/2 hour before the end of cooking time. Allspice granules or powder serve as a kitchen spice for soups, sauces (especially for boiled fish), meat dishes (e.g. of beef- or lamb ragouts), fish dishes, sea foods, game, poultry, ham, marinades, rice, fish- or meat pies, chutneys, relishes, sauerkraut and red beets. Allspice is also used as a pickling spice for cucumbers and mixed pickles [Ü1, Ü13, Ü30, Ü51, Ü54, Ü55, Ü73, Ü81].

Powdered allspice can also be added to sweet dishes like plum pudding, desserts or baked goods, especially Christmas cookies (Aachener honey biscuits, almond biscuits) [Ü51].

In the same way as clove, one can use allspice as a flavoring for mulled wine [Ü68]. In combination with clove, cardamom, cinnamon and black tea, allspice is suitable for the production of warming beverage teas [Ü73].

The food industry uses allspice as a seasoning of ketchup, pickles, sausage (especially blood sausage and liverwurst), canned meat and fish conserves [Ü73]. One particular specialty that is seasoned with allspice is Hessian bratwurst [8].

Combines well with: Bay, cinnamon, clove, ginger, juniper, nutmeg, and orange peel, but also with garlic, and onions.

As a component of spice mixes and preparations: → Bologna spice mix, → Chili powder, → Curry powder, → English pudding spice, → Fish spice, → Gingerbread spice, → Grill spice, → Mixed pickles spice, → Pickling spice, → Quatre épices, → Ras el hanout, → Roast spice → Sauce spice, → Sausage spice, → Table mustard, → Tomato ketchup, → Vegetable spice, → Venison spice, → Worcestershire sauce.

Other uses: The essential oil from allspice is used as a flavor additive for herbal liqueurs (Aromatique, Benediktiner, Chartreuse, Kartäuser, Stonsdorfer, among others) and baking oils. In the cosmetic industry, it is used as an aroma component in perfumes and soaps. The straight branches and trunks of the allspice tree are ideal for the manufacture of walking sticks and umbrella rods [Ü89, Ü92].

Medicinal herb

Herbal drug: Pimentae fructus (Amomi fructus), Allspice, contains minimum 2.5% essential oil [EB 6].

Indications: As an appetite stimulant and for the alleviation of indigestion. Today it is hardly ever used.

Similar culinary herbs

Crown allspice (bay rum tree), *Pimenta racemosa* (MILL.) J.W. MOORE (Synonym: *P. acris* (Sw.) KOSTEL.), an evergreen growing up to 10 m tall, with approximately 1 cm long and 0.5 cm wide, jug-shaped fruits with a 5-lobed calyx at the end, native to northern South America and the Antilles, cultivated in the Antilles (Puerto Rico, Dominican Republic), and also in Cameroon and India. Crown allspice fruits are used the same as allspice, but have a less appealing aroma. The essential oil content of the leaves and young twigs (Bay oil, Oleum Myricae, Oleum Pimentae acris) is 0.3 to 1%, and is used in the manufacture of cosmetic preparations, rarely also as a component of liqueurs and spice essences. The main components of Bay Oil are eugenol (about 50 to 65%) and chavicol (about 20%), furthermore it contains, among others, limonene, octane-3-one, methyleugenol (eugenol methylether), methyl chavicol, furfurol, myrcene, (−)-phellandrene and citral. Ethanolic solutions known as Bay Rum are used as hair wash, after-shave lotion or body care agents [Ü31, Ü38, Ü60, Ü89, Ü92].

Tabasco allspice (Mexican allspice, Mexico allspice, Spanish allspice, Poivre de Chiappa), 8 to 10 mm fruits of *Pimenta dioica* (L.) MERR. var. *tabasco* (*Eugenia tabasco* G. DON), native to Mexico, and used in the same way as allspice [Ü92].

Brazil allspice originates from *Calyptranthes aromatica* ST. HILL. (Myrtaceae) [8].

Jerk Pork

(Traditional Jamaican dish).
4 pork chops or tenderloin, 25 g allspice (whole), 3 spring onions (finely minced), 1 to 2 fresh chili peppers (without seeds, finely minced), 2 bay leaves, salt, freshly ground black pepper.

Place the whole allspice in a small pot on medium heat for 3 to 5 minutes while stirring; add the onions, chilies, bay leaves, pepper and salt, and prepare a thick paste. Spread the paste onto the meat and let it stand for 2 h or overnight in the refrigerator. Then, slowly grill the meat, preferably over charcoal, for 40 to 60 minutes. In order to give the meat an authentic aroma, a few whole allspice fruits are thrown into the charcoal [Ü2].

Literature

[1] Chapman G.P., Ann. Botan New Series (London) 28:451 (1964).
[2] Chung Sh. et al., Biosci. Biotechnol. Biochem. 61(1):118–123 (1997).
[3] Garcia-Fajardo J. et al., J. Ess. Oil Res. 9:181–185 (1997).
[4] Hao Y.Y. et al., J. Food Prot. 61(3):307–312 (1998).
[5] Kikuzaki H. et al., J. Nat. Prod. 63(6): 749–752 (2000).
[6] Lawrence B.M., Perfum. Flavorist 15:64 (1990).
[7] Nabney J., F. Robinson, Flavour Ind. 3:50–51 (1972).
[8] Oberdieck R., Fleischwirtschaft 69:320–330 (1989).
[9] Oya T. et al., Biosc. Biotechnol. Biochem. 61(2):263–266 (1997).
[10] Pino J. et al., Nahrung 33:717–720 (1989).
[11] Pino J.A. et al., J. Ess. Oil Res. 9(6):689–691 (1997).
[12] Rodriguez M. et al., Alimentaria (Madrid) 274:107–110 (1996), ref. CA 125: 163102y.
[13] Schulz J.M., K. Herrmann, Z. Lebensm. Unters. Forsch. 171:193–199, 278–280 (1980).
[14] Smith R., S. Beck, J. Chromatogr. 291: 424–427 (1984).
[15] Stahl E. (Hrsg.): Chromatographische und mikroskopische Analyse von Drogen, Fischer Verlag Stuttgart, New York 1978.
[16] Veek M., G. Russel, J. Food Sci. 38:1028–1031 (1973).
[17] Vösgen B., K. Herrmann, Z. Lebensm. Unters. Forsch. 170:204–207 (1980).

Literature references identified by Ü can be found in the general listing of books and monographs at the back of this book.

Angelica

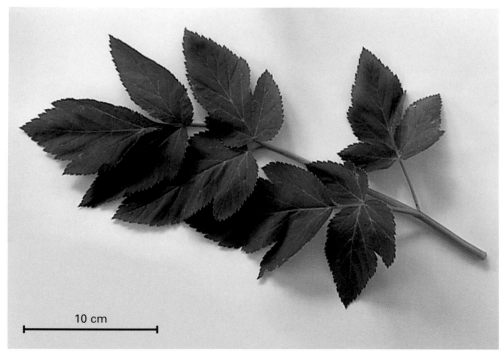

10 cm

Fig. 1: Angelica leaf

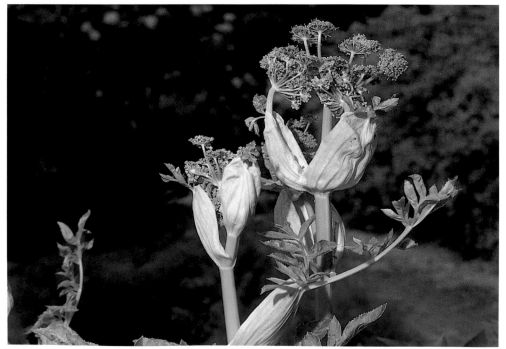

Fig. 2: Angelica (*Angelica archangelica* L.)

Plant source: *Angelica archangelica* L.

Synonyms: *Archangelica officinalis* HOFFM., *Angelica officinalis* auct.

Taxonomic classification: The species is differentiated as:
– *Angelica archangelica* L. ssp. *archangelica* with European varieties including
- - *Angelica archangelica* L. ssp. *archangelica* var. *sativa* (MILL.) RIKLI and
- - *Angelica archangelica* L. ssp. *archangelica* var. *norvegica* (RUPR.) THELL. as well as
– *Angelica archangelica* L. ssp. *litoralis* (FRIES) THELL.
For cultivation, *A. a.* ssp. *archangelica* var. *sativa* is used almost exclusively.

Family: Umbelliferous plants (Apiaceae, synonym Umbelliferae).

Common names: Engl.: angelica, garden angelica, archangel, European angelica; Fr.: archangélique; Ger.: Angelika, Engel-wurz, Erzengelwurz, Brustwurz.

Description: A biennial to quadrennial herb, up to 3 m high, forms only a rosette of basal leaves in the first year. The root is spindle-shaped, in the second year a thick, relatively short rootstock develops, look-ing as if it had been bitten off; it is sur-rounded by numerous, up to 10 mm thick, 30 to 40 cm long, light brown adventitious roots bearing yellowish latex. The stem is round and glabrous, acute angled fur-rowed, up to arm-thick at the base, reddish pruinose and pithy tube-like, bearing branches with inflorescences beginning in the mid-section. The leaves are glabrous, the lower ones up to 90 cm long, tri-fold pinnatisect, ternate-pinnate or multiple incised, the last-order leaf-sections being longish-ovate; the division of the leaves decreases towards the top, the lower leaves have a round petiole, and the upper ones situated atop very large, swollen leaf sheaths. The flowers are arranged in quasi-spherical compound umbels at the end of the branches and the stem; the diameter of the umbels is about 20 cm, bearing 20 to 40 powdery, softly pubescent rays without involucre but with numerous leaflets of the involucel. The flowers are radial, the calycinal margin barely visible, with 5 yellowish-greenish petals, 5 stamina, 2 short styles and an inferior, bilocular ovary. The fruit is a double achene that easily separates into mericarps, which are still attached to the bifurcate carpophore. The flowering period is from June to August [35, Ü21, Ü37].

Native origin: Northern Europe, but now widely distributed throughout Central- and Eastern Europe, Siberia, and Caucasia, and naturalized in North America.

Main cultivation areas: Germany (Ore Mountains, Thuringia, Franconia), France (Auvergne), Belgium, the Netherlands, Hungary, Italy, and Switzerland.

Main exporting countries: The Netherlands, Poland, and Germany.

Cultivation: The plant prefers deep, humus-rich, and moist soil, but is intolerant of stagnant moisture. Sowing occurs at the end of summer, and due to the rapid loss of germinating power, fresh or cool-stored seed is used. The rows are distanced about 50 cm apart and covered with only a thin layer of soil (needs light to germinate). To maximize root growth, small hills are often formed around each plant, and sometimes they are also decapitated. The plant is insensitive to frost but self-incompatible (cultivation pause of at least 5 years). Cultivars including, among others, 'Sächsische', 'Budakalszi' and 'Jizerka' are used for cultivation [Ü21].

Culinary Herb

Commercial forms: Angelica root: the whole or cut, dried rhizome and root (from here on referred to as roots), also as "plait ware", meaning that the adventitious roots are interwoven before drying forming a plait (due to the long adventitious roots with their high content of aromatic substance, exceptionally valuable), dried fruits, and the essential oil obtained from the roots or the fruits.

Production: The fruits are harvested starting in July of the second year by combine. If necessary, two harvests are possible in the third year. The roots are harvested in the autumn of the second year using shaker sieve diggers or complete potato harvesters, washed and dried at about 40 °C. Caution is advised for the harvesters due to the risk of photodermatosis (see below) [Ü21].

Forms used: Fresh leaves, and rarely also the dried, fresh stems, dried roots, and fresh or dried fruits.

Storage: Fresh leaves, with the stems removed, can be stored with their petioles in water or wrapped in plastic bags for a few days, (up to 8 weeks in the refrigerator, between −1 and +2 °C). The leaves can also be finely chopped and frozen in water in an ice cube tray. The candied stems are wrapped in foil and stored in a cool place but not in the refrigerator. The dried leaves, roots or fruits should be stored in well-sealed metal- or glass containers, protected from light and moisture. Particularly the dried roots are easily infested by insects.

Description. Root: The short, up to 5 cm thick rootstock is gray- or reddish brown, with transverse girdling or longitudinal grooves, bearing the remains of stems and leaf bases as well as the numerous, up to 1 cm thick, 30 cm long, cylindrical, light brown, scarcely branched secondary roots; the transverse fracture is uneven. The cross section shows the gray-white, spongy bark with the secretory ducts discernible as brown dots. Towards the inside is a light- or grayish yellow xylem, and the rhizomes show the gray- or brownish white pith [Ü37].

Fruits: Double achenes separated into mericarps, light yellow, broad-elliptic to almost rectangular, 5 to 9 mm long, 2 to 5 mm wide, compressed, with wing-like, enlarged marginal ribs [Ü37].

Leaf (Fig. 1)**:** Up to 90 cm long, 3-fold pinnatisect, the sections of last-order are ovate or ovate-lanceolate, unevenly divided, serrate or dentate, the teeth ending in sleek, thorn-like tips [Ü37].

Odor: Typical, aromatic, **Taste:** Sweet at first, then spicy, musk-like, bitter and persistently burning.

History: Angelica has been used since the 10th century in Scandinavia, and by the 14th century, it was cultivated in Central Europe, particularly in monastery gardens; since 1494, it has been grown in Bockau, Germany near the Ore Mountains. The plant played a not insignificant role as a spice and medicinal plant in medieval times [Ü92].

Constituents and Analysis

Constituents of the roots

- Essential oil: 0.3 to 1.3% with mainly monoterpenes (80 to 90%); the main components in *A. a.* ssp. *archangelica* var. *sativa* are α-pinene (14 to 32%), β-phellandrene (13 to 28%), Δ^3-carene (about 16%), α-phellandrene (2 to 14%), and other monoterpenes such as bornyl acetate, camphene, 1,8-cineole, α-copaene, *p*-cymene, limonene, *trans-p*-menth-2-ene-1-ol (possibly an artifact), myrcene, β-pinene and sabinene, the sesquiterpenes β-bisabolene and β-bisabolol, the prenylated hydroxycoumarin 7-methoxy-8-(3-methyl-2-butenyl)-2H-1-benzopyran-2-one as well as macrocyclic lactones (about 1.5%, responsible for the characteristic odor) with the main components 13-tridecanolide and 15-pentadecanolide, in addition to 12-methyl-13-tridecanolide, 16-hexadecanolide and 17-heptadecanolide, among others [1, 6, 9, 17, 18, 22, 24, 25, 29, 33]. The essential oil from the roots of *A. a.* ssp. *archangelica* var. *norvegica* contains mostly Δ⁶-carene (about 13%), α-pinene (about 10%), *p*-mentha-2,8-diene-1-ol (about 9%), limonene (about 7%) and *cis-p*-menth-2-ene-1-ol (about 5%) [2].

- Furanocoumarins: 0.5 to 1.6%, including angelicin, archangelin, bergaptene, byakangelicol, 5-β-cycloavandulyloxypsoralene, heraclenol, imperatorin, isobergaptene, isoimperatorin, marmesin, osthrutol, oxypeucedanin, xanthotoxin and xanthotoxol, as well as dihydrofuranocoumarins such as archangelicin, among others. The content of furanocoumarins rises considerably if the plant is infected by fungi [3, 7, 16, 32, Ü100].
- Hydroxycoumarins: 2′-Angeloyl-3′-isovalerylvaginate, osthenol, osthol, umbelliferone [5, 14, 15].

Constituents of the fruits

- Essential oil: 0.6% to 1.8%, with the main components hexylmethylphthalate (about 30%), α-pinene (about 12%), β-phellandrene (about 2%), β-caryophyllene (about 2.5%), camphene (about 2%), β-bisabolene (about 1.5%), macrocyclic lactones (responsible for characteristic odor), particularly 15-pentadecanolide, moreover, borneol, carvone, 1,8-cineole, limonene, *p*-cymene, myrcene, β-pinene, among others; furthermore carboxylic acids, including angelic acid and oxymyristicic acid [10, 13, 19, 22].
- Furanocoumarins: About 1.3%, with the main components imperatorin (0.5%), isoimperatorin (0.38%) and bergaptene (0.35%); furthermore, peucedanin, xanthotoxin, isopimpinellin, xanthotoxol,

among others, and the dihydrofuranocoumarin apterin [4, 7, Ü100].
- Hydroxycoumarins: Umbelliferone, among others [7].
- Fatty oil: 17 to 25%.

Constituents of the leaves

- Essential oil: About 0.1%, with the main components β-phellandrene (about 34%), α-pinene (about 27%) and β-pinene (about 24%); furthermore, myrcene, *p*-cymene, *cis*- and *trans*-β-ocimene [19].
- Furanocoumarins: About 0.2 to 0.7%, including xanthotoxin, imperatorin, oxypeucedanin, angelicin, bergaptene and isopimpinellin [7, 31, Ü100].

Tests for Identity: Organoleptic, macroscopic and microscopic analyses of the roots, according to Ph Eur (see also references in Lit. Ü37, 11, 16, 27, Ü106). The fruits are identified with TLC [34].

Quantitative assay: The essential oil content is determined volumetrically, according to Ph Eur, with dimeticon as anti-foaming agent and xylol in the graduated tube (see also DAB).

Adulterations, Misidentifications and Impurities: Adulterations and misidentification with the roots from *Angelica silvestris* L. (wild angelica) are possible. The rhizome of this adulterant, gray on the outer surface, is smaller and more fibrous than genuine angelica root; its bark has only very few red-colored secretory ducts. Misidentifications with other apiaceous roots can be detected organoleptically; for adulterations with → Lovage root, see also TLC method (phthalides!) in the Ph Eur.

Actions and Uses

Actions: The aromatic and bitter taste of angelica stimulates gastric secretions. A mixture of extracts of angelica root injected into mice significantly prevented damage from gamma irradiation (cumulative dose of 12 Gy) [23]. The essential oil has shown good spasmolytic action on the intestinal and tracheal smooth muscles of the guinea pig in vitro, surpassing that of caraway oil [26]. Extracts of the root inhibit thrombocyte aggregation [36].

Toxicology: All plant parts can cause photodermatosis after internal use or even with skin contact due to the high concentration of furanocoumarins. Photomutagenic and photocarcinogenic effects are possible [12, 36, Ü100]. After consumption of large amounts of plant parts, e.g. leaves or leaf stalks in vegetable dishes, sunbathing or use of tanning UV-lamps should be avoided.

Culinary use: Chopped young leaves can be used sparingly as a spice for soups, salads, quark, cottage cheeses, cheese preparations, custards, rhubarb- or plum compotes, as a stuffing for fish or as an ingredient used for poached seafoods. It is also used as a spice in fish boiling, e.g. of salmon or trout [Ü55, Ü74].
Young stalks, leaves and petioles are eaten, raw or blanched, as a vegetable, mainly in Scandinavia [Ü17, Ü91].
Young stalks and petioles are candied in pastry shops for decorating tortes and baked goods (Petit fours) especially in Austria and France, but are also eaten as sweets [Ü17, Ü65, Ü79, Ü91].
Angelica essential oil and extracts of the fruits and roots are used in the manufacture of herbal liqueurs such as Angelikalikör, Altvater, Bénédictine, Chartreuse, Boonekamp, Kartäuser and Stonsdorfer.

Other uses: The essential oil of angelica root serves as a component of cosmetics such as perfumes, soaps, lotions and creams [28].

13-Tridecanolide   15-Pentadecanolide   12-Methyl-13-tridecanolide

Medicinal herb

Herbal drug: Angelicae radix, Angelica root, contains minimum 2.0 ml/kg of essential oil [Ph Eur].

Indications: The root is used for loss of appetite and for dyspeptic complaints such as mild gastrointestinal cramps, bloating and flatulence. The German Commission E daily dosage is 4.5 g dried root, 1.5 to 3 g fluidextract (1:1) or 1.5 g tincture (1:5), or 10 to 20 drops of essential oil [20]. Angelica root is taken, especially, in the form of tea infusions, using 1.5 g of fine-cut dried root per cup, 30 minutes before meals [Ü106]. Because the effectiveness of preparations made from angelica fruit and herb as diuretic and diaphoretic remedies, as practiced in folk medicine, has not been substantiated, and in view of the risks (photodermatosis), the therapeutic use of these plant parts cannot be recommended [21].

Similar spices

Dong quai root (Chinese angelica root), *Angelica sinensis* (OLIV.) DIELS, is cultivated in China for use as a medicinal plant, spice and as a component of cosmetics. It contains 0.2 to 0.4% essential oil, of which the main components are phthalides (ligustilide, butylidenphthalide, butylphthalide) [Ü37].

Ashitaba, *Angelica keiskei* (MIQ.) KOIDZ., native to Japan, where it is cultivated and used similarly to *A. archangelica* [Ü61].

Greater burnet saxifrage, from *Pimpinella major* (L.) HUDS., or **Burnet saxifrage**, *Pimpinella saxifraga* L. s.l. (Apiaceae), native to nearly all of Europe, naturalized

in North America and cultivated in India. It contains 0.1 to 0.6% essential oil, of which the main component of *P. major* is the tiglic ester of *trans*-epoxypseudoisoeugenol (comprises 20 to 55%), and of *P. saxifraga*, it is epoxypseudoisoeugenyl-2-methylbutyrate (10 to 75%) [Ü99]. The oil is used as an aromatic component of liqueurs (Aromatique, Bittere Tropfen). The fresh herb is used as a salad topping, and the dried herb is also used in the manufacture of spice extracts [Ü92, Ü98].

Literature

[1] Baerheim Svendsen A., J. Karlsen, Planta Med. 14:376–380 (1966).

[2] Bernard C. et al., J. Essent. Oil Res. 9:289–294 (1997).

[3] Carbonnier J., D. Mohlo, Planta Med. 44:162–165 (1982).

[4] Ceska O. et al., Phytochemistry 26(1): 165–169 (1987).

[5] Chalchat J.C., R.Ph. Garry, J. Essent. Oil Res. 5:447–449 (1993).

[6] Chalchat J.C., R.Ph. Garry, TJ. Essent. Oil Res. 9:311–319 (1997).

[7] Cisowski W. et al., Herb. Pol. 33:233–243 (1987).

[8] Czygan F.C., Z. Phytother. 19(6):342–348 (1998).

[9] Escher S. et al., Helv. Chim. Acta 62: 2061–2072 (1979).

[10] Flath R.A. et al., Chem. Ecol. 20:1969–1984 (1994).

[11] Genius O.B., Dtsch. Apoth. Ztg. 121:386–387 (1981).

[12] Glombitza K.W., Dtsch. Apoth. Ztg. 112:1593–1598 (1972).

[13] Guenther E., in: The Essential Oils, Van Nostrand Company, Princeton New Jersey, Bd. 4, p. 553–563 (1965).

[14] Harkar S. et al., Phytochemistry 23:419–426 (1983).

[15] Härmälä P. et al., Planta Med. 58:287 (1992).

[16] Hörhammer L. et al., Dtsch. Apoth. Ztg. 106:267–272 (1966).

[17] Jacobson M. et al., J. Agric. Food Chem. 35:798–800 (1987).

[18] Kerrola K.M. et al., J. Agric. Food Chem. 42:2235–2245 (1994).

[19] Kloppenburg U., Untersuchungen über das ätherische Öl von Angelica archangelica L., Angelica silvestris L. und Carum carvi L. (Apiaceae), Dissertation, Univ. Hamburg 1977.

[20] Kommission E beim BfArM, BAnz-Nr. 101 vom 01.06.90 (1990).

[21] Kommission E beim BfArM, BAnz-Nr. 101 vom 01.06.90 (1990).

[22] Lawrence B.M., Perfumer Flavorist 21(5):57–59 (1996).

[23] Narimanov A.A., Radiobiologiia 33(2): 280–284 (1993).

[24] Nykanen I. et al., J. Essent. Oil Res. 3:229–236 (1991).

[25] Racz G. et al., Rev. Med. 24:10–12 (1978).

[26] Reiter M., W. Brandt, Arzneim. Forsch. 35:408–414 (1985).

[27] Rohdewald P. et al., Apothekengerechte Prüfvorschriften, Dtsch. Apoth. Verlag Stuttgart 1986, 1. Erg. Lfg. 1992.

[28] Schmidt E., Forum Aromather. Aromapflege E1/99:8–11 (1999).

[29] Schultz K., Ph. Kraft, J. Essent. Oil Res. 9:509–514 (1997).

[30] Shimizu M. et al., Chem. Pharm. Bull. 39:2046 (1991).

[31] Steck W., B.K. Bailey, Can. J. Chem. 47:2425–2430 und 3577–3583 (1969).

[32] Sun H., J. Jakupovic, Pharmazie 41:888–889 (1986).

[33] Taskinen J., Acta Chem. Scand. B29:637–638, 757–764 und 999–1001 (1975).

[34] Wawrzynowicz T., M. Waksmundzka-Hajnos, Liquid Chromatogr. 13:3925–3940 (1990).

[35] Weymar H., Buch der Doldengewächse, Neumann Verlag, Radebeul 1959.

[36] Zobel A.M., S.A. Brown, Can. J. Bot. 69:485–488 (1991).

Literature references identified by Ü can be found in the general listing of books and monographs at the back of this book.

Anise

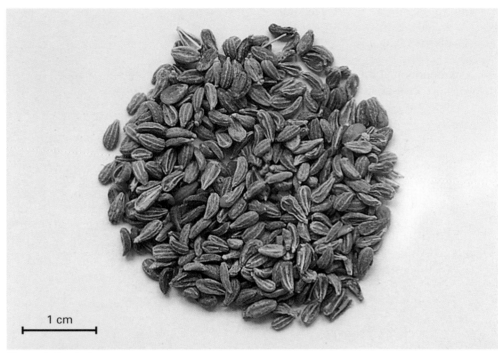

Fig. 1: Anise fruits

Plant source: *Pimpinella anisum* L.

Synonym: *Anisum vulgare* GAERTN.

Family: Umbelliferous plants (Apiaceae, synonym Umbelliferae).

Common names: Engl.: anise, aniseed; Fr.: anis vert; Ger.: Anis, Süßer Kümmel, Brotsame, Aneis, Taubenanis.

Description: A 0.2 to 0.5 m tall annual having a thin, spindle-shaped taproot, a roundish, erect, cylindrical, furrowed stem, branched in the upper part. The lower leaves are petiolate, alternate, roundish-reniform, serrate to somewhat lobed; the ones in the mid-section are pinnate, the upper ones opposite, di- to tripinnate, with lanceolate, fine tips. All parts are short, delicate and softly pubescent. The flowers are arranged in compound umbels with 7 to 15 rays; involucre is usually absent or monophyllous; one or a few filiform small involucral leaflets are present. Radially structured flowers, 5 white petals with ciliated margins and short bristly hairs on the outer surface, 5 stamina, 2 styles and an inferior, bilocular ovary. The fruit is a double achene, which is by short, appressed bristles, pubescent; is not easily detached and separates rather late into 2 mericarps, which are attached to a bifurcate carpophore and remain closed. The flowering period is from June to August [56].

Native origin: Unknown, probably native to the eastern Mediterranean region, and Anterior Asia.

Main cultivation areas: Turkey, Spain, Hungary, Italy, southern France, the Balkan countries, southern parts of the Russian Federation, India, Lebanon, China, Japan, Chile, Argentina, Mexico, Central- and South America.

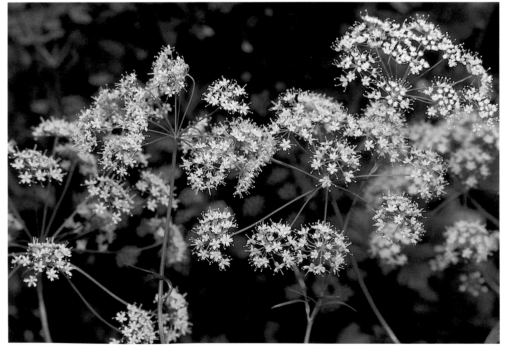

Fig. 2: Anise (*Pimpinella anisum* L.)

Main exporting countries: Turkey, followed by Spain, Hungary, Lebanon, and Egypt.

Cultivation: Sowing takes place starting in April in humus-rich, calcareous soil, in sunny locations in rows 20 cm apart. The seeds should only be lightly covered. Due to slow emergence (germination time of 25 to 30 days), in order to control weeds, it is advantageous to use a marker seeding, e.g. radishes. A frequently cultivated variety in Germany is 'Thüringer Anis'. In France, the large-fruited 'Tourraine-Anis' is cultivated [Ü46, Ü71].

Culinary herb

Commercial forms: Anise seed: dried fruits (whole, bruised or crushed), anise essential oil, and anise oleoresin.

Production: Harvest takes place when the fruits in the center of the umbel are brown and the stalk is yellow. The harvest is carried out using a swather, because the fruits fall off easily, especially with the morning dew. Post-harvest, there are secondary ripening and drying steps, followed by threshing in order to remove other plant parts.

Forms used: The whole, dried fruits (often crushed immediately prior to use), and rarely also the bruised or crushed fruits, anise essential oil, anise oleoresin, and the fresh leaves.

Storage: The dried, whole fruits are stored in well-sealed metal- or glass containers, protected from light and moisture. The fresh leaves can be packed into plastic bags and stored in the refrigerator for a few days. Anise also loses its aromatic quality relatively quickly, even under proper storage conditions. Therefore, anise should only be stored up until the next harvest. Light causes isomerization, which also occurs in anise preparations, whereby the *trans*-anethole converts partially to the relatively toxic *cis*-anethole form [3, 15, 23, 37].

Description: The **whole fruits** (Fig. 1) consist of the double achenes, mostly not yet split into their mericarps, with the thin, rigid and slightly curved pedicel, up to 12 mm long, often still attached. The double achenes are ovoid to pyriform, yellowish-green to greenish-gray, slightly compressed laterally, 3 to 6 mm long and 3 mm wide, with a stylopodium at the upper end, bearing two short, curved styles. The fruits are densely hairy (visible under lens magnification) with 5 rather indistinct ribs [Ü94]. The **powdered fruit** is greenish- or brownish-yellow. Microscopic examination reveals the conspicuous short, mostly unicellular, curved, thick-walled, whole or broken trichomes with granular (cucumber-like) cuticula (Fig. 3). Also present is the colorless, thick-walled endosperm with many very small oxalate druses, aleuron grains and oil droplets as well as flat fragments with narrow, brownish secretory ducts, sometimes tied together, and gaps consisting of colorless parenchyma; groups of parallel arranged transverse cells are situated above. Vascular bundles from the carpophore and pedicel as well as elongated, densely punctate stone cells from the commissures are rarely present.

Odor: Aromatic, **Taste:** Sweetish, reminiscent of licorice.

History: Anise has been valued since ancient times and was already mentioned in the "Papyrus Ebers" (authored in 1550 BCE). During the Roman Empire, anise was also very popular; Pliny the Elder (23 to 79 CE) praised its attributes. Benedictine monks introduced anise to Central Europe in the 8th century. In a local government decree by Karl the Great, "Capitulare de villis" (authored in about 795 CE) [1], anise is also listed. In England, it has been used since the 14th century. Tabernaemontanus (1520 to 1590) includes anise in his herbal, and it was also used as a component of the "Theriac" [10].

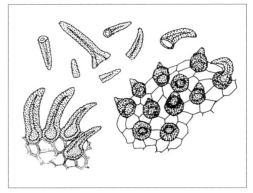

Fig. 3: Anise. Trichomes of the epidermis of the fruit wall. From Ü94.

Constituents and Analysis

DIN and ISO-Standards: ISO-Standard 7386 (Anise).

Constituents

- Essential oil: 1.5 to 6%, the main component is *trans*-anethole ((*E*)-anethole, 80 to 95%), furthermore, estragole (methylchavicol, about 1 to 4%), γ-himachalene (about 0.7 to 3%), pseudo-isoeugenyl-2-methylbutyrate (about 1 to 3.5%), epoxypseudoisoeugenyl-2-methylbutyrate (0.1 to 1.3%), anisaldehyde (0.5 to 0.9%), *cis*-anethole ((*Z*)-anethole, 0.3 to 0.4%) and the diterpene neophytoadiene. Anise oil solidifies between 15 and 19 °C due to the high melting point of anethole (21 °C) [8, 13, 14, 25–28, 30, 41, 47].

---

[1] "Capitulare Caroli Magni de villis vel curtis imperialibus", an imperial government decree regulating agricultural practices, was authored by the Benedictine monk Abbot Ansegis in about 795 CE per request of Karl the Great (742 to 814); this document called for the cultivation of 24 medicinal plants and culinary herbs by monasteries and imperial leasehold estates, e.g. anise, black cumin, celery, chervil, chives, dill, fennel, garlic, leek, lovage, mint, mustard, onions, parsley, poppy, rosemary, sage, shallot, southernwood, tarragon, watercress [Ü23, Ü44, Ü92].

trans-Anethole   Estragole   Pseudoisoeugenol-2-methyl-butyrate   Epoxypseudoisoeugenol-2-methylbutyrate

γ-Himachalene   Neophytadiene

- Phenylacrylic acids: Caffeic acid derivatives, particularly chlorogenic acid (about 0.1%), other caffeoyl quinic acids, p-coumaroyl- and feruloyl quinic acids [11].
- Flavonoids: Apigenin-7-O-glucoside, luteolin-7-O-glucoside, quercetin-3-O-glucuronide, rutin, isoorientin, isovitexin, among others [12, 29].
- Furanocoumarins: Bergaptene, among others [9, 23].
- Hydroxycoumarins: Umbelliferone, among others [23].
- Fatty oil: About 30%, composed of about 65% of petroselinic acid [23, 55].

The essential oil from the herb contains only about 30% trans-anethole, but 20% of both pseudoisoeugenol isomers (see above), about 15% germacrene D, about 12% β-bisabolene and 3% γ-himachalene [28].

Tests for Identity: Organoleptic, macroscopic, microscopic and TLC analyses [52, Ph Eur] as well as TAS [32], HPLC [19, 36] and GC assays of the essential oil [Ph Eur].

Quantitative assay: The content of essential oil can be determined volumetrically with steam distillation and xylol in the graduated tube [Ph Eur]. The quantification of the essential oil components can be carried out with GC [Ph Eur].

Adulterations, Misidentifications and Impurities: Admixtures of toxic hemlock fruits from *Conium maculatum* L. are rare. The adulterant is separated into mericarps, and the individual fruits are glabrous with distinctly undulating ribs. The powder shows the occurrence of characteristic cup-like cells with a prominent, ribbed structure [Ü37].

Anise oil is also obtained from → Star anise (*Illicium verum* HOOK. f.). The Ph Eur allows for both species as raw materials. The considerably less expensive essential oil from star anise is characterized by its fenchone content; the pseudoisoeugenol isomers are absent. Synthetic anethole has also been observed as an adulterant of anise oil; it contains up to 15% cis-anethole, and can be differentiated from genuine anise oil by GC [Ph Eur] or TLC [44, 48].

Actions and Uses

Actions: On the basis of its aromatic taste, anise and anise oil are appetite stimulating and digestion promoting.

Anethole, in concentrations from 10 to 25 mg/l, caused contractions in the small intestine of the mouse in vitro, yet at higher doses (50, 75, 200 mg/l), it led to relaxation of the intestines [21]. 200 mg/l of anise oil showed antispasmodic action by antagonizing a carbachol-induced spasm in the intestinal and tracheal smooth muscles of the guinea pig [43]. In mice, the essential oil suppressed tonic and clonic convulsions induced by pentylenetetrazole or maximal electroshock [40]. Moreover, anise oil has shown secretolytic and expectorant activity [24, 39, 45, overview in Lit. 58].

In anesthetized guinea pigs, the oral application of an ethanolic solution of anise oil (12%, 10 to 50 mg/kg body weight) caused a 3- to 6-fold increase in the fluid quantity in the respiratory tract [6]. Similar results were obtained in experiments with rats [5] and cats [7]. In anesthetized cats, two drops of the essential oil stimulated movement of the mobile fibers of the ciliated epithelium, which had been inhibited from a dose of opium [54].

Anise oil has also demonstrated antimicrobial action [20, 34, 35, 41, 50]. Moreover, anise has, similar to fennel, shown mild estrogenic activity due to its anethole content [1].

Toxicology: Based on existing data, there is no acute or chronic toxicity with the regular use of this herb as a spice [2, Ü37]. With higher dosages, an estrogenic effect, due to the content of anethole, similar to that of → Fennel could be expected [49]. The sensitization potential is small [53, 57, Ü39]. Occasionally, allergic reactions of the skin, respiratory or gastrointestinal tract have been observed [24]. The IgE-type antibodies of the affected persons show cross-reaction with allergens from other Apiaceae (coriander, fennel, Roman caraway). The proteins involved are suspected to be similar to birch pollen allergens (birch-profilin), among others [22, 51].

Culinary use: In India, anise is used as a spice in soups, stews and fish recipes. The roasted, and then mildly nut-like tasting fruits are also chewed in Southeast Asian countries. The Romans used anise fruits, covered with sugar, as a digestive-aid after eating rich meals.

Anise is milled or crushed with a mortar. In Europe, anise fruit is used predominantly as a cookie- or biscuit spice, especially during Christmas (e.g. anise cookies, anise pretzels (Bavaria), ginger bread, Guetzli and Chräbeli; traditional Swiss Christmas cookies), but it is also used similarly to caraway as a bread spice. Likewise, it is well suited as a spice for fruit compotes, fruit salads, fruit soups, and plum marmalade. Anise is also used as a component of sweet and sour sauces, soups, fish dishes, vegetable dishes (e.g. cauliflower, carrots, and red cabbage), salads, boiled potatoes, and pumpkin. It can be used as a component of marinades for fish, meat and crustaceans. Similarly, anise is used as a pickling spice, e.g. for cucumbers, red beets, and sauerkraut.

The essential oil of anise is a component of liqueurs: in Greece of Ouzo or Mastika, in France of Pastis (Pernod, Ricard, Berger) or Anisette, in Spain of Pacharan, in Turkey of Raki, in Russia of Allasch, in Germany of Abtei, Bénédictine, Boonekamp, Küstennebel, Stonsdorfer, and Goldwasser. Anise oil is also used, however, instead of anise fruit as a flavor component of baked goods and sweets (anise bonbons).

Anise liqueur is also used in the kitchen, e.g. as a spice for sauces, fish soups or beurre pour escargots [46, Ü13, Ü45, Ü55, Ü59, Ü70, Ü73, Ü79]. The young leaves can be used as an ingredient in cabbage- or fruit salads, fresh cheeses as well as fish soups.

Combines well with: Chervil, coriander or rosemary.

As a component of spice mixes and preparations: → Bologna spice mix, → Bread spice, → Curry powder, → Gingerbread spice, → Herbes de Provence, → Pastry spice, → Poultry spice.

Other uses: Anise essential oil serves as a flavor component of toothpastes, mouthwashes, soaps, perfumes, creams and lotions. It is also used as an aroma component of pipe tobacco. Anise water is used, in India, similarly to that of 'Kölnisch Wasser' (eau de Cologne). Pigeon breeders place anise fruit or anise oil in the pigeon house in order to entice their (or someone else's) pigeons.

Medicinal herb

Herbal drugs: Anisi fructus, Aniseed, contains not less than 20 ml/kg of essential oil [Ph Eur], Anisi aetheroleum, Anise Oil, may also be obtained from Star anise fruit (*Illicium verum* HOOK. fil.) [Ph Eur, requirements → Star anise, Constituents].

Indications: Anise fruit and/or anise oil are used internally for dyspeptic complaints, and internally or externally for catarrhs of the respiratory tract. The German Commission E average daily dose for internal use is 3.0 g of aniseed or 0.3 g essential oil, or corresponding preparations. The single-dose is 0.5 to 1.0 g. For internal use, the cut or crushed dried fruit is prepared as a tea infusion (1 to 2 teaspoons per 1 cup of boiled water) or aqueous-ethanolic extracts (alcohol content minimum 50%). For external use, lipophilic ointments or oily preparations, containing 5 to 10% essential oil, are used as rubs or as inhalants. For bronchial catarrh, 1 cup of freshly prepared tea is drunk in the morning and the evening. For the treatment of dyspepsia, 1 tablespoon of the tea is taken several times daily, and for infants and toddlers, 1 teaspoon. Anise schnapps also has appetite stimulating and digestion promoting effects. In the southwestern United States and in Mexico, anise fruit is used for menstrual complaints. In folk medicine, anise and anise schnapps are believed to be aphrodisiacs and lactagogues. Pliny the Elder (23 to 79 CE) had already reported these effects in the 1st century (possibly due to an estrogenic effect) [1, 2, 10, 31, 46].

Other culinary spices with an anise-like aroma

Anise-hyssop, *Agastache foeniculum* (PURSH) KUNTZE (Lamiaceae), native to North America; in the USA, it is cultivated as a forage plant for bees. The main components of the essential oil, depending on the variety, are estragole (methylchavicol, comprising up to 75%), limonene (up to 57%) or myrcene (up to 59%). The leaves are used as a spice. Its use is not advised due to the toxicologically high estragole content of some varieties [16, 18, 33, 38, Ü61].

Chinese giant hyssop (Korean mint)**,** *Agastache rugosa* (FISCH. et C.A. MEYER) KUNTZE (*Lophanthus rugosus* FISCH. et MEYER, Lamiaceae), native to China, Eastern Siberia, Korea and Japan [Ü61]. The main components of the essential oil are estragole (comprising about 80%), furthermore anisaldehyde, *p*-methoxy cinnamic aldehyde and limonene [17] or methyleugenol (eugenol methyl ether) [Ü43]. The leaves are used as a spice [Ü92]. Its use is not advised due to the toxicologically high estragole content.

Pimpinella anisetum BOISS. et BAL. (Apiaceae), native to Turkey, where it is cultivated exclusively for the production of essential oil. The main components of the fruit's essential oil are *trans*-anethole (about 77%) and estragole (about 22%) [4, Ü61].

Likewise, the following also have an anise-like aroma → Fennel, → Star anise, → Sweet cicely.

Anise cookies
3 eggs, 280 g confectioner's sugar, 1 package of vanilla sugar, 200 g flour, 100 g food starch, 1 heaping teaspoon of ground anise.

Mix the eggs, confectioner's and vanilla sugar in a bowl until it reaches a creamy consistency; then mix the flour with the food starch and anise, incorporating the flour mixture continuously in small portions into the cream. Using a teaspoon, drop small amounts of the cookie dough onto an aluminum foil-lined cookie sheet and let them stand overnight in a warm room. Bake the cookies 30 to 40 minutes, at 160 to 180 °C until they are lightly browned [Ü23].

Literature

[1] Albert-Puleo M., J. Ethnopharmacol. 2(4): 337–344 (1980).

[2] Anonym, Anisi fructus, ESCOP Monographs (1997).

[3] Baerheim-Svendsen A., H.M.J.A. Koning, Sci. Pharm. 51:409–414 (1983).

[4] Baser K.H.C. et al., J. Essent. Oil Res. 11:445–446 (1999).

[5] Boyd E.M., Pharmacol. Rev. 6:521–542 (1954).

[6] Boyd E.M., G.L. Pearson, Am. J. Med. Sci. 211:602–610 (1946).

[7] Boyd E.M., E.P. Shephard, J. Pharmacol. Exp. Therap. 163:250–256 (1968).

[8] Burkhardt G. et al., Pharm. Weekbl. Sci. 8(3):190–193 (1986).

[9] Ceska O. et al., Phytochemistry 26(1): 165–169 (1987).

[10] Czygan F.C., Z. Phytother. 13(3):101–106 (1992).

[11] Dirks U., K. Herrmann, Zeitschr. Lebensm. Unters. Forsch. 179:12–16 (1984).

[12] El-Moghazi A.M. et al., Fitoterapia 50:267–268 (1979).

[13] El-Wakeil F. et al., Seifen – Öle – Fette – Wachse 112:77–80 (1986).

[14] Embong M.B. et al., J. Canad. Plant Sci. 57:681–689 (1977).

[15] Fehr D., Pharm. Ztg. 125:1300–1303 (1980).

[16] Fuentes-Granados R.G. et al., J. Essent. Oil Res. 12:581–591 (2000).

[17] Fujita Y., Botan. Mag. (Tokyo) 64:165 zit. bei Ü43 (1951).

[18] Fujita Y., T. Ueda, CA 53:22754 zit. bei Ü43 (1959).

[19] Gracza L., Dtsch. Apoth. Ztg. 120: 1859–1863 (1980).

[20] Ibrahim Y.K.E, M.S. Ogunmodele, Pharm. Acta Helv. 66:286–288 (1991).

[21] Imaseki I., Y. Kitabatake, Yakugaku Zasshi 82:1326–1328 (1962).

[22] Jensen-Jarolim E. et al., Clin. Exp. Allergy 27(11):1299–1306 (1997).

[23] Kartnig T., G. Scholz, Fette, Seifen, Anstrichm. 71(4):276–280 (1969).

[24] Kommission E, BAnz. 122 vom 06.07.88 (1988).

[25] Kraus A., F.J. Hammerschmidt, Dragoco Report 27:31 (1980).

[26] Kubeczka K.H., Acta Horticulturae 73:85 (1978).

[27] Kubeczka K.H. et al., Z. Naturforsch. 31b:283–284 (1976).

[28] Kubeczka K.H., et al., in: E.J. Brunke (ed.) Progress in Essential Oil Research, Walter de Gruyter & Co, Berlin 1986, p. 279–298 (1986).

[29] Kunzemann J., K. Herrmann, Z. Lebensm. Untersuch. Forsch. 164:194–200 (1977).

[30] Lawrence B.M., Perfumer Flavorist 12:67–68 (1987).

[31] Linares E., R.A. Bye, J. Ethnopharmacol. 19:153–183 (1987).

[32] Lipták J. et al., Pharmazie 35(9):545–546 (1980).

[33] Manjarrez A., V. Mendoza, Perfumery Essent. Oil Record 57:561 zit. bei Ü43 (1966).

[34] Maruzella J.C., M. Freundlich, J. Am. Pharm. Assoc. 48:356–358 (1959).

[35] Maruzella J.C., A. Sicurella, J. Am. Pharm. Assoc. 49:692–694 (1960).

[36] Miething H., Pharm. Ztg. 125:1081–1082 (1987).

[37] Miething H. et al., Phytotherapy Res. 4:121–123 (1990).

[38] Mikus B. et al., Drogenreport 10(18):68–73 (1997).

[39] Müller-Limroth W., H.H. Fröhlich, Fortschr. Med. 98:95–101 (1980).

[40] Pourgholami M.H. et al., J. Ethnopharmacol. 66(2):211–215 (1999).

[41] Ramadan F.M. et al., Chem. Mikrobiol. Technol. Lebensm. 2:51–55 (1972).

[42] Reichling J. et al., Z. Naturforsch. 40c: 465–468 (1985).

[43] Reiter M., W. Brandt, Arzneim. Forsch. 35:408–414 (1985).

[44] Saukel J., Sci. Pharm. 53:62–64 (1985).

[45] Schilcher H., Dtsch. Apoth. Ztg. 124(29): 1433–1442 (1984).

[46] Scholz H., Natürlich (12):31–36 (1998).

[47] Schultze W. et al., Dtsch. Apoth. Ztg. 127:372–378 (1987).

[48] Seger V., Untersuchungen zu Inhaltsstoffen der Früchte von Pimpinella anisum L. und Illicium verum Hook. f., Dissertation Freie Universität Berlin 1985.

[49] Sharaf A., N. Goma, J. Endocrinol. 310:289–290 (1964).

[50] Shukla H.S., S.C. Tripathi, Agric. Biol. Chem. 51:1991–1993 (1987).

[51] Stäger J. et al., Allergy 46:475–478 (1991).

[52] Stahl E. (Hrsg.) Chromatographische und mikroskopische Analyse von Drogen, Fischer Verlag Stuttgart, New York 1978.

[53] Stricker W.E. et al., J. Allergy Clin. Immunol. 77:516–519 (1986).

[54] Van Dongen K., H. Leusink, Arch. Int. Pharmacodyn. 93:261–276 (1953).

[55] Van Loon J., Z. Lebensm. Unters. Forsch. 153:289–293 (1973).

[56] Weymar H., Buch der Doldengewächse, Neumann Verlag, Radebeul 1959.

[57] Wüthrich B., R. Dietsch, Schweiz. Med. Wochenschr. 115:358–364 (1985).

[58] Zänglein A., W. Schultze, Z. Phytother. 10(6):191–a202 (1989).

Literature references identified by Ü can be found in the general listing of books and monographs at the back of this book.

Annatto

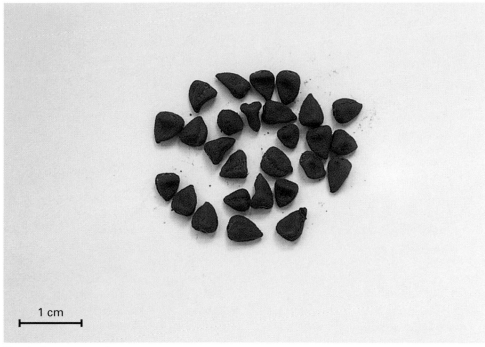

Fig. 1: Annatto seeds

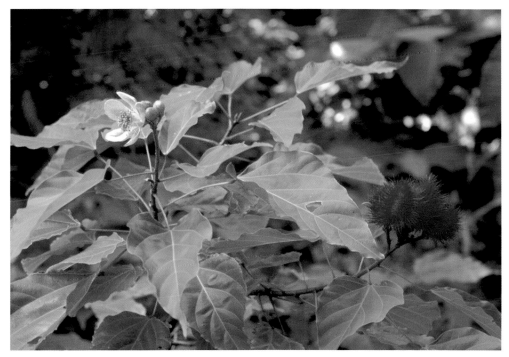

Fig. 2: Annatto (*Bixa orellana* L.)

Plant source: *Bixa orellana* L.

Synonyms: *Orellana americana* KUNTZE, *Bixa urucurana* WILLD.

Family: Annatto plants (Bixaceae).

Common names: Engl.: an(n)atto-tree, atsuete, achiote tree, lipstick tree; Fr.: rocouyier; Ger.: Annatto, Orlean(a)-strauch, Orlean(a)baum, Orangenraute, Rukubaum, Ach(i)ote, Onoto, Pumacuja, Urucu, Rocouyer.

Description: Shrub or up to 10 m high tree with spirally arranged foliage. The single leaves are 15 to 32 cm long, with an entire margin, palmately veined, acuminate, rarely with a narrowed base. The flowers are arranged in panicles, similar to wild roses, with 5 light pink petals and 5 sepals which fall off upon anthesis; numerous stamina situated on a convex disk, superior ovary, 2 carpels. The fruit is a monolocular, bivalved dehiscent, brownish-red capsule, walnut-sized, with soft, pliable prickles, containing 36 to 48 very hard seeds with a pith-like, soft and pulpy sarkotesta (also considered an arillus or endocarp by a few authors) that solidifies upon storage and has a vanilla-like odor [3, Ü42, Ü92].

Native origin: Caribbean Islands and tropical South America. Through cultivation, it has been naturalized in the tropics worldwide.

Main cultivation areas: Tropical America and worldwide in the tropics, also cultivated as a supportive plant in vanilla plantations, and as an ornamental- and shade tree, or as a protective hedge.

Main exporting countries: South- and Central America, East Africa, India, Peru, Panama, Ecuador, and Jamaica.

Cultivation: Cultivation of this evergreen shrub or tree is only possible in tropical zones. Propagation is carried out by seed.

Culinary herb

Commercial forms: Annatto seed (whole or crushed), annatto extract (annatto, oil- or aqueous extracts of the seeds; oil-extracted annatto is liquid, and the aqueous extract is a paste, formed into cakes or rolls), sodium or potassium salts of norbixin.

Production: The fruits are harvested when ripe. The seeds are removed and either dried (annatto seed) or they are processed into an orange-red product (annatto extract) by stirring the seeds in hot water, filtering and drying, after which the settled precipitate or the total extract are dried [Ü42]. Extraction of the coloring matter can also be carried out with fatty oil or with supercritical CO_2 [5].

Forms used: Whole or powdered annatto seeds, annatto extract.

Storage: Store the seeds in well-sealed porcelain-, glass- or suitable metal containers, protected from light and moisture in as cool an environment as possible. Under these conditions, annatto seeds or annatto extract can be stored for a very long time.

Description. Whole seed (Fig. 1): The reddish-brown, irregularly triangular rounded annatto seeds are hard, acuminate on one side, 4 to 6 mm long and 3 mm wide, with a longitudinal groove. They produce a brick-red streak on white paper [Ü60]. Annatto is a soft, malleable, orange-red mass with a salty-bitter taste and sometimes with disagreeable odor; it turns reddish-brown and odorless when drying out and takes on a hard and brittle consistency [Ü60].

Powdered seed: Microscopic examination reveals, in particular, the roundish cells of the epidermis, filled with pigment, and a palisade cell layer underneath [Ü60].

Odor: Vanilla-like when fresh, later odorless, **Taste:** Astringent, pepper-like.

History: The annatto shrub was already used in tropical America in pre-Columbian times and probably also cultivated [Ü61].

Constituents and Analysis

Constituents

- Diapocarotenoids, apocarotenoids, carotenoids: 3.5 to 6% (up to 13%), the main component is bixin (about 80%), α-bixin, methyl-9′Z-6,6′-diapocarotene-6,6′-dioate, annatto pigment, monomethylester of α-norbixin, red, fat-soluble, alkali salts are water soluble, easily transforms in the stable all-trans form β-bixin (= isobixin); furthermore, α- and β-norbixin, methyl bixin (dimethylester of norbixin), the apocarotenoid methylapolycopenoate as well as other minor diapocarotenoids, apocarotenoids and carotenoids [8, 11, 12, 13].

- **Essential oil:** 0.25 to 0.85%, the main component is ishwaran [8, 9].
- Fatty oil [8].
- Starch [8].

Tests for Identity with TLC [14] or HPLC [10, 17].

Quantitative assay of bixin, see Lit. [9, 7, 4, 1, 10, 17].

Actions and Uses

Actions: In in-vitro experiments, bixin (100 µg/ml) has shown cytostatic activity [18].

Toxicology: Based on existing data, there is no acute or chronic toxicity with the regular use of annatto as a food colorant. In animal experiments (rats, pigs), water- and fat-soluble annatto extracts showed no toxic effects even in long-term administration (in rats over 3 generations) and dosage levels well above those used in food colorants [6].
Applications of oily extracts of the drug, or trans-bixin, to anesthetized dogs in dosages corresponding to the ethnomedical

Bixin   R = CH₃
Norbixin   R = H

Methyl-9′Z-apo-6′-lycopenoate

Ishwaran

marginal ridges and attached to a bifurcate carpophore. The flowering period is from March to April [Ü37, Ü45, Ü60, Ü76]. *Ferula foetida* has a similar habitus but is only 1 m tall, and the petals are white [Ü37].

Native origin: *F. assa-foetida* is native to eastern Iran, and *F. foetida* is also native to western Afghanistan, Iraq, Turkmenistan, Pakistan, and India (Indus region).

Main cultivation areas: The oleo-gum-resin is only obtained from plants in the wild (see below).

Main exporting countries: Iran, Afghanistan, and to a lesser extent, India, Iraq, and Pakistan.

Cultivation: None.

Culinary Herb

Commercial forms: Asafetida: in grains (in agglutinated tears, in lacrimis, in granis), in clumps (in masses of tears, in massis); commercial varieties Chadda (best quality), Hing (or Ching) and Hingra (or Chingra, both are good quality grades), Kambulidans and Schabandi (inferior quality); different origins: e.g. Afghanistan: Pathani, Iran: Irani Hing, Bandhani Hing (cut with Gummi arabicum, rice flour, etc.); Pakistan: Herra Hing. In the retail spice trade, especially in Indian specialty shops, asafetida powder is frequently offered, which is prevented from agglutinating through the admixing of rice meal, starch or powdered fenugreek seed [Ü37, Ü92].

Production: In April, the upper part of the root is laid bare. After about 30 to 40 days, an incision is made at the top of the root-stock, sometimes the entire aerial stem is also cut off, and after a few days, the thick, gummy exudate oozes out. This procedure is repeated in intervals of 2 to 3 days by making new incisions or by cutting off a thin slice of the root crown. With these methods, one plant produces a total of about 1 kg of gum resin in a 2 to 3 month period [18, Ü60, Ü76, Ü81].

Forms used: Powdered asafetida.

Storage: In well-sealed metal- or glass containers, protected from light and moisture. The whole drug can be stored for several years while the asafetida powder has only a short shelf life due to the rapid loss of aroma.

Description. Whole gum-resin (Fig. 1): Loose pea to hazelnut-sized grains, more or less stuck together, or larger clumps; dough-like and sticky when fresh, with a pale gray color, hardening upon storage and turning from light- to dark brown, with lighter-colored grains embedded. The fracture is porcelain-like, first white, brown on the edges, then turning red and later brown [Ü37, DAB 6].

Odor: Alliaceous and penetrating, **Taste:** Bitter and pungent.

History: Asafetida was already used in ancient times in India as a medicinal and spice plant (in old Sanskrit writings mentioned as "hingu"). It is claimed that asafetida was brought to Greece by Alexander the Great (336–323 BCE). In the Roman Empire, asafetida was in high demand but also very expensive. In the cookbook "De re coquinaria" which is attributed to the gourmet Marcus Gavius Apicius [1]), asafetida was recommended. In the 19th century, this spice was often used in southwestern Germany, for example for roasted lamb dishes, liver- or blood sausages [Ü81].

---

[1]) The most extensive Roman cookbook, "De re coquinaria", appeared in 10 volumes in the 3rd or 4th century and is attributed to the gourmet Marcus Gavius Apicius who lived during the reign of emperor Tiberius (42 BCE to 14 CE). He apparently committed suicide after spending all his fortunes because he feared that he could not continue his lavish lifestyle.

Constituents and Analysis

Constituents

- Essential oil: 5 to 25%, the odoriferous and aromatic constituents are mainly alkyldi-, alkyltri- and alkyltetrasulfides (comprising 30 to 60%, in English language literature, these compounds are also called alkylpolysulfans). The proportion of essential oil components varies greatly depending on the origin. The essential oil from Iranian material consisted of about 23% 2-butyl-*trans*-prop-1-enyl-disulfide, about 11% 2-butyl-*cis*-prop-1-enyl-disulfide, about 3% 1-(methylthio)propyl-*trans*-prop-1-enyldisulfide, about 3% 1-(methylthio)propyl-*cis*-1-prop-1-enyldisulfide and about 30% monoterpenes, particularly (*Z*)- and (*E*)-β-ocimene, α- and β-pinene as well as α- and β-phellandrene. The essential oil from Pakistani material contained 11% 2-butyl-*trans*-prop-1-enyl-disulfide, about 38% 1-(methylthio)propyl-*trans*-prop-1-enyldisulfide, about 18% 1-(methylthio)propyl-*cis*-prop-1-enyldisulfide and only 0.5% monoterpene hydrocarbons [13, 18, 20, 21, 23, Ü92].
- Resin: A mixture collectively referred to as asarin, 40 to 65%, consisting mostly of umbelliferone ethers with acyclic sesquiterpenes, for example with umbelliprenin and its hydroxyderivatives or with monocyclic- or bicyclic sesquiterpenes, respectively (farnesiferols A, B and C, possibly artifacts, asacoumarins A and B, assaroetidine, ferocolicin, among others) as well as ferulic esters of asaresitannol [3, 4, 7, 8, 11, 12, 13, 17, 21].
- Mucilage: 20 to 30% [8].

Tests for Identity: Organoleptic and TLC [Ü101], GC or GC/MS [18, 23] analyses. Other tests for identity include dabbing the fresh fracture with concentrated sulfuric acid (the surface of the fracture turns red or reddish-brown) or concentrated nitric acid (the fracture turns green). The whitish suspension, which is obtained when grinding asafetida in water, turns greenish-yellow upon addition of alkali [Ü60].

2-Butyl-*trans*-prop-1-enyl-disulfide   2-Butyl-*cis*-prop-1-enyl-disulfide   1-(Methylthio)propyl-*trans*-prop-1-enyldisulfide

Quantitative assay: Determination of the ethanol-soluble fraction, usually 55 to 75% [Ü60]. The essential oil can be determined oxidimetrically [1].

Adulterations, Misidentifications and Impurities have been observed, most often with other apiaceous gum resins, e.g. galbanum and ammoniacum. Such adulterants can now be detected by TLC. Due to frequent admixtures with sand and other minerals as a result of the harvesting method, or intentional adulteration with e.g. gypsum, testing for ash residue is recommended (max. 15%, according to DAB 6).

Actions and Uses

Actions: On the basis of its bitter and acrid taste, and also due to the stimulating effect of its essential oil on the gastric mucosa, asafetida has appetite stimulating and digestion promoting action. Feeding rats with a diet with asafetida (0.25% in the feed) over an eight-week period, led to an increase in the activity of their pancreas lipase, pancreas amylase, and of chymotrypsin. Single doses had no effect [19]. Asafetida has carminative and expectorant activity [5, Ü60]. The essential oil from the gum resin has demonstrated antimicrobial activity [10]. An aqueous extract of the gum resin has shown good anthelminthic action in mice [14]. The concomitant topical application to the skin of mice of an aqueous extract of asafetida gum resin together with a carcinogen (7,12-dimethylbenzanthracene) and a co-carcinogen (Croton oil), showed, compared with a control group, which was treated with the carcinogen and the co-carcinogen alone, a

reduction of tumor induction of about 80%. With oral administration of the extract, the survival time of tumor-bearing mice was lengthened by over 50% [25].

Toxicology: Dosages of 3 g are considered non-toxic [6]; even dosages of 15 g are reported to be free of any side effects [9]. After the intake of very high dosages, gastrointestinal complaints such as belching, stomach pain, diarrhea and bloating as well as headaches and dizziness occur [8, Ü58]. In one case, after the intake of an asafetida-glycerine preparation by an infant, methemoglobinanemia with concurrent cyanosis, respiratory stimulation and lethargy were observed [15]. In the AMES-test, a very weak mutagenic effect was observed with an ethanolic extract [24]. An aqueous extract was not mutagenic in a test on the fruit fly (*Drosophila melanogaster*) [2]. Administration of asafetida to male mice above a dosage of 50 mg/kg/body weight over 32 days caused chromosomal changes in the spermatozoa, and sterility [26].

Culinary use: Asafetida is used as a spice, especially in anterior, central, and southern Asia. The main consumer of asafetida is India, where it is used, among other uses, in the vegetarian cooking of members of the Brahmin- and Jain castes, who also, on religious grounds, do not eat *Allium* species (e.g. garlic and onion). Asafetida is also, however, frequently used in western- and southern India as spice for legumes, vegetables, pickles and sauces as well as for meats, especially mutton. It is also used in Iranian, Afghani and Kurdish cooking as a spice for roasted meat dishes as well as for fresh or salted fish [Ü20, Ü81].

Used for seasoning are the typical commercial powder, containing admixed filling material, a self-prepared powder or a suspension prepared by dissolving pieces or grains of the gum resin in warm water. To make the powder, small pieces of the gum resin are pulverized together with starch flour using a mortar and pestle. By chilling first (in the freezer compartment), pulverizing the gum resin will be made easier. Use of the alcoholic extract is also typical, although very sparingly dosed.

In Europe, asafetida is used, although rarely, as a spice for fish, vegetables, legumes, chutneys, pickles and roasted meat sauces [16, Ü13, Ü20, Ü55, Ü68, Ü73, Ü92].

In Iran, the pulp from the stalks and leaves is eaten as a vegetable.

As a component of spice mixes and preparations: → Chat masala, → Curry powder, → Sambhar powder.

Other uses: In the perfume industry, it is used as a fixative and aroma component, and as a repellant, e.g. for cats, dogs, and mice, but also for termites and threadworms [16].

Similar tasting spices: → Garlic, → Ramsons.

Medicinal herb

Herbal drug: Asafetida, Gummiresina asa foetida [DAB 6, ChinP IX, BHP 83] is no longer listed in newer European pharmacopoeias.

Indications: The British Herbal Pharmacopoeia 1983 (BHP 83, removed in BHP 90) recommended the use of asafetida for colic-like flatulence, irritable colon, bronchitis, pertussis, nervous conditions and hysteria (dosage: 0.3 to 1.0 g powdered gum resin, t.i.d., or 2 to 4 ml tincture daily). Asafetida is also used as an anthelminthic [22]. In folk medicine, it was formerly used for asthma, amenorrhea, menopausal syndrome, cramps and epilepsy, among other uses [Ü37].

Literature

[1] Abraham K.O. et al., Flavor Ind. 4:301–302 (1973).

[2] Abraham S.K., P.C. Kesavan, Mutat. Res. 136:85–88 (1985).

[3] Appendino G. et al. Phytochemistry 35(1): 183–186 (1994).

[4] Banerji A. et al., Tetrahedron Letters 29(13):1557 (1988).

[5] Bhat et al., Indian J. Pharm. 17:9 (1955).

[6] Bordia A. et al., Indian Med. Res. 63:707–711 (1975).

[7] Caglioti L. et al., Helv. Chim. Acta 41:2278–2292 (1958).

[8] De Smet P.A.G.M. et al. (eds.), in: Adverse Effects of Herbal Drugs, Springer Verlag Berlin, Heidelberg, New York 1992, Bd. 1, p. 91–95 (1992).

[9] Duke I.A., in: CRC-Handbook of Medicinal Herbs, 3. Print, CRC-Press, Boca Raton 1986, p. 194.

[10] Fariq S.R. et al., Pak. J. Sci. Ind. Res. 38(9–10):358–361 (1995, ref. CA 126: 303577e.

[11] Fujita M. et al., J. Pharm. Soc. Japan 78:395 (1958).

[12] Hofer O. et al., Monatsh. Chem. 115: 1207–1218 (1984).

[13] Kajimoto T. et al., Phytochemistry 28: 1761–1763 (1989).

[14] Kavianpour M. et al., Planta Med. 62, Abstracts of the 44th Ann. Congress of GA, 52 (1996).

[15] Kelly K.J. et al., Pediatrics 73:717–719 (1984).

[16] Leung A.Y, in: Encyclopedia of common natural ingredients used in food, drugs and cosmetics, John Wiley & Sons, Cichester, Brisbane, Toronto 1980, p. 37.

[17] Nassar M.I. et al., Pharmazie 50(11):766–767 (1995).

[18] Noleau I. et al., J. Essent. Oil Res. 3:241–256 (1991).

[19] Platel K., K. Srinivasan, Nahrung 44(1): 42–46 (2000).

[20] Rajanikanth B. et al., Phytochemistry 23: 899–900 (1984).

[21] Samini M.N., W. Unger, Planta Med. 36(2):128–133 (1979).

[22] Schulze G., Forum Aromather. Aromapflege 15/99:26–28 (1999).

[23] Sefidkon E. et al., J. Essent. Oil Res. 10:687–689 (1998).

[24] Shashikanth K.N., A. Hosono, Agric. Biol. Chem. 50:2947–2948 (1986).

[25] Unnikrishnan M.C., R. Kuttan, Cancer Lett. 51:85–89 (1990).

[26] Walia K., Cytologia 38:719–724 (1973).

Literature references identified by Ü can be found in the general listing of books and monographs at the back of this book.

Basil

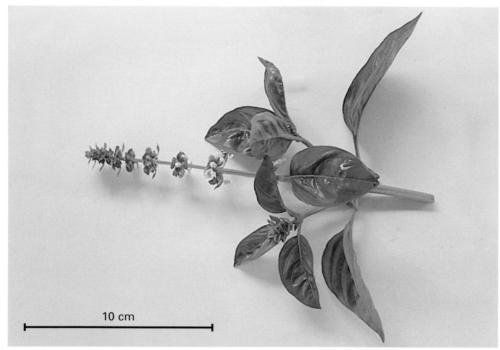

Fig. 1: Basil flowering tops

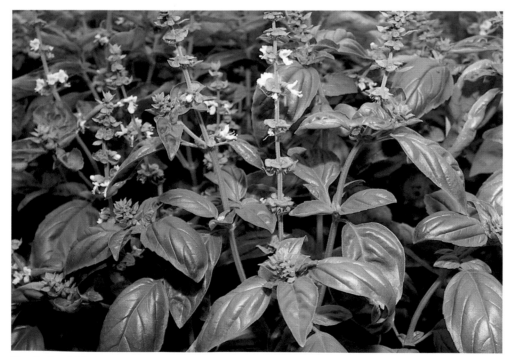

Fig. 2: Basil (*Ocimum basilicum* L.)

Plant source: *Ocimum basilicum* L.

Taxonomic classification: The species is morphologically and chemically quite heterogenic, and is subdivided into many, not clearly differentiated varieties (*O. b.* var. *basilicum*, var. *difforme* BENTH., var. *glabratum* BENTH., var. *majus* BENTH., var. *minimum* (L.) ALEF., var. *purpurescens* BENTH., var. *thyrsiflorum* BENTH.). Approximately 60 varieties are in cultivation.

Family: Plants of the mint family (Lamiaceae, synonym Labiatae).

Common names: Engl.: basil, sweet basil; Fr.: basilic, grand basilic; Ger.: Basilikum, Basilienkraut, Deutscher Pfeffer, Königskraut, Hirnkraut, Herrenkraut, Löffelbasilikum, Schmöckkraut, Suppenbasil, Braunsilge, Bäsigla.

Description: An annual herb with a single or branched, quadrangular stem, glabrous or sparsely hairy, up to 60 cm high (some cultivars only up to 25 cm). The leaves are alternate arranged, petiolated, ovoid or ovoid-oblong, obtuse or acuminate, up to 7 cm long and up to 3 cm wide, entire-margined or more or less dentate, often with hairy margin, lamina glabrous, vaulted and wavy, blistered or curly contracted, winered in some varieties. The flowers are situated in the upper part of the stem and the branches, arranged in axial false whorls; bilabiate corolla with an upwards recurved, 4-lobed upper lip, lower lip undivided, white to reddish, calyx clearly bilabiate, upper lip undivided, spoon-shaped, lower lip 4-toothed, 4 stamina, superior ovary, biphyllous, quadrilocular. The fruit disintegrates into 4 nutlets, with one seed each. The flowering period is from June to July [Ü60].

Native origin: Not known with certainty, probably native to northwestern India.

Main cultivation areas: The Netherlands, Hungary, southern France, Belgium, Spain, Italy, the Czech Republic, Germany, India, Turkey, Morocco, the USA (California), and the Russian Federation.

Main exporting countries: Egypt, France, Italy, the Balkan countries, Hungary, the Netherlands, and Morocco.

Cultivation: Basil prefers humus rich, sandy loam soil in warm, sunny locations. The plants are started in the greenhouse (light requirements for germination) around mid-March. It is possible to transplant the plantlets in the field by the end of May. In Europe, direct sowing can take place by the beginning of June, although at this latitude, it is not advisable, because then there will only be a very short vegetation period. The plant is very sensitive to frost (it dies already at 0 °C). Basil should not be cultivated for several years in the same location. During dry spells, it must be irrigated sufficiently, but not excessively. The plant attracts snails. The author has found that the plant does not thrive during cold and damp summers. Therefore, for personal use, it is recommended to grow the plants in pots in the windowsill. Varieties cultivated in Europe include, among others, the green-leaved varieties 'Genoveser', 'Großer Grünes' (both suitable for growing in pots), 'Lemon' (so-called lemon basil, with a citrus-like aroma), 'Bavires', 'Bubikopf', 'Feinblättriges', 'Kleinblättriges', 'Mammouth', 'Sperlings Balkonstar' and 'Salatblättriges', as well as the red-leaved varieties 'Dark Opal', 'Opal', 'Purple Ruffles', 'Rothaut' and 'Rubin'. Varieties cultivated in southeastern Asia include, among others, 'Horapha' (Thai basil), 'Cinnamon' (cinnamon basil) and 'Anise' (anise basil), and in northern Africa, the variety 'African Blue' is cultivated [Ü14, Ü21].

Culinary herb

Commercial forms: Basil leaf: the dried, rubbed herb; in the culinary herb trade as fresh, bundled herb or in herb pots; basil essential oil, basil oleoresin.

Production: In commercial cultivation, the first cutting takes place at the start of the flowering period using a sickle bar type mower with adjustable cutting height. Weather permitting, a second cutting is possible in September. Post-harvest, the crop is rapidly dried at 30 °C. Coarse-stemmed herb material is rubbed [Ü21]. To fulfill immediate demands, the leaves can be harvested throughout the entire vegetation period, as soon as the plant has become strong enough. A few leaves should always be left on the plant in order to assure regrowth.

Forms used: Fresh leaves, fresh or dried herb, basil essential oil, basil oleoresin.

Storage: The fresh leaves or the fresh herb can be stored in plastic bags in the refrigerator for a few days or stored as a purée with water in the deep freezer. It is possible to layer the fresh leaves, lightly salted, into glasses with a screw cap and to fill them up with olive oil. Preservation using vinegar is also practiced. The dried leaves are stored in a cool place in airtight porcelain-, glass or metal containers, protected from light and moisture; the loss of essential oil is high (about 60% within 6 months).

Description. Whole herb (Fig. 1): See description of the whole plant.

Powdered leaf: Characteristic are, besides the glandular scales typical for Lamiaceae, the sparsely occurring uniseriate covering trichomes, composed of 2 or 3, occasionally up to 6 cells, and the relatively numerous capitate glands with unicellular stalks and mono- or bicellular heads [Ü94].

Odor: Depending on the variable essential oil composition, e.g. lemon-, anise-, cinnamon- or clove-like, **Taste:** Spicy, sometimes peppery and cooling.

History: Basil was already cultivated in Southeast Asia and Egypt 3000 years ago. It is claimed that the Greeks already brought this herb to the West during the conquests of Alexander the Great (356–323 BCE). Cultivation in Central Europe has been documented since the 12th century [6].

Constituents and Analysis

DIN and ISO-Standards: ISO-Standard 11 163 (Dried basil).

Constituents

- Essential oil: In the fresh leaves 0.02 to 0.5%, in the dried herb 0.2 to 2.7%; the main components are, depending on the chemotype, linalool (up to 85%), estragole (up to 91%), citral (up to 90%), (E)-methyl-cinnamate (up to 82%), eugenol (up to 80%) or methyl eugenol (eugenol-methylether, up to 44%), in mixed chemotypes mostly linalool + geraniol, linalool + estragole, linalool + eugenol, linalool + (E)-methyl cinnamate, linalool + eugenol + (Z,Z)-α-farnesene + τ-cadinol, estragole + methyleugenol, estragole + linalool, (E)-methylcinnamate + linalool, (E)-methylcinnamate + eugenol, linalool + estragole + eugenol, estragole + citronellal, including, among others, rarer components such as geranyl acetate (up to 44%), geraniol (up to 27%), methylisoeugenol (up to 26%), 1,8-cineole (up to 20%), α-bulnesene (up to 20%), δ-cadinol (up to 20%), bergamottene (up to 13%), α-muurolol (up to 11%), β-caryophyllene (up to 10%), β-elemene (up to 6%), γ-cadinene (up to 5%) and α-terpineol (up to 5%) [4, 11, 15, 18, 20, 21, 26, 31, 35, 36, 40, 42, Ü43, Ü83; for a review of main components in various chemotypes, see Lit. 25].
- Hydroxycinnamic acid derivatives (labiate tannins): 2 to 3.5%, mostly rosmarinic acid (about 2%) [20].
- Flavonoids: 0.5 to 0.7%, quercetin- and kaempferol glycosides, xanthomicrol (5,4′-dihydroxy-6,7,8-trimethoxyflavone), on the leaf surface salvigenin and nevadensin, among others [9, 12, 20].

- Triterpenes, sterols: β-Sitosterin and oleanolic acid, among others [Ü43].
- Fatty oil: The seeds are high in linolenic acid [32].

Tests for Identity: Sensoric, macroscopic and microscopic examinations as well as TLC analyses of extracts [Ü102], the essential oil [2] or GC analysis of the essential oil [27, 38]. The German standard license describes a TLC assay for the detection of linalool and eugenol [Ü12].

Quantitative assay: Following the Ph Eur procedure for the volumetric quantification of essential oils in vegetable drugs, using steam distillation with xylol in the graduated tube. The German standard license requires a lower essential oil limit of 0.4% [Ü12]. The rosmarinic acid content can be determined with HPLC [10] or after silylation with GC [29].

Adulterations, Misidentifications and Impurities: Not known.

Actions and Uses

Actions: On the basis of its aromatic and slightly pungent taste, it has appetite stimulating and digestion promoting activity.
The powdered herb and the methanolic or aqueous extracts inhibited the occurrence of acetylsalicylic acid-induced gastric ulcers in rats [1]. Basil oil showed good spasmolytic action in isolated guinea pig intestinal smooth muscles [28]. It has also shown anthelmintic, insecticidal and antimicrobial activity [3, 14, 19, 30, 39]. The antiviral action of aqueous basil extracts, as observed in vitro [41], was dependent on their rosmarinic acid content, and occurred only with topical application.
The fatty oil of the seeds has shown good antiphlogistic and antiulcerogenic properties [32, 33, 34].

Toxicology: Based on existing data, there is no acute or chronic toxicity with the regular use of this herb as a spice. The sensitization potential is not known.

Culinary use: Basil is popular especially in French, Italian, Greek, Transcaucasian, and Thai cooking, however its popularity in Central Europe has been growing for a few years.
Basil should be used sparingly, and added to the meal only shortly before completion. When cooked, it loses its aroma and becomes bitter.
Freshly picked leaves, plucked to pieces, or dried, powdered herb serve as a spice for salads (especially tomato salads in every known combination, e.g. with mozzarella cheese, but also of green salad), sauces (e.g. pesto sauce, sauce vinaigrette), soups (e.g. soupe au pistou, turtle soup, oxtail soup), mayonnaise, eggplant, potatoes, rice, legumes, spinach, mushrooms, egg dishes, noodle dishes, meat dishes (e.g. mutton and pork dishes, meat loaf), fish dishes (e.g. Hamburg eel soup), pizzas, cottage cheese, yogurt, soft cheese, vinegar, butter, liverwurst, pumpkin, cucumbers and sauerkraut. The freshly picked leaves, plucked to pieces, can be mixed with butter and spread on steaks before serving [40, Ü1, Ü46, Ü51, Ü56, Ü65, Ü70, Ü79, Ü86, Ü107].
The dried herb is used industrially, especially as a spice for canned fish.
Basil essential oil serves as an aromatic component of liqueurs, e.g. Chartreuse [6, Ü17, Ü30, Ü55, Ü74, Ü92], and also of foods (see Chapter 13.2).

Combines well with: Coriander, garlic, onion, oregano, paprika, parsley, pepper, rosemary, saffron, sage, savory, tarragon, and thyme [Ü55].

As a component of spice mixes and preparations: → Curry, → Egg spice, → Fines Herbes, → Fish spice, → Herb oil, → Herb seasoning salt, → Herb vinegar, → Herbes de Provence, → Meat spice, → Poultry spice, → Roast spice, → Soup spice, → Vegetable spice.

Other uses: In the perfume industry.

Medicinal herb

Herbal drugs: Basilici herba, Basil herb [DAC], Basilici aetheroleum, Basil oil.

Indications: Basil herb is used for supportive treatment of bloating and flatulence, as well as to stimulate appetite, facilitate digestion, and as a diuretic. Because the essential oil of some chemotypes may contain high levels of estragole, it should not be used in therapeutic doses during pregnancy, while nursing, in infants and toddlers as well as for long-term durations. On this basis and because its efficacy has not been conclusively substantiated, the German Commission E did not approve its therapeutic use. There is no safety concern with regard to its use as an aroma or flavor enhancer at up to 5% of a preparation [16]. Basil herb is taken in the form of unsweetened tea infusions (2 to 4 g per cup of water, 2 to 3 times daily, no longer than 8 days) [Ü106]. In folk medicine, it is also used as a lactagogue, aphrodisiac, for common cold conditions, headaches and inflammations of the urogenital tract.
Basil oil, which in combination with other essential oils, is used predominantly for rheumatic complaints, arthralgia and muscular tenseness. Likewise, the Commission E gave basil oil a negative evaluation for the same reasons as stated above for basil herb [17].

Other Ocimum-species used as culinary herbs

Hoary basil (American basil) *Ocimum americanum* L., is grown in tropical zones of Asia and Africa. The main components of its essential oil, depending on the chemotype, are estragole 1,8-cineole, citral, linalool + terpinenol-4 or linalool + terpinenol-4 + camphor + 1,8-cineole [7, 13, 23, 25].

Camphor basil (Hoary basil), *Ocimum canum* SIMS (also classified as synonymous to *O. americanum* L.), is grown in tropical zones of Asia and Africa. It contains 0.1 to 0.6% essential oil, of which the main components, depending on the chemotype, are linalool, camphor, *(E)*-methylcinnamate, terpinenol-4 or citral [13, 22, 40, Ü43].

African basil (East Indian basil, fever plant), *Ocimum gratissimum* L., is grown in Africa, southern France, southeastern Asia, and Brazil. It contains 0.4 to 1.2% essential oil, of which the main components, depending on the chemotype, are eugenol, ethylcinnamate, thymol + *p*-cymene or citral + geraniol [7, 13, 22, 37, 40, Ü43].

Camphor basil (Kapoor-tulsi), *Ocimum kilimandscharicum* BAKER ex GÜRKE, is grown in India, Nepal, and Turkey. The main components of its essential oil, depending on the chemotype, are eugenol, camphor or linalool + camphor + 1,8-cineole [13, 25, Ü61].

Albahaca (Alfavaca), *Ocimum micranthum* WILLD., is grown in Ecuador. The main components of its essential oil are elemene, 1,8-cineole, β-caryophyllene and β-selinene [5].

Holy basil (Sacred basil, Tulsi), *Ocimum tenuiflorum* L, (Syn.: *O. sanctum* L.), is grown in southern Asia, northern South America, the Dutch Caribbean Islands, and Africa. The main components of its essential oil, depending on the chemotype, are citral, eugenol + methyleugenol, estragole + linalool + 1,8-cineole or chavibetol + eugenol [13, Ü43].

African basil, *Ocimum suave* WILLD., is grown in a few African countries and in Sri Lanka. The main components of its essential oil are eugenol (about 72%), and *cis*-β-ocimene (about 14%), followed by, among others, β-cubebene, β-bisabolene and β-caryophyllene [23].

Literature

[1] Akhtar M.S., M. Munir, J. Ethnopharmacol. 27(1/2):163–176 (1989).
[2] Anonym, Caelo Sortiments- und Preisliste 97–99, Caesar & Loretz GmbH, Hilden 1997, p. 260 (1997).

Grilled Basil-Tomatoes with Cheese
The tops of 8 medium-sized tomatoes are removed to form lids, and the tomatoes are then hollowed out. The tomato pulp and the finely chopped "lids" are mixed with 2 tablespoons of breadcrumbs, 2 finely grated garlic cloves, a bundle of basil (finely plucked), some pepper and salt, and then, the mixture is filled into the hollow tomatoes. Place the tomatoes next to each other in a buttered casserole and distribute the remaining filling mixture around them. 150 g grated Swiss cheese (Emmentaler), 2 eggs and $^1/_4$ l of milk and a pinch of pepper are mixed and spread over the tomatoes. Bake at 180 °C in a preheated oven until golden brown (about 25 min). The dish can be served with green salad and farmer's bread [Ü86].

[3] Basilico M.Z., J.C. Basilico, Lett. Appl. Microbiol. 29(4):238–241 (1999).
[4] Chalchat J.C. et al., J. Essent. Oil Res. 11:375–380 (1999).
[5] Charles D.J. et al., J. Agric. Food Chem. 38:120–122 (1990).
[6] Czygan F.Ch., Z. Phytother. 18(1):58–66 (1997).
[7] Demissew S., J. Essent. Oil Res. 5:465–479 (1993).
[8] Drinkwater N.R. et al., J. Nat. Cancer Inst. 57:1323–1331 (1976).
[9] Fatope M.O., Y. Takeda, Planta Med. 1988:190 (1988).
[10] Gracza L., P. Ruff, Arch. Pharmaz. 317:339–345 (1984).
[11] Grayer R.J. et al., Phytochemistry 43:1033–1039 (1996).
[12] Grayer R.J. et al., Phytochemistry 43:1041–1047 (1996).
[13] Gupta S.C., J. Essent. Oil Res. 8(3):275–279 (1996).
[14] Jain M.L., S.R. Jain, Planta Med. 22(1):66–70 (1972).
[15] Junghanns W., K. Hammer, Herba Germanica 2(2):92–94 (1994).
[16] Kommission E, BAnz. 54 vom 18.03.92.
[17] Kommission E, BAnz. 54 vom 18.03.92.
[18] Kumar S. et al., J. Med. Aromat. Plant Sci. 21:46 (1999).
[19] Lachowicz K.J. et al., Lett. Appl. Microbiol. 26(3):209–214 (1998).
[20] Lemberkovics É., Planta Med. 59(7):A700 (1993).
[21] Marotti M. et al., J. Agric. Food Chem. 44:3926–3929 (1996).
[22] Martins P.A. et al., Planta Med. 65(2):187–189 (1999).
[23] Mikus B. et al., Drogenreport 10(18):68–73 (1997).
[24] Miller E.C. et al., Cancer Res. 43:1124–1134 (1983).
[25] Pasquier B., J.C. Chalchat, RIV Ital. EPPOS (Spec. Num., 15th Journees Internationales Huiles Essentielles, 1996): p. 544–550 (1997).
[26] Pérez-Alonso M.J. et al., J. Essent. Oil Res. 7(1):73–75 (1995).
[27] Qaisar M. et al., J. Chem. Soc. Pak. 18(4):331–335 (1996).
[28] Reiter M., W. Brandt, Arzneim. Forsch. 35:408–414 (1985).
[29] Reschke A., Z. Lebensm. Unters. Forsch. 176:116–119 (1983).
[30] Sattar A.A. et al., Pharmazie 50(1):62–65 (1995).
[31] Sheen L.Y. et al., J. Agric. Food Chem. 39:939–943 (1991).
[32] Singh S., Indian J. Exp. Biol. 36(10):1028–1031 (1998).
[33] Singh S., Indian J. Exp. Biol. 37(3):248–252 (1999).
[34] Singh S., Indian J. Exp. Biol. 37(3):253–257 (1999).
[35] Tateo F., J. Essent. Oil Res. 1:137–138 (1989).
[36] Thoppil J.E., Acta Pharm. (Zagreb): 46(3):195–199 (1996).
[37] Vahirua-Lechat I. et al., Riv. Ital. EPPOS 1997 (Spec. Num., 15th Journees Internat Huiles Essentielles, 1996): p. 704–711 (1997).
[38] Vernin G., I. Metzger, Perfumer and Flavorist 9:71–86 (1984).
[39] Wan J. et al., J. Appl. Microbiol. 84(2):152–158 (1998).
[40] Yagi E. et al., J. Essent. Oil Res. 13:13–17 (2001).
[41] Yamasaki K. et al., Biol. Pharm. Bull. 21(8):829–833 (1998).
[42] De Vasconcelos Silva M.G. et al., J. Essent. Oil Res. 10(5):558–560 (1998).

Literature references identified by Ü can be found in the general listing of books and monographs at the back of this book.

Bay

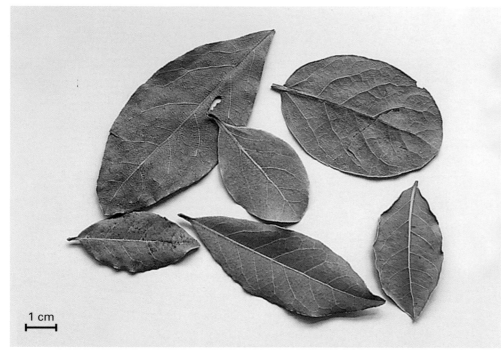

Fig. 1: Bay leaf, dried

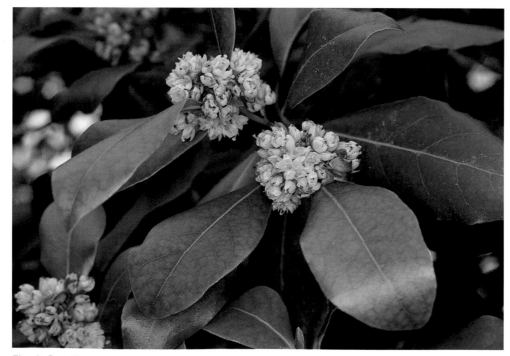

Fig. 2: Bay (*Laurus nobilis* L.)

Plant source: *Laurus nobilis* L.

Taxonomic classification: This species can be subdivided into several varieties especially on the basis of the different shapes of the leaves and sizes of the fruits. For the production of bay leaves for the spice trade, however, there is no distinction made between these varieties.

Family: Laurel (Lauraceae).

Common names: Engl.: bay, bay laurel, Grecian laurel, sweet bay, true bay; Fr.: laurier noble, laurier commun, laurier sauce, laurier d'Apollon, laurier franc, laurier à jambon; Ger: Lorbeer, Lorbeerbaum, Gewürzlorbeer.

Description: Up to 15 m tall tree with black bark, mostly kept as a shrub in cultivation to facilitate harvest, evergreen, dioecious. The leaves alternate, lanceolate, about 10 cm long, 3 to 5 cm wide, pointed at both ends, short-petiolate, leathery, often slightly sinuous, with gristly, turned down margin, dark green and shiny upper surface. The flowers are arranged in axillary, tufted false umbels or short panicles, with 4-lobed perigone, fused at the base; male flowers whitish-green mostly with 8 to 12 stamina, bearing in their middle a sessile gland each, the anthers open with two upwards lifting lids; female flowers with 4 staminodes, ovary with short stalk and triangular, blunt stigma. The fruit is a deep black berry, up to 2 cm long. The blooming period is March until May [Ü42].

Native origin: Probably native to Asia Minor, today it occurs throughout the Mediterranean region, in the Republics of the former Yugoslavia and in India.

Main cultivation areas: Italy, Greece, Republics of the former Yugoslavia,

Turkey, Syria, Spain, Morocco, Albania and France, furthermore, among others, the Russian Federation (Black Sea region), as well as in Central- and South America.

Main exporting countries: Mediterranean countries, especially Turkey.

Cultivation: The plants prefer well drained, nutrient- and humus rich soil in full sunny, wind protected places, but they can also thrive in the shade. Propagation is carried out in the spring by seed or semi-ripe cuttings (to root in soil under plastic cover), which germinate or root best at 20 °C. Because it is not winter hardy, in Central Europe bay is cultivated in tubs, which during the growth period must be sufficiently watered and fertilized about every 2 to 3 weeks. A continuous water shortage is tolerated just as little as standing water. When temperatures drop below –5 °C, the plants must be brought indoors, where they should only be watered sparingly. They should be repotted every 3 to 4 years. Formative pruning is well tolerated [Ü2, Ü32, Ü 66].

Culinary herb

Commercial forms: Bay leaf: Whole, rarely the dried and ground leaves, bay essential oil.

Production: The leaves can be harvested throughout the entire year. The small bay twigs can be clipped, and then hung up in a dry, dark, ventilated place. After drying, the leaves can be removed from the twigs. In order to prevent the leaves from rolling up, they can be dried between 2 layers of blotting paper.

Forms used: Fresh or dried leaves, whole or in large pieces, powdered bay leaf.

Storage: Fresh leaves can be stored wrapped in plastic bags in the refrigerator for a few days. Dried leaves are stored in well-closed porcelain-, glass- or suitable metal containers protected from light and

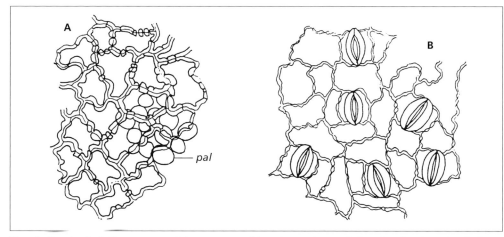

Fig. 3: Bay leaf. **A** Fragments of the upper epidermis, underneath it pal palisade cells, **B** Fragments of the lower epidermis. From Ü48.

moisture. The supply should be replenished with new material every two years. Powdered leaves lose their aroma quickly.

Description. Whole leaf (Fig. 1): See description of whole plant.

Cut leaf: Beneath the upper leaf epidermis, a double or triple layer of palisade tissue is discernible, containing numerous, spherical oil cells that are also present in the spongy parenchyma. The surface section of the upper epidermis shows the polyhedral cells with stout walls, their radial cell walls are jagged-undulate, appearing beaded-punctate with increased depth of focus [Ü29].

Powdered leaf: Characteristic are the shreds of the upper leaf epidermis, which, in top view, show the irregularly shaped cells with thickened walls looking beaded due to their large pits; also present are shreds of the lower epidermis with less-thickened cell walls and numerous paracytic stomata (Fig. 3), as well as lignified fibers, mostly associated with vascular tissue, stone cells and large, ovoid oil cells [Ü48].

Odor: Upon rubbing of the fresh leaves, sweetish, balsamic and somewhat piquant, **Taste:** Fresh leaves aromatic and slightly bitter; dried leaves aromatic.

History: Bay leaves were already cultivated in Mediterranean regions during antiquity; they were highly valued by the Greeks and Romans. In the 3rd century cookbook, "De re coquinaria", named after the Roman gourmet Apicius (see footnote in → Asafetida monograph), bay leaves and flowers were mentioned. Pictures of bay leaf trees have been found in old Pompeii [Ü42, Ü61, for mythology 11, 36, Ü97].

Constituents and Analysis

DIN- and ISO-Standards: ISO-Standard 6576 (Laurel (*Laurus nobilis* Linnaeus) – Whole and pounded leaves – Specification).

Constituents

- Essential oil: About 0.8 to 4% (up to 10% in fall), the main component is usually 1,8-cineole (12 to 71%, mostly 25 to 50%); the co-constituents are qualitatively and quantitatively variable depending on origin, race and time of harvest: Linalool (6 to 30%), *p*-cymene (0 to 20%), α-phellandrene (0 to 20%), geraniol (0 to 20%), eugenol (traces to 19%), linalyl acetate (1 to 16%), α-pinene (2 to 16%), sabinene (4 to 13%), α-terpinyl acetate (0 to 12%), methyl eugenol (eugenol methylether, 2 to

12%), α-terpineol (7 to 9%), β-pinene (3 to 5%) and terpinenol-4 (1 to 5%); furthermore, camphene, citral, myrcene, β-pinene, and γ-terpinene, among others [2, 3, 7, 18, 20, 23, 27, 30, 32, 33]. A batch from Sicily was found to contain 46.5% 1,8-cineole, 11.8% α-terpinyl acetate, 7.3% sabinene, 5.7% α-pinene, 4.3% β-pinene, 2.4% terpinenol-4 [5]. Bay leaves from Egypt contained, among other components, 37.6% 1,8-cineole, 19.8% p-cymene, 7.1% α-terpinyl acetate, 4.7% myrcene, 3.7% β-pinene, 3.7% terpinenol-4, 3.5% α-terpineol and 2.8% linalool [40].

- Isoquinoline alkaloids: Aporphine- and nor-aporphine type (about 0.1%), including, among others, (+)-actinodaphnine, (+)-boldine, (+)-cryptodorine, (+)-isodomesticine, (+)-launobine, N-(+)-methylactinodaphnine, (+)-nandigerine, (+)-neolitisine and (+)-reticuline [28].
- Sesquiterpene lactones: Dehydrocostuslactone (up to 65% of the compounds of this group), costunolide (up to 35%), as well as, among others, artemorine, eremanthine, desacetyllaurenobiolide, laurenobiolide, reynosine, santamarine, verlotorin and zaluzanine. The constituents are likely to be responsible for the bitter principles, which are lost during the drying process [14, 41, 42, 44].
- Flavonoids: Mainly rutin, isoquercitrin, hyperoside and kaempferol-3-rhamnoglucoside, furthermore quercitrin, quercetin-3-arabinoside, kaempferol-3-glucoside, -3-galactoside, -3-rhamnoside and –3-arabinoside [19, 24]. Kaempferol-3-rhamnoside is in part linked to 1 or 2 p-coumaroyl moieties [15].
- Catechins: Proanthocyanidins [35, 37].
- Lignan glycosides: (+)-5´-Methoxyisolariciresinol-9´-O-xyloside, (+)-5´-sec-oisolariciresinol-9´-O- xyloside and schizandraside [48].
- Phenylacrylic and phenolcarboxylic acids: Free or bound, including, among others, p-coumaric acid, ferulic acid, sinapic acid, gentisinic acid and vanillic acid [38].

Tests for Identity: Macroscopic and microscopic examination. A number of GC/MS methods for the analysis of the essential oil have been described [5, 33, 40].

Quantitative assay: The content of essential oil is determined gravimetrically with steam-distillation [EB 6], or volumetrically, according to Ph Eur. The composition of the distilled oil is analyzed with GC [7].

Adulterations, Misidentifications and Impurities are possible, with the leaves of *Laurus azorica* (SEUBERT) FRANCO, Azores bay, having strongly pubescent young leaves, or *Prunus laurocerasus* L., cherry laurel, with a serrate leaf-margin [Ü37].

Actions and Uses

Actions: Due to its aromatic taste, bay leaf has appetite stimulating and digestion promoting action.

Extracts of bay leaf lowered the blood glucose levels in animals with experimentally induced diabetes mellitus [4]. In rats that were administered ethanol, the extracts were able to retard the elevation of blood alcohol levels. The effect could be traced back to a delay in stomach emptying and absorption. The sesquiterpene lactones with exocyclic methylene groups, costunolide, dehydrocostuslactone and santamarine, among others, were determined to be active constituents [25, 49]. Aqueous extracts of the seeds and their fatty oil protected rats against gastric ulcers [1].

Insect repellent action against the flour beetle and the bean bruchid (bean seed beetle) has been demonstrated for bay leaves, extracts thereof and components of the essential oil [31, 34]. Components of the essential oil, especially 1,8-cineole or geraniol can expel cockroaches [46]. The essential oil has moderate antimicrobial and antioxidative activity [5, 40].

Toxicology: Based on existing data, there is no acute or chronic toxicity with the normal use of bay leaves as a seasoning.

Based on the content of sesquiterpene lac-

tones with exocyclic methylene groups [Ü100], bay leaves have a moderate sensitization potential. The allergenic constituents are also present in bay oil and bay butter (see below). Cross-reactions occur with many Compositae (Asteraceae), e.g. feverfew, *Tanacetum parthenium* (L.) SCH. BIP., and elecampane, *Inula helenium* L. Cases of contact dermatitis have been observed especially with exposure to bay butter or bay oil, but also with bay leaves, for example in kitchen personnel, vegetable handlers and housewives. Cooking does not eliminate allergenic activity. Hence, allergic symptoms, e.g. swollen lips, stomatitis, can also occur with internal exposure to foods that have been prepared with bay leaves or products thereof [10, 12, 13, 16, 17]. People, who are allergic to Compositae, should avoid contact with bay leaves and foods containing them.

Culinary use: Bay leaves are especially popular in the Mediterranean region and in France. They are cooked whole or in large pieces with meals and then removed before serving. For Central Europeans, $1/2$ to 1 leaf per dish is usually sufficient, but in the Mediterranean countries considerably larger amounts are added. If one tears the leaf edges, the aroma will be released better. Powdered bay leaf should only be added at the very end of the cooking process. Dried, but preferably fresh bay leaves, are well suited as a spice for sauces (e.g. of tomato sauce for noodles or other pastas), soups, meat dishes (pot roast, sauerbraten, mutton, venison, boiled ham, salt meat, fricassee), fish dishes (steamed fish, but also fried fish), rice dishes, vegetable dishes (carrots, sauerkraut, red cabbage), peas pudding, dishes made from mollusks and crustaceans (crabs, shrimp, prawns, mussels), brawns, mushrooms, pickled vegetables (mixed pickles, red beets, tomatoes, sauerkraut, cucumbers) as well as milk puddings or dessert creams. For the preparation of béchamel sauce and for the flavoring of vanilla- or rice pudding, bay leaves are cooked in milk. When grilling meats, bay leaves can also be placed on the coals, and for grilling kebabs bay leaf can be placed in between the pieces of meat on the skewer [Ü13, Ü30, Ü46, Ü55, Ü68, Ü70, Ü73, Ü81, Ü95].

For the preparation of oily extract, oil is poured over fresh or dried bay leaves and allowed to soak completely for a few days. The bay oil obtained from this process (not to be confused with official bay oil, see below) is well suited for refining Italian salads [Ü1].

The essential oil of bay leaf (bay oil) is used as a spice for fish conserves and for the production of spice- and liqueur essences as well as soup spices [Ü92].

Combines well with: Black pepper, clove, juniper berries, marjoram, parsley, tarragon, and thyme.

As a component of spice mixes and preparations: → Bouquet garni, → Cocktail sauce, → Garam masala, → Herb vinegar, → Masala, → Meat spice, → Mélange classique, → Mixed pickles spice, → Parisian pepper, → Pickling spice, → Sauce spice, → Vegetable spice, → Venison spice.

Other uses: The fruit, in ground form, is occasionally used as an ingredient for spice mixtures [Ü98]. The essential oil from bay leaves is a component of a few perfumes for men [Ü39]. It is claimed that bay leaves, added to stored flour, repel weevils [Ü66]. The wood is valued for the manufacture of furniture [Ü42].

Medicinal herb

Herbal drugs: Lauri folium, Bay leaf [Lorbeerblatt EB 6], from *Laurus officinalis*, Lauri fructus, Bay fruit [Lorbeeren DAB 6, Ph Helv VI], Lauri Oleum, Bay butter or Bay oil, a mixture of fatty and essential oil, obtained by hot pressing of the fruits [DAB 6, ÖAB, Ph Helv V].

Indications: Bay is used for loss of appetite and digestive complaints. In the folk medicine of the plant's countries of origin, tea infusions made from bay leaves are taken as a carminative, expectorant, diuretic, antispasmodic emmenagogue and diaphoretic remedy [8].

Similar culinary herbs

Indonesian bay leaf (Indonesian: daun salam; also called Indian bay leaf, a holdover from when Indonesia was known as "East India"), *Syzygium polyanthum* (WIGHT) WALP. (Synonym: *Eugenia polyantha* WIGHT, Myrtaceae), a tree that reaches up to 25 m in height, native to the Indian union territory of the Nicobar Islands, Myanmar, Thailand, Malaysia and Indonesia, where it is also cultivated. It is used as a spice for rice dishes and kerri sauces, and as a component of East Asian spice mixes [Ü92, Ü98].

The dried leaves of croton, *Codiaeum variegatum* (L.) BL., (Euphorbiaceae), are also called Indian bay leaf and used similarly. The plant is native to the Moluccas Islands and is cultivated outdoors but in Central Europe it is grown in pots or tubs as an ornamental plant [Ü92]. It contains toxic and allergy inducing constituents (possibly the phorbol ester) and should not be used as a spice [Ü84].

Myrtle leaf (wax myrtle), *Myrtus communis* L. (Myrtaceae), native origin unknown but widely distributed from the Mediterranean region up to the northwestern Himalayas, is also cultivated as an ornamental- and hedge plant [Ü61]. The leaves contain 0.1 to 0.8% essential oil, of which the main components are α-pinene (15 to 75%), 1,8-cineole (12 to 45%), limonene (5 to 19%), linalool (2 to 19%), myrtenol (0.7 to 5%) and myrtenyl acetate (1 to 35%) [6, 9, 21, 22, 29, 39, 45]. The main components of the essential oil from the berries are 1,8-cineole (20 to 31%), α-pinene (8 to 25%), limonene (8 to 18%) and myrtenyl acetate (10 to 20%) [21, 26]. The leaves are used in the same way as bay leaves, together with thyme herb, as a meat spice, e.g. for roasted pork or grilled lamb, and for venison, and combined with fennel as a grill spice, a few twigs are laid on the burning coals. In southern Italy, fresh cheese is wrapped in myrtle leaves to intensify the aroma. The essential oil of the fresh leaves is used in the perfume industry. The bilberry-like fruits are used as a spice for sauces and meats. In Corsica, a stomachic liqueur (Myrtéi) is made with myrtle [Ü66, Ü74, Ü98].

Boldo leaf, *Peumus boldus* MOL. (Monimiaceae), an evergreen tree native to Chile, and cultivated in Algeria [Ü61]. It contains 2 to 3% essential oil, of which the main components are *p*-cymene (2 to 14%), limonene (traces up to 17%), ascaridol (1 to 42%), 1,8-cineole (0 to 12%), β-phellandrene (about 8%) and sabinene (about 6%), as well as 0.2 to 0.5% aporphine type isoquinoline alkaloids (according to Ph Eur, not less than 0.1% calculated as boldine) [47, Ü99]. Boldo leaves are used therapeutically as cholagogue. As a spice, they are used similarly as bay leaves, but measured carefully [Ü78].

Potatoes with bay leaves
(Serves 4 to 6)
1 kg peeled potatoes, cut into 1.5 cm thick slices, 2 large garlic cloves, minced, 4 bay leaves, olive oil, salt, freshly ground black pepper, 450 ml chicken broth (can also be prepared from instant broth cubes).

A flat casserole is brushed with olive oil. Layer half the amount of potato slices, garlic and bay leaves into the dish, season to taste with salt and pepper; add two tablespoons of olive oil. Prepare the other half of the ingredients the same way. Pour the chicken broth over the dish and let it simmer or slightly boil for 25 to 30 minutes, until the potatoes are done and the liquid has mostly evaporated. Pour off the remaining liquid and remove the bay leaves before serving [Ü55].

Literature

[1] Afifi F.U. et al., J. Ethnopharmacol. 58(1):9–14 (1997).

[2] Agkül A. et al., J. Ess. Oil Res. 1:277–280 (1989).

[3] Anac O., Perfumer Flav. 11:73–75 (1986).

[4] Ashajeva L.A. et al., Farmacija (Moskwa) 33(2):49–51 (1984).

[5] Baratta Z.M. et al., J. Ess. Oil Res. 10:618–627 (1998).

[6] Boelens M.H., R. Jimenez, J. Ess. Oil Res. 4:349–353 (1991).

[7] Borges P. et al., Nahrung 36:494–496 (1992).

[8] Boulous L: Medicinal Plants of North Africa, Reference Publications, Inc., Michigan 1983.

[9] Chalchat J.C. et al., J. Ess. Oil Res. 10:613–617 (1998).

[10] Cheminat A. et al., Arch. Derm. Res. 276: 178–181 (1984).

[11] Czygan F.C., Dtsch. Apoth. Ztg. 135(51/52):4707–4711 (1995).

[12] De Smet P.A.G.M. et al. (Eds.), in: Adverse Effects of Herbal Drugs, Springer Verlag Berlin, Heidelberg, New York 1992, Bd. 1, p. 249–254.

[13] Ebner H., H. Stöger, Wien Klin Wschr. 83:901–905 (1973).

[14] El-Feraly F.S., D.A. Benigni, J. Nat. Prod. 43:527–531 (1980).

[15] Fiorini Ch. et al., Phytochemistry 47(5): 821–824 (1998).

[16] Hausen B.M., Dtsch. Apoth. Ztg. 131(20): 987–996 (1991).

[17] Hausen B.M., Dtsch. Med. Wochenschr. 110:634–638 (1985).

[18] Hokwerda H. et al., Planta Med. 44:116–119 (1982).

[19] Knackstedt J., K. Herrmann, Z. Lebensm. Unters. Forsch. 173:288–290 (1981).

[20] Lawrence B., Perfum. Flavorist 6:59 (1981).

[21] Lawrence B.M., Perfumer Flavorist 15:63, 65–66 (1990).

[22] Lawrence B.M. et al., Am. Perfum Cosmet. 85:53–55 (1970).

[23] Lin Z.K. et al., Acta Botanica Sinica 32: 878–882 (1990).

[24] Makarov V.A., Khim. Prir. Soedin (2):203 (1971).

[25] Matsuda H. et al., Bioorg Med. Chem. Lett. 9(18):2647–2652 (1999).

[26] Mazza G., J. Chromatogr. 264:304–311 (1983).

[27] Müller-Ribau F.J. et al., J. Agric. Food Chem. 45(12):4821–4825 (1997).

[28] Pech B., J. Bruneton, J. Nat. Prod. 45(5): 560–563 (1982).

[29] Peyron L., Plantes Méd. Phytothér. 4:279–285 (1970).

[30] Pino J., P. Borges, E. Roncal, Nahrung 37:592–595 (1993).

[31] Regnault-Roger C., A. Hamraoui, Stored Prod. Res. 29:259–264 (1993).

[32] Riaz M. et al., Pak. J. Sci. Res. 32:33–35 (1989).

[33] Roque O.R., J. Ess. Oil Res. 1:199–200 (1989).

[34] Saim N., C.E. Meloan, Stored Prod. Res. 22:141–144 (1986).

[35] Sakar M., R. Engelshowe, Z. Lebensm. Unters. Forsch. 180:494–495 (1985).

[36] Scholz H., Natürlich 20(2):42–49 (2000).

[37] Schulz J.M., K. Herrmann, Z. Lebensm. Unters. Forsch. 171(4):278–280 (1980).

[38] Schulz J.M., K. Herrmann., Z. Lebensm. Unters. Forsch. 171:192–199 (1980).

[39] Shikiev A.S. et al., Chem. Nat. Comp. 14:455–456 (1978).

[40] Soliman F.M. et al., Bull. Fac. Pharmacy 32:387–389 (1996).

[41] Strack D. et al., Z. Naturforsch C, Biosci. 35C:915 (1980).

[42] Tada H., K. Takeda, Chem. Pharm. Bull. 24:667–671 (1976).

[43] Tattje D.H.E. et al., Planta Med. 44(2): 116–119 (1982).

[44] Tori H. et al., Chem. Pharm. Bull. 24:667 (1976).

[45] Vanhaelen M., Vanhaelen-Fastre, Planta Med. 39:164–167 (1980).

[46] Verma M., C.E. Meloan, Am. Lab. 13:66–69 (1981).

[47] Vila R. et al., Planta Med. 65(2):178–179 (1999).

[48] Yahara S. et al., Shoyakugaku Zasshi 46:184–186 (1992), ref. CA 118:35873u.

[49] Yoshikawa M. et al., Bioorg. Med. Chem. 8(8):2071–2077 (2000).

[50] Zola A. et al., Plant. Med. Phytother. 11: 241–246 (1977).

Literature references identified by Ü can be found in the general listing of books and monographs at the back of this book.

Black cumin

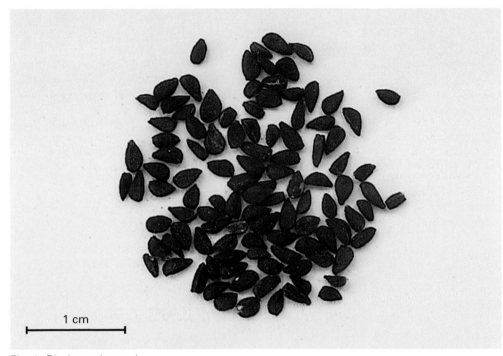

Fig. 1: Black cumin seeds

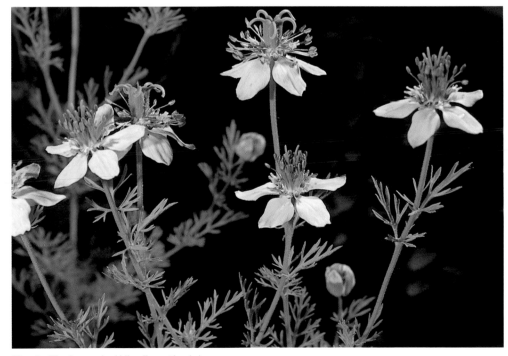

Fig. 2: Black cumin (*Nigella sativa* L.)

Plant source: *Nigella sativa* L.

Family: Crowfoot family (Ranunculaceae).

Common names: Engl.: black cum(m)in, blackseed, small fennel, wild onion seed; Fr.: nielle, nigelle, poivrette, cumin noir, toute épice, cheveux de Venus; Ger.: Schwarzkümmel, Echter Schwarzkümmel, Schwarzer Kreuzkümmel, Schwarzer Kümmel, Schwarzer Koriander, Römischer Koriander, Brotwurz, Schabasamen, Zwiebelsamen.

Description: An annual herb, about 30 to 60 cm in height. The leaves are multiple pinnate and the leaflets are narrow-lanceolate to linear. The small flowers bear 5 white petals and numerous stamina with a circular arrangement of 5 to 10 nectorial petals in between, and 4 to 7 fused ovaries. The ripe follicles contain numerous black seeds [Ü106].

Native origin: Mediterranean region and Western Asia.

Main cultivation areas: Cultivated in India, to a lesser extent in Pakistan, in the Mediterranean region (Egypt and Turkey, among others), in the Sudan, Ethiopia, Syria, Iraq, Iran, in the Balkan countries, and the Russian Federation.

Main exporting countries: India, Egypt, Central Asia, Southern Europe, and Russian Federation.

Cultivation: This hardy plant prefers sandy loam soils in warm, not too damp locations. Propagation is carried out by direct seeding usually in April with row spacing of 20 to 30 cm. In gardens, seeds can also be sown in September to November. The seeds must be covered with soil (dark germinator!). There are no cultivars [Ü21].

Culinary herb

Commercial forms: Black cumin: ripe seeds, whole or ground (in Indian spice shops also described as black onion seed, kalonji or kala jeera), black cumin oil (fatty oil).

Production: The harvest takes place when the capsules begin to turn brown, around the middle of August, either through combine harvesting or cut with a swather and aged for a few days at the threshing yard and then dried [Ü21].

Forms used: Whole or ground seeds, black cumin oil (fatty oil).

Storage: The seeds are stored in a dry and cool place, protected from light and moisture, in air-tight porcelain-, glass- or suitable metal containers; the fatty oil is stored in completely filled, tightly closed containers in a cool place (below 25° C), protected from light.

Description. Whole seed (Fig. 1): The seeds are dull black, 2 to 3.5 mm long, up to 2 mm thick, with an ovoid or sphenoidal outline, 3- to 4-angled, flattened, somewhat arched on the dorsal side, with slightly reticulate venation or finely granular surface [EB 6].

Powdered seed: Gray-black. The chloral hydrate preparation shows the fragments of the testa epidermis with up to 100 μm large, radially elongated, thick-walled cells with black-brown walls and black-brown content whose outer walls are extended to a truncated, cone-shaped papilla. Besides the above mentioned epidermis cells, there are also small-celled tissue fragments with stout, reticulately striated walls and brown content as well as large-celled, stout-walled tissue of the endosperm with aleuron grains [Ü60, EB 6].

Odor: Spicy when rubbed, caraway-like (nutmeg-like, camphor-like), **Taste:** First bitter then slightly pungent and spicy.

History: Black cumin was already cultivated in antiquity by the Egyptians, Arabs and Indians, who used it as a spice and medicinal plant; it was introduced later to a number of European countries. It was mentioned in the imperial decree "Capitulare de villis" (authored about 795, see footnote → Anise), regulating agricultural practices. In Germany, the plant was formerly cultivated in Erfurt and Söflingen (near Ulm) [Ü61].

Constituents and Analysis

Constituents

■ Essential oil: About 0.4 to 2.5%, the main components are *p*-cymene (about 38%), thymoquinone (about 30%), α-pinene (5 to 14%), β-pinene (about 5%) and limonene (about 4%). Thymohydroquinone was also isolated from the essential oil. As oxidation products of the thymoquinones (distillation artifacts?), dithymoquinone and its oligomers (nigellone) occur [19, 27, 28, Ü44]. Based on differing data, the main components are limonene (about 60%) and α-thujene (about 15%) besides α-pinene, γ-terpinene, sabinene and methylbenzoate [16] or *p*-cymenone (about 77%), citronellyl acetate (5%), carvone (4%) and limonene (4%), respectively (chemical races?) [Ü92].

■ Fatty oil: 30 to 35%, as acid components of the triacylglycerols, 50 to 60% linoleic acid, 18 to 25% oleic acid, 10 to 15% palmitinic acid, 3 to 4% stearinic acid, 2 to 3% eicosadienoic acid, furthermore small amounts of myristic-, palmitoleic-, stearic-, α-linolenic-, arachic-, eicosenic- and eicosapentadienoic acid [1, 9, 28, 45]. The fatty oil obtained by cold pressing contains the components of the essential oil (up to 0.2% thymoquinone, among others) and therefore has a spicy taste [27].

■ Alkaloids: The pyrazole alkaloids nigellidine and nigellicine, the isoquinoline-alkaloids nigellimine and nigellimine-*N*-oxide [12, 26, Ü44].

■ Tocopherols: α-, β-, γ-, δ-Tocopherol [45].

■ Sterols: β-Sitosterol, stigmasterol, campesterol, isofucosterol, stigmastanol [1, 45].

■ Triterpene saponins: About 1.5% melianthine (mixture?), aglycone hederagenin (melianthigenin) [11, 35].

■ Anthraquinone derivatives (?) [6].

p-Cymene   Thymoquinone   Thymohydroquinone

Nigellidine   Nigellicine   Nigellimine

Tests for Identity: Based on morphological and anatomical characteristics of the seeds.

Quantitative assay: The fatty acids of the fatty oil are analyzed with TLC or GC [27]; thymoquinone, dithymoquinone, thymohydroquinone and thymol in the fatty oil are quantified with HPLC [23], thymoquinone in the fatty oil with GC [27], and components of the essential oil with capillary-GC and GC/MS [33].

Adulterations, Misidentifications and Impurities are possible with the seeds of wild fennel, *Nigella arvensis* L., love-in-a-mist, *N. damascena* L., corncockle, *Agrostemma githago* L., or Jimson weed, *Datura stramonium* L. They are characterized by smaller gray, dark-brown, reniform or larger seeds, respectively, with a coarsely granular surface [EB 6].

Actions and Uses

Actions: Due to its aromatic taste, black cumin has appetizing and digestion promoting action.

Spasmolytic action: The essential oil has a relaxing effect in vitro in the isolated guinea pig trachea and ileum (EC$_{50}$ 46 and 74 mg/l) [36].

Analgesic and antiphlogistic action: The fatty oil and pure thymoquinone both inhibited cyclooxygenase and 5-lipoxygenase and thereby inhibited thromboxane and leucotriene formation in vitro in rat peritoneal lymphocytes. The authors suggest that the results provide clarification for the antiphlogistic effect (used for asthma and rheumatism!) [27]. Nigellone can inhibit in vitro the release of histamine from mast cells induced by compound 48/80 and calcium-ionophore A23187 [15]. Using mice as experimental animals in various test models analgesic effects of the seeds have been demonstrated [30], of high doses of the fatty oil (50 to 400 mg/kg body weight) or of thymoquinone (2.5 to 10 mg/kg body weight, p.o.). The effect was suppressed by naloxone [2].

Anthelmintic action: The seeds have anthelmintic activity [4]. In animal experiments (goats and sheep) it has been demonstrated that the glycoside fraction of the seeds definitely contributes to the anthelmintic action against tapeworms (cestodes). The isolated saponins alone were ineffective [6]. In children, it was also shown that a single oral administration of the seeds (40 mg/kg body weight) or an equivalent amount of an ethanolic extract of the seeds reduced the fecal excretion of tapeworm eggs, which was comparable to the reduction caused by niclosamide (50 mg / kg body weight) [7].

Gastroprotective action: The administration of black cumin oil inhibited by about 50% the formation of ethanol-induced gastric ulcers in rats. At the same time, the mucin and glutathione content in the stomach elevated and the histamine level dropped [21].

Hepatoprotective action: In animal tests (mice), thymoquinone (100 mg/kg body weight, single dose, p.o.) can avert carbon tetrachloride-induced liver damage. This effect is attributed to the antioxidative action (preventing lipid peroxidation). Similar results could also be shown in rats [8, 20, 34].

Anticholesterolemic action: Supplementing the rat diet with black cumin oil (800 mg/kg body weight over 4 weeks) led to a significant drop of the cholesterol, LDL and triacylglycerols levels as well as to an increase the level of HDL in the blood [20].

Immunostimulant action: Injections (i.p.) of black cumin oil in mice infected with cytomegaloviruses significantly reduced the virus titer in the liver and spleen, and at the same time increased the serum level of IFN-γ and the number of CD4(+)-cells. In contrast to the controls, the treated mice were free of the viruses after 10 days [37]. Other studies also suggest an immunostimulant effect of black cumin [25, 40].

Antitumor action: The induction of gastric tumors after internal application of Benzo[a]pyrone in mice could be inhibited by 70% by thymoquinone (0.01% in the drinking water). The studies point to a potentiation of the detoxification function of the liver (increased production of glutathione-S-transferase, thereby elevating the glutathione level) [13]. The occurrence and growth of skin tumors after external application of dimethylbenz[a]anthracene /croton oil or 20-methylcholanthrene was also reduced by extracts from the seeds (100 mg/kg body weight, i.p.) [38]. Ethanolic extracts of the seeds are more strongly cytotoxic in vitro against tumor cells than against human umbilical cord endothelial cells [40]. Thymoquinone and dithymoquinone are also lethal against cytostatic resistant (doxorubicin, etoposide) tumor cells [43].

Antimicrobial action: The essential oil, the fatty oil, extracts of the dried seeds and isolated thymohydroquinone or thymoquinone (e.g. MIC for *Staphylococcus aureus* 8 µg/ml) have shown good antimicrobial activity, also against *Shigella* spp., *Vibrio cholerae* and *Escherichia coli* as well as against numerous other antibiotic-resistant bacteria [3, 19, 22, 24, 32].

Other actions: Black cumin essential oil (4 to 21 µl/kg body weight) and thymoquinone (0.2 to 1.6 mg/kg body weight) led to a drop in blood pressure in rats [18]. Following a 15-day treatment with black cumin extract (0.6 ml/kg body weight) in rats, diuresis increased by about 16%. At the same time the blood pressure decreased by about 22% [44]. The seeds are also supposed to have a galactagogue effect [5]. The essential oil has good antioxidative activity [14].

Toxicology: Based on existing data, there is no acute or chronic toxicity with the use of black cumin as a normally dosed spice. Hexane extracts of the seeds (2 g/kg body weight) fed to rats, post coitum, from day 1 to 10, inhibited gestation [29]. The intake of 20 g seeds caused vomiting in humans and abortion in pregnant women [Ü58].

Aqueous extracts of the seeds applied in rats p.o. for 14 days led to liver damage (increase of serum-γ-glutamyl-transferase levels, degenerative changes of the hepatocytes) [41].

The sensitization potential of black cumin is low but allergic contact dermatitis after topical application of black cumin oil has been observed [39].

Culinary use: The seeds are used whole or ground, especially in the countries of the Near East and Turkey, sometimes mixed with sesame seeds as a bread seasoning (added with the flour or sprinkled on the bread before baking), bakery products, sweets, quark, cheese, sauces and soups. In India, the seeds are used whole, often pre-roasted, added to dishes made from legumes and vegetables and as an ingredient for sour preserves and chutneys. They are also sprinkled over naan-bread (bread baked in a very hot oven, a so-called Tandoori-oven, about 1.5 cm thick, drop-shaped, rolled out into approximately 15 cm long flat cakes). In Egypt, the seeds are ground with coffee to add flavor. In France, the powdered seeds are used the same as pepper. In Central Europe, black cumin is rarely used as a seasoning [42, Ü55, Ü68, Ü73].

The seeds can be roasted briefly in a pan (without fat) in order to strengthen their aroma. They are best ground in a coffee- or pepper mill.

The seeds are suitable, whole or ground, added directly to vegetables (e.g. eggplant, cabbage, spinach), legumes, yogurt, cottage cheese, salads (tomato-, cucumber salad), braised/roast lamb and poultry, fish dishes, pickles and chutneys. Roasted seeds can be added to buttered vegetables, such as cabbage or zucchini. Before placing on the grill, steaks or brats can be smeared with the seeds [Ü2, Ü13, Ü68, Ü81, Ü111].

Rolls, pretzels or other baked goods can be sprinkled with black cumin before baking [Ü81].

The seeds are also used as a seasoning for the pickling of cucumbers and pumpkins [Ü81].

The flavoring of coffee with the ground seeds (6 teaspoons coffee + 1 teaspoon black cumin) is recommended [42].

Combines well with: Ajowan, allspice, coriander, garlic, peppermint, summer savory, and thyme.

As a component of spice mixes and preparations: → Panch phoron, → Ras el hanout.

Other uses: The fatty oil is used as a cooking oil, especially in India.

Medicinal herb

Herbal drug: Nigellae semen, Black cumin seed [EB 6].

Indications: Formerly used for intestinal catarrh, diarrhea, jaundice, dysmenorrhoea and for pulmonary disorders, as a diuretic remedy and to promote breast milk production (single dose 1 g) [Ü60, Ü68].

In India, black cumin seeds are used for digestive disorders, menstrual problems, bronchial catarrhs and as an anthelmintic, especially for tapeworms in children. A paste made from the seeds is applied topically for the treatment of abscesses, hemorrhoids and inflammation of the testicles [6, 16]. In Egypt the fatty oil is used as an antasthmatic [19]. In Saudi Arabia, it is used for stiffness and joint pain, for asthma and eczema [27]. Due to its high linoleic acid content, it is also used as a dietary supplement (1.5 to 3 g/d) [10, 31].

Similar spice herbs

Wild fennel, *Nigella arvensis* L., occurs in Southern- and Central Europe, cultivated in Iran, the herb is used as a seasoning for soups, the seeds are used in the same way as cumin [Ü61].

Damascus black cumin (love-in-a-mist), *Nigella damascena* L., cultivated in Southern Europe, the seeds contain, among others, essential oil and 0.1 to 0.3% damascenin (3-methoxy-*N*-methylanthranilic acid-methyl ester, during steam distillation it goes into the essential oil and makes it fluorescent blue) in addition to damascinin (3-hydroxy-4-methylamino-*N*-methylanthranilic acid-methyl ester) [17]. The seeds are used in the same way as black cumin. The fatty oil is used preferably in the cosmetic industry [Ü98].

Spicy Cucumber Salad
(Serves 2 to 4)
1 cucumber (finely minced), salt, 250 g thick yogurt, $1/2$ teaspoon black cumin, 1 teaspoon fresh mint (finely minced), lettuce for garnishing.

The diced cucumber pieces are placed onto a flat bowl and seasoned to taste with salt. Add the yogurt, black cumin and mint; mix the ingredients well. Serve on chilled plates, garnished with lettuce. The salad should be mixed with the yogurt and spices immediately before serving otherwise the diced cucumber will water down the dressing [Ü55].

Literature

[1] Abd Alla El-Sayed A.M. et al., Dtsch. Lebensm. Rundsch. 93(5):149–152 (1997).

[2] Abdel-Fattah A.M. et al., Eur. J. Pharmacol. 400(1):89–97 (2000).

[3] Aboul Ela M.A. et al., Pharmazie 51(12): 993–994 (1996).

[4] Agarwal R. et al., Indian J. Exp. Biol. 17(11): 1264–1265 (1979).

[5] Agrawala I.P. et al., Indian J. Med. 25(8):535–537 (1971).

[6] Akhtar M.S., M. Aslam, Pak. J. Pharmacol. 14(2):7–14 (1997).

[7] Akhtar M.S., S. Riffat, J. Pak. Med. Assoc. 41(8):185–187 (1991).

[8] Al-Gharably N.M. et al., Res. Commun. Pharmacol. Toxicol. 2(1/2):41–50 (1997).

[9] Al-Jassir M.S., Food Chem. 45:239–242 (1992).

[10] Anonym, Dtsch. Apoth. Ztg. 137(45): 4098 (1997).

[11] Ansari A.A. et al., Phytochemistry 27: 3977–3979 (1988).

[12] Atta-Ur-Rahman et al., J. Nat. Prod. 55(5):676–678 (1992).

[13] Badary O.A. et al., Eur. J. Cancer Prev. 8(5):435–440 (1999).

[14] Burits M., F. Bucar, Phytother. Res. 14(5): 323–328 (2000).

[15] Chakravarty N., Ann. Allergy 70(3):237–242 (1993).

[16] Chana J.S., Forum Aromather. Aromapflege 10/96:52–55 (1996).

[17] Döpke W., G. Fritsch, Pharmazie 25(1): 69–70 (1970).

[18] El Thahir K.E. et al., Gen. Pharmacol. 24:1123–1131 (1993).

[19] El-Alfy T.S. et al., Pharmazie 30(2): 109–111 (1975).

[20] El-Dakhakhny M. et al., Arzneim. Forsch. 50(9):832–836 (2000).

[21] El-Dakhakhny M. et al., J. Ethnopharmacol. 72(1/2):299–304 (2000).

[22] Ferdous A.J., S.N. Islam, Phytother. Res. 6(2):137–140 (1992).

[23] Ghosheh O.A. et al., J. Pharm. Biomed. Anal. 19(5):757–762 (1999).

[24] Hanafy M.S., M.E. Hatem, J. Ethnopharmacol. 34(2/3):275–278 (1991).

[25] Haq A. et al., Immunpharmacology 30(2):147–155 (1995).

[26] Hata K. et al., Chem. Pharm. Bull. 26: 2279 (1978), ref. Ü43.

[27] Houghton P.J. et al., Planta Med. 61(1): 33–36 (1995).

[28] Karawya M.S. et al., J. Pharm. Sci. 3(2): 49–57 (1994).

[29] Keshri G. et al., Indian J. Physiol. Pharmacol. 39(1):59–62 (1995).

[30] Khanna T. et al., Fitoterapia 64:407–410 (1993).

[31] Lauterbacher L.M., Dtsch. Apoth. Ztg. 137(50):4602–4603 (1997).

[32] Morsi N.M., Acta Microbiol. Pol. 49(1): 63–74 (2000).

[33] Mozaffari F.S. et al., J. Ess. Oil Res. 12: 36–38 (2000).

[34] Nagi M.N. et al., Biochem. Mol Biol. Int. 47(1):153–159 (1999).

[35] Paris R.R., Compt. Rend. 250:2925 (1960), ref. Ü43.

[36] Reiter M., W. Brandt, Arzneim. Forsch. 35:408–414 (1985).

[37] Salemal M.L., M.S. Hossainb, Int. J. Immunpharmacol. 22(9):729–740 (2000).

[38] Salomi M.J. et al., Nutr. Cancer 16:67–72 (1991).

[39] Steinmann A. et al., Contact Dermatitis 36(5):268–269 (1997).

[40] Swamy S.M., B.K. Tan, J. Ethnopharmacol. 70(1):1–7 (2000).

[41] Tennekoon K.H. et al., J. Ethnopharmacol. 31(3):283–289 (1991).

[42] Vonarburg B., Natürlich 18(6):65–68 (1998).

[43] Worthen D.R. et al., Anticancer Res. 18(3A):1527–1532 (1998).

[44] Zaoui A. et al., Therapie 55(3):379–382 (2000).

[45] Zeiton M.A.M., W.E. Neff, Ol., Corps Gras, Lipides 2(3):245–248 (1995), ref. CA 124:085284x.

Literature references identified by Ü can be found in the general listing of books and monographs at the back of this book.

Borage

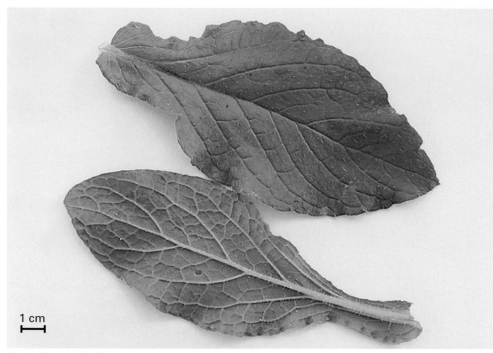

Fig. 1: Borage leaf

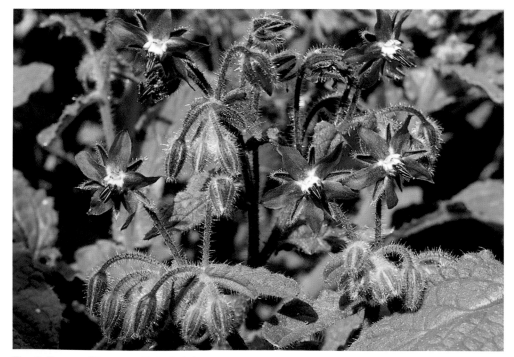

Fig. 2: Borage (*Borago officinalis* L.)

Plant source: *Borago officinalis* L.

Family: Forget-me-not or borage family (Boraginaceae).

Common names: Engl.: borage, talewort; Fr.: bourrache, bourroche; Ger.: Borretsch, Borgel, Gurkenkraut, Gurkenkönig, Himmelsstern, Wohlgemut.

Description: Annual herb, up to 1 m tall, with a single or branched, fleshy stem, bearing stinging bristles. The leaves are alternate, 3 to 20 cm long and 2 to 7 cm wide; the lower ones are elliptic and narrowing towards the stem, and the upper leaves are half-amplexicaul, ovate-oblong, entire-margined and rough due to bristly hairs. The drooping flowers have long pedicels arranged in leafy, umbellate-paniculate inflorescences; the calyx is divided into roughly pubescent tips with a fused base; the corolla is coalescent, with a well-shaped dilated margin with 5 pointed tips and 5 faucal scales at the base, cerulean blue to reddish, rarely white, 1.5 to 2.5 cm wide; the 5 stamina are fused to the corolla, having a broad filament and a violet, horn-like appendix. The anthers are black, the style is filiform with capitate stigma, and the ovary is diphyllous and superior, later forming a fruit which separates into 4 elongated, ovate, 4 to 7 mm long, light-brown nutlets (loculi) with a rough surface and characteristic appendices (rich in fat), which originate from the receptacles. Flowering period is from May to August [22, Ü37, Ü41].

Native origin: Native to the northeastern Mediterranean region, and introduced to Western-, Central- and Eastern Europe, as well as Asia, and America.

Main cultivation areas: Cultivated, almost exclusively on a small scale or in gardens, throughout most of Europe (especially the UK and France), the USA and Canada, India, China, and New Zealand.

Main exporting countries: No export trade of the fresh flowers and leaves. For the medicinal herb (dried), republics of the former Yugoslavia, Bulgaria, and Turkey.

Cultivation: Borage thrives in almost any soil type, however it does especially well in nutritionally rich, fairly moist soil, but with good drainage. Propagation occurs through direct sowing from April until June (darkness requirements for germination). For personal use, one or two plants are sufficient, which, because they produce a substantial amount of fruits, spread rapidly in the garden. The perennial species *B. pygmaea* (DC.) CHATER et GREUTER (*B. laxiflora* POIR.) can also be cultivated, although it requires protection from severe winter frost. The variety 'Alba' has white flowers [Ü41, Ü46, Ü96].

Culinary herb

Commercial forms: Rarely commercially traded. In the vegetable trade, the fresh leaves are occasionally offered, and for medicinal use, the fatty oil of the seeds. Dried borage herb is not traded as a culinary herb due to the rapid loss of its aroma, color and flavor.

Production: For medicinal end-use, the herb or flowers are harvested during the flowering period and dried. To obtain the nutlets, the herb is harvested in August, as soon as the plant begins to turn brown. After drying, it is threshed. For personal use, the young leaves and flowers can be plucked and used fresh [Ü41].

Forms used: The fresh young leaves, fresh flowers, and for dietetic purposes, the fatty oil, and very rarely for medicinal purposes, the dried herb and the dried flowers.

Storage: The leaves should always be harvested while they are still fresh since they wilt quickly. The dried herb loses its aroma

after a short time; it should be stored in a cool place, protected from light and moisture, in porcelain-, glass- or suitable metal containers.

Description. Whole leaf (Fig. 1): The fresh leaves for culinary use and the dried inflorescences for medicinal applications; see description of the whole plant.

Odor and **Taste** of the fresh leaves and flowers are cucumber-like.

History: Borage was probably first cultivated by the Arabs, probably predominantly for medicinal purposes. In antiquity, the plant was believed to have antidepressant effects. By the Middle Ages, it reached Europe, and since the 16th century, it has been a popular culinary herb [Ü56, Ü92].

Constituents and Analysis

Constituents

▪ Essential oil: Very small amounts, containing n-nona-2,6-dienal and n-nona-2,6-diene-1-ol [Ü92].
▪ Mucilage: About 10%, mostly galactoarabinoglucans [3].
▪ Pyrrolizidine alkaloids: 0.0001 to 0.001%, consisting of amabiline, supinine and the stereoisomeric pairs lycopsamine and intermedine as well as 7-acetyllycopsamine and acetylintermedine [9, 10, 16, 18, Ü100].
▪ Silicic acid: Partially in form of water-soluble salts; 1.5 to 2.2% [Ü37].
▪ Cyanogenic glycosides: Trace amounts [21].
▪ Hydroxycinnamic acid derivatives ("labiate tannins"): About 1.7%, rosmarinic acid (0.05 to 0.7%) and chlorogenic acid, among others [4, 8].
▪ Flavonoids [4].
▪ Hydroxycoumarins: Scopoletin [4].
The fruits, which are not used as a spice, contain, among others, fatty oil (30 to 40%) with a high amount (about 20%) of nutritionally important γ-linolenic acid [2, 6, 15, 19].

Tests for Identity based on macroscopic and microscopic analyses. The alkaloids can be detected, according to Ph Fr, after extraction with methanol, evaporation to dryness, redissolving the residue in sulfuric acid and precipitation with potassium tetraiodomercurate (Mayer's reagent) or potassium iodobismuthate (Dragendorff's reagent).

Quantitative assay: Spectrophotometric determination of the unsaturated pyrrolizidine alkaloids [11, 12]; determination of the rosmarinic acid content with GC after silylation [14].

Adulterations, Misidentifications and Impurities can be excluded due to the characteristic habitus and morphology of the plant.

Actions and Uses

Actions: On the basis of its aromatic taste, appetite-stimulating effects should be assumed. Other scientifically substantiated actions are not known.

Toxicology: Pyrrolizidine alkaloids with double bonds at position 1,2 of the necine-structure and esterification at the C-1 hydroxymethyl-group, containing branched carboxylic acids with at least 5 C-atoms, have hepatotoxic, pneumotoxic and carcinogenic effects. Esterification of the OH-group at position 7 of the necine ring intensifies this effect [17, 20, Ü100]. The pyrrolizidine alkaloids in borage have all these structural requirements for toxicity. Five leaves contain about 1 to 10 μg of alkaloids. 1 μg is the official upper daily limit for medicinal applications (limited to a 6 weeks dosage regimen) [1, 5]. The toxicologically relevant limit can therefore be exceeded with the use of this herb as a spice.

Culinary use: Borage leaves should not be cooked with foods. They are added to warm meals shortly before serving. Due to the stinging, bristly hairs, the leaves must be chopped very finely.

Freshly picked, young, chopped leaves are used as a spice for salads, especially cucumber salads, but also tomato-, zucchini- and potato salads, for stews (e.g. potato soup), vegetables in butter, noodle stuffing, meat sauces, salsa, mustard sauces, egg dishes, yogurt, sour cream, cottage cheese, soft cheese, herb butter, and summer beverages, as well as for pickling cucumbers.

Young, chopped leaves are also eaten raw as salad, and, like chives, as a bread topping or cooked as a vegetable (often together with mangold: Ligurian risotto) [Ü63, Ü70, Ü95]. Because, in this way, one consumes relatively large amounts of the herb, this type of use for borage is not advisable.

Freshly plucked flowers serve as a spice and garnish for salads (added just before serving because it wilts and loses its color rapidly), cold fruit and vegetable soups, chilled summer beverages, and to add a blue color to herb vinegars. They can also be candied [Ü55, Ü74, Ü79].

The dried herb and dried leaves have almost no aroma.

Even though the probability of harm to human health from the use of borage is extremely low, a residual risk from its use cannot be completely ruled out. Nonetheless, for those who just cannot do without borage, it should be used sparingly and not too frequently due to its content of toxic pyrrolizidine alkaloids (see above).

Combines well with: Anise, dill, garlic, lemon balm, and salad burnet.

As a component of spice mixes and preparations: → Frankfurter green sauce, → Herb butter, → Salad spice.

Medicinal herb

Herbal drugs: Boraginis herba (sommité fleurie de bourrache) [Ph Fr 2000], Boraginis flos (fleur de bourrache) [Ph Fr 2000].

Indications: In folk medicine, borage is used as an expectorant (due to mucilage), as an anti-inflammatory remedy for kidney- and bladder ailments (due to soluble silicic acid), for menopausal syndrome and for venous inflammations, among other uses [Ü37]. Because its efficacy has not been substantiated and due to its content of toxic pyrrolizidine alkaloids, the German Commission E did not approve the medicinal use of borage herb or flowers [7].

Similar spice herbs

Comfrey, *Symphytum officinale* L. (Boraginaceae), is often mentioned in the popular scientific literature as a spice or vegetable, although, the young leaves especially, which contain a relatively high level of pyrrolizidine alkaloids (up to 0.009%), should not be used as an edible spice or vegetable. The same holds true for other *Symphytum*-species (*S. tuberosum* L., *S.* × *uplandicum* NYM., *S. asperum* LEP.) [13, Ü100].

Literature

[1] Anonym, Z. Phytother. 13(5):8 (1992).
[2] Anonym, Dtsch. Apoth. Ztg. 139(3): 268–271 (1999).
[3] Franz G., Planta Med. 17(3):217–220 (1969).
[4] Gudej J., M. Tomczyk, Herb. Pol. 42(4): 252–256 (1996).
[5] Habs M. et al., Dtsch. Apoth. Ztg. 132(38): 1939 (1992).
[6] Ippen H., Z. Phytother. 16(3):167–170 (1995).
[7] Kommission E beim BfArM, Anz.-Nr. 127 vom 12.07.1991.
[8] Lamaison J.L. et al., Ann. Pharm. Franc. 48:103–108 (1990).
[9] Larson K.M., F.R. Stermitz, J. Nat. Prod. 47(4):747–748 (1984).
[10] Luethy J. et al., Pharm. Acta Helv. 59(9/10):242–246 (1984).
[11] Mattocks A.R., Anal. Chem. 39:443–447 (1967).
[12] Mattocks A.R., Anal. Chem. 40: 1749–1750 (1968).
[13] Mütterlein R., C.G. Arnold, Pharm. Ztg.-Wissensch. 138(5/6):119–125 (1993).
[14] Reschke A., Z. Lebensm. Unters. Forsch. 176:116–119 (1983).
[15] Richter Th., Z. Phytother. 19(2):102 (1998).
[16] Röder E., Dtsch. Apoth. Ztg. 132(45): 2427–2435 (1992).
[17] Röder E., Current Organic Chemistry 3:557–576 (1999).
[18] Röder E., Pharmazie 50(2):83–98 (1995).
[19] Sun Q., Zhongcaoyao 26(9):456–457 (1995), zitiert in CA 124:112372h.
[20] Teuscher E., U. Lindequist in: R. Saller, H. Feiereis (Hrsg.): Erweiterte Schulmedizin. Anwendung in Diagnostik und Therapie Bd. 1, H. Marseille Verlag, München 1993, p. 68–76.
[21] Van Valen F., Prod. K. Ned. Akad. Wet., Ser. C, 82(2):171–176 (1979).
[22] Weymar H., Buch der Lippenblütler und Rauhblattgewächse, Neumann Verlag, Radebeul 1961.

Literature references identified by Ü can be found in the general listing of books and monographs at the back of this book.

Caper

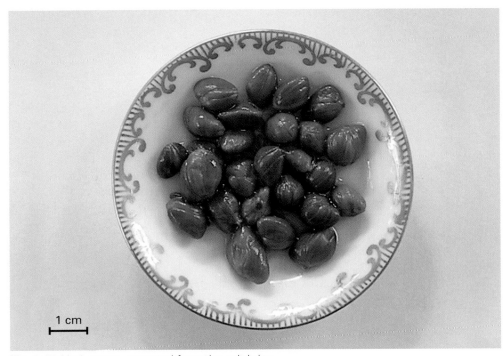

Fig. 1: Pickled capers, removed from the salt brine

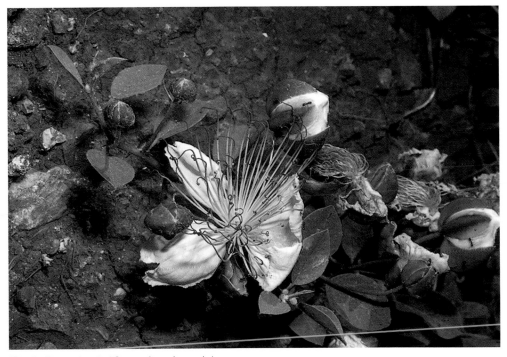

Fig. 2: Caper bush (*Capparis spinosa* L.)

Plant source: *Capparis spinosa* L.

Taxonomic classification: There are numerous subspecies, varieties or forms of *C. spinosa*, some of which are also considered to be separate species (e.g. *C. rupestris* SIBTH. et SM., *C. aegyptica* LAM., *C. mucronifolia* BOISS.).

Family: Caper family (Capparaceae, synonym Capparidaceae).

Common names: Engl.: caper, caper-bush, caper-plant; Fr.: câprier; Ger.: Kapern, Echter Kapernstrauch, Kapperstrauch.

Description: Up to 1 m tall shrub, branched, often climbing. Leaves with 2 backwards pointing thorns on each base, alternate, short petiolate, simple, round, mostly reddish pruinose at the veins, petioles and young twigs. Large flowers with long stalks, arranged singly in the axils of the leaves; 4 free sepals, 4 free, large, whitish to reddish petals, numerous stamina with small anthers and long, reddish-purple filaments, ovary with nearly sessile stigma and long gynophore. The fruit is a berry with many seeds, plum-sized, at first 5 cm long and 3 cm wide and cucumber-like, later developing into a 2-valved capsule [Ü42].

Native origin: Mediterranean region to the Caucasus, Turkestan, Tibet, Africa up to the Sahara, India, and Southeastern Asia.

Main cultivation areas: Mediterranean region, especially Southern France, the Balearic Islands and Cyprus, Spain, Algeria, Morocco and Italy, as well as in the southern Russian Federation, and in the USA (especially California).

Main exporting countries: Spain, France, Morocco, Italy, and Algeria.

Cultivation: The caper shrub needs over-winter temperatures of at least 8 °C, and thus can only be grown in countries with relatively warm winter temperatures, e.g. in the Mediterranean region. It is propagated by suckers. The first harvest is already possible one year after planting. The highest yields come from 6 to 8 years old shrubs. A caper tree remains productive until about 50 years. The annual yield per shrub amounts to about 0.5 to 3.0 kg [Ü89, Ü92].

Culinary herb

Commercial forms: Capers: Pickled in vinegar, brine or oil, closed flower buds, classified in six categories depending on their size: **Nonparailles** (4 to 7 mm, tightly closed, round, mild), **Surfines** (7 to 8 mm, mostly tightly closed), **Capucines** (8 to 9 mm, mostly tightly closed), **Capotes** (9 to 10 mm, mostly tightly closed), **Fines** (12 to 13 mm, mostly tightly closed) and **Hors calibres** (Communes, 13 to 15 mm, mostly tightly closed). The smaller the bud, the higher the quality. [Ü13, Ü98]. Italian varieties include **Capperone**, **Capres commune** (both large), and **Capres en races** (not sorted). Spanish varieties include **Comun** and **Malloquinqua**. The unripe fruits, fermented in brine, are rarely traded, mainly in Spain (**Caper berries**, Fr. cornichons de câprier; Ger.: Kaperngurken), usually with an about 5 cm long gynophore.

Production: It is possible to pick the unopened flower buds daily, before sunrise, when they are still relatively small, from the end of May until the beginning of September. Post-harvest they are washed and then after wilting for one day, usually in the shade, they are sorted according to size using screens. Then they are preserved either in 5% vinegar with the added cooking salt or in the first instance fermented in water for 4 to 7 days and afterwards in 10 to 12% common salt solution, and after a few days in 15 to 18% common salt solution (lactic fermentation). Preservation is done by placing the buds in a salt solution (6%) with acetic acid (1%), in oil or imbedding them in salt [2, 18, Ü30, Ü42, Ü92].

Forms used: Flower buds, whole or chopped, pickled in salt or vinegar brine.

Storage: In the refrigerator, always immersed in brine. Shelf life is 2 to 3 years.

Description. Whole flower bud (Fig. 1): Flower buds, up to 1.5 cm long, up to 0.7 cm wide, roundish-tetragonal, oblique-ovoid, somewhat flattened; they should be small (the small buds are especially valued), olive-green to blue-green, lightly pointed, hard, not soft and not sap-green [Ü30]. For more information see description of the whole plant.

Taste of capers pickled with vinegar: Somewhat sourish, salty, weakly pungent, **Odor:** Sourish.

History: The caper bush was already mentioned in the Bible (Old Testament) and was also known to the ancient Egyptians. In Mediterranean regions, it has been a popular spice for centuries [Ü92].

Constituents and Analysis

Constituents

- Glucosinolates: In the flower buds (as well as in the leaves and seeds), the main component is glucocapparin. Catalyzed by the enzyme myrosinase, which is stored in the myrosine cells, mustard oils are formed due to cleavage of the glucosinolates after tissue damage (Fig. 12, General Section) glucocapparin is converted to methyl mustard oil (methylisothiocyanate, with pungent taste, volatile). After fermentation, other constituents have also been detected in the steam distillate, including isopropyl mustard oil (isopropylisothiocyanate) and sec.-butyl mustard oil (sec.-butylisothiocyanate) [2, 12, 15]. In the leaves (and roots), indole glucosinolates also occur, particularly glucobrassicin (3-indolylmethylglucosinolate), which presumably is also present in the flower buds. Glucobrassicin converts after cleavage to 3-hydroxymethylindole and thiocyanic acid (see Fig.: → Mustard) [19].
- Essential oil: Among others, linalool, cis-linalool oxide and aliphatic hydrocarbons [2].
- Phenolcarboxylic acids: Including, among others, p-methoxy benzoic acid [13].
- Flavonoids: Especially rutin (about 0.5%, in the leaves about 4%) as well as kaempferol-3-O-glucoside, kaempferol-3-O-rutinoside and kaempferol-3-O-rhamnorutinoside [8, 17, 20].
- Polyterpenes: Aliphatic polyprenols with 12, 13 or 14 isoprene units: cappaprenol-12, cappaprenol-13 and cappaprenol-14 [21].
- Elementary sulfur [9].

Tests for Identity: Analysis of the essential oil constituents with TLC, GC or GC-MS [1].

Quantitative assay: The content and fingerprint of the glucosinolates can be determined with HPLC (detection of the desulfoglucosinolates) [14, 19, → Watercress].

Adulterations, Misidentifications and Impurities are possible, especially with pickled flower buds from scotch broom, lesser celandine, marsh marigold or → Garden nasturtium, (these species are described below). The flowers of these

Glucocapparin   Methyl mustard oil   Isopropyl mustard oil R = H
sec.-Butyl mustard oil R = CH$_3$

plants are quinate. Sometimes, pickled capers also contain fruits of the plant in form of longish berries with many seeds; they can, however, be differentiated from genuine capers by their characteristic appearance. Occasionally, to increase coloration the illegal addition of copper ions as a fining agent has been noted (perceptible by deep green color!).

Actions and Uses

Actions: Due to their pungent taste, they are appetizing and digestion promoting.
In animal tests (carrageen edema in rats), extracts of the plants have shown antiphlogistic action [2]. The polyterpenes are considered to be the antiinflammatory active principles [21]. *p*-Methoxybenzoic acid isolated from the plant has good antihepatotoxic activity. It provided protection to rats with carbon tetrachloride- and paracetamol-induced liver damage [13]. Aqueous extracts of the plant (15 µg/ml nutrient medium) completely inhibited the growth of a few fungi (*Microsporium canis, Trichophyton violaceum*) [3].

Toxicology: Based on existing data, there is no acute or chronic toxicity with the normal use of capers by healthy individuals. Due to the skin and mucous membrane irritating effects of the mustard oils, an irritating effect on renal tissue is possible in predisposed patients with kidney disease. After the intake of large amounts, gastrointestinal disturbances are possible even in healthy individuals.
The sensitization potential appears to be low. Contact dermatitis has been described in one case of cutaneous application of the plant as a wet compress [4].

Culinary use: Capers, usually chopped, serve as a spice in piquant sauces (caper-, caper tomato-, caper-chives-, ravigote-, tuna fish-, tapénade-, among others), remoulade, mayonnaise and marinades, which are served mainly with fish and fish salads as well as cold beef or poultry. Especially popular are German Königsberger meatballs and the Italian vitello tonnato (cold veal with tuna fish caper sauce). Capers are also well suited as a spicy side dish with steak tartar, chicken fricassee, calf fricassee, fish ragout, salads (egg salad, meat salad, rice salad, herring salad, tuna fish salad, sausage salad, cheese salad), fish dishes (e.g. salmon dishes, fried fish), egg dishes, roll of ham, quark, pâté, Italian hors d'oeuvres (antipasti, e.g. sweet-sour eggplant salad) and pizzas. To meals that must be cooked, capers should be added after the end of the cooking process due to the volatility of the methyl mustard oil [Ü2, Ü30, Ü56, Ü68, Ü80, Ü95, Ü111]. Caper berries are suitable as a side dish with cheese and sausage plates [Ü13].

Combines well with: Black pepper, cooking mustard, dill, horseradish, and onions.

As a component of spice mixes and preparations: → Meat spice, → Mixed pickles spice, → Tartar sauce.

Medicinal herb

Herbal drug: Capparidis flos, Caper flowers, or flower buds preserved in vinegar, common salt or oil.

Indications: In the Arab countries, the herb is decocted for treatment of arthritic pains [21].

Similar culinary spices

The flower buds of *Capparis rupestris* SIBTH. et SMITH, native to Greece, *C. aegyptica* LAM. (Both species are also understood to be subspecies or forms of *C. spinosa*), native to Egypt, *Capparis ovata* DESF. (Syn. *C. herbacea* WILLD., today often also included in the species *C. spinosa* L.), native to the Caucasus region, the Crimea as well as Turkey, and *C. aphylla* ROTH, Pakistan, used in the same ways as *C. spinosa* L. [Ü42].

Pilewort buds (lesser celandine), buds of *Ranunculus ficaria* L. (Ranunculaceae), pickled in vinegar, the plant is native to and wild collected in Europe, the Near East and Northern Africa. A main constituent is ranunculin, which breaks down in bruised plant tissue by enzyme action to release protoanemonin (pungent tasting, see General Chapter 2, Fig. 13) [7, Ü100].

Marsh marigold buds, buds of *Caltha palustris* L. (Ranunculaceae), pickled in vinegar, the plant is native to and wild collected in Europe, Asia Minor, Central Asia, Northern Asia, Eastern Asia and North America. A main constituent is ranunculin, which breaks down in bruised plant tissue by enzyme action to release protoanemonin (pungent tasting, see General Chapter 2, Fig. 13). Furthermore, it contains triterpene saponins and small amounts of aporphine alkaloids, especially corytuberin [5, 6, 10, 11]. Although the quantity of protoanemonin that is formed is very low, there is one case described in the older literature of poisoning after ingestion of large quantities of the plant (the leaves eaten as a salad) [Ü58].

Scotch broom buds (goat capers), buds of *Cytisus scoparius* (L.) LINK (*Sarothamnus scoparius* (L.) WIMM., Fabaceae), the plant is native to and wild collected in Western-, Southern- and Central Europe, northward up to southern Sweden, eastward up to the Ukraine, and naturalized along the American coast. Constituents include tyramine (up to 2%), quinolizidine alkaloids (0.004%), of which the main alkaloid is (-)-sparteine [16]. Its use is not recommended due to the high content of tyramine (about 100 mg can cause a migraine headache attack) [Ü100].

Bladder nut buds, buds of *Staphylea pinnata* L. (Staphyleaceae), pickled in vinegar, the plant is native to and wild collected in Central Europe to southern Italy, Bulgaria, western Ukraine and southwestern Asia. Grown in gardens, especially in Georgia (Europe) and northern Armenia, it is used as a spice [Ü61].

Unripe fruits of garden nasturtium → Garden nasturtium.

Tapénade (Sauce Provençal).
2 tablespoons of drained capers, 4 anchovy filets, 4 to 5 black, pitted olives, 200 ml olive oil, lemon juice, black pepper.

Crush the capers, anchovies and olives in a mortar, and slowly add the oil to the paste. Season to taste with lemon juice and black pepper. This sauce is a perfect condiment for hardboiled eggs, cold fish and meat salads [Ü55].

Caper spurge fruits, fruits of *Euphorbia lathyris* L. (mole plant, Euphorbiaceae), occasionally pickled in vinegar, and used as a substitute for capers. They contain, among others, the strong skin- and mucous membrane irritating and likely cocarcinogen ingenol-3-hexadecanic acid esters. Their use should absolutely be avoided [Ü34].

Literature

[1] Afsharypuor S. et al., Pharm. Acta Helv. 72(5):307–309 (1998).

[2] Ageel A.M. et al., Agents Actions 17:383 (1985).

[3] Ali-Shtayeh M.S., S.I. Ghdwib, Mycoses 42(11/12):665–672 (1999).

[4] Angelini G. et al.. Contact Dermatitis 24(5):382–383 (1991).

[5] Bhandari P. et al., Planta Med. 53(1):98–100 (1987).

[6] Bonora A. et al., Phytochemistry 26:2277 (1987), ref. in Ü100 (1987).

[7] Bonora A. et al., Biochem. Physiol. Pflanz. 183:443, ref. in Ü100 (1988).

[8] Brauns D.H., Arch. Pharm. 242:556 (1904), ref. in Ü43.

[9] Brevard H. et al., Flavour Fragrance J. 7:313–321 (1992).

[10] Bruni A. et al., J. Nat. Prod. 49(6): 1172–1173 (1986).

[11] Czygan F.Ch., Dtsch. Apoth. Ztg. 139(42): 4032–4034 (1999).

[12] Delaveau P., Bull. Soc. Botan. France 105:225 (1958), ref. in Ü43 (1958).

[13] Gadgoli C., S.H. Mishra, J. Ethnopharmacol. 66(2):187–192 (1999).

[14] Hrncirik K. et al., Z. Lebensm. Unters. Forsch. A 206:103–107 (1997).

[15] Kjaer A. et al., Acta Chem. Scand. 14: 1226 (1960), ref. in Ü43.

[16] Murakoshi I. et al., Phytochemistry 25: 521–524 (1986).

[17] Rodrigo A. et al., J. Food Sci. 57:152–154 (1992).

[18] Sanchez A. et al., J. Food Sci. 57:675–678 (1992).

[19] Schraudolf H., Phytochemistry 28: 259–260 (1989).

[20] Tuerkoez S. et al., J. Fac. Pharm. Gazi. Univ. 12(1):17–21 (1995), ref. in CA 124:025571d.

[21] al-Said M.S. et al., Pharmazie 43(9): 640–641 (1988).

Literature references identified by Ü can be found in the general listing of books and monographs at the back of this book.

Caraway

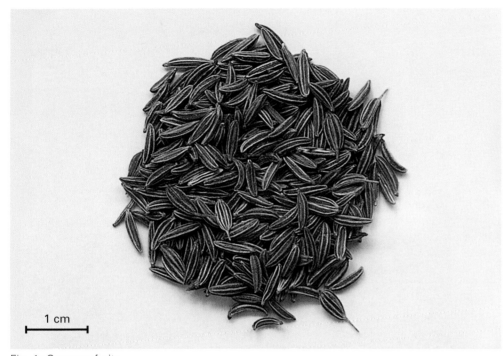

Fig. 1: Caraway fruits

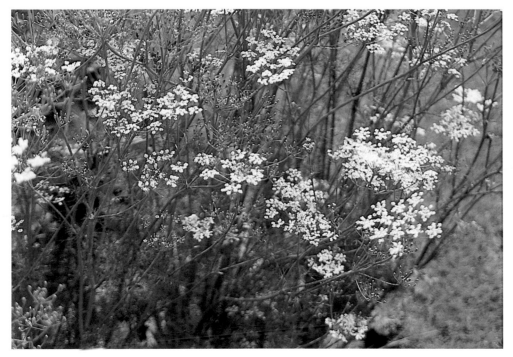

Fig. 2: Caraway (*Carum carvi* L.)

Plant source: *Carum carvi* L.

Family: Umbelliferous plants (Apiaceae, synonym Umbelliferae).

Common names: Engl.: caraway (sometimes also inaccurately referred to as → Cumin); Fr.: semence de carvi, cumin de prés, anis des Vosges; Ger.: Kümmel, Wiesen-Kümmel, Feld-Kümmel, Echter Kümmel, Carve.

Description: Biennial to perennial herb, 0.3 to 1.0 m in height, with spindle-shaped taproot, forming only one basal rosette in the 1st year; in the 2nd year 1 to 3 flowering stalks emerge. The leaves are alternate, petiolate, sheath-like at the base, glabrous, 2-fold, partially 3-fold pinnate; main and secondary stems each bearing a terminal, composite umbel with 8 to 16 rays, involucre and small involucres mostly absent. Flowers are radial with 5 petals, white to light pink, 5 stamina, 2 styles, inferior ovary, bilocular; the fruits are double achenes (cremocarps), which are separated into their mericarps, attached to a bifurcate carpophore. Flowering period is from May to June [32].

Native origin: Probably native to temperate Asia, caraway is now widely distributed, in North- and Central Europe, Siberia, the Caucasus region, the Near East, the Himalayas, Mongolia and Morocco, among others, and has been naturalized in North America, New Zealand, and in some parts of South America.

Main cultivation areas: Egypt, Poland, Denmark, Hungary, Turkey, the Netherlands, the Czech Republic, Spain, the Russian Federation, Morocco and the USA, and furthermore it is cultivated in, among other countries, Yugoslavia, England, Germany, France, Norway, Sweden, Finland, India, and Central Asia.

Main exporting countries: Poland, the Netherlands, Hungary, and Egypt.

Cultivation: Caraway prefers damp, humus soil (but not with standing moisture), if possible chalky, but under no circumstances acidic soil, in sunny or half shade locations protected from wind. Seeds can be sown from March to May or at the beginning of August, spaced in rows of 30 cm. The seeds should only be lightly covered (germination is light dependent), and after the plants emerge they can be thinned out to about 15 cm apart. From biennial forms, the first harvest takes place in July of the second year. Cultivars grown in Germany and Austria include, among others, 'Arterner', 'Bleija', 'Konczewicki', 'Niederdeutscher', 'Record', 'Sylvia' and 'Volhouden', and occasionally annual varieties of caraway are cultivated (e.g. 'Karzo') [Ü14, Ü17, Ü21]. There are cultivation experiments with annual caraway that have not, up to this point, attained satisfactory quality [21].

Culinary herb

Commercial forms: Caraway seeds: dried mericarps, whole, coarsely ground or crushed. Fruits originating from Holland are larger, and caraway from Eastern European countries are smaller ("straw caraway") than those grown in Central Europe. The darker the color of the fruit, the lower the commercial value. Caraway essential oil and caraway oleoresin are also commercially traded.

Production: Caraway is harvested, usually with a field swather and combine, when the seeds begin to turn brown. The fruits are dried on floor-level, turned over frequently, in a cold ventilated facility or in warm air (max. 35 ºC) [Ü21]. When growing caraway in the garden, the infructescences should be cut off and stored to mature in a shady, aerated location, and

then the fruits are scraped off and dried in a thin layer.

Forms used: The whole, dried fruits, crushed fruits, and rarely also the broken or ground fruits. The fresh leaves and roots are rarely used.

Storage: The fresh leaves and roots can be stored wrapped in plastic bags in the refrigerator for a few days. The dried fruits are kept in tightly sealed metal- or glass containers, protected from light and moisture; the shelf life is several years. Ground caraway loses its aroma rapidly.

Description. Whole fruit (Fig. 1): Gray-brown, glabrous, mostly crescent-shaped, 3 to 7 mm long, 1 to 2 mm wide mericarps with 5 prominent, lighter-colored ribs, which give the cross-section of the single fruit an irregular, pentagonal shape. In the grooves between ribs, there is a secretory canal; the commissural surface contains two oil streaks. The white endosperm fills the entire seed.

Caraway powder is dark brown and contains many fragments of the mostly brown secretory canals with long, transversal cells, numerous cells of the endosperm with aleuron grains, oil droplets and small

calcium oxalate rosettes; also present are single stone cells from the upper part of the ribs as well as fragments of the vessels with sclerenchymatic fibers (Fig. 3). Stout fibers with over 20 µm thick vessels (from the stems and the rays of the umbels) and starch must be absent [Ü49].

Odor: Aromatic, **Taste:** Spicy, slightly pungent.

History: Caraway is probably one of the oldest spices. Discoveries found in Neolithic lake dwellings along the sub-alpine zone indicate its early use. Caraway was also found in the tomb of Tutankhamen (born in 1336 or 1337 BCE). In Central Europe, its first use has been documented in the imperial decree by Karl the Great ("Capitulare de villis", authored in about 796 CE, see footnote under → Anise). At the beginning of the 12th century, caraway was cultivated by the Arabs in Morocco and Spain. Later, in the 13th century, it also reached England. Hieronymus Bock, in his herbal compendium (1546), considered caraway the most useful Arabian spice and medicinal plant for its frequent use in cooking, baking and as a medicinal remedy [Ü92].

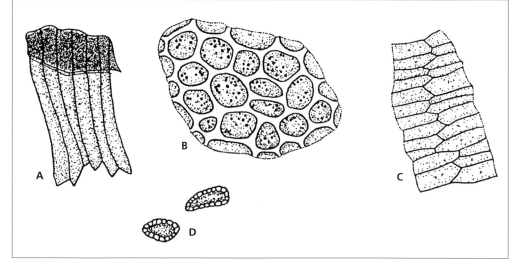

Fig. 3: Caraway. **A** Transversal cells with secretory canal underneath, **B** Cells from the endosperm with minute calcium oxalate rosettes, **C** Transversal cells, **D** Stone cells from the upper part of the ribs. From Ü49

Constituents and Analysis

DIN and ISO-Standards: ISO-Standard 5561 (Caraway).

Constituents of the fruits

- Essential oil: 3 to 8%, high content in materials from humid, maritime climates in the temperate zones (such as the Netherlands, Northern Germany and Scandinavia); low content in annual varieties. The main constituents are (*S*)-(+)-carvone (D-carvone, as the main odoriferous compound, 50 to 80%) and (*R*)-(+)-limonene (up to 49%). Carvone and limonene make up 90 to 98% of the total essential oil content. Also present are myrcene, α-phellandrene, *p*-cymene, β-caryophyllene, *cis*- and *trans*-carveol, *cis*- and *trans*-dihydrocarvone, *trans*-dihydrocarveol, terpinolene [4, 7, 20, 24–26, Ü30]. Caraway from Egypt was found to contain mostly carvone (81%) and *p*-cymene (16%) [13].
- Phenylacrylic acids: Phenolcarboxylic acids (about 0.35%), particularly caffeic acids, in part ester-like bound with quinic acid (chlorogenic acid, 4-caffeoylquinic acid, 3-caffeoylquinic acid); also present are *p*-coumaroyl- and feruloylquinic acids [2].
- Flavonoids: About 0.4%, mainly isoquercitrin and quercetin-3-(*O*-caffeoyl)-glucoside; furthermore, quercetin-3-*O*-β-D-glucuronide (miquelianin) and astragalin (kaempferol-3-*O*-glucoside) [10, 17].
- Furanocoumarins (in traces): Bergaptene and xanthotoxin, among others [Ü37].
- Fatty oil (10 to 22%), with up to 25% petroselinic acid bound in the triacylglycerols [Ü37].
- Protein (about 25%).
- Polysaccharides (about 13%): Particularly β(1→4)-mannans; starch is absent [11].

Constituents of the leaves

- Essential oil: Mostly composed of sesquiterpenes, including β-caryophyllene, elemene, α-caryophyllene (humulene), cadinene and germacrene, among others [Ü37].

Constituents of the roots

- Essential oil: Containing predominantly aliphatic aldehydes [Ü37].

Tests for Identity: Organoleptic, macroscopic and microscopic analyses as well as TLC of the extract [31, Ph Eur] or the essential oil [8, 12, Ü101], using GC [1, 9] or HPLC [15, 23].

Quantitative analysis: The essential oil content can be determined volumetrically with steam distillation and xylol in the graduated tube [Ph Eur]. For analysis of the extract see [16].

Adulterations, Misidentifications and Impurities: Unlikely. Due to the characteristic appearance and typical odor adulterations are excluded. Indian caraway (*Carum gracile* LINDLE) looks similar but has a different odor. Impurities from the seeds and fruits of weeds and unripe caraway fruits are sometimes encountered.

Actions and Uses

Actions: Caraway increases the secretion of saliva and gastric juice as well as bile excretion and intestinal motility and therefore has appetizing and digestion promoting action [19, 27, 28]. Caraway has shown a distinctive spasmolytic effect in animal experiments (guinea pig ileum). Aqueous-ethanolic extracts of caraway fruit (2.5 or 10 ml/liter) counteracted the spasmodic action of acetylcholine and histamine, similar to atropine [5, 6]. Likewise, caraway essential oil showed a relaxant effect on isolated guinea pig trachea (ED$_{50}$ 27 mg/liter) [22]. Carvone-enantiomers were more strongly active than the essential oil [29].

In mice, carvone and limonene have been shown to induce the production of the detoxifying enzyme glutathione S-transferase, which suppresses the biotransformation of carcinogenic substances to their active forms [34]. Similar to all essential oils, caraway oil has antimicrobial action. Effective dilutions with an effect on bacteria range from, depending on the species, 1 : 150 (V/V, for *Pseudomonas aeruginosa*) and 1 : 2600 (V/V, for *Bacillus subtilis*) [18].

Toxicology: Based on existing data, there is no acute or chronic toxicity with the normal use of caraway as a spice. The intake of high amounts of caraway extracts (for example in form of caraway tea as an abortive) or of caraway essential oil (in caraway spirits) can lead to irritation of the kidneys. The sensitization potential is small. Allergic reactions are possible however, in individuals who are allergic to other Apiaceae plants (e.g. celery, carrots, parsley, anise, fennel, cumin, coriander) or mugwort, a plant of the aster family (celery-mugwort-spice-syndrome) [30, 33, Ü39].

Culinary use: The greatest consumption of caraway is in German and Austrian cooking. But it also plays a big role in the cooking of temperate Asia, Arabia, Egypt, Scandinavia and Russia. In Ireland, caraway is an integral component of Irish stew.

For the best taste impact the fruits are ground in a spice mill immediately before use. Caraway should be added to the meal about 10 minutes before the cooking is finished. In order to use caraway in cooking without actually eating the seeds, they can be placed in a tea ball or in a cloth herb sack. Because some people find caraway completely distasteful, it is appropriate to ask your guests in advance before preparing a meal with caraway. Caraway is used as a topping spice on rolls, pretzels and pretzel sticks, as a spice for bread (farmer's bread, caraway bread, pain d'épices in France, pumpernickel bread), quark and cheese (e.g. Liptauer style cheese spread, Limburger cheese), vegetable dishes (especially braised white cabbage and sauerkraut, red beets, carrots, celery, wild parsnip, parsley roots, onion soup and potato soup), boiled peeled potatoes (add caraway chopped), potatoes boiled unpeeled (add caraway to water in which vegetables have been boiled), fried potatoes, baked potatoes, noodles, sausage products (e.g. for Chümmischüblige, popular in Switzerland), meat dishes (especially pork, but also lamb, calf, goose, and duck), cooking brew from crawfish, lobster and crabs, sauces (especially fish sauces), dips, salads (especially cabbage salad) and as a pickling spice for cucumbers and tomatoes.

Caraway is also recommended as a spice for sweet dishes such as rhubarb marmalade, compotes, apple cake and baked apples. In Great Britain, caraway cake is popular, especially at harvest time. In addition to the usual ingredients (wheat flour, butter, sugar, eggs, baking powder), it contains the pulp of vanilla pod and caraway.

Young caraway leaves, finely chopped, are used in the same way as parsley, as a component of herb butter, as a topping for cream sauces, venison dishes, green salads, vegetable soups and stews. They are added to the dish at the end of the cooking process.

Caraway root can be used as a spice in vegetable soups, but it can also be cooked, similar to wild parsnip, and be prepared as a vegetable with light sauce. In Russia, the roots are marinated and cooked with honey and sugar.

Caraway essential oil is used in the production of liqueurs (Allasch, Aquavit, Bommerlunder, Cloc, Eiskümmel, Kristallkümmel, Gilka-Kümmel, Goldwasser, Maltese Cross) [Ü10, Ü13, Ü19, Ü20, Ü23, Ü51, Ü53, Ü55, Ü56, Ü59, Ü71, Ü73, Ü78, Ü81, Ü90].

Combines well with: Bay leaf, chilies, chives, clove, coriander, garlic, juniper berries, onions, parsley and pepper, but is used predominantly as a separate spice.

As a component of spice mixes and preparations: → Arabian spice mix, → Bologna spice mix, → Bread spice, → Chili con carne spice, → Curry powder, → Fish spice, → Grill spice, → Harissa, → Meat spice, → Quark spice, → Table mustard, → Tunisian spice mix, → Vegetable spice.

Other uses: Caraway essential oils are used in the perfume industry and as a germination-inhibiter for stored potatoes.

Medicinal herb

Herbal drugs: Carvi fructus, Caraway fruit, contains not less than 30 ml/kg of essential oil [Ph Eur], Carvi aetheroleum, Caraway oil, contains not more than 50.0% D-carvone [USP-NF], or 50 to 65% D-carvone [DAB], Aetheroleum Carvi [ÖAB].

Indications: Caraway is used for digestive problems, especially for mild spasms of the gastrointestinal tract, flatulence, bloating, nervous heart-stomach complaints and Roemheld's syndrome. Caraway is used in the form of tea infusions (1 to 5 g freshly crushed or ground fruits per cup; adult daily dose: 1.5 to 6.0 g; children 1 to 4 years: 1 to 2 g; children under 1 year: 1 g), the essential oil (1 to 2 drops on a sugar cube; daily dose: 5 to 6 drops) or prepared medicinal products (usually in combination with fennel essential oil, anise essential oil and/or with aqueous-ethanolic extracts of chamomile flowers) [3, 14, Ü12]. Caraway is used to improve the digestibility of flatulence-causing foods such as cabbage or fresh bread.

In folk medicine, caraway tea is used by nursing mothers to promote the flow of milk (lactagogue) and also to bring on menstruation (emmenagogue).

Similar Spices

Genuine mountain laserwort fruits (from *Laserpitium siler* L., sermountain-laserwort, Apiaceae, also from *Laser trilobum* (L.) BORKH., gladich, three-lobed sermountain), grown in Turkey, where it is used the same as → Cumin, is rarely applied today in Central Europe. It contains about 8% essential oil, of which the main components are limonene (about 60%) and perillaldehyde (about 32%) [Ü61, Ü93].
→ Cumin.
→ Black cumin.

Caraway soup
40 g butter (or margarine), 50 g flour, 1 teaspoon finely cut caraway, 1 garlic clove, 125 g finely shredded Emmentaler cheese, 3 tablespoons of milk, salt, pepper, nutmeg.

Mix melted butter (or margarine) and the flour and brown the mixture in a pan, add 1 l of water while stirring and the garlic clove and season to taste with salt, nutmeg and pepper. Simmer for $1/2$ hour. Stir the Emmentaler cheese with 3 tablespoons of milk and add the soup. Serve with dark bread sprinkled with sugar [Ü59].

Literature

[1] Benecke R., H. Thieme, Zentralbl. Pharm. Pharmakother. Laboratoriumsdiagn. 115(2):155–161 (1976).
[2] Dirks U., K. Herrmann, Zeitschr. Lebensm. Unters. Forsch. 179:12–16 (1984).
[3] ESCOP, ESCOP Monographs, Carvi fructus Caraway (1997).
[4] Fehr D., Pharm. Ztg. 125:1300–1303 (1980).
[5] Forster H., Z. Allgemeinmed. 59:1327–1331 (1983).
[6] Forster H.B. et al., Planta Med. 40(4): 309–319 (1980).
[7] Galambosi B., P. Peura, J. Ess. Oil Res. 8:389–397 (1996).
[8] Glasl H., H. Wagner, Perfum. Flavorist 5(4):6–16 (1980).
[9] Glasl H., H. Wagner, Dtsch. Apoth. Ztg. 114:146 (1974).
[10] Harborne J.B., C.A. Williams, Phytochemistry 11:1741–1750 (1972).
[11] Hopf H., O. Kandler, Phytochemistry 16:1715–1717 (1977).
[12] Hörhammer L. et al., Dtsch. Apoth. Ztg. 104:1398 (1964).
[13] Janssen A.M. et al., Pharm. Weekbl. 10: 277–280 (1988).
[14] Kommission E beim BfArM., BAnz 22a vom 01.02.1990.
[15] Kovar K.A., E. Bock, J. Chromatogr. 160: 199 (1983).
[16] Krüger H., B. Zeiger, Drogenreport 6(10):31–32 (1993).

[17] Kunzemann J., K. Herrmann, Z. Lebensm. Untersuch. Forsch. 164: 194–200 (1977).

[18] Maruzzella J.C., M. Freundlich, J. Am. Pharm. Assoc. 48(6):356–358 (1959).

[19] Micklefield G.H. et al., Phytother. Res. 14(1):20–23 (2000).

[20] Opdyke D.L.J., Food Cosmet. Toxicol. 11:1051 (1973).

[21] Pank F., Herba Germanica 3(3):87–95 (1995).

[22] Reiter M., W. Brandt, Arzneim. Forsch. 35:408–414 (1985).

[23] Ross M.S.F., J. Chromatogr. 160:199 (1978).

[24] Rothbächer H., F. Suteu, Pharmazie 27(5):340–341 (1972).

[25] Salveson A., A. Baerheim Svendsen, Planta Med. 30:93–96 (1979).

[26] Salveson A., A. Baerheim Svendsen, Sci. Pharm. 46(2):93–100 (1978).

[27] Schilcher H., Therapiewoche 36:1100–1112 (1986).

[28] Schilcher H., Dtsch. Apoth. Ztg. 124(29): 1433–1442 (1984).

[29] Schuster K.P., Wirkungsstärke und Wirkungsverluste spasmolytisch wirksamer Arzneidrogen, galenischer Zubereitungen und Arzneifertigwaren, geprüft am isolierten Darm des Meerschweinchens und am Darm der Katze in situ, Dissertation Ludwig-Maximilian-Universität München 1971.

[30] Stäger J. et al., Allergy 46:475–478 (1991).

[31] Stahl E. (Hrsg.), Chromatographische und mikroskopische Analyse von Drogen, Fischer Verlag Stuttgart, New York 1978.

[32] Weymar H., Buch der Doldengewächse, Neumann Verlag, Radebeul 1959.

[33] Wüthrich B., T. Hofer, Dtsch. Med. Wschr. 109:981–986 (1984).

[34] Zheng G.Q. et al., Planta Med. 58(4): 338–341 (1992).

Literature references identified by Ü can be found in the general listing of books and monographs at the back of this book.

Cardamom

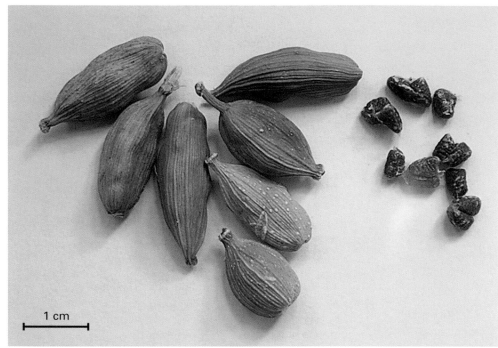

Fig. 1: Cardamom fruits and seeds removed from the capsules

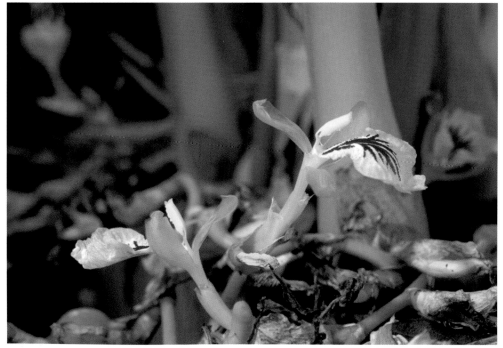

Fig. 2: Cardamom (*Elettaria cardamomum* (L.) MATON)

Plant source: *Elettaria cardamomum* (L.) MATON.

Synonyms: *Elettaria cardamomum* (L.) MATON var. *miniscula* BURKHILL, *Alpinia cardamomum* ROXB., *Amomum cardamomum* L. non ROXB. nec auct. mult.

Taxonomic classification: The true cardamom is supplied by *E. cardamomum* (L.) MATON var. *miniscula* BURKHILL cv. 'Malabar' and cv. 'Mysore'. Fruits of *E. cardamomum* (L.) MATON var. *betamajor* THWAITES (also understood to be a separate species: *E. major* SMITH, see below) is regarded as an adulterant [9].

Family: Ginger family (Zingiberaceae).

Common names: Engl.: cardamom, Chester cardamom; Fr.: cardamomier; Ger.: (der or das) Kardamom, Malabar-Kardamom.

Description: Rhizomatous perennial, 2 to 3 m in height, the 2 to 2.5 cm thick, bulbous, rhizome bears dense, regularly ringed leaf scars and long, strong roots. The sterile pseudo-stalks, 2 to 3 m high, are formed from the long sheaths of the leaves. The up to 75 cm long leaves, are two-rowed arranged, entire-margined, lanceolate and distinctly acuminate and have each other embracing sheaths, the upper leaf surface is softly pubescent and the lower surface has silky hairs and translucent dots. The scapes are up to 60 cm long, running almost parallel to the ground, with densely arranged, ovate leaves at the base, bearing erect inflorescences. The solitary flowers are mostly situated in panicles of 4, in the axils of the upper bracts. Outer perigone (calyx) is tubular, bluntly tridentate, greenish, inner perigone (corolla) greenish-white, tubular in the lower part, expanding towards the top, with a 3-partite fringe, falling off, 6 stamina, the outer whorl forming a petal-like, white lip with yellowish rim and purple or blue, fan-like striations; within the inner whorl, one stamen is fertile, the two other ones are forming threads situated on the inferior, trilocular ovary; the style is filiform with a funnel-shaped, fringed stigma. The fruit is a 6 to 20 mm long, ovoid to oblong, trilocular capsule.

Native origin: Occurs in the southern part of western coastal India ("Malabar Coast" and "Pepper Coast") in damp forests at elevations between 750 and 1,500 m.

Main cultivation areas: India (Mysore, Kerala, Madras, Karnataka, Tamil Nadu), Sri Lanka, Guatemala, Tanzania, Madagascar, and Papua New Guinea.

Main exporting countries: Guatemala, India and Indonesia, as well as Sri Lanka, and Thailand.

Cultivation: The plant requires consistently warm and humid climate as well as deep, well-soaked clay soil. It grows where the annual precipitation is about 2,500 mm. The plant prefers shade and therefore thrives well in forest glade areas. Propagation is carried out mostly with rhizome pieces, and rarely seedlings are used. The seeds have only a low germinating power and require 1 to 2 months to germinate. After growing in planter beds for 10 to 12 months, they are transplanted in suitable forest glade areas or under shade trees. The first bloom takes place in the third year after planting. The best yield is attained after 6 years. The harvest period extends to over 3 to 4 months per year because of the uneven time of ripening of the fruits. The plants are productive for 10 to 15 years [9, Ü89].

Culinary herb

Commercial forms: Cardamom: Closed, dried, mature fruit capsules; varieties include **Green** (artificially dried, green), **Sun dried** (dried in the sun, beige to beige-brown), and **Bleached** (chemically bleached), whole or ground (cardamom ground in the seed coat), **Cardamom seeds:** whole, crushed or coarsely ground. The commercial variety "Allepey Green" is supplied by *E. c.* var. *miniscula* BURKHILL cv. 'Mysore', and the varieties "Coorg Green" and "Coorg Bleached" are supplied by *E. c.* var. *miniscula* BURKHILL cv. 'Malabar'. Cardamom essential oil and cardamom oleoresin are also commercially traded [for details see Lit. 9].

Production: The fruits are harvested shortly before ripening to avoid opening of the capsules. Either the whole panicles or the individual fruits are clipped off with a shears. Afterwards they are washed and often they are stored in heaps for final ripening for a few days, and then sun dried on mats or in drying kilns (so-called curing houses, the first 3 hours at 70 °C, and then at 60 °C until dry). In order to prevent fading during drying, they are pre-treated with a sodium bicarbonate solution. Pieces of fruit stalks and the remains of flower parts are mechanically removed. Leaving the seeds in the fruit capsules should prevent volatilization of the essential oils during transport and storage and also makes it easier to differentiate between high quality grades and inferior grades. In contrast to the green fruits (Greens) that are harvested unripe, the ripe, yellow fruits (Yellows) are always sun dried. White cardamom is produced by bleaching with sulfur dioxide or hydrogen peroxide [11, 13, Ü89].

Forms used: Dried, whole or crushed seeds, and in Southeastern Asia, the whole fruits as well.

Storage: In a cool, dry place, protected from light, in well-closed glass-, porcelain- or suitable metal containers. Storage of the seeds is not recommended due to high essential oil loss by evaporation (30% in 8 months). Cardamom powder should only be stored for a short time (according to DAC, not longer than 24 hours).

Description. Whole fruit and seeds (Fig. 1): Fruits are 0.6 cm to 2.0 cm long, up to 1 cm wide, ovoid or oblong capsules with leather-like, yellowish-green to brownish-gray, up to 1 mm thick walls having distinctly parallel, longitudinal striations (vascular bundles). The blunt end of the capsule bears a small, 1 to 2 mm long, tubular, beak-like projection or the remains of the perigone, usually with a short piece of the pedicel at the base. The seeds are situated inside the capsule in 3 double rows separated by thin partition walls. In each compartment are 4 to 8 angular, reddish-gray to black seeds, 2 to 3 mm long, first attached but easy to separate from each other, covered with an easily removable skin-like membrane (arillus) [DAC].

Powdered seed: The slide preparation with water shows the microscopically distinct starch aggregates which have been released from the perisperm, as well as free starch grains, 1 to 5 μm in diameter. The chloral hydrate slide preparation shows the fragments of the elongated, thick-walled epidermal cells of the testa with a layer of delicate transversal cells beneath and fragments of the palisade-shaped, yellowish or dark-brown stone cell layer as well as thin-walled parenchyma of the perisperm (Fig. 3), fragments of the layer of oil cells, in the shreds of the perisperm, calcium oxalate crystals, 10 μm in diameter, and thin-walled parenchyma of the endosperm and of the embryos [Ü29]. In material which has been ground with the capsules, large parenchyma cells of the fruit wall with almost table-shaped oxalate crystals and interspersed, rather small secretory cavities with yellowish-brown content as well as sclerenchymatic fibers with narrow slit-like pits [Ü49].

Odor: Faintly camphor-like, **Taste:** Aromatic, slightly pungent, spicy, mildly burning.

History: As evidenced by the clay tables from the Nineveh produced during the era of the reign of emperor Assurbanipal (669 to 627 BCE), cardamom was already known to the Babylonians around 700 BCE. It was also mentioned in old Indian literature as "Ela". Theophrastus (372 to

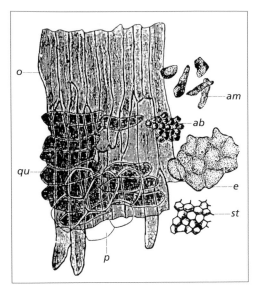

Fig. 3: Cardamom: Shreds of the testa, **o** epidermis, **qu** transverse cell layer, **p** parenchyma, **st** fragments of the layer of stone cells from the testa, **e** pieces of perisperm, **ab** starch granules, **am** starch aggregates. From Ü25.

280 BCE), Dioscorides (2nd half of the 1st century) and Plinius the Elder (23 to 79 CE) described its use as well. Cardamom was the preferred and recommended spice in the Roman cookbook "De re coquinaria", which is attributed to the Roman gourmet Apicius (see footnote in → Asafetida). The first Chinese texts documenting its use were dated 720 CE. It was introduced to Central Europe in the late Middle Ages, and in 1559, it was mentioned, for example, in the city ordinance of Cologne, regulating the trade with cardamom [9, Ü76].

Constituents and Analysis

DIN- and ISO-Standards: DIN-Standard 10206 (Cardamom, technical specifications), ISO-Standard 882-1 (Whole cardamom), ISO-Standard 882-2 (Ground cardamom), ISO-Standard 4733-1981 (Cardamom oil).

Constituents

- Essential oil: In the fruits 3 to 7.5% (lower content in the yellow variety), in

the seeds 4 to 10%. Over 120 constituents have been detected. The composition strongly depends on the region of origin, variety and degree of ripeness. The main components are usually monoterpenes: α-terpinyl acetate (28 to 50%), 1,8-cineole (2 to 44%), sabinene (3 to 5%), limonene (2 to 14%), menthone (up to 6%), linalyl acetate (1.6 to 7.7%), linalool (0.4 to 3.7%), β-phellandrene (3%), β-terpineol (0.7 to 2.1%), furthermore, among others, α-terpineol, α-pinene, myrcene, *p*-cymene, geraniol, nerol, nerolidol, borneol and 2-methylhept-2-ene-6-one. The most important odoriferous components are α-terpinyl acetate, 1,8-cineole, linalyl acetate and linalool [6–9, 14, Ü37].
- Hydroxycinnamic acid derivatives [9].
- Starch: 20 to 45% [9].
- Fatty oil: 1 to 4%, in the seeds 10% [9].

Tests for Identity: Organoleptic, macroscopic and microscopic examinations as well as TLC [9, Ü102] or GC [9, 10].

Quantitative assay: Determination of the essential oil content of the crushed seeds, which have been separated from the capsule walls, using steam distillation with xylol in the graduated tube [DAC].

Adulterations, Misidentifications and Impurities are possible, with Ceylon-cardamom, which are the fruits of *E. cardamomum* (L.) MATON var. *betamajor* THWAITES, up to 4 cm long, up to 1 cm wide, with dirty brown coloration and a diameter of up to 5 mm (see also below).

Actions and Uses

Actions: Due to its aromatic odor and spicy, slightly pungent taste, cardamom has gastric juice and bile secretion promoting action and therefore appetizing and digestive action. In an animal test, an acetone dry extract of cardamom was shown to increase bile secretion, although only at very high doses (100 mg extract/kg body weight) [Ü37]. Dry extracts of cardamom, which probably also contained no essential

oil, have caused a reduction in gastric juice production in animal tests [12]. In animals given doses of about 250 µl of the essential oil per kg body weight, good antiinflammatory, analgesic and antispasmodic effects were observed [2, 5].

Toxicology: Based on existing data, there is no acute or chronic toxicity with regular use of cardamom as a spice.

Culinary use: Cardamom plays a large role as a spice, especially in Arab countries (Kuwait, Saudi Arabia), India, Thailand, and Indonesia, but also in Sweden and Finland. In the USA, cardamom is less well known but it is a component of popular Indian chai teas, which are now served in most coffeehouses and cafés.

In order to obtain the seeds, it is helpful to crush the capsule in a mortar and pestle and remove the capsule remains. Due to its very high flavor intensity, cardamom should be measured carefully: About 1 seed per kg of a dish, and for sweet dishes $1/2$ seed per 1 liter liquid. Ground cardamom should be added immediately before the completion of heating a dish. Unground seeds can be added about 5 minutes before completion. The capsule can be cooked with the meal. To enhance their aromatic contribution to a meal, the seeds can be lightly browned in a pan (without fat) prior to use.

Powdered cardamom is used primarily to improve the taste of cakes and pastries, e.g. fruit tarts, and especially Christmas season baked goods such as ginger bread, almond biscuits, honey biscuits and stollen, creams for fruit tarts, confectioneries, fruit salads and compotes (especially made from pears or apples), sweet pumpkin dishes, chewing gum, ice cream, mulled wine, punch and liqueurs. Rarely, and very carefully measured, cardamom is used as a flavor component of marinades, rissoles, chicken fricassee, pea soup, rice pudding, potato salad, pickles, pickled herrings and sauces for fish as well as rice dishes.

Cardamom is an indispensable component of Swedish punch and Swedish cardamom bread.

In the Orient and in parts of Africa, cardamom is used as a flavor component in coffee (cardamom coffee, 1 to 2 crushed seeds per cup or also an opened capsule placed in the spout of the coffeepot) or tea (cardamom tea, 12 whole, broken open capsules and 2 to 3 tablespoonfuls black tea leaf per 1.5 liter boiling water). In Europe, people sometimes make their coffee with a pinch of cocoa powder, a couple of grains of salt and a pinch of powdered cardamom. In East Frisia, tea is given a special note by the addition of cardamom. In many parts of Asia, cardamom is used as a component of betel chew. It is also chewed to improve the breath.

The essential oil of cardamom serves as a flavoring component of cakes and pastries and liqueurs (Abtei, Angostura, Cassia, Chartreuse, Cordial Medoc, Curacao, Goldwasser; Halb-und-Halb) [13, Ü3, Ü13, Ü45, Ü51, Ü55, Ü59, Ü73, Ü108, Ü111].

Combines well with: In sweet dishes with cinnamon, clove, ginger, saffron, and star anise; in salty dishes, with allspice, black pepper, clove, coriander, garlic, and onions; together with nutmeg as a spice in fish dishes.

As a component of spice mixes and preparations: → Almond biscuit spice, → Arabian spice mix, → Baharat, → Bologna spice mix, → Curry powder, → Fish spice, → Five-spice-mix, → Garam masala, → Gingerbread spice, → Grill spice, → Masala, → Mulled wine spice, → Pastry spice, → Plum jam spice, → Poultry spice, → Ras el hanout, → Sausage spice, → Seven seas spice, → Soup spice, → Stollen spice, → Table mustard, → Zhug.

Other uses: The essential oil is used in the perfume industry.

Medicinal herb

Herbal drug: Cardamomi fructus, Cardamom, contains not less than 4% essential oil [DAC]. Although the fruits are commercially traded, only the seeds are used medicinally.

Indications: For indigestion, average daily dose is 1.5 dried ground seed, 1 to 2 g tincture (according to EB 6), or equivalent preparations [4].

Fruits or seeds of ginger family plants that are used the same as cardamom

Wild cardamom (Ceylon cardamom, brown cardamom, long cardamom), *Elettaria cardamomum* (L.) MATON var. *betamajor* THWAITES (*Elettaria major* SMITH), occurs wild in Sri Lanka, the dried fruits are 2 to 4 cm long, 1 cm wide, dark brown, strongly grooved, 4 to 5% essential oil with camphoraceous odor of which the main components are *p*-cymene (about 35%) and terpinenol-4 (about 30%). It is only rarely used as a spice, and used as an adulterant to true cardamom [9].

Bengal cardamom, *Amomum aromaticum* ROXB., native to India (Sikkim), its seeds are occasionally traded as false cardamom [9, Ü61].

Round cardamom (Siam cardamom, Java cardamom), *Amomum compactum* SOLAND. ex MATON (*A. cardamomum* ROXB. non L., *A. kepulaga* SPRAGUE et BURKHILL), native to the Malay Peninsula where it is cultivated as well as in Java and Sumatra. The seeds contain about 2.4% essential oil, of which the main components are camphor and borneol. It has value as a spice in Java and Sumatra, and is also exported to southeastern Asian countries [9].

Chinese cardamom (Bitter cardamom, black cardamom, round Chinese cardamom), *Amomum globosum* LOUR., native to southern China, Vietnam, Cambodia, Laos, northern Thailand, the fruits are round, dark brown, and contain 3 to 6% essential oil [9].

Cambodian cardamom (Indochina cardamom, Chinese cardamom, white-fruit amomum), *Amomum krervanh* PIERRE ex GAGNEP., native to Southeastern Asia where it is also cultivated [Ü61].

Java cardamom, from *Amomum maximum* ROXB., native to the Malay Peninsula, and cultivated in Java [Ü61].

Indian cardamom (Greater- or Nepal cardamom), from *Amomum subulatum* ROXB., native to Nepal, where it is cultivated as well as in India, the seeds are costate, dark red when mature, dark brown when dried, containing about 1% essential oil [9, Ü61].

False cardamom, from *Amomum xanthioides* WALL., native to Southeastern Asia, cultivated in India and China [Ü61].

Madagascar cardamom (Cameroon cardamom), from *Aframomum angustifolium* (SONN.) K. SCHUM., native to Madagascar, Zanzibar, Pemba, and Seychelles [9, Ü61].

Cameroon cardamom, from *Aframomum daniellii* (J.D. HOOKER) K. SCHUM. or *A. letestuanum* GAGNEP., native to tropical Africa [Ü92].

Korarima cardamom (Nutmeg cardamom, Guragi spice), from *Aframomum korarima* (PEREIRA) ENGL., native to Ethiopia and Somalia, where it is also cultivated, containing 1 to 2% essential oil, with a camphoraceous odor [9, Ü61].

Almond Biscuits ("Spekulatius")

100 g soft butter, 100 g sugar, 1 egg, 1/2 of an organic lemon, 50 g peeled, finely ground almonds, 1 teaspoon baking powder, 1/2 teaspoon cardamom powder, 1/2 teaspoon cinnamon powder, 1 knife tip of clove powder, 250 g whole wheat flour.

Mix the butter, sugar and egg to a foamy consistency, add the rubbed lemon peel and the squeezed lemon juice. Incorporate the almonds, baking powder and spices, and mix well. At the end, add the whole-wheat flour to prepare the dough. Let it stand for about 1 h in a cool place. Roll out the dough to a thickness of 4 cm and use a cookie cutter to cut the cookies. Place the cookies on a paper-lined baking sheet and bake in a preheated oven at 180 °C for about 15 minutes [3].

Literature

[1] Al-Zuhair H. et al., Pharmacol. Res. 34(1/2):79–82 (1996).

[2] Badd A.Z.M., Chem. Mikrobiol. Technol. Lebensm. 14:177–182 (1992).

[3] Buhmann C., Natürlich 19(12):43–44 (1999).

[4] Kommissiom E beim BfArM., BAnz-Nr. 223 vom 30.11.86, Berichtigung 13.03. 1990 und 01.09.1990

[5] Kubo J. et al., J. Agric. Food Chem. 39: 1984–1986 (1991).

[6] Lewis Y.S. et al., Perfum Ess. Oil Res. 57:623–628 (1966).

[7] Menut C. et al., Flavour Fragrance 6:183–186 (1991).

[8] Noleau I. et al., Flavour Fragrance 2:123–127 (1987).

[9] Oberdieck R., Fleischwirtschaft 72:1657–1663 (1992).

[10] Rajapakse-Arambelewa et al., J. Sci. Fodd. Agric. 30:521–527 (1979).

[11] Rivals P., A.H. Mansour, J. Agric. trop. Bot. appl. 21:37–43 (1974).

[12] Sakai K. et al., Chem. Pharm. Bull. 37: 215–217 (1989).

[13] Scholz H., Natürlich 19(12):40–44 (1999).

[14] Variyar P.S., Bandyopadhyay C., PAFAI J. 17(1):19–25 (1995).

Literature references identified by Ü can be found in the general listing of books and monographs at the back of this book.

Celery

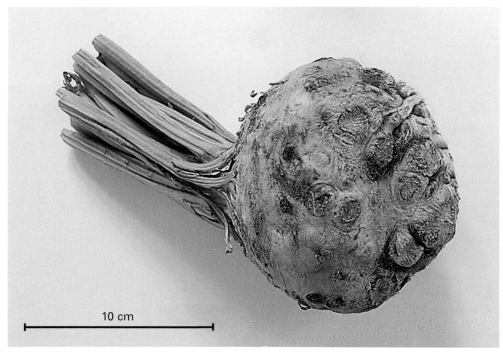

Fig. 1: Celery tuber

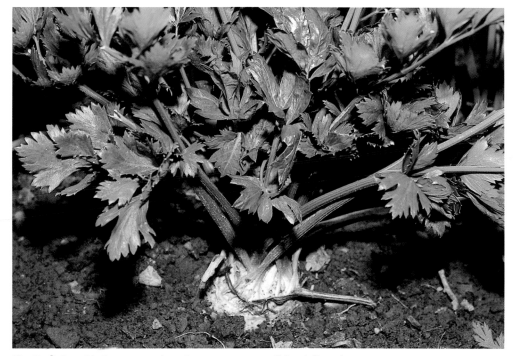

Fig. 2: Celery (*Apium graveolens* L. var. *rapaceum* (MILL.) GAUD.)

Plant source: *Apium graveolens* L.

Taxonomic classification: The species can be subdivided as follows:
Apium graveolens L. var. *graveolens*, wild celery, marsh celery,
Apium gravcolens L. var. *rapaceum* (MILL.) GAUD., celeriac, turnip-root celery,
Apium graveolens L. var. *dulce* (MILL.) PERS., pole celery, salad celery, blanched celery,
Apium graveolens L. var. *secalinum* ALEF., cutting (soup) celery.

Family: Umbelliferous plants (Apiaceae, synonym Umbelliferae).

Common names: Engl.: celery, celeriac (turnip-root celery); Fr,: céleri, ache; Ger.: Sellerie, Eppich.

Description: Celery is an apiaceous biennial plant, up to 1 m high. The foliage leaves are 1 to 2 times pinnate with usually three-lobed, rhombic leaflcts. The small whitish flowers with 5 petals, 2 stamina and 2 styles appear on robust rays of compound umbels with no involucres and small involucres. The ripe fruits are small, grayish green to brownish, ovate double achenes, sometimes split into their mericarps [Ü106].
The fleshy rounded tuber of turnip-root celery, up to 15 cm in diameter, develops from the root, the hypocotyl and the lower part of the stem axis. It bears fleshy secondary roots, thick as fingers.
The elongated, thickened, ribbed leaf stalks, being blanched or becoming blanched by darkening of the lower part of the stalks, are storage organs of pole celery.
Cutting celery resembles the wild form. Some cultivars of cutting celery have curled leafs.

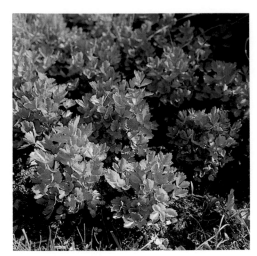

Fig. 3: Cutting celery (*Apium graveolens* L. var. *secalinum* ALEF.)

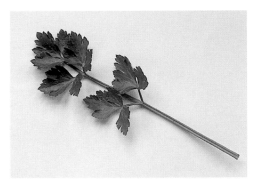

Fig. 4: Leaf of cutting celery

Native origin: The wild form was probably first taken into cultivation in Egypt. Today it is widely distributed in damp, nutrient rich, argillaceous, saliferous regions in all of Europe, of Western Asia to Eastern India, in North- and South Africa, as well as South- and North America. The other varieties are known in cultivation only.

Main cultivation areas: Germany (especially Bavaria and North Rhine-Westphalia), France, Holland, as well as in other European countries, Asian countries, and North America.

Main exporting countries: Germany, France, followed by Holland, former Yugoslavia, Poland, and Hungary, and for celery fruits also India.

Cultivation: Celery needs nutrient-rich, calcareous, deeply loosened-up soils, a sunny to half-shade location and a high rainfall, humid climate. Sowing takes place in January to March indoors under glass at a temperature of at least 16 °C. The seed stock should not be covered (light germinator!). After pricking out the seedlings into 5- to 8 cm pots, they are placed in a hotbed. After the last frost, they can be transplanted outdoors (spaced at about 40 × 40 cm). Cutting celery can be sown directly in the open field in March to April. Greening of blanched celery is prevented by covering the stalk ends with straw. However, there are also new so-called self-blanching varieties, whose stalks also do not green without this procedure. In order to harvest the fruits, the tubers must overwinter in a cool frost-free location and must be planted out again in the second year.

Turnip-root celery varieties with white tubers include, among others, 'Alba', 'Anita', 'Bergers weiße Kugel', 'Brilliant', 'Cesar', 'Diamant', 'Dolvi', 'Frigga', 'Galina', 'Kojak', 'Mars', 'Mentor', 'Monarch', 'Ortho', 'Prinz', 'Radiant', 'Regent' and 'Topa'. Self-blanching blanched celery varieties include 'Golden Spartan', 'Goldgelber', 'Selfira' and 'White Pascal'. 'Tall Utah' is a good variety that remains green and is not blanched. Good varieties of cutting celery are 'Aromatischer', 'Gewöhnlicher Schnitt', and 'Wiener Markt' [Ü5, Ü15, Ü96].

Culinary herb

Commercial forms: Celery seed: the dried fruits, celery seed oleoresin, the dried, peeled or unpeeled tubers, dried leaves, in the vegetable trade the fresh tubers, fresh leaf stalk of blanched celery, fresh leaves of cutting (soup) celery.

Production: The harvest of the tubers takes place September to October, blanched celery can be harvested after August. Leaf celery leaves can be harvested fresh as needed.

Forms used: The fresh or dried leaves of cutting- or turnip-root celery, the tubers of turnip-root celery, the fresh stalks of blanched celery, and the dried fruits.

Storage: Celery root tubers with the leaves cut off, can be stored for a few weeks in the vegetable drawer of the refrigerator, or, until spring, in a cool, humid basement, placed in moderately humid sand so that the bulbs do not touch each other. Blanched celery stalks can be kept in perforated plastic bags for one week in the refrigerator or in humid sand in the basement for a couple of weeks. The fresh leaves, with the cut stems immersed in water, or wrapped in plastic bags, can be stored for several days (at –1 to +2 °C, up to 8 weeks) in the refrigerator. The leaves can be finely chopped and placed in the ice-tray with some water or frozen in a freezer bag in the deep freezer, respectively; they can also be stored in dried form [Ü4, Ü96].

Description. Tuber (Fig. 1): Greenish-brownish, cream-white on the inside, sometimes hollow, roundish to napiform, irregular surface due to scars of the leaf stalks and roots, with remains of the leaf stalks at the apex and attached root fiber bundles, diameter 10 to 15 cm, weight 0.5 to 1.0 kg, spicy taste, somewhat sweet, odor characteristic and spicy.

Fruit: Gray-green to brownish, sometimes separated into oval mericarps, mericarp 0.8 to 1.5 mm long, about 1.7 mm wide, 0.5 to 1.2 mm thick, with 3 dorsal, narrow, light-colored to whitish, very prominent ridges. The powder shows double layers of particularly distinct narrow, transversal cells; also present are fragments of the cuticula with colorless, irregularly striated cells and numerous stomata, dark-brown fragments of the oil ducts, elongated stone cells of the mesocarp, cells of the endosperm with aleuron grains, oil drops and small oxalate rosettes as well as spiral and annular vessels associated with ligneous fibers. Starch is absent [Ü37, Ü48]. The odor upon bruising is characteristic, spicy, taste somewhat bitter.

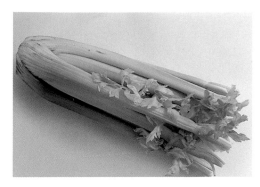

Fig. 5: Blanched celery

Leaf (Fig. 4): Dark-green, shiny, glabrous, basal leaves of the 1-year old plant 10 to 60 cm long, petiolate, pinnate, with cuneiform, up to 3-lobed, dentate, wide tips, in blanched celery (Fig. 5) the stalks are elongated, thickened, ribbed white, reddish or light-green, in the lower part up to 2.0 cm wide. Upon rubbing, a characteristic aromatic odor appears, taste is slightly sweet, aromatic, bitter and somewhat pungent.

History: Celery was already valued in Egypt and ancient Greece. In classical Rome it was a popular vegetable. As a medicinal plant, it was listed in imperial government decree "Capitulare de villis" (authored 795, see footnote → Anise). It was only later in the 18th century, when turnip-root celery was established in the German and northern cuisine under the influence of the French cuisine. Blanched celery is especially used in Southern Europe and England [Ü45, for mythology Ü56].

Constituents and Analysis

DIN- and ISO-Standards: ISO Specification 6574 (Celery seed).

Constituents of the tuber (celeriac)

- Essential oil: 0.01 to 0.15%, the main components are R-(+)-limonene (9 to 30%) β-pinene (8 to 18%), cis-β-ocimene (5 to 8%) and 3-methyl-4-ethyl-hexane (11 to 17%), significantly

contributing to the odor are the phthalides sedanenolide (about 13%), trans-sedanolide (about 7%), cis-sedanolide (about 5%), (Z)-ligustilide (about 4%), 3-butylidenephthalide and 3-butylphthalide [22, 29, Ü37].

- Flavonoids: About 0.05%, mainly apiin (apigenin-7-O-apiosylglucoside), besides luteolin-7-O-apiosylglucoside [18].
- Furanocoumarin derivatives (about 0.5 mg/100 g fresh weight), content varies considerably, upon fungi infection of the plant but also fungicide treatment, their content increases temporarily (phytoalexins!): Xanthotoxin, bergaptene, isopimpinellin, psoralene, imperatorin and angelicin [24, 26, 39].
- Hydroxycoumarins: Scopoletin, aesculetin [25, Ü37].
- Polyines: Falcarinol, falcarindiol [9].
- Hydroxycinnamic acid derivatives: Chlorogenic acid (3-caffeoylquinic acid), 3-p-coumaroylquinic acid, 3-feru-

loylquinic acid, spectrum very specific to varieties and origins [10].

- Monosaccharides, oligosaccharides, sugar alcohols: Glucose (1 to 5%), saccharose (7 to 21%), mannitol (10 to 29%) [10].

Constituents of the leaves

- Essential oil: 0.1 to 0.8%, the main components are R-(+)-limonene (60%), myrcene (about 10%), β-caryophyllene (about 14%), β-selinene (about 8%), as well as phthalides (10 to 35%), which, aside of β-selinene, also contribute significantly to the odor: 3-Butylphthalide, sedanolide, 3-butylidenephthalide, sedanenolide and 3-isovalerylidene-3a,4-dihydrophthalide; also present are, among others, α- and β-pinene, α-selinene, α-terpineol, γ-terpinene, 1-pentylcyclohexa-1,3-diene, pentylbenzene, carveol, cis-β-ocimene, hex-3-ene-1-ol, dihydrocarvone and apiol [5, 22, 23, 33]. In three varieties of cutting cel-

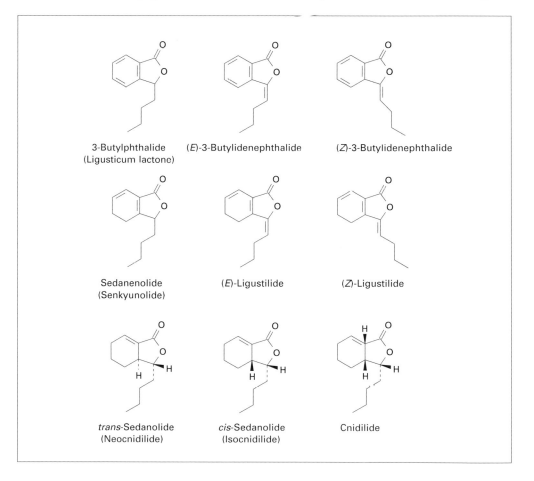

3-Butylphthalide (Ligusticum lactone)

(E)-3-Butylidenephthalide

(Z)-3-Butylidenephthalide

Sedanenolide (Senkyunolide)

(E)-Ligustilide

(Z)-Ligustilide

trans-Sedanolide (Neocnidilide)

cis-Sedanolide (Isocnidilide)

Cnidilide

ery of Egyptian origin, the following components have been identified: Limonene (13 to 15%), myrcene (10 to 13%), β-selinene (8 to 10%), (E)-β-farnesene (6 to 9%), cis-allo-β-ocimene (6 to 10%), α-caryophyllene (humulene, 5 to 9%), β-pinene (5 to 9%), α-pinene (4 to 7%), trans-sedanolide (5 to 7%), sedanenolide (3 to 10%), apiol (2 to 8%), cis-β-ocimene (2 to 8%) and γ-terpinene (2 to 6%) [17, 34].

- Flavonoids: About 0.15%, the main components are apiin (apigenin-7-O-apiosyl glucoside), furthermore, luteolin-7-O-apiosylglucoside, apigenin-7-O-glucoside and a chrysoeriol glucoside [18, 19].
- Furanocoumarin derivatives: About 0.2%, bergaptene, xanthotoxin, isopimpinellin, psoralene, strongly elevated levels upon fungi infection, tissue injury and fungicide treatment (phytoalexins!) [6, 13, 26, 32, 37, Ü100].
- Hydroxycoumarins: Scopoletin [25].
- Caffeic acid derivatives: Chlorogenic acid, among others [25].
- Steroids: β-Sitosterol, stigmasterol, campesterol [14, 43].

Constituents of the fruit

- Essential oil: 1.9 to 3%, the main components are R(+)-limonene (about 60%) and β-selinene (up to 13%), phthalides (responsible for the aroma besides β-selinene), particularly trans-sedanolide (about 16%), 3-butylenephthalide (1.5 to 8%), 3-butylphthalide (0.2 to 10%), sedanolide (about 3%) and 3-isobutylidene-3a,4-dihydrophthalide (0.7 to 6.5%), furthermore, α-pinene, β-pinene, myrcene and β-caryophyllene [4, Ü37].
- Flavonoids: 1 to 2.5% luteolin-7-apiosylglucoside, chrysoeriol-7-apiosylglucoside and apiin [15, 20].
- Furanocoumarin derivatives: About 0.2%, including, among others, bergaptene, isoimperatorin, isopimpinellin and seselin, dihydrofurocoumarins: including, among others rutaretin, nodakenetin, and (–)-2,3-dihydro-2(1-hydroxy-1-hydroxymethylethyl)-7H-furo[3,2g][1]-benzopyran-7-one, as well as

furanocoumarin glycosides such as apioside and celereoside [12, 21, 26, Ü100].
- Fatty oil (5 to 30%), with 40 to 60% petroselinic acid [Ü37].

Tests for Identity: The identity of celery plant parts can be determined with organoleptic, macroscopic and microscopic analysis, as well as with GC of the essential oil [16, 29] or TLC of the flavonoids [Ü37].

Quantitative assay: The content of essential oil is determined volumetrically with steam distillation, according to the European Pharmacopoeia, using a prefilled graduated tube with xylol [Ph Eur].

Adulterations, Misidentifications and Impurities: Celeriac, blanched celery and cutting celery are rarely misidentified due to their characteristic appearance, odor and taste. Accidental adulteration of the fruits, particularly in powder form, can be detected with TLC.

Actions and Uses

Actions: Due to its aromatic and slightly bitter taste, a stimulant effect on salivation, secretion of gastric juice, excretion of bile and intestinal motility must be accepted. For the frequently postulated diuretic effect, there is no conclusive evidence.
Animal studies (mice, rats) demonstrated sedative effects (extension of the pentobarbital- and ethanol- sleeping time) for higher doses of the essential oil of celery fruits (100 to 300 mg/kg body weight, i.p.) and for isolated phthalides (25 to 100 mg/kg body weight, i.p.) [8, Ü37]. In mice, a dose-dependent anodyne effect (hot plate test, writhing test after subcutaneous injections of acetic acid) was observed from ethanolic extracts of the drug [3].
Methanolic extracts of celery fruits showed hepatoprotective effects in rats that were given the hepatotoxic substances paracetamol and thioacetamide, determined by measuring blood levels of serum-transaminases (SGOT and SGPT) and other liver enzymes [12, 36].

In rats that received a high-fat hyperlipidemic diet, the application of aqueous celery extracts reduced the elevation of total cholesterol, LDL and triacylglycerols content in the blood. The triacylglycerols content in the liver increased however [38]. Similar to most essential oils, celery essential oil, especially its high-boiling fraction, has antimicrobial action [1, 5, 30, 31].

Toxicology: Based on existing data, there is no acute or chronic toxicity if used as a normally dosed spice.
After the intake of celery plants, which have been seriously damaged or infected with fungi and/or treated with fungicides, and thus have high levels of furanocoumarins, and subsequent exposure of the skin to sunlight, photodermatosis may occur [7, 24, Ü39].
The consumption of raw or cooked celery has caused allergic reactions such as contact urticaria of the oral mucous membrane and even anaphylactic shock. People who are also allergic to mugwort pollen (celery-carrot-mugwort-syndrome) and/or birch pollen (birch-celery-syndrome) were particularly affected [11, 40, 42]. Api g1 and Api g4 have been isolated as allergens. Api g4 (14.3 kDa) shows great structural similarity (71 to 82%) to the so-called profilins of other plants, e.g. birch-profilin Bet v 1 and cross-reacts immunologically with it [35].

Culinary use: The use of celery in Central European cooking is relatively new. It wasn't until the beginning of the 19th century that it was used here to a large extent. The leaves are used mainly in French and in North American cooking. The tubers are used, cut into strips, sliced or rubbed, eaten fresh or cooked with the meal. The leaves are chopped and added just before the end of the cooking process. It is cooked with some dishes, e.g. legumes. The fruits are crushed before use. Celery easily predominates the flavor, so it should be measured sparingly.
The tubers of turnip-root celery are used as a vegetable, raw or prepared. In so-called → Soup greens they are cut into thumb-sized strips, and along with leeks,

carrots and parsley, are used as a seasoning of soups and stewed dishes. The raw tubers are added to salads, cold soups, especially in combination with tomatoes and potatoes as well as vegetable purées [Ü81].

The leaves of cutting celery, but also of turnip-root- and blanched-celery, are suitable fresh or dried to improve the taste of salads, soups, sauces, vegetable broths, vegetables (e.g. carrots), legumes, chopped meat, liver, stewed meat, grilled dishes and tomato juice [Ü45, Ü46, Ü73]. The leaf stalks of blanched celery serve as a vegetable, raw or cooked. They are also used prepared as a seasoning for soups, sauces, stews, noodle dishes, quark, tofu, omclcts and rice [Ü73]. The juice obtained from an electric kitchen juicer can be drunk cold [Ü20].

The crushed fruits are added to poached vegetables or farces, salad dressing, marinades or sauces (mainly barbecue sauce, cheese sauces, and sauces with tomatoes) and fish pastes. It is also used as a seasoning of party snacks, crackers and bread. It is a component of the cocktail "Bloody Mary" (see below) [Ü1, Ü2, Ü55].

Combines well with: Garlic or onions.

As a component of spice mixes and preparations: → Barbecue spice (fruit), → Bouquet garni (herb), → Celery salt, → Herb butter, → Herb salt, → Meat spice, → Pickling spice, → Poultry spice, → Quark spice, → Salad seasoning, → Seven-seas spice, → Soup greens (tuber), → Tomato ketchup.

Other uses: The essential oil and sedanolide are used in the perfume industry.

Medicinal herb

Herbal drugs: Apii fructus, Celery fruit, Apii herba, Celery herb, Apii radix, Celery root, Apii graveolentis aetheroleum ex fructibus, Celery fruit oil.

Indications: Celery fruit and leaf are only used occasionally in folk medicine as a stomachic and carminative for digestive disorders, as a diuretic for bladder and kidney disorders and for gout and rheumatic complaints. To prepare a tea infusion, 1 g of the fruits should be crushed immediately before use. 1 to 4 g is the recommended daily dose. It should not be used for kidney disease because of the kidney irritant effect of its essential oil. The juice of celery tubers cooked with sugar also serves as a cough remedy. The German Commission E of the BfArM did not approve the therapeutic use of any celery plant parts due to unsubstantiated efficacy and the possibility of the occurrence of allergic reactions [28].

Bloody Mary

50 ml Vodka, 10 ml lemon juice, freshly ground pepper, celery salt, 2 squirts of Tabasco, 3 to 5 squirts Worcestershire sauce, 120 ml tomato juice.

Fill the ice cubes into a longdrink glass and then add the spices, lemon juice and Vodka. Add the tomato juice and stir well with a bartender's spoon [2].

Literature

[1] Afzal H., M.S. Aktar, J. Pak. Med. Assoc. 31:230–232 (1981).
[2] Anonym, Internet: www.foodnews.ch (2001).
[3] Atta A.H., A. Alkofahi, J. Ethnopharmacol. 60(2):117–124 (1998).
[4] Bartschak D., A. Mosandl, GIT Labor-Fachz. 41(9):874–876 (1997).
[5] Bauermann U. et al., Drogenreport 6(10): 24–30 (1993).
[6] Beier R.C. et al., Food Chem. Toxicol. 21(2):163–165 (1983).
[7] Birmungham D.J. et al., Arch. Dermatol. 83:73–87 (1961)
[8] Bjeldanes L.F., I.S. Kim, J. Food Sci. 43: 143–144 (1978).
[9] Bohlmann F., Chem. Ber. 100:3454–3456 (1967).
[10] Brandl W. et al., Z. Lebensm. Unters. Forsch. 177:325–327 (1983).
[11] Breiteneder H. et al., Eur. J. Biochem. 233(2):484–489 (1995).
[12] Ceska O. et al., Phytochemistry 26(1): 165–169 (1987).
[13] Chaudhary S.K. et al., J. Agric. Food Chem. 33:1153–1157 (1985).
[14] Claus R., H.O. Hoppen, Experientia 35: 1674–1675 (1979).
[15] Farooq M.O. et al., Naturwissenschaften 45:265 (1958).
[16] Fehr D., Pharmazie 34:658–662 (1979).
[17] Fehr D., Pharmazie 29:349 (1974).
[18] Galensa R., K. Herrmann, Z. Lebensm. Unters. Forsch. 169:170–172 (1979).
[19] Galensa R., K. Herrmann, J. Chromatogr. 189:217–224 (1980).
[20] Garg S.K. et al., Planta Med. 38:363–365 (1980).
[21] Garg S.K. et al., Planta Mcd. 43:306–308 (1981).
[22] Gijbels M.J.M. et al., Fitoterapia 56:17 (1985).
[23] Gold H.J., C.W. Wilson, J. Food Sci. 28:484 (1963).
[24] Heath-Paglioso S. et al., Phytochemistry 31:2683–2688 (1992).
[25] Herrmann K., Z. Lebensm. Unters. Forsch. 106:341–348 (1957).
[26] Innocenti G. et al., Planta Med. 29(2): 165–170 (1976).
[27] Ivie W., New Scientist 92:370 (1981).
[28] Komm. E. beim BfArM., BAnz. 127 vom 12.07.1991.
[29] Mac Leod G., J.M. Ames, Phytochemistry 28(7):1817–1824 (1989).
[30] Maruzella J.C., M. Freundlich, J. Am. Pharm. Assoc. 48:356–358 (1959).

[31] Maruzella J.C., L. Ligouri, J. Am. Pharm. Assoc. 47:250–254 (1958).

[32] Nigg H.N. et al., J. Agric. Food Chem. 45(4):1430–1436 (1997).

[33] Pino J.A. et al., J. Ess. Oil Res. 9:719–720 (1997).

[34] Saleh M.M. et al., Pharm. Weekbl. Sci: 13(6):277–279 (1985).

[35] Scheurer S. et al., Clin. Exp. Allergy 30(7): 962–971 (2000).

[36] Singh A., S.S. Handa, J. Ethnopharmacol. 49(3):119–126 (1995).

[37] Trumble J.T. et al., Acta Hortic. 1994: 381(Intern. Symp. on Nat. Phenols in Plant Resistance, Vol. 2):596–599 (1994), ref. CA 126:209561y.

[38] Tsi D. et al., Planta Med. 61(1):18–21 (1995).

[39] Uecker S. et al., Pharmazie 46(8): 599–601 (1991).

[40] Vallier P. et al., Clin. Allergy 18(5): 491–500 (1988).

[41] Weymar H., Buch der Doldengewächse, Neumann Verlag, Radebeul 1959.

[42] Wüthrich B., R. Dietschi, Schweiz. Med. Wochenschr. 115:358–364 (1985).

[43] Zlatanov M., St.A. Ivanov, Fett Wiss. Technol. 97(10):381–383 (1995).

Literature references identified by Ü can be found in the general listing of books and monographs at the back of this book.

Chervil

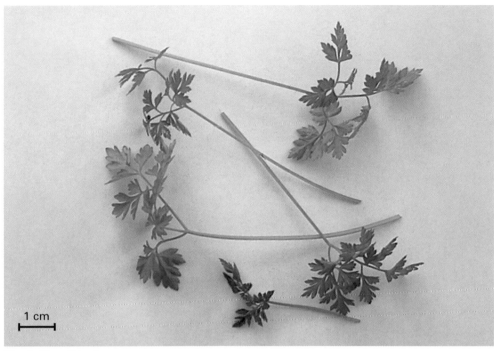

Fig. 1: Chervil leaf

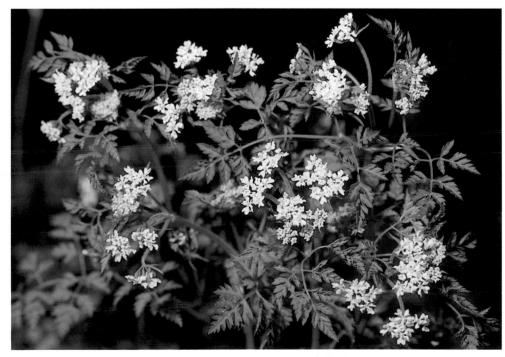

Fig. 2: Chervil (*Anthriscus cerefolium* (L.) HOFFM. ssp. *cerefolium*)

Plant source: *Anthriscus cerefolium* (L.) HOFFM. ssp. *cerefolium*.

Synonym: *Anthriscus cerefolium* (L.) HOFFM. var. *sativus* (LAM.) ENDL.

Family: Umbelliferous plants (Apiaceae, synonym Umbelliferae).

Common names: Engl.: chervil, charvil; Fr.: cerfeuil; Ger.: Kerbel, Echter Garten-Kerbel, Körfel, Körbel, Korbel, Kufel.

Description (Fig. 2): Annual plant, sometimes over-wintering, up to 70 cm high, with thin roots, spindle-shaped; thin, branched stems, with angular furrows at the base, finely grooved in the upper parts, softly pubescent above the nodes. Lower leaves petiolate, the upper ones are sitting on sheaths with skin-like margins, thin, 2 to 4 times pinnatisect with fringed leaflets, tip lanceolate, short mucronate or almost pinnatisect. The main axis and lateral branches with one terminal, composite umbel each, having 3 to 5 densely tomentose rays, involucre mostly absent, small involucres 1- to 4-foliate. Flowers radial, 5 white petals, 5 stamina, 2 styles, inferior ovary, bilocular. The fruit is a double achene (cremocarp), separating into 2 black, glabrous and shiny, 7 to 11 mm long mericarps, which remain closed and have a long, beak-like projection, the commissural surface is curled having a deep longitudinal furrow. Flowering period is from May to August (5).

Native origin: Only known to be cultivated, its wild relative is probably *Anthriscus cerefolium* (L.) HOFFM. ssp. *trichospermus* (WIMM.) ARCANG., native to southern Europe, and southwestern Asia.

Main cultivation areas: Europe, Northern Africa, Eastern Asia, North- and South America.

Main exporting countries: Chervil is mostly used fresh and commercial trade rarely occurs.

Cultivation: Chervil prefers loose-packed, consistently damp soil and half-shaded locations. In order to have a continuous supply of herb to harvest, it should be planted in intervals of 2 to 3 weeks from March through August in rows 20 to 25 cm apart. The seeds should not be covered (germination is light dependent). Sowing the plant after July suppresses flowering. Planting seed in September to overwinter is also effective. Then the harvest can begin already in March. In order to optimize herb formation, the umbels should be removed. Growing chervil in pots or planter beds, under plastic film until the plants reach a height of 5 cm, enables the harvest of fresh herb during the winter. In addition to the smooth-leafed varieties ('Glattblättriger', 'Einfacher') curly-leafed varieties are also cultivated ('Benarys Krauskopf', 'Struwwelpeter') [6, Ü2, Ü21, Ü41, Ü65, Ü86].

Culinary herb

Commercial forms: Chervil leaf: dried herb, rubbed, deep frozen fresh herb, the fresh herb is rarely traded in the vegetable market.

Production: The herb can be harvested beginning 6 to 8 weeks after planting up until the formation of buds.

Forms used: The young, fresh, finely chopped herb, and rarely the dried, ground herb.

Storage: The herb or the leaves can be stored in the refrigerator for a few days, kept in water or wrapped in a plastic bag. The leaves can also be stored finely chopped and salted or immersed in water and frozen in the ice tray. Drying leads to almost complete aroma loss and is not recommended.

Description. Whole herb (Fig. 1): See description of the whole plant.

Odor: Sweetish and aromatic, **Taste:** Anise-like and spicy in the fresh plant.

History: There is not much known about the early history of chervil. The Romans were probably responsible for spreading the plant into Central Europe. In a local government decree by Karl the Great, "Capitulare de villis" (authored in about 795 CE, see footnote, → Anise), its cultivation was made mandatory. In medieval herb books, chervil was noted also for its useful attributes [Ü56].

Constituents and Analysis

Constituents

- Essential oil: About 0.3 to 0.9%, the main components are estragole (methylchavicol, 60 to 80%), 1-allyl-2,4-dimethoxybenzene (16 to 30%) and undecane (5 to 10%), furthermore, in very small amounts chavibetol (contributing to the odor), limonene, *p*-cymene, *trans*-anethole and 1,8-cineole, among others [2–4, 7].
- Flavonoids: Apiin, among others.
- Furanocoumarins: Apterin, among others.

Tests for Identity: Organoleptic examination in addition to macroscopic and microscopic analysis, as well as GC or GC-MS assays of the essential oil [2].

Quantitative assay: Volumetric determination of the essential oil in the fresh, cut or freshly ground material, following the Ph Eur procedure with xylol in the graduated tube.

Adulterations, Misidentifications and Impurities: Caution! Do not collect or use plant materials from the wild. Toxic herbs such as hemlock (*Conium maculatum* L.), rough chervil (*Chaerophyllum temulum* L.) or fool's parsley (*Aethusa cynapium* L., toxicity unclear) are possibly mistaken for chervil.

Actions and Uses

Actions: On the basis of its aromatic odor and spicy taste, chervil has gastric juice- and bile secretion promoting effects and therefore appetizing and digestive. Extracts of chervil have shown good antioxidative activity in vitro in the test model "ascorbic acid induced lipid peroxidation in rat brain homogenates" [1]. Other studies on the efficacy of chervil are not known.

Toxicology: Based on existing data, there is acute or chronic toxicity with the normal use of chervil as a spice.
Estragole has shown hepatocarcinogenic effects in animal tests (see Lit. → Fennel). Whether high doses pose a risk to humans is not known. Due to the low doses used as a spice and the low content of essential oil in the herb, any negative health effects are unlikely. The ingested amount of estragole is significantly lower compared to the therapeutic dose of → Fennel. Phototoxic reactions are possible [Ü39].

Culinary use: Chervil is an indispensable culinary herb in French cooking. But it is also very popular in Dutch and English cooking.
The chopped, fresh herb is used. Due to rapid volatilization, chervil should be added just before serving (cooked for maximum 1 minute) or it should be sprinkled over the finished dish. The uncut leaves can also be used as a garnish.
The fresh herb serves as a spice for fresh salads which lack full flavor on their own, mushroom salads, cooked fish, meat dishes (chicken, veal, lamb) and egg recipes (e.g. omelets and scrambled eggs), to improve the taste of sauces (yogurt-based chervil sauce for asparagus, Sauce hollandaise, Sauce béarnaise, béchamel-, ravigote- and fish sauce), herb mayonnaise, bouillons and soups (tomato soup, potato soup) as well as for preparing herb soups

(chervil soup), herb quark, herb fresh cheese, buttermilk, yogurt and herb butter. Chervil is also used as a spice in green beans, carrots, kohlrabi, savoy cabbage, potatoes, stewed cucumbers, spinach and mushrooms [Ü2, Ü59, Ü71, Ü79, Ü86, Ü90, Ü95].
Dried, ground herb can be added as a spice in grilled or cooked fish, egg dishes, sauces for poultry dishes, herb butter and quark [Ü23].

Combines well with: Parsley, saffron, and tarragon.

As a component of spice mixes and preparations: → Bouquet garni, → Egg spice, → Fines herbes, → Frankfurter green sauce, → Herb butter, → Salad spice, → Soup spice, → Tartar sauce.

Medicinal herb

Herbal drug: Cerefolii germanici herba, Chervil herb.

Indications: Used only in folk medicine as a diuretic.

Chervil soup
50 g butter or margarine, 50 g flour, 1 liter broth (made from beef or bouillon cubes), 1/8 to 1/2 liter of sweet cream, 2 yolks, salt, lemon juice, 1 pinch of nutmeg, 1 cup of washed, finely chopped chervil leaves.

Mix melted butter (or margarine) and the flour and brown the mixture in a pan, add the broth while stirring and let it boil for a short time. Mix the cream with the yolks and add it to the soup; season to taste with salt, lemon juice, nutmeg and then carefully incorporate the chervil. Sprinkle with large roasted bread crumbs made in butter and garnish with a few chervil leaves [Ü59].

Similar culinary herbs

Bulbous chervil (turnip-rooted chervil, garden chervil, parsnip chervil, *Chaerophyllum bulbosum* L. ssp. *bulbosum*, Apiaceae) native to Central- and Eastern Europe, Turkey, Iran, the Caucasus up to the Urals, Altai, today only rarely cultivated in Central- and Southeastern Europe. The cooked roots are eaten as a vegetable, the young leaves are used as a spice or as salad [Ü61].

Literature

[1] Fejes S. et al., Phytother. Res. 14(5):362–365 (2000).
[2] Lemberkovics E. et al., J. Ess. Oil Res. 6:421–422 (1994).
[3] Petri G. et al., Vortragsrcf., Abstract in Drogenreport 7:58 (1993).
[4] Simandi B. et al., J. Ess. Oil Res. 8(3):305–306 (1996).
[5] Weymar H., Buch der Doldengewächse, Neumann Verlag, Radebeul 1959.
[6] Würmli A., Natürlich 20(2):58–59 (2000).
[7] Zwaving J.H. et al., Pharm. Weekblad 106(12):182–189 (1971).

Literature references identified by Ü can be found in the general listing of books and monographs at the back of this book.

Chives

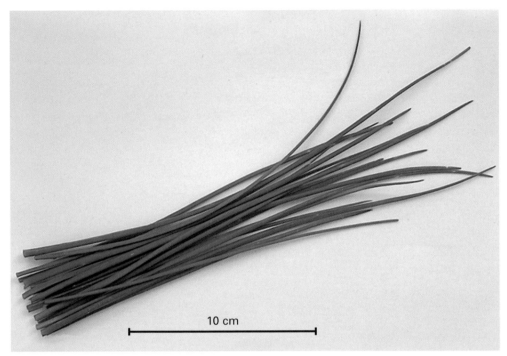

Fig. 1: Chives

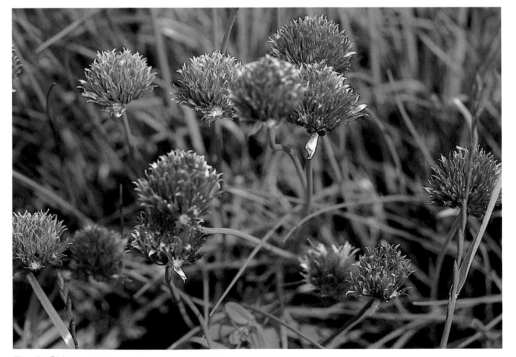

Fig. 2: Chives (*Allium schoenoprasum* L.)

Plant source: *Allium schoenoprasum* L.

Taxonomic classification: On the basis of its very large diversity of shape, the species can be divided into several varieties, including, among others, *A. schoenoprasum* var. *schoenoprasum*, garden chive, and *A. schoenoprasum* var. *sibiricum* (L.) GARCKE, alpine chive, Siberian chive.

Family: Allium plants (Alliaceae; in older literature this species was placed in the lily family, Liliaceae).

Common names: Engl.: chives, cive garlic, cives, civet; Fr.: ciboulette, civette, petit porreau, fausse échalote; Ger.: Schnittlauch, Binsenlauch, Brieslauch, Graslauch, Jakobszwiebel, Pankokenkraut, Preseloak, Prieslauch, Schnittling, Schnittzwiebel, Spaltlauch, Suppenlauch.

Description: Perennial plant, up to 30 cm (seldom 40 cm) tall, tufted because of its branched rhizome, foliage leaves rising from the ground axis are erect, tubular and terete, with their thickened sheaths forming incomplete bulbs, inflorescence axis is as long as the leaves, leafy in the lower part only. The inflorescence is a multiflorous pseudoumbel. Brood bulbs are not formed. The flower has 6 almost bluishred perigone leaves. The ovary is three-chambered. The seeds are black and trigonous. It flowers from June to August [Ü42, Ü85].

Native origin: Widely distributed throughout almost all of Eurasia and North America.

Main cultivation areas: Cultivated mostly in gardens in almost all countries, field cropping also to a small extent for industrial processing.

Main exporting countries: No meaningful world trade.

Cultivation: Chives grow with good water supply in almost all, humus loamy soils, but especially well in calcareous soils in sunny or half shade locations. It is cold resistant. Sowing is carried out in the early spring with spacing between rows of 30 to 40 cm, as soon as the soil conditions permit. Thereby attention should be paid to the sowing depth in a loose, fine crumbly substrate. A vinyl covering will accelerate the emergence of seedlings. In gardens, propagation by purchased ball-rooted seedlings or stock divisions is also possible in spring or autumn. During drought, chives should be watered sufficiently. Crops remain productive for 2 to 4 years. Afterwards the foliage leaves become much finer and the plant grows only scantily. Forced cultivation and pot planting are important for supply in winter and early spring. For personal demand, before the first frost a few clumps should be dug out and reset in pots on the windowsill or in the veranda. The most frequently open field grown cultivars are the fine- or medium coarse- fistulous varieties including, among others, 'Grolau', 'Wielau', 'Welta' and 'Polycross', and in forced cultivation the coarse-leaved varieties including, among others, 'Treibnoris' [Ü14, Ü21, Ü33, Ü96].

Culinary Herb

Commercial forms: Chives: freeze-dried, cut leaves (tubular cut or in flakes), fresh leaves, quick-frozen, cut leaves, in the vegetable trade in small herb pots.

Production: The harvest for the fresh market is done by cutting with a shears or knife 2 to 3 cm above the soil (in order to save the regrowing leaves), for industrial processing harvesting is done when the leaves are at least 15 cm long with a loader combine or with a spinach complete (combine) harvester. After the 2nd year, 3 to 5 cuts annually are possible. For personal demand, the leaves can be removed anytime of year. Even if there is no demand,

the leaves should be cut, in order to prevent the occurrence of flowers and old, hard leaves. In all cases, the largest section of the inflorescence should be clipped off [Ü21].

Forms used: Mainly the fine cut fresh or quick-frozen, and rarely the freeze-dried leaves. Dried leaves have very little flavor.

Storage: The leaves should be used as fresh as possible; if immersed in water immediately, they can be stored in the refrigerator for a few days, or wrapped in plastic bags, for 1 to 2 weeks. It is also possible to store them for longer as deep-frozen leaves in plastic bags or chopped and frozen with water in the ice-tray. Drying leads to considerable aroma loss.

Description. Whole leaf (Fig. 1): See description of the whole plant.

Odor: Almost odorless if unbruised, after bruising, an alliaceous odor, **Taste:** Pungent, spicy, cepaceous.

History: In Central Asia, chives have been used for several thousand years. In Europe, it was probably cultivated for the first time in Italy, at the end of the Middle Ages [Ü66, Ü97].

Constituents and Analysis

Constituents

- Alliins (*S*-alk(ene)ylcysteine sulfoxides), from the composition of the volatile fraction, it can be concluded must be present in the unbruised plant: *S*-methyl-L-cysteine sulfoxide, *S*-propyl-L-cysteine sulfoxide, *S*-prop-1-enyl-L-cysteine sulfoxide and *S*-pentyl-L-cysteine sulfoxide.
- Alliaceous oils: The non-volatile alliins come into contact with the enzyme allinase and are transformed to the volatile alk(en)ylsulfenic acids, which spontaneously transform to their alliaceous smelling, odoriferous breakdown products, the alk(en)yl-alkane/alkene-thiosulfinates (Fig. 10, General Section). Detected were, among others, propyl-propanethiosulfinate (57%), (*E,Z*)-prop-1-enyl-propanethiosulfinate (25%) and propylmethanethiosulfinate (7%) [2] as well as their secondary products dipropyl-disulfide, prop-1-enyl-propyl-disulfide, methyl-propyl-disulfide, methyl-pentyl-disulfide, pentylhydrodisulfide and 3,5-diethyl-1,2,4-trithiolan [6, 8, 14].
- Saponins [Ü60].
- Vitamin C (70 to 100 mg/100 g dry weight) [Ü98].

Methyl-L-cysteine sulfoxide   R = CH₃
Propyl-L-cysteine sulfoxide   R = CH₂CH₂CH₃
Prop-1-enyl-L-cysteine sulfoxide   R = CH=CH₂CH₃

Propyl-propanethiosulfinate   Prop-1-enyl-propanethiosulfinate   Propyl-methanethiosulfinate

Dipropyldisulfide   Prop-1-enylpropyldisulfide   Methylpropyl-disulfide   3,5-Diethyl-1,2,4-trithiolane

Tests for Identity: → Onion.

Quantitative assay: → Onion.

Actions and Uses

Actions: Due to the pungent taste of chives as well as the irritant effect of the alliaceous oils on the gastric mucosa, they have appetizing and digestion promoting action. Besides these and the fungistatic effect of chives [15] there are no other known experimentally proven actions. It is quite probable, however, that it has similar actions as other alliaceous oil producing plants (→ Garlic, → Onion).

Toxicology: Based on existing data, there is no acute or chronic toxicity with the use of regular doses of chives by healthy individuals. It can be assumed that high doses can lead to gastric irritation in sensitive people.

Culinary use: Chives are used today in almost all European, but also in Chinese, Indian and North American cooking. It should be cut just prior to use and never cooked or fried with the dish (change- and loss of aroma!). Chives are best cut in form of small bundled rolls with shears or with a sharp knife and should never be chopped or ground. Before serving, they are sprinkled over the meal and mixed under.
Fine cut fresh or quick-frozen chives are used as a seasoning of soups (especially for beef broth with liver dumplings, semolina dumpling soup and frittatas, and of cheese soups), white stock and cream sauces (especially those with an egg-, yogurt-, quark- or cream base), mayonnaises, dips, quark, cream cheese, butter (chive butter, as a bread spread or as an accompaniment with steak), salads (especially tomato-, cucumber-, lettuce-, meat-, noodle- and potato salad), egg dishes (e.g. scrambled eggs, omelets), meat dishes (e.g. cooked beef with horseradish and cream sauce, roast pork, young chicken), fish dishes (sea- and freshwater fish), vegetable dishes (e.g. of spinach), mushroom dishes, potato dishes (e.g. of hash browns and oven-baked potatoes filled with sour cream) and as a topping for buttered bread or overbaked toasts [Ü1, Ü2, Ü13, Ü17, Ü45, Ü56, Ü70, Ü71, Ü79, Ü95]. The fresh flowers can be used as a garnish for salads [Ü90]. It provides a pink color to herb vinegar [Ü79].

Combines well with: Chervil, cress, hyssop, lemon balm, parsley, and onions, combined with parsley, tarragon and chervil for → Fines herbes [Ü74].

As a component of spice mixes and preparations: → Bouquet garni, → Café de Paris spice mixture, → Fines herbes, → Frankfurter green sauce, → Herb butter, → Pickling spice, → Quark spice, → Vegetable sauce.

Medicinal herb

Herbal drug: Allium-schoenoprasum-leaves, Chive leaves.

Indications: In folk medicine it is used for helminth affection.

Similar culinary herbs

Arabian chive (Egyptian leek), *Allium kurrat* SCHWEINF. ex K. KRAUSE, only known in cultivation, grown and used especially in Egypt. The leaves are cut several times annually and are used in the same way as chives [5].

Chinese chives (Nira, garlic chive, Oriental garlic, *Allium chinense*, → Mild chives, and *A. ramosum* L., cultivated in China, are also designated as Chinese chives), *Allium tuberosum* ROTTLER ex SPRENG. (*A. angulosum* LOUR. non L., *A. senescens* MIQ. non L.), native from Japan to India, cultivated in Japan, China, Myanmar, India, Indonesia, Malaysia, and in the Philippines. The main constituents are *S*-methyl-L-cysteine sulfoxide, *S*-allyl-L-cysteine sulfoxide and their decomposition products, mainly methyl-methanethiosulfinate (74%), (*Z,E*),-prop-1-enyl-methanethiosulfinate (13%) as well as the derivative mono- and oligosulfides, particularly dimethyldisulfide and dimethyltrisulfide, furthermore, among others, dimethylsulfide, diallylsulfide, methylallyldisulfide, methylallyltrisulfide and dimethyltetrasulfide [2, 7, 10] as well as steroid saponins [13]. The small cut young leaves are used as a seasoning for quark, tofu, eggs, noodles and wok dishes with ox or shrimp, sprinkled on butter bread or as a salad, salad ingredient or eaten blanched as a vegetable. In China, the young inflorescences are used for making soups [5, Ü51, Ü61, Ü74].

Mild chives (Rakkyo), *Allium chinense* G. DON (*A. bakeri* REGEL), native origin is uncertain, only occurs in the wild escaped from gardens, some small scale cultivation in China, Japan and Cuba. The main constituents are *S*-(prop-1-enyl-L-cysteine sulfoxide, *S*-allyl-L-cysteine sulfoxide and *S*-methyl-L-cysteine sulfoxide, the γ-glutamyl-derivatives of the corresponding alk(en)ylcysteine-derivatives and alliaceous oils are methyl-methanethiosulfinate, propyl-propanethiosulfinate, propyl-prop-2-enthiosulfinate, propyl-methanethiosulfinate as well as allyl-methanethiosulfinate and as their decomposition products di-, tri- and polysulfides, furthermore steroid saponins [1, 3, 4, 9, 11, 12]. The garlic-like smelling leaves are in the vegetable trade like chives, and the small bulbs marinated just like so-called → Pearl onion (See: → Onion, Similar onion species) [Ü61].

Rocambole, sand leek, giant leek, Spanish garlic, *Allium scorodoprasum* L. (2 subspecies), native to Central- and Southern Europe, Asia Minor, cultivated to a small extent in Europe, China, and Korea, the leaves and flower stalks are used in the same way as chives [Ü61].

Knolau, a general name for some plants with garlic-like smelling leaves, which are used in the same way as chives: among others hybrid of *Allium schoenoprasum* × *A. sativum* [Ü92], cultured varieties of *A. chinense*, → Mild chives (see above) [Ü98] and of *Allium tuberosum*, → Chinese chives (see above). Cultivated in European gardens [Ü96].

**Schnittlauchtrunk
à la Lechthaler**
100 ml double-strength broth, 100 g
natural yogurt, chives, salt, pepper.

Quickly mix the ingredients with 2
ice cubes in a blender and season to
taste; pour the mixture in a pre-
chilled glass, and garnish with 2
chive flowers, if available [Ü57].

Literature

[1] Baba M. et al., Biol. Pharm. Bull. 23(5): 660–662 (2000).

[2] Block E. et al., J. Agric. Food Chem. 40:2431–2438 (1992).

[3] Fenwick G.R. et al., CRC Crit. Rev. Food Sci. Nutr. 22:199–377 (1985).

[4] Freeman G.G., R.J. Whenham, J. Sci. Food Agric. 26:1869 (1975), ref. Ü43.

[5] Hanelt P., Drogenreport 7(11):17–25 (1994).

[6] Hashimoto S. et al., Food Sci. 48:1858 (1983).

[7] Iida H. et al., J. Food Sci. 48:660–661 (1983).

[8] Kameoka H., S. Hashimoto, Phytochemistry 22:294–295 (1983).

[9] Kuroda M. et al., Phytochemistry 40(4): 1071–1076 (1995).

[10] Mackenzie I.A., D.A. Ferns, Phytochemistry 16:763 (1977).

[11] Matsuura H. et al., Chem. Pharm. Bull. 37:1390–1391 (1989).

[12] Saghir A.R., Proc. Am. Soc. Hort. Sci. 84:386–398 (1964).

[13] Sang S. et al., J. Nat. Prod. 62(7):1028–1029 (1999).

[14] Wahlroos Ö., A.I. Virtanen, Acta Chem. Scand. 19:1327 (1965), ref. Ü43.

[15] Yin M.C., S.M. Tsao, Int. J. Food Microbiol. 49(1/2):49–56 (1999).

Literature references identified by Ü can be found in the general listing of books and monographs at the back of this book.

Cinnamon

Plant source: *Cinnamomum verum* J.S. PRESL.

Synonym: *Cinnamomum zeylanicum* auct.

Taxonomic classification: A subdivision of cultivated plants of this species is sometimes made into the varieties *C. verum* J.S. PRESL. var. *verum* and *C. verum* J.S. PRESL. var. *subcordatum* NEES.

Family: Laurel (Lauraceae).

Common names: Engl.: cinnamon, cinnamom, cinnamon tree, Ceylon cinnamon; Fr.: canellier, canelle de Ceylon; Ger: Zimt, Ceylon-Zimt, Kaneel.

Description: Up to 10 m tall, evergreen trees with dense foliage. In plantations, they are mostly kept as bushes by coppicing. The ovate-lanceolate entire leaves are opposite, coriaceous, up to 20 cm long, acuminate, nearly parallelinervate. The little inconspicuous flowers, about 0.5 cm in diameter, having a whitish-green 5-leaved perianth, 9 stamina and 3 staminodes are arranged in loose, silky pubescent panicles. The fruit is berry-like, lilac-black, up to 1.7 cm long, partially enclosed from the adnate calyx [Ü106].

Native origin: Southwestern India and Sri Lanka.

Main cultivation areas: Sri Lanka, as well as India, China, Seychelles, Madagascar, Indonesia (Java), Jamaica, Martinique, French Guiana, and Brazil.

Main exporting countries: Indonesia, Sri Lanka, Madagascar, in addition to China, Seychelles, and Brazil.

Cultivation: Cinnamon needs deep, loose soil in damp, but not waterlogged posi-

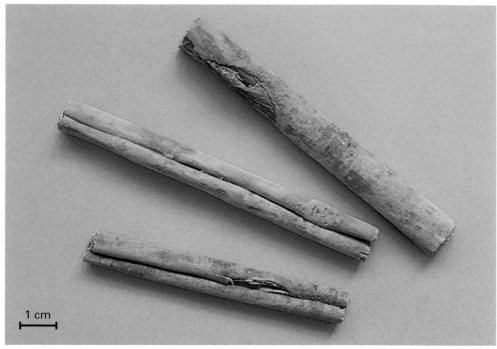

Fig. 1: Ceylon cinnamon

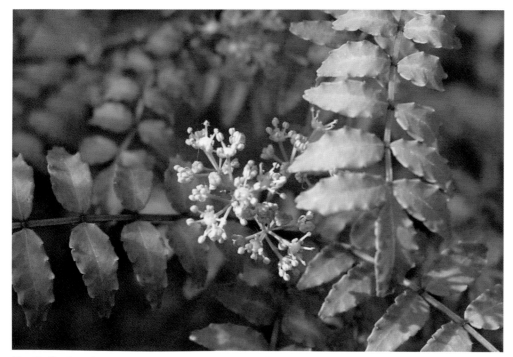

Fig. 2: Ceylon cinnamon (*Cinnamomum verum* J.S. PRESL.)

tions with average temperatures of about 26 to 28 °C. The annual rainfall amount should be about 2500 mm. Propagation is carried out by seed or cuttings in nursery beds, and transplantation to the final location can occur after about one year. Cutting back the main axis encourages the development of root suckers and coppice shoots. After 5 to 6 years the plant is ripe for the first cutting [Ü30, Ü89].

Culinary herb

Commercial forms: Cinnamon (Ceylon cinnamon, true cinnamon; Ger.: Ceylon-Zimtrinde, Echter Zimt, Echter Kanehl, Kahnel, Canehl, Caneel, Kaneel, Madagaskar-Zimt, as well as Java-Zimt and Seychellen-Zimt, see below): 8 to 10 cm long rolls, featherings, ground cinnamon, cinnamon essential oil, cinnamon oleoresin (oil- or water-soluble). Thin, light barks in thin rolls are of the best quality. The thickness of the walls of bark pieces are graded according to "ekelle" (center of cultivation in Sri Lanka): 00000 = up to 0.2 mm, 000 = up to 0.25 mm, 00 = up to 0.3 mm, 0 = up to 0.5 mm thickness. Varieties with wall thickness over 0.5 mm are classified with Roman numerals of I to IV, I = up to 0.7 mm, IV > 2.0 mm) [47, Ü30, Ü89, Ü92].

Production: The cutting of thumb-size, 1 to 2 year old root suckers and coppice shoots is done twice annually at the end of the rainy season, thereby the plant maintains a good sap level and the bark is more easily peeled. After cutting, the young shoots of leaves and lateral branches are removed. Then the outer bark is scraped down to the sclereid, rubbed with a brass rod, which makes loosening of the remaining inner bark easier, circular and slit longitudinally from one end to the other of the shoot and removed from the wood. 2 to 4 pieces of bark are placed one inside another around a brass rod. After removing the rod, the bark now assuming the shape of a quill is filled with smaller pieces of bark. Afterwards they are dried [47]. According to another source, the fresh peeled-off pieces of bark are wrapped inside of a mat and fermented, then, placed over a rounded wooden bar while the primary cortex is pulled off all the way down to the layer of stone cells, and with a twisting motion, separated from the mucilaginous remains of the cambium. Next the bark is shade-dried, followed by sun-drying to bleach it. During drying, the pieces of bark roll up. The dried cinnamon is later sorted according to color and thickness, and then 6 to 10 pieces of bark are inserted into one another to form rolls (quills) [Ü89]. The rolls are reduced to about 75 cm long and shipped in cylindrical bales. The 8 to 10 cm long pieces are commercially traded. The small pieces of bark (chips) and thin inner pieces of bark (featherings) left after preparing the quills are used to make cinnamon powder or distilled for cinnamon oil [Ü89].

Forms used: Dried cinnamon bark, whole or ground.

Storage: Cinnamon is stored protected from light and moisture in airtight porcelain-, glass- or suitable metal containers. Cinnamon sticks keep their aroma for 3 to 4 years under suitable storage conditions. Cinnamon powder loses its aroma quickly.

Description. Whole bark (Fig. 1): Yellowish-brown, smooth, 8 to 10 cm long, up to 1 cm thick rolls or double rolls, consisting of channeled 0.2 to 0.8 mm thick bark pieces whose surface is covered with fine whitish, sinuate longitudinal striations, which are interrupted by 1 to 1.5 cm large, roundish and dark-brown areas (leaf scars and scars of the branches). The fracture is short and fibrous [Ü92, Ph Eur].

Microscopic description: The microscopic image of the cross section reveals, just below the shreds of brown parenchyma cells, the still intact circle of stone cells, which is sometimes associated with primary bast fibers on the outside. Below it, is a starch-rich parenchyma with embedded bast fibers, mucilage cells and oil cells, which is traversed by uniseriate or biseriate medullary rays that contain calcium oxalate needles [Ü29].

Powdered bark: The powder is yellowish to reddish, consisting mostly of parenchyma rich in starch. The chloral hydrate preparation shows the numerous, prominent and colorless bast fibers, whole or fragmented, with narrow lumen and thick, lignified, sparsely punctuate walls, groups of roundish stone cells with moderately thick, punctate and furrowed walls as well as parenchymatic cells with small calcium oxalate needles and embedded oil cells (Fig. 4) [Ü29, Ü49, Ph Eur].

Odor: Agreeable balsamic-spicy, **Taste:** Spicy, sweetish-mucilaginous, only slightly harsh.

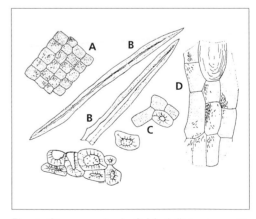

Fig. 3: Cinnamon twig with fruits

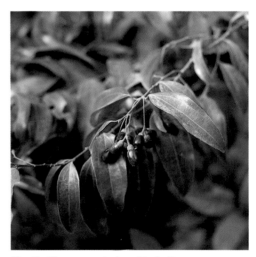

Fig. 4: Cinnamon bark. **A** Medullary rays with small needles of calcium oxalate, **B** Bast fibers, **C** Stone cells, **D** Parenchyma with oil cells and small oxalate needles. Ü49

History: Chinese cinnamon was first mentioned almost 5000 years ago. In the herbal of the Chinese emperor Shen Nung (about 2700 BCE), its use was described. Cinnamon was highly valued in Chinese cooking, particularly by the imperial courts. The bible and old Sanskrit texts mention this spice repeatedly. From China, its use spread following the trade routes through the kingdoms along the Euphrates and Tigris to Mediterranean regions. In ancient Rome, cinnamon was highly valued and used extensively. After the sea routes to India were established, Ceylon cinnamon was brought to Europe by the Portuguese, whom, in 1505, had secured their own trade monopoly. After the Portuguese were replaced as the dominating power in Ceylon (Sri Lanka) by the Dutch in 1658, the latter established commercial plantations. After the British conquered Ceylon in 1795/96, they took over the trade with cinnamon. The French brought *C. verum* to the Seychelles in the middle of the 18th century. After the interest in cinnamon cultivation had vanished, the plantations on the islands were increasingly neglected [45, 47, Ü31, Ü89, Ü97].

Constituents and Analysis

DIN- and ISO-Standards: DIN-Standard 10202 (Cinnamon, technical delivery conditions), ISO-Standard 6538 and 6539 (Cinnamon).

Constituents

- Essential oil: 0.2 to 2.5% (up to 4%), the main component is cinnamic aldehyde (42 to 82%), also present are, among others, eugenol (1 to 11%), cinnamic alcohol (about 8%), cinnamic acid (up to 10%), cinnamyl acetate, *o*-methoxycinnamic aldehyde, benzyl benzoate, linalool and safrole (up to 2%, in a specific chemotype up to 10%). During storage, the content of cinnamic aldehyde increases while the content of cinnamyl acetate decreases [2, 11, 23, 33, 41, 56]. In the trunk bark of chemical races from Northeast India, 85% benzylbenzoate [36] was detected, while cinnamon from Madagascar contained about 74% eugenol and only 4% cinnamic aldehyde [34].
- Proanthocyanidins: About 2%, mono-linked tri- to pentamers [22, 38].
- Phenolcarboxylic acids: Protocatechuic acid, among others [46].
- Diterpenes: Cinnzeylanol, cinnzeylanin (acetylcinnzeylanol) [18].
- Sterols: β-Sitosterol, among others [18].
- Sugar alcohols: Mannitol (up to 1.8%) [Ü37].
- Mucilage: 2 to 4%, arabinoxylans, glucans [16, 44].
- Starch: 5 to 10%.

Essential oil from the leaves contains 55 to 95% eugenol and only a small amount of cinnamic aldehyde [7], in some chemical races up to 40% safrole [23], about 40% cinnamic aldehyde, and 10% eugenol [34], or 65% benzylbenzoate [36]. The essential oil obtained from the flowers is dominated by cinnamyl acetate (about 42%), *trans*-α-bergamottene (about 8%), and β-caryophyllene epoxide (about 7%) [20].

Tests for Identity: The identity of Ceylon cinnamon bark can be determined with macroscopic and microscopic analysis as well as with TLC [40, 51, Ü77, Ü102, Ph Eur]; Ceylon cinnamon oil is identified with TLC [Ph Helv, DAC 86].

Quantitative assay: The content of essential oil is determined after steam distillation with xylol in the graduated tube [Ph Eur]; the content of cinnamic aldehyde is measured with GC [48], or fluorometrically [53]. The carbonyl constituents are analyzed acidimetrically after reaction with hydroxylamine hydrochloride [Ph Helv, ÖAB, DAC 86], the components of the cinnamon oil are assayed with GC, GC/MS [36] or HPLC [13], respectively.

Adulterations, Misidentifications and Impurities are possible with Chinese cinnamon, which has a considerably thicker bark with cork cells, or, with the bark of other Cinnamomum species, characterized by their high coumarin content (more than 0.03%). Within 2 to 3 minutes after moistening with 10% barium hydroxide solution, the adulterants show an intense yellowish-green fluorescence at UV 366 (in contrast to Ceylon cinnamon with only faint blue-green color). Moreover, Chinese cinnamon can be detected by the absence of eugenol [Ü93, U106]. Other impurities and adulterants of Ceylon cinnamon powder observed in the past, included, for example, starch, flour, dried ground bread, sawdust, tree bark, shells of walnuts, hazelnuts and coconuts [Ü29].

Actions and Uses

Actions: Due to its aromatic taste, cinnamon bark has appetizing and digestive promoting action. Aqueous solutions saturated with cinnamon oil administered through a catheter in dogs decreased motility of the stomach and increased intestinal motility [39]. However in isolat-

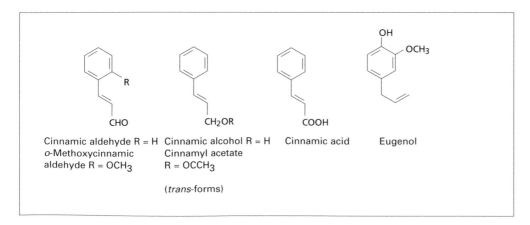

Cinnamic aldehyde R = H
o-Methoxycinnamic
aldehyde R = OCH₃

Cinnamic alcohol R = H
Cinnamyl acetate
R = OCCH₃

Cinnamic acid

Eugenol

(*trans*-forms)

ed guinea pig ileum, cinnamon oil showed a relaxant effect (ED_{50} 41 and 12 mg/litre). Cinnamic aldehyde (0.1 mg/ml in organ bath) also showed a papaverine-like spasmolytic effect [17, 42].

Ethanolic extracts of Ceylon cinnamon have demonstrated an anodyne effect in various test models with mice [4]. A methanolic dry extract of Chinese cinnamon (50 to 200 mg/kg body weight, p.o.) has antiphlogistic action. In mice, it inhibited the rise of acetic acid-induced capillary permeability, the development of Carrageenan-induced edema, ear edema induced by arachidonic acid, and granuloma induced by implantation of cotton pellets [26]. Extracts of the drug have shown antipyretic action in animal tests (mice infected with influenza viruses). Active principles that have been isolated include cinnamic acid ethyl ester, cinnamyl acetate, 4-allylanisol, 7-hydroxycoumarin, 2-hydroxy cinnamic acid and 2´-hydroxy acetophenone. As the mechanism of action it can be ascertained that the first four constituents listed above suppress production of interleukin-1α [27].

Extracts of cinnamon bark have shown in vitro good antioxidative capacity [6, 10, 11, 24, 30, 32, 57]. Growth of and urease activity of *Helicobacter pylori* was also inhibited by extracts of cinnamon [37, 52].

The intake of cinnamon (1 to 6 g daily) has been shown to reduce the mean fasting serum glucose of people with diabetes 2 (18 to 29%) [22a].

Cinnamon oil also repels cockroaches [1]. The isolated diterpenes of cinnamon bark have insecticidal activity [19].

Toxicology: Based on existing data, there is no chronic or acute toxicity with the use of cinnamon bark and cinnamon oil at normal doses [11].

After the intake of large amounts of cinnamon bark, vomiting has been reported [11]. Large doses of Chinese cinnamon, misused as an abortifacient, led to methemoglobinuria, hematinuria, albuminaria and nephritis [Ü58]. Also observed were spastic fits, tachycardia, increased gastrointestinal peristalsis, respiration and perspiration, followed by CNS-sedative effects with somnolence and depression [Ü106].

Oral administration of an ethanolic cinnamon extract (100 mg/kg body weight per day, for 90 days) in mice, led to hypertrophy of the reproductive organs, increased sperm motility and sperm count as well as a decrease of the blood hemoglobin content [49].

Cinnamon bark has a moderate sensitization potential. The main allergen is cinnamic aldehyde, which is mostly responsible for perfume or cosmetic allergies. Numerous case reports exist. Allergic reactions of the skin and mucous membranes have been observed in baking personnel and after the use of cinnamon-oil containing chewing gum, toothpastes or ointments. In workers processing cinnamon for export, asthma, skin inflammations and hair loss have been observed. Cross-reaction has been observed in individuals who are allergic to Peru balsam [9, 14, 15, 54, Ü39]

Food law regulations: The acceptable-daily-intake (ADI) for cinnamic aldehyde in finished products is 1.25 mg/kg [3].

Culinary use: Cinnamon is an important spice in the cooking of Arabia, the Orient and Southeast- and Eastern Asia. There it is used predominantly for salty dishes, as a seasoning of lamb, e.g. in Moroccan tagine and Iranian khorak, or as a filling of fruits of eggplants. In India it is a component of pilaws, curries, biryanis and kormas. In China and Korea, roast pork is flavored with cinnamon.

It is most favorable to add the whole pieces of cinnamon bark to season cooked dishes about 10 minutes before the end of the cooking process and then remove them prior to serving. Putting broken pieces of the bark in a metal tea infuser is also recommended. For the seasoning of salty dishes one must measure the cinnamon very carefully. Keep in mind that cinnamon is refused by many people!

Ceylon cinnamon bark serves as a seasoning of sweet dishes, rice pudding, cream soups, semolina pudding, omelets, cookies and cakes (e.g. gingerbread, almond biscuits, cinnamon crumpets, apple cakes, pancakes), compotes (e.g. pumpkin-, pear-, apple-, apricot-, plum-, orange- compotes), fruit salads, baked apples, chocolate desserts, toasted bread (sprinkled with 3 parts sugar and 1 part cinnamon powder, then toasted again for 1 min), but also of salty dishes such as soups, sauces (e.g. for meat dishes), meat- and fish dishes, sweet yeast dumplings, fillings for roast goose and duck, red cabbage, bulb vegetables and vegetable pancakes [45, Ü1, Ü2, Ü55, Ü65, Ü73, Ü91, Ü98, Ü109].

Cinnamon is also used as a beverage spice, e.g. of hot drinks such as mulled wine, punch, hot chocolate, but also of coffee (combined with grated chocolate as a flavoring of cappuccino), as well as of cold soft drinks such as cola and punches [Ü98]. In the liqueur industry, cinnamon is used as a flavoring of herbal liqueurs. Cinnamon oil serves as a flavoring of bakery products, confectionaries and liqueur but due to its intense inherent smell only to a limited extent.

Combines well with: Allspice, clove, coriander, nutmeg, and vanilla.

As a component of spice mixes and preparations: → Almond biscuit spice, → Apple cake spice, → Baharat, → Char masala, → Chilli spice, → Curry powder, → Egg spice, → English pudding spice, → Five-spice mix, → Garam masala, → Gingerbread spice, → La kama, → Masala, → Mulled wine spice, → Plum jam spice, → Quatre épices, → Ras el hanout, → Salsa comum, → Sausage spice, → Scappis spice mix, → Seven-seas spice, → Stollen spice, → Table mustard, → Tomato ketchup.

Other uses: The essential oil of the leaves is mostly used as a component of toothpastes, oral care products, but also of perfumes as well as for the production of eugenol [Ü24].

Medicinal herb

Herbal drugs: Cinnamomi cortex, Cinnamon bark, contains minimum 12 ml essential oil/kg [Ph Eur], Cinnamomi zeylanici cortices aetheroleum, Cinnamon oil, [Ph Eur: 55 to 75% *trans*-cinnamic aldehyde].

Indications: For loss of appetite, dyspeptic complaints such as mild spasmodic complaints in the gastrointestinal tract, bloating and flatulence (daily dose 2 to 4 g cinnamon bark, usually in the form of cinnamon tincture [Ph Eur], rarely in the form of tea infusions or 0.05 to 0.2 g cinnamon essential oil). Cinnamon bark should not be used during pregnancy or in cases of gastric- and intestinal ulcers [24]. In folk medicine, cinnamon bark is used internally also for diarrhea, common cold conditions and verminosis and diabetes, externally for treatment of wounds [55], and cinnamon oil is used for dysmenorrhea [Ü106].

Similar culinary herbs

Chinese cinnamon (Fig. 5, Cassia cinnamon, Cassia lignea; Ger.: Chinesischer Zimt, Kassia-Zimt, Zimtkassia, Holzkassia, Kaneel, Gemeiner Zimt, Mutter-Zimt, Canton-Zimt, Kwantung-Zimt, Kwangsi-Zimt, China junk-Zimt, Holz-Zimt, Englischer Zimt, Indischer Zimt), the bark of *Cinnamomum aromaticum* NEES (Synonym: *C. cassia* BL.), Cinnamon cassia, Chinese cinnamon tree, native to Southern China, Myanmar, Vietnam and Laos, cultivated in tropical Southeastern China, and to a lesser extent in Vietnam and in Java, it is exported predominantly to the USA [Ü61, Ü93]. The bark is obtained similarly to that of Ceylon cinnamon (see above). Because up until 6 years, the thick and often not entirely straight branches are used to obtain the bark, and the phellem is only coarsely scraped off, the bark pieces are irregular and thicker (1 to 3 mm) than those of Ceylon cinnamon and are therefore not placed one inside another. The commercially traded quills are 25 to 40 cm long. Names of commercial varieties include "Cassia lignea whole selected", "C.l. broken", "C.l. whole scraped" and "C.l. broken scraped". It is also differentiated according to qualities: Cassia lignea (stem bark), Cassia vera prima, Cassia vera secunda and Cassia vera tertia or Alba, Continental (C 00000 Special to C 0), Mexican (M 00000 special to M 0000) and Hamburg (H 1, H 2, H 3). The content of essential oil ranges from 1 to 4%, of which the main component is cinnamic aldehyde (80 to 95%), as well as, among others, *o*-methoxycinnamic aldehyde (1.5 to 3.8%), coumarin (up to over 1%), cinnamic alcohol and cinnamic acid [8, 21, 28, 43], eugenol and linalool are mostly absent. Chinese cinnamon is used therapeutically in the same way as Ceylon cinnamon. As a seasoning it is less commonly used in Europe than Ceylon cinnamon. It serves as a seasoning of, among others, mulled wine, Christmas cookies, plum sauce, game dishes and pickles [25, Ü51]. Shortly before the tree ceases to bloom, the unripe dried fruits are harvested. The so-called cassia buds (cassia flowers, clove cinnamon, Cassiae flos) serve as a spice and, today although rarely, are used as a flavoring of liqueurs. They contain 1.5% essential oil with cinnamic aldehyde as the main component. Cassia oil is obtained from the leaves, which finds use in the food industry [Ü61, Ü89, Ü92].

Saigon cinnamon (Vietnam cinnamon, Japanese cinnamon, Danang cinnamon, Tonki cinnamon, Malabar cinnamon, also cinnamon lignea or Annam cinnamon), bark of *Cinnamomum loureirii* NEES, native to the Southeast Asian mainland, grown almost exclusively in Vietnam and exported predominantly to the USA. Saigon cinnamon is a highly valued spice in Japan and China. It contains 2 to 7% essential oil, of which the main component is cinnamic aldehyde and eugenol also occurs [Ü37, Ü61, Ü93, Ü98].

Padang cinnamon (Batavia cinnamon, Java cinnamon, Batavia cassia, Indonesian cinnamon, Myanmar cinnamon, Korintji cassia, Macassar cinnamon, Timor cinnamon, also Malabar cinnamon, cinnamon lignea or Cassia vera), the bark of *Cinnamomum burmanii* (NEES) BL., native to the Malaysian Archipelago where it is cultivated as well as in the Philippines. The

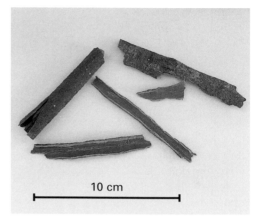

Fig. 5: Chinese cinnamon bark

main producer is Indonesia. The material of commerce originates partly from cultivation and partly from wild collection. Quality grades are AA, A, B, C, and D. Padang cinnamon contains about 4% essential oil with up to 77% cinnamic aldehyde, as well as coumarin (0.05%). Eugenol and *o*-methoxycinnamic aldehyde are absent [21, Ü37, Ü89, Ü93, Ü98].

Annam cinnamon, the bark from *Cinnamomum obtusifolium* NEES, native to the Eastern Himalayas, the Khasia mountains, Assam, Myanmar and Andaman, cultivated in Vietnam [Ü61, Ü98].

The following species are of less economic value and only of regional importance:

Culilawan cinnamon (Lavang cinnamon), the bark of *Cinnamomum culilawan* (L) BL., native to the Malay Archipelago, cultivated in Malaysia (Penang) and India (Calcutta). It contains 3.5 to 6% (up to 9%) essential oil, of which the composition is strongly dependent on the origin. The eugenol-type contains about 70% eugenol, and the eugenol-safrole type 85 to 97%, with both components at about the same proportions; the safrole-type is dominated by safrole and cinnamic aldehyde should be absent [50, Ü37, Ü61, Ü92, Ü98].

Malabar cinnamon (Indian cassia lignea), the bark of *Cinnamomum tamala* (BUCH.-HAM.) NEES et EBERM. (Synonym: *C. cassia* D. DON non BL.), native to India, Bangladesh and Myanmar, cultivated in India (Assam) and Myanmar, the leaves are also used as a spice [Ü61, Ü98].

Bark of *Cinnamomum iners* REINW. ex BL. (wild cinnamon), native to Southeast Asian mainland, Indonesia and the Philippines, where it is frequently cultivated [Ü61].

Bark of *Cinnamomum deschampsii* GAMBLE, native to Malacca, cultivated in Malaysia (Penang) [Ü61, Ü98].

Seychelles cinnamon (Madagascar cinnamon), the usually unscraped bark of *Cinnamomum verum* J.S. PRESL., which is produced in the Seychelles or in Madagascar, today often originating from trees escaped from cultivation. It contains 0.6 to 1.3% essential oil of which about 32% is cinnamic aldehyde, of low quality [Ü37, Ü92, Ü98].

Philippine cinnamon, the bark of *Cinnamomum philippinensis* MERR. [Ü92].

American cinnamon, fruit calyx of *Ocotea quixos* (LAM.) KOSTERM. ex O.C. SCHMIDT (Lauraceae), native to Brazil, cultivated in South America, the main components in the essential oil are cinnamic aldehyde, furthermore *o*-methoxycinnamic aldehyde, cinnamic acid and methyl cinnamate [35, Ü61].

Clove cinnamon (clove bark, clove cassia, black cinnamon), the bark of *Dicypellium caryophyllatum* (MART.) NEES (Lauraceae), native to Brazil and Guiana, eugenol is the main component of its essential oil [Ü60].

White cinnamon (white kaneel), the bark of *Canella winterana* (L.) GAERTN. (Synonym: *C. alba* MURR., *Winterana canella* L., Canellaceae), native to the Islands of the West Indies and Southern Florida, it contains 0.8 to 1.3% essential oil, of which

the main component is eugenol, furthermore, among others, 1,8-cineole, β-caryophyllene and β-pinene [Ü60, Ü92].

Winter's cinnamon (winter's bark), the bark of *Drimys winteri* J.R. et G. FORST. (Synonym: *Wintera aromatica* DESCOURT., Winteraceae), native from Chile to Tierra del Fuego, the main components of its essential oil are the sesquiterpenes drimenol (6% in the dried bark), drimenin (2%) and confertifoline (3.8%), also occurring is the pungent tasting sesquiterpene dialdehyde polygodial [5, Ü37, Ü92].

Bark of *Nectandra cinnamoides* NEES (Lauraceae), native to tropical South America, cultivated in Ecuador. The flower calyx is also used as a spice [Ü61].

Cinnamon apple

4 apples, 1 tablespoon ground cinnamon, 60 g butter, 2 tablespoons sugar, 60 g walnuts, 60 g nougat, 1/8 l white wine, 1/8 l whipped cream, 1 sachet vanilla sugar or 1 peeled vanilla pod.

Wash the apples, cut them in half and remove the core. Place the apple halves in a greased oven form. Sprinkle the apples with cinnamon powder and place the butter flakes on the top of them. Mix the sugar, chopped walnut and nougat pieces for use as topping. Pour white wine over the apples, cover with aluminum foil or parchment paper and bake at 220 °C for up to 30 minutes. Place whipped cream on top of each apple piece [Ü109].

Literature

[1] Ahmad F. et al., Insect Sci. Its Appl. 16(3/4):391–393 (1995), ref. CA 128: 150622e (1995).
[2] Angmor J.D. et al., Planta Med. 35(4): 342–347 (1979).
[3] Anonym: Natural flavouring substances, their sources and added artificial flavouring substances, Council of Europe, Strasbourg 1973, ref. Lit. 11.(s.u.).
[4] Atta A.H., A. Alkofahi, J. Ethnopharmacol. 60(2):117–124 (1998).
[5] Barrera A.F. et al., J. Ess. Oil Res 12: 685 688 (2000).
[6] Beuchat L.R., Food Preserv. 1994:167–179 (1994).
[7] Chalchat J.C. et al., Riv. Ital. EPPOS (Spec. Num.):729–740 (1998).
[8] Chowdhury M.A., J. Pharm. Pharmacol. 16:347 (1964), zit. Ü37.
[9] Collins F.W., Contact Dermatitis 2:167 (1975), zit. Ü39 (1975).
[10] Conner D.E., L.R. Beuchat, J. Appl. Bacteriol. 59:49–55 (1985).
[11] De Smet P.A.G.M. et al. (Eds.): Adverse Effects of Herbal Drugs, Springer Verlag Berlin, Heidelberg, New York 1992, Bd. 1, p. 105–114 (1992).
[12] Dhuley J.N., Indian J. Exp. Biol. 37(3): 238–242 (1999).
[13] Ehlers D. et al., Z. Lebensm. Unters. Forsch. 200(4):282–288 (1995).
[14] Fisher A.A., Hautarzt 21:295–297 (1970).
[15] Futrell J.M., R.L. Rietschel, Cutis 52(5): 288–290 (1993).
[16] Godwa D.C., C. Sarathy, Carbohydr. Res. 166:263–269 (1987).
[17] Harada M., S. Yano, Chem. Pharm. Bull. 23:941–947 (1975).
[18] Isogai A. et al., Agric. Biol. Chem. 40: 2305–2306 (1976).
[19] Isogai A. et al., Agric. Biol. Chem. 41: 1779–1784 (1977).
[20] Jayaprakasha G.K. et al., J. Agric. Food Chem. 48(9):4294–4295 (2000).
[21] Karig F., Dtsch. Apoth. Ztg. 46:1781–1784 (1975).
[22] Kaul R., Pharmazie i.u. Zeit 25(4): 175–185 (1996).
[22a] Khan A. et al., Diabetes Care 26(12): 3215-3218
[23] Koketsu M. et al., Cienc. Tecnol. Aliment. 17(3):281–285 (1998), ref. CA 128: 261630a.
[24] Kommission E beim BfArM., BAnz-Nr. 22a vom 01.02.1990.
[25] Kommission E beim BfArM., BAnz-Nr. 22a vom 01.02.1990.

[26] Kubo M. et al., Biol. Pharm. Bull. 19(8): 1041–1045 (1996).

[27] Kurokawa M. et al., Eur. J. Pharmacol. 348:45–51 (1998).

[28] Lockwood G.B., Planta Med. 36(4): 380–381 (1979).

[29] Lugasi A. et al., Spec. Publ. – R. Soc. Chem. 179 (Agri-Food Quality):372–375 (1996) , ref. CA 125:216961m.

[30] Mabrouk S.S., N.M. El-Shaheb, Z. Lebensm. Unters. Forsch. 171:344–347 (1980).

[31] Mancini-Filho J. et al., Boll Chim. Farm. 137(11):443–447 (1998).

[32] Mastura M. et al., Cytobios 98(387): 17–23 (1999).

[33] Miller K.G. et al., Chromatographia 42(11/12):639–646 (1996).

[34] Möllenbeck S. et al., Flavour Fragrance J:12(2):63–69 (1997).

[35] Naranjo P. et al., J. Ethnopharmacol. 4(2): 233–236 (1981).

[36] Nath S.C. et al, J. Ess. Oil Res. 8(3): 327–328 (1996).

[37] Neeman I. et al., Eur. Pat. Appl. EP 689,842(Cl. A61K35/78), 3. Jan. 1996, Appl. 94/401,473, 29 Jun. 1994, ref. CA 124:156022y.

[38] Nonaka J. et al., J. Chem. Soc. Perkin. Trans. 1:2139–2145 (1983).

[39] Plant O.H., G.H. Miller, J. Exp. Pharmacol. Ther. 27:149–164 (1926).

[40] Poole S.K. et al., J. Planar Chromatogr. Mod. TLC 8(4):257–268 (1995).

[41] Prasad S. et al., PAFAI J. Oct.–Dec.:35–37 (1989), zit. Lit. 7 (s.o.).

[42] Reiter M., W. Brandt, Arzneim. Forsch. 35:408–414 (1985).

[43] Sagara K. et al., J. Chromatogr. 409:365–370 (1987).

[44] Sarathy C., D.C. Gowda, Indian J. Chem, Sect. B, 27B:694–695 (1988), zit. Ü37.

[45] Scholz H., Natürlich 17(12):44–49 (1997).

[46] Schulz J.M., K. Herrmann, Z. Lebensm. Unters. Forsch. 171:193–199 (1980).

[47] Seidemann J., Drogenreport 11(20):68–75 (1998).

[48] Senanayake U.M., T.H. Lee, J. Chromatogr. 116:468–471 (1976).

[49] Shah A.H. et al., Plant Foods Hum. Nutr. 52(3):231–239 (1998).

[50] Spoon W., D. Spruit, Chem. Weekbl. 54:580 (1958), zit. Ü37.

[51] Stahl E. (Hrsg.): Chromatographische und mikroskopische Analyse von Drogen, Fischer Verlag Stuttgart, New York 1978.

[52] Tabak M. et al., J. Appl. Bacteriol. 80(6): 667–672 (1996).

[53] Tsai S.Y., S.C. Chen, J. Nat. Prod. 47: 536–538 (1984).

[54] Uragoda C.G., Br. J. Ind. Med. 41(2): 224–227 (1984).

[55] Vohora S.B., J. Ethnopharmacol. 16:201–211 (1986).

[56] Wijesekera R.O., CRC Crit. Rev. Food Sci. Nutr. 10:1–30 (1978).

[57] Yousef R.T., G.G. Tawil, Pharmazie 35: 698–701 (1980).

Literature references identified by Ü can be found in the general listing of books and monographs at the back of this book.

Citrus-species

Plant sources: Mainly the fruit peels, the fruit juice and the essential oil obtained from the peels, flowers and leaves of the following species are used as spice ingredients:
Citrus aurantium L., bitter orange,
Citrus limon (L.) BURM. f., lemon,
Citrus medica L., citron.

Taxonomic classification: Citrus-species are characterized by their typical fruits, which are multilocular berries. Their fruit pulp consists of juice-filled emergences, which grow from subepidermal tissue of the inner side of the pericarp into the loculi.

Due to selective breeding and the strong tendency towards mutative changes and hybridization, a quite considerable variability in forms has manifested, which makes their classification into species extraordinarily difficult. Depending on the botanical authority, there are 16 (according to SWINGLE), 36 (according to MANSFELD), or 145 different species (according to TANAKA). The demarcation between the *Citrus*, *Fortunella* and *Poncirus* genera is also unclear [Ü26, Ü61].

Family: Rue family (Rutaceae).

Description: Shrubs or trees, up to 15 m high. Leaves leathery and alternate, mostly with a rimmed or winged leaf stalk, entire, rarely trifoliate, ovate-lanceolate to lanceolate, entire-margined or irregularly crenate or serrate, evergreen, often with thorn-shaped axillary shoots; flowers single or in groups in the axils of the leaves, or more rarely, in corymbs terminal on the branches, hermaphrodite or male. The sweet-scented flowers have 3 to 5 sepals, usually fused to a cup with 3 to 5 teeth; 4 to 8 petals, thickish and lineally elongated, white or reddish, glandular; stamina mostly in groups of 20, rarely only 5, with a thick pillow- or ring-like disk, superior ovary, 5- to multi-locular with 4 to 8 ovules. The whole fruit is a roundish to oblong berry with a fruit wall (pericarp) consisting of a yellow, orange-red to red outer layer (flavedo, zedra), rich in schizolysigenous glands filled with essential oil, a white inner layer, more or less spongy (albedo) and the skin-like endocarp. Juice-filled, tubular vesicles (emergences), originating from the mesocarp, are enclosed by the membranous endocarp and form the edible part of the fruit. Embedded in the juice-filled vesicles are a few seeds with a thick, white testa; in some varieties seeds are absent [Ü26, Ü42].

Native origin: Southern Asia (India, southern China, the Malay Archipelago); the wild form is probably originally native to New Guinea and Melanesia.

Cultivation: Citrus plants are frost sensitive (critical lower temperature limit of –2° to –3° C). Subtropical zones are best suited for its cultivation. Fruits harvested in the tropics have a less aromatic taste and are mostly consumed locally. Propagation is carried out by vegetative means. The seeds, especially from cultivated orange-, lemon- or *Poncirus*-species, serve as the stocks for grafting (usually done by budding). The stocks have a significant influence on fruit yield, fruit quality, and pest-, frost- and drought resistance. The plants require much sun, good wind protection with stone embankments or protective windbreak plant walls, and sufficient irrigation in regions with annual total rainfall of less than 1200 mm. The first yield occurs in 3 to 5 years after grafting. Depending on the variety, the tree produces a full yield for 20 to 40 years, but can also be productive for over 100 years [Ü42, Ü82]. It is possible to grow the trees in a bucket. In the summer, the trees should be placed in a sunny, warm location that is protected from continuous rain. They can overwinter at 5 to 10 °C [Ü56].

Culinary Herb

Production: Citrus fruits must be harvested ripe, because a natural after-ripening of these low-starch fruits does not take place. Occasionally, however, green fruits are harvested and artificially ripened through an ethylene treatment. Fruits treated in this way have a lower sugar content and not as complete of an aroma (often discerned in the green calyx). After harvest, the fruits are washed, artificially colored, and sometimes they are dipped in a fungicide bath (2% sodium orthophenylphenolate + 1% hexamine) and waxed. The waxing process closes the pores and slows down desiccation and oxidative processes, e.g. the breakdown of vitamin C [Ü98].

History: The first time Europeans came into contact with Citrus species was during the conquests of Alexander the Great in Media (an ancient kingdom in northwestern Iran) in the 3rd century BCE. The Greeks learned the cultivation of Citrus species from Persian horticulturists. Theophrastus of Eresos (372–288 BCE) first documented a citrus fruit for medicinal use, in the form of a lemon with low acidity and a thick peel. Palladius first reported citrus cultivations in Sicily and Naples during the 4th century. Citrons were first grown in Palestine in the 6th century, and by the year 1000, they were cultivated in Salerno. Bitter orange cultivars reached southern Europe in the 9th century via the Sunda Islands, Hindustan, Arabia and North Africa. The cultivation of bitter oranges in Southern Europe can be traced back to the 16th century. The first plantations were established in 1792 in Spain, in

1870 in Italy, in 1922 in Morocco and by the 18th century, orange trees reached Central America. The first successful cultivation in the southern states of the USA occurred in 1815, and by 1842, bitter oranges were grown in California. Grapefruits were first grown in 1885 in California, Arizona and Florida. North of the Alps, Citrus species were first cultivated in the 16th century in buckets and special glass houses (orangeries) [Ü26, Ü31, Ü42].

Constituents and Analysis

Constituents of the fruits

- Essential oil: The main components are usually limonene and citral (a mixture of neral and geranial), which mainly contribute to the odor; furthermore, mostly β-pinene, γ-terpinene, α-terpineol and terpinenol-4.
- Flavonoids: In the fruit peel and pulp of the bitter variety, flavone neohesperidosides (neohesperidose=2-O-α-L-rhamnopyranosyl-β-D-glucopyranose), such as naringin and neohesperidin, as well as highly methoxylated, lipophilic analogs.
- Limonoids (modified triterpenes): Particularly in the seeds but also in the pulp and fruit wall; some of them are strongly bitter and insect repellent. In some citrus juices (e.g. navel oranges and grapefruits), some hours after squeezing a conversion of the non-bitter precursor limonate A-ring-lactone to the bitter limonoid limonin occurs due to the formation of an additional lactone ring at pH levels below 6.5 (delayed bitterness); the reaction is catalyzed by the enzyme limonin-D-ring-lactone-hydrolase [21].
- Hydroxycoumarins and furanocoumarins.

R^1 = OH,   R^2 = H   Naringin
R^1 = OCH$_3$, R^2 = OH   Neohesperidin

Rha

Limonate A-ring-lactone

Limonin

Limonin-17β–D-glucoside

Nomilin-17β–D-glucoside

- Vitamin C: In the juice 20 to 90 mg/100 ml, in the albedo up to 200 mg/100 g and in the flavedo up to 380 mg/100 g (calculated with reference to the fresh fruit) [37].

Other Citrus-species whose essential oils are used as aroma and flavor ingredients

The essential oils of other Citrus-species are used in the food-, liqueur- and perfume industries. This includes the essential oil of *Citrus sinensis* (L.) OSBECK, Sweet orange: Oleum Aurantii dulcis, Sweet orange peel oil (Portugal oil), of *Citrus bergamia* RISSO et POIT., Bergamot orange: Oleum Bergamottae, Bergamot oil, of *Citrus aurantifolia* (CHRISTM. et PANZ.) SWINGLE, Lime (see below): Oleum Limettae, Lime oil, and of *Citrus myrtifolia* RAF., Chinotto orange, Chinotto orange oil.

Literature See Lemon Lit page.

Bitter orange

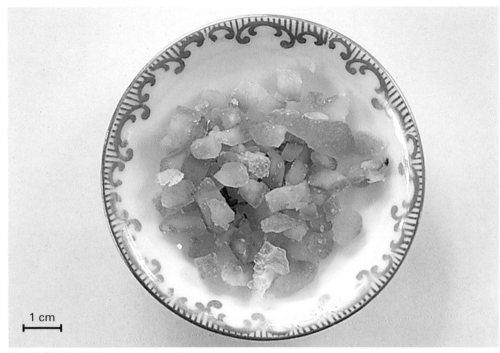

Fig. 1: Candied bitter orange peel

1 cm

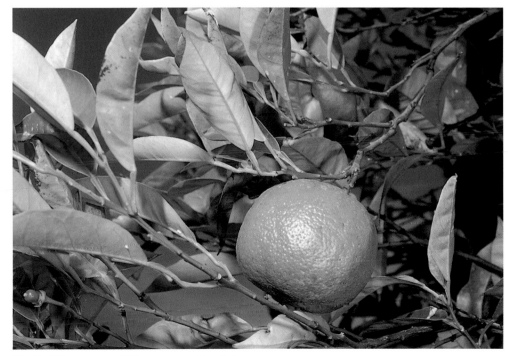

Fig. 2: Bitter orange (*Citrus × aurantium* L.)

Plant source: *Citrus × aurantium* L.

Synonyms: *Citrus aurantium* L. ssp. *aurantium*, *C. aurantium* L. ssp. *amara* ENGL., *C. bigaradia* RISSO et POIT.

Family: Rue family (Rutaceae).

Common names: Engl.: bitter orange, sour orange, bitter Seville orange; Fr.: bigaradier, orange amère; Ger.: Pomeranze, Bittere Orange, Bitter-Orange, Bigarad(i)e.

Main cultivation areas: Paraguay, Morocco, and Spain.

Main exporting countries: Spain, Portugal, Israel, Greece (Crete), and the West Indies.

Culinary herb

Commercial forms: Orange succade: candied orange peel, also the dried bitter orange peel and orange essential oil (oil of bitter orange).

Production: The peels of the ripe fruits are mechanically peeled off or manually peeled split into four pieces, mostly freed from the white spongy tissue (albedo) and dried (bitter orange peel). The peels are candied (bitter orange succade) by placing them in cane sugar solutions with gradually increasing concentrations (today this is often done under vacuum). The essential oil of bitter orange is expressed from the peel, after removal of the fruit pulp, by machine (today it is only rarely done manually with a sponge), or after mechanically rupturing the oil cavities of the peel and centrifuging. Steam distillation yields little essential oil with shorter shelf life.

Forms used: Bitter orange succade (candied outer fruit peel), fresh or dried outer fruit peel, essential oil of bitter orange peel.

Storage: The candied bitter orange peels are stored in a dry and cool place. The fresh peel can be stored in the refrigerator for a few days. The dried peels are stored in well-sealed porcelain-, glass or suitable metal containers, protected from light and moisture. The essential oil from bitter oranges should be stored in tightly closed, appropriately sized containers (to avoid too much air in the headspace), protected from light and heat.

Description. Whole peel: The dried outer layer of the fruit wall (flavedo) consists of the 5 to 8 cm long, 3 to 5 cm wide and about 1.5 mm thick, elliptical pieces, which are acuminate on both ends and more or less curved or bulgy. The peel fragments are yellowish to reddish brown with a distinctly knobby outer surface and a whitish yellow, coarsely punctate inner surface [DAB].

Cut peel (Fig. 1): The candied bitter orange peels of commerce occur usually with an orange-yellow surface, in the form of glass-like cubes with a diameter of about 5 to 10 mm.

Odor: Aromatic, **Taste:** Spicy and bitter; the candied peels are bittersweet.

Constituents and Analysis

Constituents of the fruit wall

- Essential oil: About 1.2 to 3%, the main components are (+)-limonene (about 85 to 90%, with a weak lemon-like aroma) and esters (about 2.5%, with the odoriferous constituents linalyl-, geranyl-, citronellyl acetate, decylpelargonate, anthranilic acid methyl ester), free alcohols (about 0.4%: linalool, α-terpineol, among others), aliphatic aldehydes (about 0.8%, including citral, nonanal, decanal, duodecanal, contributing to the odor); furthermore, myrcene, α-

and β-pinene, p-cymene [9]. In the expressed oil from Cuban oranges, limonene (about 86%) and myrcene (about 5%) were detected; no other components above the 1% level were documented [41]. The expressed bitter orange oil also contains hydroxy-coumarins, furanocoumarins and lipophilic flavonoids.

- Flavonoids: 7-O-Neohesperidosides of the flavanons narigenin and hesperitin, which include naringin and neohesperidin (responsible for the bitterness); furthermore, hesperidin, rutin and eriocitrin, as well as higher methoxylated flavonoids such as sinensetin, nobiletin, tangeretin, 3,5,6,7,8,3′,4′-heptamethoxyflavone and quercetogenin [9, 15, 32].
- Hydroxycoumarins: Meranzin, auraptenol, isomeranzin (possibly an artifact of auraptenol), osthol and columbianetin-O-β-glucoside [31, 32].
- Furanocoumarins: Bergaptene, epoxy-bergamottin, auraptene and 5-(6′,7′-dihydroxy-3′,7′-dimethyl-2-octenyloxy) psoralene [32].
- Carotenoids.
- Pectin.

Constituents of the seeds (which also occur in the peel and fruit pulp):

- Limonoids: Limonin glucoside, nomilin glucoside, desacetylnomilin glucoside, desacetylnomilinic acid glucoside, obacunone glucoside, isolimonic acid and ichangin [6].

Tests for Identity following the TLC assays of the Ph Eur or Ph Helv; see also Lit. [8, 40, 50, Ü77, Ü102].

Quantitative assay: Volumetric determination of the essential oil content from the ground peelings with steam distillation and xylol in the graduated tube [Ph Eur, Ph Helv]. The content of furanocoumarins, hydroxycoumarins and lipophilic flavonoids in the essential oil can be determined with HPLC [32].

Adulterations, Misidentifications and Impurities can occur with peelings from other Citrus species; they can be recog-

nized by their lower bitterness values (for bitter orange peels, not less than 600, according to DAB 1996).

Actions and Uses

Actions: On the basis of its bitter-aromatic taste, bitter orange peel has appetite stimulating and digestion promoting action. Extracts of bitter orange peel have shown an antispasmodic effect in isolated guinea pig intestine [2, 47].
Numerous citrus-flavonoids have antitumor activity. A few polymethoxylated flavonoids, particularly tangeretin and nobiletin, inhibited the mutagenicity of various mutagens (e.g. 2-aminofluorene, benzo[a]pyrene, among others) in the Salmonella/microsome assay [8], inhibited the partition of human breast cancer cells [11] as well as of other tumor cells [27], the invasive growth of tumor cells [53], and promoted apoptosis (self destruction) of leukemic cells in vitro (without damaging normal lymphocytes) [22]. Heptamethoxyflavone inhibited activation of the Epstein-Barr virus, carcinogenesis and mouse skin tumor promotion [23]. The screening of citrus-flavones and citrus juices as potential cancer chemopreventors has been discussed [24]. Additionally, a few monoterpenes of the essential oil, e.g. limonene, prevented the genesis of mammary-, liver-, lung-, and gastric tumors in rodents and showed chemotherapeutic activity against rodent mammary and pancreatic tumors [14].
Citrus-flavonoids have anti-hyperlipidemic activity. In animal experiments, in rats fed a cholesterol-rich diet, naringin or naringenin (0.1% in feed) lowered the plasma cholesterol level through inhibition of the 3-hydroxy-methylglutaryl-coenzymes A-reductase and acylcoenzyme A: cholesterol acyltransferase [29, 48].
Moreover, antiviral, antiphlogistic, analgesic, diuretic, antihypertensive, antithrombogenic and antiarteriosclerotic activities of citrus-flavonoids have been reported [5, 17, 19].
Essential oil of bitter orange has antimicrobial action [16].

Toxicology: There is no acute or chronic toxicity with the use of bitter orange peels, and its essential oil as a spice.

Due to the content of furanocoumarins intensive skin contact with fresh fruits or expressed bitter orange oil may cause photosensitization. In this case after exposure of the sensitized areas to sunlight erythema and eventually edemas may occur.

Culinary use: Bitter orange succade is used as a baking spice, e.g. in ring-shaped poundcake and in quick breads. Moreover, it also serves as a spice for sweet dishes (e.g. uncooked puddings), sauces and fillings (e.g. for fowl- or fish dishes) [Ü81].

The essential oil of bitter orange is used primarily in the liqueur industry as a flavoring component of Curaçao and of aperitifs, among other uses.

Unripe, dried bitter orange fruits (orangettes) are used for the manufacture of bitter liqueurs [Ü92, Ü98].

As a component of spice mixes and preparations: → Cumberland sauce, → Gingerbread spice mix.

Other uses: The fruit pulp serves as a component of marmalades (orange marmalade, Seville marmalade), and the fruit juice serves as a component of refreshing beverages (orangeade). The so-called Orange-Petit-Grain oil is an essential oil obtained from the leaves, young twigs and unripe fruits, and Neroli oil (Nafa oil, Essence of Neroli) is an essential oil obtained from the flowers. Both are used in the perfume and soap industry. The fatty oil of the seeds is used in the production of soaps [Ü61, Ü92, Ü98].

Medicinal herb

Herbal drugs: Aurantii amari epicarpium et mesocarpium, Bitter-orange epicarp and mesocarp, contains minimum 20 ml/kg of essential oil [Ph Eur], and Aurantii amari flavedo, which is the outer layer of the fruit wall (flavedo), mostly freed from the spongy white tissue (albedo), containing minimum 30 ml/kg essential oil, and a bitterness value of not less than 1500 [Ph Helv], Aurantii amari floris aetheroleum, Bitter-orange-flower oil [Ph Eur], Aurantii amari flos, Bitter-orange flower, contains minimum 8.0% of total flavonoids [Ph Eur], and Aurantii fructus immaturi, Immature bitter orange fruit [Fructus Aurantii immaturus PPRC 2000], which is now rarely used in Europe but widely used in China.

Indications: Dried bitter orange peel is used for loss of appetite and digestive complaints in tincture form (Aurantii amari epicarpii et mesocarpii tinctura Ph Eur) (daily dose: 2 to 3 g), extract form (daily dose: 1 to 2 g), as a tea infusion (daily dose: 4 to 6 g) or as a syrup (one teaspoonful, t.i.d., after meals) [28, 54]. Essential oil of bitter orange (1 to 2 drops, t.i.d.) is used in folk medicine for treatment of kidney- and bladder problems and also as a cholagogue, among other uses [54].

Literature see → Lemon.

Citron

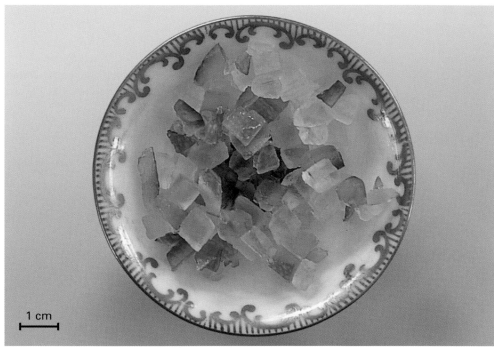

Fig. 1: Candied citron peel

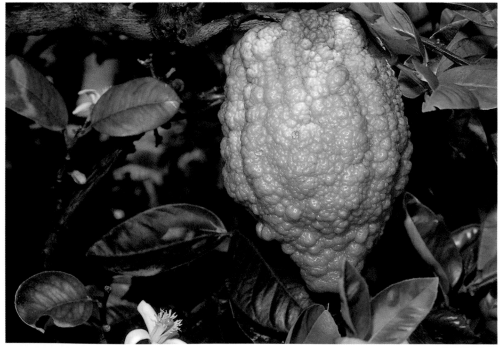

Fig. 2: Citron (Citrus medica L. var. medica)

1 cm

Plant source: *Citrus medica* L. var. *medica*.

Taxonomic classification: The species can be subdivided into the following varieties, among others:
C. medica L. var. *medica*, Citron, fruit peels used for the production of candied citron peel,
C. medica L. var. *ethrog* ENGL., Ethrog (esrog, etrog), cultivated in Israel and in Corfu, and used for ritual purposes in Israel,
C. medica L. var. *sarcodactylis* (HOOLA VAN NOOTEN) SWINGLE, Flesh-finger citron (Buddha's hand), cultivated in South- and East Asia, where the fruits are used to scent clothing and rooms.

Family: Rue family (Rutaceae).

Common names: Engl.: citron; Fr.: cédrat, cédratier; Ger.: Zitronatzitrone, Zedratzitrone, Zedernfrucht.

Main cultivation areas: Italy, Greece, Corsica, California, West India, and Brazil.

Main exporting countries: Italy and Greece (Crete).

Culinary herb

Commercial forms: Candied citron peel (succade): candied fruit peel, essential oil (citron oil, frequently also mixed with bergamot oil, lemon oil, and sweet orange peel oil).

Production: The 15 to 25 cm long, 5 to 10 cm wide and 1 to 2.5 kg fruits are picked when green. The fruits are separated from the sour pulp, which makes up only about 30% of the fruit weight. The fruit peels are preserved by cooking them in 3% salt water or sea water and, usually only in the countries of consumption, soaked for several days and candied through a several week treatment with sugar solutions of increasing concentrations. Today, this is often done under vacuum. After a two-month storage period, the candied peels are ready for market [Ü92].

Forms used: Candied fruit peels.

Storage: Candied lemon peel should be stored in a cool and dry place.

Description. Whole pieces: Greenish to yellowish and glassy pieces of the thick, mostly wrinkled and candied fruit wall.

Cut pieces (Fig. 1): The candied citron peel of commerce mostly occurs in cube-like pieces with a side length of 5 to 10 mm, and a light green, glass-like outer surface.

Odor: Aromatic, **Taste:** Bitter-aromatic and sweet.

Constituents and Analysis

Constituents of the fruit peel

- Essential oil: Its composition depends strongly on the cultivar and subspecies; the main components of the essential oil from the fruit peel of fresh citrons are limonene (about 60 to 80%, high concentrations in *C. m.* var. *ethrog*), γ-terpinene (5 to 32%, high concentrations in *C. m.* var. *sarcodactylis*, low levels in *C. m.* var. *ethrog*) and β-pinene (in cv. 'Rugosa' up to 15%); furthermore citral (1% to 20%, high concentrations are reached with pressed oils) [42, Ü60].
- Flavonoids: Hesperidin, among others.

Actions and Uses

Actions: On the basis of the bitter-aromatic taste of citron, it has appetite stimulating and digestion promoting effects. There are no known pharmacological studies available on citron.

Toxicology: There is no acute and chronic toxicity with the regular use of candied citron peel as a spice.

Culinary use: As a flavor component of baked goods, especially in Christmas baking, fruit cakes (stollen), spice cakes, English cakes, cakes and pastries (with a long shelf life), cereal dishes for breakfast, sweet dishes, confectionaries and spice sauces [Ü92].

Candied citron peels are likewise used as a component of poultry fillings (goose, turkey, duck) [Ü45].

Other uses: The fruit flesh is used for the manufacture of marmalades and to make fruit juice.

Medicinal herb

Herbal drug: Citri medicae pericarpium, Citreum, the fresh pericarp, today no longer used.

Literature see → Lemon.

Lemon

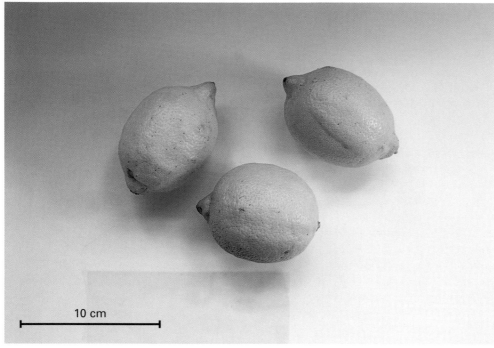

Fig. 1: Lemons

Plant source: *Citrus limon* (L.) BURM. f.

Synonyms: *Citrus limonum* RISSO, *C. medica* L. var. *limonum* (RISSO) WIGHT et ARN.

Taxonomic classification: A species with a wide variety of forms, slightly to prominently thorny edges and usually with non-winged petioles.

Family: Rue family (Rutaceae).

Common names: Engl.: lemon; Fr.: citron, citronnier, limonier; Ger.: Zitrone, Sauer-Zitrone.

Main cultivation areas: California, Italy (Sicily), Spain, Greece, and Northern Africa.

Main exporting countries: Spain, African countries, and the Caribbean.

Culinary herb

Commercial forms: Fresh lemon fruits, particularly from the cultivars 'Eureka', 'Lisbon', 'Verna' and 'Villafranca', dried lemon peels, usually in ribbons, candied lemon peels, and essential oil of fresh lemon peel.

Production: Lemons are harvested several times per season, for example, in Sicily they are harvested from September to November, December to May and from June to September. They are ripe when the green part of the peel is shiny. The first harvest can take place in the 5th year after grafting. A 15 to 20 year old tree produces about 1,000 fruits and a fully-grown tree up to 2,000 fruits. The essential oil is obtained by mechanical means or by manual expression of the fresh peels (using a

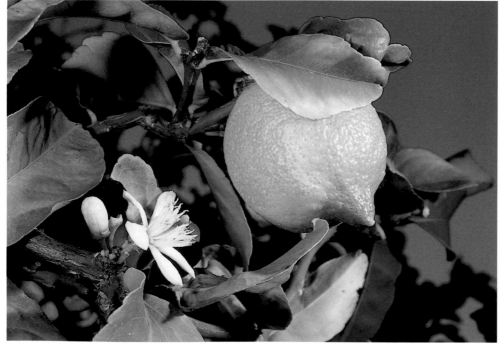

Fig. 2: Lemon (*Citrus limon* (L.) BURM. f.)

sponge to suck in the essential oil pressed out), which is only rarely practiced today, or of the mechanical produced abrasion, furthermore through fulling of the whole fruits between roller conveyors or metal discs, by centrifugation after homogenization of the whole fruits, by extraction with light liquid solvents or more rarely by steam distillation, usually under vacuum. Steam distillation under normal air pressure yields a less aromatic and less shelf-stable oil. Distillation under vacuum produces a higher quality oil. Fractional distillation can remove the less intense smelling terpene hydrocarbons. Oil produced by fractional distillation contains up to 50% citral and 25% esters (calculated as linalyl acetate). Lemon petitgrain oil is produced by steam distillation of the twigs, leaves and unripe fruits (containing about 15% citral and 10% geranyl- or neryl-acetate or -geraniate) [Ü26, Ü31].

Forms used: Fresh lemon peels, candied lemon peels, lemon juice, and lemon essential oil.

When purchasing lemons from which the peels are to be used as a spice, it is important to make sure that the fruits were not treated with insecticides or pesticides. When in doubt, blanch the fruits for 1 minute in boiling water [Ü55].

Storage: The fruits can be stored at room temperature for about a week and in the refrigerator for about a month. Lemon oil should be stored, protected from light, in tightly sealed containers of appropriate size (to minimize the oxygen amount in the headspace).

Description. Whole fruit (Fig. 1): Ovate fruits, with a nipple-like, acuminate and often tumid apex, yellow, 7 to 10 cm long, with an average weight of about 150 g. The peel is about 2 to 3 mm thick, light yellow when fresh, brownish-yellow when dry, with numerous punctate depressions and a whitish inner surface [DAB 6]

Cut peel: The candied lemon peel of commerce usually consists of yellow, glass-like, about 5 to 10 mm wide cubes.

Odor: Aromatic and characteristic, **Taste:** The peel is pungent, the candied peel is sweet, and the fruit juice is intensely sour.

Constituents and Analysis

Constituents of the fruit wall

- Essential oil: 0.2 to 0.6% in the dried peel, 1.2 to 1.5% in the fresh peel; the main components are (+)-limonene (65 to 70%, with a faint lemon-like odor), citral (1 to 5%, significantly contributing to the odor), β-pinene (4 to 9%), γ-terpinene (9 to 12%) and linalool (1.5%). Also present are 1,8-cineole, geranyl acetate, nonanal, citronellal, α-phellandrene, α-terpineol, terpinenol-4, camphene and (Z)-α-bisabolene, among others [3, 9, 12].
- Flavonoids: Hesperidin, diosmin, eriocitrin, rutin, naringenin-7-rhamnoglucoside, limocitrol, isolimocitrol, limocitrol- and isolimocitrol-3-glucosides, limocitrin-3-glucoside, apigenin-6,8-di-C-glucoside, luteolin-7-rhamnoglucoside, luteolin-6,8-di-C-glucoside, 2-O-glucosylvitexin, isovitexin and chrysoeriol-8-C-glucoside, among others; some cultivars also contain neohesperidin, naringin and poncirin [4, 33, 52, Ü43, Ü60].
- Carotenoids [39].
- Hydroxycoumarins: 5-Geranyl-oxy-7-methoxycoumarin, 5,7-dimethoxy-coumarin, byakangelicin and limettin derivatives [4, 43, 44].
- Furanocoumarins: Psoralene, 5-methoxypsoralene, oxypeucedanin, isoimperatorin, isopimpinellin, bergaptol, 8-geranyloxypsoralene and 5-geranyloxypsoralene (bergamottin) [36].
- Phenyl propane derivatives: p-Coumaroyl glucaric acid, diferuloyl glucaric acid, citrusin A [4,34].
- Pectin [43].

Constituents of the pulp

- Fruit acids: Citric acid, about 5 to 8% [Ü60].
- Flavonoids: Eriocitrin, hesperidin [33, 45].
- Vitamin C: 0.03 to 0.08% [Ü60].

Constituents of the seeds

- Limonoids: Limonin, nomilinic acid, limoninic acid and limonin-17β-D-glucoside [4].

Tests for Identity: To identify lemon fruits the peel should be analyzed for its carotenoid profile [20]. The lemon oil is identified with TLC based on the detection of citral and specific coumarin derivatives (e.g. bergamottin) [50, Ü77, Ph Eur], characteristic flavonoids [45] or by its physico-chemical parameters and UV spectrum [Ph Eur].

Quantitative assay: Volumetric determination of the essential oil content with steam distillation and xylol in the graduated tube [DAB, Ph Helv]; the lemon oil is evaluated quantitatively for its content of carbonyl constituents using a titrimetric method [Ph Eur]; a densitometric TLC assay determines the citral content [45].

Adulterations, Misidentifications and Impurities: Lemon juice can be adulterated with other citrus juices or artificial ingredients. Impurities, freshness and quality can be evaluated with CE (Capillary-Electrophoresis) [10].

Actions and Uses

Actions: Due to the aromatic taste of lemon peel and the acidic-aromatic taste of lemon juice, it has appetite stimulating and digestion promoting effects.

In animal experiments, lyophilized lemon juice (5 g/kg body weight over 15 d or 30 d in drinking water) lowered levels of cholesterol, LDL and triacylglycerols in the blood of rats with diet-induced hypercholesterolemia and led to an elevated HDL level (orange juice had a similar effect) [51]. Similar results were attained with hesperidin [35].

6,8-Di C-glucosylapigenin has shown a hypotensive effect following i.v. administration in rats. Diosmin, in the form of its aglycone diosmetin, which is formed in the intestines, has shown a vasotonic effect [7, 13, Ü106]. Coumarin derivatives isolated from lemon peels inhibited in vitro 12-O-tetradecanoylphorbol-13-acetate (TPA)-induced Epstein-Barr virus activation in Raji cells and thereby inhibited tumor promotion. Furthermore, they suppressed TPA-induced superoxide generation in promyelocytic leukemia cells and reduced lipopolysaccharide (LPS)- and interferon-alpha (IFN-α)-induced nitric oxide (NO) generation in macrophage cells [34]. Lemon juice inhibited in vitro the formation of carcinogenic nitrosamines from dimethylamine and sodium nitrate (determination of the formed N-nitrosodimethylamine), vegetable juice had a moderate inhibitory effect, and comparable concentrations of vitamin C had almost no effect [1].

Lemon oil has antimicrobial activity [49].

Due to similar constituents, the pharmacological actions of lemons are comparable to those of → Bitter orange.

Toxicology: There is no acute or chronic toxicity with the regular use of lemon peel, lemon juice and lemon oil as a spice, beverage and food ingredient.

Frequent consumption of citrus fruits or citrus juice containing beverages can lead to chemical erosion of the tooth enamel. In order to avoid lasting damage, teeth brushing should not occur immediately after intake of citrus fruits. For drinking lemon or orange juices, the use of a straw is recommended [30].

Close skin contact with fresh lemons or pressed lemon oil can lead to photosensitization due to the presence of furanocoumarins. Exposure to sunlight causes erythema and edema of the sensitized areas [36]. Citral and citronellal are the potentially sensitizing agents [Ü39]. Autoxidation products of limonene can also trigger allergic reactions [26].

Culinary use: Lemon filets (fruit pieces, freed from peel, skin and seed) serve as garnishes and flavor components of fish and meat dishes, of pastries, ice cream, marmalades and sweets. Quartered lemons or fruit slices are also used as garnishes and flavor components (e.g. in fish dishes) [Ü55].

Lemon julienne (about 1 mm thick, noodle-like cut strips of lemon peels) serves to embellish sweet as well as piquant dishes, e.g. ice creams, tortes and pastries. Lemons can be peeled in a spiral form by using a zester or a peeler [Ü55].

Lemon juice is used for the production of refreshing beverages (citron pressé) and as a flavor component of beverage teas. A few splashes of the juice gives a fruity aroma to fruit salads. Leaf salads can also be improved with lemon juice. It is also used as a component of baked goods, e.g. lemon meringue gateau, marmalades and jellies. To obtain the juice, the fruit is rolled back and forth under pressure with the hands on a firm base, in doing so causing the rupture of the juice-filled, tubular vesicles of the fruit, which increases the juice yield during pressing [Ü13].

Thin slices of raw meat or fish can be tenderized with lemon juice. In Latin America, raw fish that is marinated in lemon juice is called "ceviche" (thin strips of fish placed in lemon juice together with chilies, onions and some spice herbs for five to six hours, after which the dish is ready to eat). A combination of lemon juice with orange juice, garlic and ginger makes a good marinade for grilled chicken or pork loin.

Dabbing some lemon juice on cut fruit and vegetable sections (e.g. apples, celery, artichokes) slows down the discoloration of their cut surface area [Ü2, Ü55].

Grated peels from lemons, untreated with fungicides or insecticides, adds a piquant aroma to marinades, fillings, salads, compotes, quark puddings, cakes (e.g. butter cake), baked puddings or sauces. It also serves to round off Provençal meat stews and the Italian dish ossobucco in cremolata with chopped parsley and garlic strewn over the dish before serving.

In order to flavor a dessert, a sugar cube that has been rubbed against the peel of an untreated lemon can be added [Ü2, Ü55]. Candied lemon peel is used as a baking spice, e.g. in English cakes [Ü2].

Lemon oil is used in the manufacture of baking flavor oils, fruit essences, refreshing beverages, baked goods and sweets [Ü92].

Combines well with garlic and rosemary; lemon juice, grated lemon peel, rosemary leaf, garlic mixed with olive oil makes for a universal meat spice.

As a component of spice mixes and preparations: → Mulling wine spice, → Sauce spice.

Other uses: Lemon oil is used in the cosmetic industry for the manufacture of soaps, face lotions, perfumes (eau de cologne) and bath salts. The fatty oil of the seeds is used in the manufacture of soaps. The remains of the fruit peels left over from the production of essential oil can be used to make pectin [Ü61].

Medicinal herb

Herbal drugs: Limonis flavedo recens, Fresh lemon peel: the fresh, outer peel (flavedo) of the ripe fruit obtained by removing the white, spongy tissue (albedo), contains minimum 1.2% essential oil [Ph Helv], Limonis aetheroleum, Lemon oil: obtained by suitable mechanical means without the aid of heat, contains 2.2 to 4.5% carbonyl compounds, calculated as citral [Ph Eur].

Indications: Lemon peel is used for digestive complaints (daily dose 1 g of the dried peel) [Ü60]. Lemon juice is used in folk medicine, diluted in warm water and sweetened with raw sugar or honey, for the prophylaxis of respiratory tract infections (juice of one lemon about twice an hour) [55].

Similar spices

Lime (key lime), the fruits of *Citrus aurantiifolia* (CHRISTM. et PANZ.) SWINGLE (Rutaceae) serve as a substitute for lemon especially in hot regions. The main components of the essential oil of the fruit peel are limonene (about 40%), β-pinene (about 28%), geraniol (about 7%) and citral (about 7%). Furthermore, it contains α-terpineol, terpinenol-4 and (E)-β-farnesene, among others [25]. The sour juice is slightly bitter and is used mainly for souring foods, chutneys or pickles. In western countries, it is used in the form of sweetened juice syrups and in liqueurs. In the Middle East, dried limes are added to hotpot. The peels are used for the flavoring of sorbets and ice creams [Ü2, Ü92].

Kaffir lime (Indian lime, combava), *Citrus hystrix* DC. (Rutaceae), the grated peels and leaves are used, which have a strongly lemon-like pleasant aroma. The main components of the fruit peel oil are β-pinene (about 48%), limonene (about 15%), citronellal (about 12%) and terpinenol-4 (about 9%), and of the leaf oil are citronellal (about 72%), citronellol (about 7%) and citronellyl acetate (about 4%) [25]. The oil is commonly used especially in Thailand and Indonesia in soups, and in curry-, fish-, chicken-, and wok dishes. It is well suited as a spice in western hot-pots and pot roasts. The commercially available dried peels are soaked in water before use. The leaves can be added during cooking in the same manner as bay leaves. The fruit peels and leaves are removed before serving the meal. Various Indonesian spice mixes contain the leaf (→ Bomboe, → Sambal). The fruit peels are also traded in cut and dried or candied forms (papeda peels, combava peels). The leaves can be stored for two to three weeks in the refrigerator and also freeze well [Ü68, Ü74, Ü98].

Calamondin, the fruit peels of *Citrus madurensis* LOUR. (*C. microcarpa* BUNGE, *C. mitis* BLANCO, from some authors integrated in *Fortunella japonica*, see below, Rutaceae), cultivated mainly in the Philippines. The main component of the essential oil is limonene (about 95%) [25]. It is used in the manufacture of fruit essences and as a flavor component of sauce spices [Ü61, Ü92].

Kumquat, the fruit of *Fortunella japonica* (THUNB.) SWINGLE (*Citrus japonica* THUNB., Rutaceae), cultivated especially in Brazil. The diameter of the sphere-shaped or oval, orange-colored fruit is only 1.5 to 3.0 cm. The main component of the essential oil is limonene (up to 88% [38]). The fruit is well suited to be cooked along with roasted duck, pork dishes and sauces for ham dishes. They can also be eaten raw, e.g. added as an ingredient of fruit salads, or consumed cooked with the peels, candied or in syrup. The fruits of the Malaysian kumquat (*F. polyandra* (RIDL.) TANAKA), cultivated on the Malaysian Peninsula, and of the Hong Kong kumquat (*F. hindsii* (CHAMP.) SWINGLE), cultivated in China and Japan, are used similarly [Ü2, Ü61, Ü55].

Hesperethusa fruit, of *Hesperethusa crenulata* (ROXB.) ROEM (*Limonia crenulata* ROXB., *L. acidissima* auct. non L., Rutaceae), native to Southeastern Asia, cultivated in Java and India. It is used as a spice for fish and meat dishes [Ü61].

Literature

[1] Achiwa Y. et al., Nippon Shokuhin Kagaku Kogaku Kaishi 44(1):50–54 (1997), ref. CA 126:198762m.

[2] Ammon H.P.T, Z. Phytother. 10(6):167–174 (1989).

[3] Ayedoun A.M. et al., J. Ess. Oil Res. 8:441–444 (1996).

[4] Baldi A. et al., J. Chromatogr. A 718(1):89–97 (1995).

[5] Benavente-García O. et al., J. Agric. Food Chem. 45:4505–4515 (1997).

[6] Bennett R.D. et al., Phytochemistry 30:3803–3805 (1991).

[7] Boukskela E., Donyo K.A., Angiology 48:391–399 (1997).

[8] Calomme M. et al., Planta Med. 62(3):222–226 (1996).

[9] Calvarano I., Essenze Deriv. Agrum. 36:5 (1966).

[10] Cancalon P.F., J. Assoc. Off. Anal. Chem. Int. 82(1):95–106 (1999).

[11] Carroll K.K. et al., Antiox. Health Dis. 7 (Flavonoids in Health and Disease), Marcel Dekker, Inc. 1998, ref. CA: 128:135952u.

[12] Chamblee Th.S. et al., J. Agric. Food Chem. 39:162–169 (1991).

[13] Codignola A. et al., Planta Med. 58 (Suppl. 7):A628 (1992).

[14] Crowell P.L., J. Nutr. 129(3):775S–778S (1999).

[15] Del Río J.A. et al., Planta Med. 64(6):575–576 (1998).

[16] Fariq S.R. et al., Pak. J. Sci. Ind. Res. 38(9–10):358–361 (1995), ref. CA 126:303577e.

[17] Franke G., Nutzpflanzen der Tropen und Subtropen, Hirzel, 2. Aufl. Verlag, Leipzig 1975, Bd. II, p. 202–244.

[18] Galati E.M. et al., Farmaco 40(11):709–712 (1994).

[19] Galati E.M. et al., Farmaco 51(3):219–221 (1996).

[20] Gross J., Chromatographia 13:572 (1980).

[21] Hasegawa Sh., M. Miyake, Food Rev. Int. 12(4):413–435 (1996).

[22] Hirano T. et al., Brit. J. of Cancer 72:1380–1388 (1995).

[23] Iwase Y. et al., Cancer Lett. 154(1):101–105 (2000).

[24] Iwase Y. et al., Cancer Lett. 139(2):227–236 (1999).

[25] Jantan I. et al., J. Ess. Oil Res. 8:627–632 (1996).

[26] Karlberg A.T., A. Dooms-Goossens, Contact Dermatitis 36(4):201–206 (1997).

[27] Kawaii S. et al., Biosci. Biotechnol. Biochem. 63(5):896–899 (1999).

[28] Kommission E beim BfArM, BAnz-Nr. 193 vom 15.10.87, Berichtigung vom 13.3.90.

[29] Lee S.H. et al., Ann. Nutr. Metab. 43(3):173–180 (1999).

[30] McAndrew R., S. Kourkouta, J. Periodontol. 66(6):443–448 (1995).

[31] McHale D. et al., Phytochemistry 26:2547 (1987).

[32] McHale D., J.B. Sheridan, J. Ess. Oil Res. 1:139–149 (1989).

[33] Miyaka Y. et al., Food Sci. Technol. 3(1):84–89 (1997).

[34] Miyake Y. et al., J. Agric. Food Chem. 47(8):3151–3157 (1999).

[35] Monforte M.T. et al., Farmaco 50(9):595–599 (1995).

[36] Naganuma M. et al., Arch. Derm. Res. 278:31 (1985).

37] Nagy S., J. Agric. Food Chem. 28(1):8–18 (1980).

[38] Nguyen Manh Pha et al., J. Ess. Oil Res. 8(4):415–416 (1996).

[39] Noga G., F. Lenz, Chromatographia 17:139 (1983).

[40] Pachaly P., Dtsch. Apoth. Ztg. 139(11):1181–1182 (1999).

[41] Pino J.A., A. Rosado, J. Ess. Oil Res. 12:675–676 (2000).

[42] Poiana M. et al., J. Ess. Oil Res. 10(2):145–152 (1997).

[43] Postorino C.E. et al., Essenze Deriv. Agrum. 52:367 (1982).

[44] Risch B., K. Herrmann, Z. Lebensm. Unters. Forsch. 187:530–534 (1988).

[45] Robards K. et al., J. Sci. Food Agric. 75(1):87–101 (1997).

[46] Rossini C. et al., J. Planar Chromatogr.-Modern. TLC 4:259 (1991).

[47] Schuster K.P., Wirkungsstärke und Wirkungsverluste spasmolytisch wirksamer Arzneidrogen, galenischer Zubereitungen und Arzneifertigwaren, geprüft am isolierten Darm des Meerschweinchens und am Darm der Katze in situ, Dissertation Ludwig Maximilian-Universität München (1971).

[48] Shin Y.W. et al., Int. J. Vitamin Nutr. Res. 69(5):341–347 (1999).

[49] Siddiqui R.F. et al., Pak. J. Sci. Ind. Res. 38(9–10):358–361 ref. CA 126:303577e (1995).

[50] Stahl E. (Hrsg.), Chromatographische und mikroskopische Analyse von Drogen, Fischer Verlag, Stuttgart, New York 1978.

[51] Trovato A. et al., Phytomedicine 2: 221–227 (1996).

[52] Tsiklauri G., Soobshch. Akad. Nauk. Gruz. 152(2):401–404 (1997) zit.: CA 127: 290576x.

[53] Vermeulen S. et al., Pathol. Res. Practice 192:694–707 (1996).

[54] Vonarburg B., Natürlich 16(1):56–60 (1996).

[55] Vonarburg B., Natürlich 19(1):56–61 (1999).

Literature references identified by Ü can be found in the general listing of books and monographs at the back of this book.

Clove

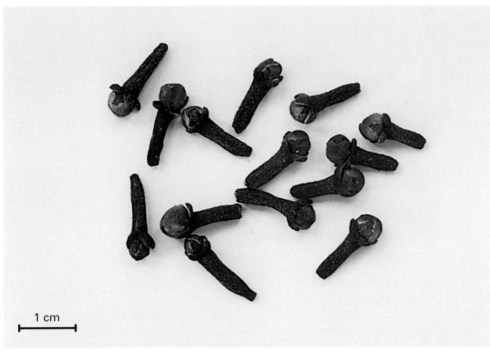

Fig. 1: Clove

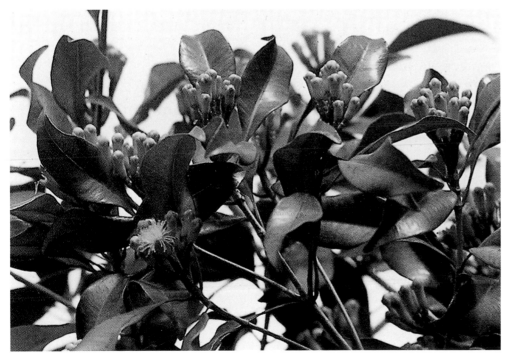

Fig. 2: Clove tree (*Syzygium aromaticum* (L.) MERR. et L.M. PERRY)

Plant source: *Syzygium aromaticum* (L.) MERR. et L.M. PERRY.

Synonyms: *Caryophyllus aromaticus* L., *Eugenia aromatica* (L.) BAILL. non O.C. BERG, *E. caryophyllata* THUNB., *E. caryophyllus* (SPRENG.) BULL. et HARR., *Jambosa caryophyllus* (SPRENG.) NIEDENZU.

Family: Myrtle family (Myrtaceae).

Common names: Engl.: clove, clove tree; Fr.: giroflé, clous de giroflé, giroflier; Ger: Gewürznelke, Gewürznelkenbaum.

Description: Up to 20 m tall, evergreen tree with pyramid-shaped top. The petiolated leaves are leathery, elliptic to lanceolate, 9 to 12 cm long, 3.5 cm to 4.5 cm wide. The terminal flowers are arranged in tripartite paniculate corymbs. Flowers 10 to 14 mm long, with 2 scale-like prophylls, tubular calyx 1 to 1.5 cm long, 4 thick sepals, 4 petals, whitish pink to carmine-red, numerous stamina, inferior ovary, which is partially enclosed by and fused with a tubular hypanthium (cup-like structure of the flower axis). The fruit is a dark red berry, 2.5 cm to 3 cm long, 1.3 to 1.5 cm wide, crowned by 4 curved sepals and containing 1, rarely 2 seeds [Ü37, Ü45, Ü76].

Native origin: Moluccas Islands (Ternate, Tidore, Mare, Moti, Makian).

Main cultivation areas: Indonesia (especially in Ambon), Tanzania (in Zanzibar = Unguja, and Pemba), Madagascar and Malaysia (Penang), as well as in South India, Sri Lanka, Réunion, Mauritius, Comoros, Martinique, Dominican Republic as well as Jamaica, Gabonese Republic, and French Guiana.

Main exporting countries: Tanzania, Madagascar, Comoros and Malaysia, followed by Sri Lanka, Indonesia, Brazil, and the Antilles.

Cultivation: Clove trees prefer nutrient rich, well moistened but permeable soil in damp warm lowlands of the inner tropics near the coast. In areas with high winds, the trees require wind protection. Propagation is carried out almost exclusively by seeds, which very rapidly lose their viability, and therefore, immediately after harvest, they must be put into damp, shaded seedbeds. After 2 years the plants reach about 1 m in height and will be transplanted to their final location. The first harvest is possible after 6 to 8 years. Highest productivity occurs around the 25th year, although trees over 100 years old can still produce a good yield [49, Ü31]. Only chemotypes with a high eugenol content in the essential oil are cultivated. Wild forms occur in the Moluccas Islands with essential oil that is dominated by 2,4,6-trimethoxybenzyl acetone (eugenone) and 2-methyl-5-hydroxy-7-methoxy chromone (eugenine) and only traces of eugenol [Ü43].

Culinary herb

Commercial forms: Cloves: dried, unopened flower buds. Varieties include Amboina-cloves (Moluccas cloves, about 15 mm long, light brown, high essential oil content, very good quality), Zanzibar- and Pemba-cloves (about 12 mm long, dark brown, graded according to stem content, 2%, 4% or over 5%, the latter is used only for oil production), as well as Madagascar-, Réunion- and Mauritius-cloves (low quality). Clove oil is traded as clove flower oil (clove flower bud oil, official in the Ph Eur as Clove oil: Caryophylli floris aetheroleum), as well as clove stem oil and clove leaf oil.

Production: From the ground or on ladders, the branches are pulled down with hooks, after which the still closed flower buds with already reddened petals are hand picked. Stems and attached petals are removed by hand or mechanically. The buds are sun-dried on mats or on cement surfaces or rarely in metal pans over a low flame until they turn reddish-brown. There are typically 2 harvests per year (July to October, and December) [49, Ü92].

Forms used: Cloves, whole or ground.

Storage: The whole flower buds can be stored for up to 2 years, in tightly closed porcelain or glass containers, protected from light and moisture. The powdered material loses its aroma very rapidly during storage.

Description. Whole flower buds (Fig. 1): The flower buds are reddish brown, consisting of a quadrangular, stalk-like, 10 to 12 mm long and 2 to 3 mm wide hypanthium, which is crowned by 4 divergent lobes enclosing a spherical head, 4 to 6 mm in diameter. The head shows 4 overlapping petals, which enclose numerous, inwardly bent stamina and a short, erect style. In the upper part of the hypanthium a bilocular ovary with numerous ovules is contained. Upon bruising with the fingernail, the hypanthium exudes essential oil (fingernail test) [Ü29, Ph Eur].

Powdered flower buds: The chloral hydrate slide preparation shows the wall fragments of the partially burst anthers and, beneath their epidermis, a layer of fibrous cells; also present are numerous, not fully developed, tetrahedral pollen grains with 3 pores at edges as well as shreds of the parenchyma with the remains of the secretory cavities (Fig. 3). Other characteristic features include the small bundles of sclerenchymatous fibers which are thick-walled, lignified and pitted, and the rows of calcium oxalate clusters adjacent to the vascular bundles. Starch is absent [Ü49, Ph Eur].

Odor: Characteristic, warm, spicy-sweet, **Taste:** Spicy and burning.

History: Clove trees were first cultivated on the Moluccas Islands (Ambon and

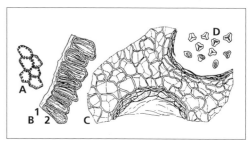

Fig. 3: Cloves. Fragments from the wall of an anther **A** Fibrous cells, top view **B** Side view, 1 epidermis, 2 fibrous cells, **C** Fragments of the parenchyma with the remains of two secretory cavities which are lined with secreting cells, **D** Pollen grains. From Ü49.

Seram). Cloves were already described in an Ayurvedic text from about 1500 BCE. By 220 BCE, they had been documented in China. Between 313 and 337 CE, the emperor Constantine sent "Caryophylla" to the Pope Sylvester I. In the 7th century, the Arabs introduced clove to Mediterranean trade routes. In 1524, the Portuguese conquered the Moluccas Islands and eliminated the transit trade by the Arabs, Venetians and Genoese and established their own trade business with cloves. After the Dutch invaded the Moluccas Islands in 1605, they destroyed most of the clove tree cultivations and, in order to secure their trade monopoly, they started plantations on the islands of Ternate and Ambon. Finally, in 1769, the French were able to smuggle young clove trees to Mauritius; in 1793, it was cultivated in French Guiana and in 1818, on Zanzibar [13, 49, Ü42, Ü61, Ü97].

Constituents and Analysis

DIN- and ISO Standards: DIN-Standard 10205 (Cloves, trade specifications), ISO-Standard 2254 (Cloves).

Constituents

- Essential oil: 15 to 17% (up to 21%), the main constituents (about 99% of the essential oil) are eugenol (70 to 90%), acetyleugenol (eugenyl acetate, up to

17%) and β-caryophyllene (5 to 12%). Numerous other components occur in very small amounts of which heptane-2-one (methylamyl ketone) and octane-2-one (methylheptyl ketone) significantly contribute to the odor. Eugenol also occurs to a small amount in its glycosidic form [18, 27–29, 35, 36, 41, 61]. During extended storage, the undesirable aroma component methyl acetate is formed from the side chains of acetyl eugenol [28].

Eugenol   Acetyleugenol   β-Caryophyllene   Heptane-2-one   Octane-2-one

- Acetophenone derivatives: 2,6-Dihydroxy-4-methoxy-acetophenone and its 4-O-methyl derivative [38].
- Flavonoids: About 0.5%, particularly the quercetin- and kaempferol glycosides kaempferol-3-O-glucoside, quercetin-3-O-glucoside, quercetin-3-O-galacatoside, quercetin-3,4-O-diglucoside [58].
- Chromone glycosides: Biflorin (5,7-dihydroxy-2-methylchromone-8-C-β-D-glucoside), isobiflorin (5,7-dihydroxy-2-methylchromone-8-C-β-D-glucoside) [64].
- Tannins: About 10% gallic acid derivatives, including, among others, the ellagitannin eugeniin (1,2,3-trigalloyl-4,6-hexahydroxydiphenoyl-β-D-glucose) [15].
- Hydroxycinnamic acid derivatives: 3- and 4-caffeoyl-, p-coumaroyl- and 3-feruloyl quinic acids [15].
- Phenolcarboxylic acids: p-Hydroxybenzoic acid, salicylic acid, syringic acid, vanillic acid, gentisinic acid, protocatechuic acid [15, 50].
- Triterpenes, sterols: Oleanolic acid (1 to 2%), and among others, 2α-hydroxyoleanolic acid (crataegolic acid, maslinic acid, 0.15%), β-sitosterol-β-D-glucoside [5, 48].

Eugenol is also the main essential oil component of clove pedicles (4 to 8%) and clove leaves (2 to 3%). The content of acetyleugenol is very low in the essential oil from clove pedicles and older leaves, but relatively high in very young leaves.

The now rarely used essential oil from the unripe berries of clove trees (known as mother cloves or Anthophylli, with an oil content of 2 to 8%) also contain mostly eugenol, in addition to about 35% 2-hydroxy-4,6-dimethoxy-5-methylacetophenone [23].

Tests for Identity: Organoleptic, macroscopic and microscopic assays as well as TLC analysis of the extract [55, Ü102, Ph Eur] or the essential oil [Ü77, Ü101, Ph Eur].

Quantitative assay: The content of essential oil can be determined with steam distillation, following the Ph Eur procedure with xylol in the graduated tube; eugenol, β-caryophyllene and acetyleugenol levels are determined with GC [40, Ph Eur].

Adulterations, Misidentifications and Impurities: Admixtures of other clove tree plant parts such as flower stalks, pedicles, petioles, flower buds without petals or stamina, ("cloves without head"), unripe or ripe fruits (up to 2.5 cm long, up to 8 mm thick) and/or improperly dried flower buds with a pale brown color and mealy surface (so called "Khoker" cloves, little aroma) are possible. The Ph Eur limits the content of impurities to 4% and the content of discolored flower buds to 2%. Spent, extracted cloves occurred occasionally in the spice trade; they can be recognized with the "fingernail test", or by the fact that they float on the surface of water horizontally, while the unspent cloves with a high content of essential oil (density: 1.030 to 1.063) sink to the bottom or float vertically (density test in water) [Ü29].

Actions and Uses

Actions: Due to the aromatic taste, cloves have appetite stimulating and digestion promoting activity.

Clove oil and eugenol are carminative [12, 13, 59, 60]. In animal experiments, saturated, aqueous solutions of clove oil in intestinal preparations (duodenum, ileum, jejunum) inhibited spasms induced by acetylcholine, carbachol, barium chloride, histamine or nicotine [12, 46]. It is assumed that the mechanism for these actions is a blockade of the calcium channel [51]. Eugenol and acetyl eugenol have cholagogue action. In animal experiments (rats), these compounds triggered a long-lasting increase of bile flow [24].

In animal tests, clove inhibited the formation of gastric ulcers and positively influenced healing by stimulating the production of mucus [22, 63].

Cloves and their essential oil may protect the organism from carcinogenic substances. The feeding of cloves to mice (0.5 to 2% in feed) led to elevated levels of SH-group compounds in the liver, the detoxifying enzyme glutathione S-transferase and cytochrome-b_5 [33]. Similar effects were achieved in mice with components of clove oil (α- and β-caryophyllene, α- and β-caryophyllene oxide) [65].

Clove oil, eugenol and acetyl eugenol inhibit thrombocyte aggregation. They limited the generation of thromboxane A_2 in blood platelets in vitro (measured as the content of its breakdown product thromboxane B_2) [54].

Eugenol has antiphlogistic action. With local application in rats, it inhibited the formation of experimentally induced carrageenan-edema, and in rabbits an antiinflammatory effect was shown in the Arthus reaction model [14]. The antiphlogistic action is possibly due to an interference of prostaglandin biosynthesis [13]. In rats, an inhibition of anaphylactic reactions has been shown, probably due to an inhibited histamine release from rat peritoneal mast cells [26].

Eugenol inhibited the vasoconstrictive effects of noradrenaline, histamine and sympathetic nerve stimulation in isolated central rabbit ear artery [53]. In patients with migraine, oral administration of clove oil (100 mg) led to a reduction of pain intensity [42].

Extracts of clove and clove oil have good antimicrobial activity [4, 6, 9, 13, 16, 21, 44]. They also inhibit the growth of *Helicobacter pylori*, but have no influence on urease-activity [3]. For their effect against pathogenic mouth bacteria, e.g. *Prevotella intermedia*, the flavones kaempferol and myricetin probably contribute to the antibacterial action [10]. The growth of mycotoxin forming fungi and mycotoxins was completely suppressed by only 0.1% clove powder in substrate [39]. Aqueous extracts of clove inhibit the reproduction of Herpes simplex- and Cytomelago viruses in vivo and in vitro [34, 62].

Clove extracts have shown good radical scavenging properties [11, 43]. These extracts or eugenol inhibit the rancidity development of fats, e.g. in fatty meat dishes [25, 52, 57].

Clove oil has insect repellent activity, e.g. against mosquitoes and cockroaches [1]. Clove oil ointment, applied to insect bites, diminishes inflammatory reactions [2].

For an overview of clove pharmacology see Lit. [13].

Toxicology: The U.S. FDA permits eugenol as a food ingredient at a level of 2.5 mg/kg body weight, ADI (= acceptable daily intake) [13]. At very high dosages, which likely exceed the detoxifying capacity of the liver, clove oil or eugenol lead to hepatotoxic effects [8, 17, 56]. There is one case report of serious liver damage after a child ingested 5 to 10 ml clove oil [20]. In undiluted form, clove oil is a tissue irritant [31] and neurotoxic agent [7].

Eugenol has a low to moderate sensitization potential [13, Ü39]. Allergic reactions occurred especially after contact with dental materials and in root canal procedures but not with root canal fillings containing zinc oxide and clove oil [19, 32]. People with eczema of the hands and allergies to cosmetics and perfumes often show a positive skin reaction to eugenol, isoeugenol and clove oil [Ü39].

Culinary use: Cloves have a very penetrating taste, and therefore should be measured carefully when adding to food. Frequently, only the less intense-tasting heads (buds or caps) are used for spicing cakes, pastries and sweet dishes. Whole cloves are either cooked with or heated up with (in marinades and pastries), or added 3 to 5 minutes (in soup stocks, soups, and compotes) or 10 to 15 minutes (in meat dishes) before completion. They are usually removed before serving [Ü81].

Cloves are used as a spice for sweet dishes, cakes and pastries, e.g. spice bread and cakes (see below), drinks such as punch, mulled wine (glogg) or burnt punch, plum jam, fruit preserves, especially pears, apples and plums, baked apples, fruit juices and fruit compotes [49, Ü2, Ü55, Ü73, Ü90].

In small amounts (for dishes that serve 4 persons, 1 or 2 cloves are usually sufficient), cloves are suitable for spicing of meat broths, marinades (of mushrooms, meat, vegetables, fruits, and less often fish), soups, roast venison, roast pork, roast lamb, roast beef and roast duck, and dishes made from smoked or pickled meat, ham dishes, cooked bacon, ragouts and fish (eel, carp) as well as cabbage dishes (especially red cabbage, sauerkraut, but also green cabbage), vinegar marinades (e.g. for pickles, pumpkin, red turnips) and sweet-sour pickled herring. It is also used to round off brown sauces. Cloves are not suitable as a spice in chicken or turkey because they will overpower their fine aroma [49, Ü1, Ü2, Ü51, Ü55, Ü73, Ü95].

For roasting fatty meat or pork with rind, the cloves are stuck into square shaped incisions into the fat- or rind layer. For preparation of soup broths, e.g. clear chicken broth of fish stock, an onion with 1 to 2 bay leaves attached with cloves is added [Ü1, Ü23, Ü55, Ü95]. For making punch, apple- or orange squares are larded with cloves [Ü1].

In North America, cloves are also used for larding of hams [Ü55, Ü74], and in England as a spice in bread sauces [Ü55].

Clove oil is used as an aromatic component in liqueurs, especially stomach bitters, e.g. Abtei, Alpenkräuter, Angostura, Aromatique, Boonekamp, Goldwasser and Stonsdorfer [49, Ü92].

Combines well with: Bay leaf, garlic, onion, parsley, pepper, and thyme, in sweet dishes with anise, cardamom, cinnamon, ginger, and nutmeg.

As a component of spice mixes and preparations: → Apple cake spice, → Arabian spice mix, → Baharat, → Barbecue spice, → Char masala, → Chili powder, → Curry powder, → English pudding spice, → Fish spice, → Garam masala, → Ginger bread spice, → Meat spice, → Mélange classique, → Pastry spice, → Pickling spice, → Plum jam spice, → Quatre épices, → Ras el hanout, → Salsa comum, → Sambal badjak, → Sausage spice.→ Scappis spice mix, → Seven seas spice, → Spiced biscuit spice, → Stollen spice, → Tomato ketchup, → Vegetable spice, → Venison spice.

Other uses: At the end of the 19th century, the tobacco industry in Indonesia introduced crushed cloves as an additive (up to 1/3) for tobacco. The cigarettes made from this type of tobacco make a crackling noise when smoked and are therefore appropriately called "Kreket" cigarettes. Cloves are also used to flavor betel chews. Clove oil is used in the perfume and soap manufacturing industry. Eugenol is a raw material for the semi-synthetic production of vanillin.

Similar spices: → Allspice.

Medicinal herb

Herbal drugs: Caryophylli flos, Clove, contains not less than 150 ml/kg essential oil [Ph Eur], Caryophylli floris aetheroleum, Clove oil, contains 75 to 88% eugenol, 5 to 14% β-caryophyllene and 4 to 15% acetyleugenol [Ph Eur].

Indications: Clove oil is used today in stomatology, although only rarely, due to its good antiseptic, slightly caustic and anesthetic effect, as a component of root canal fillings (with zinc oxide, it solidifies to zinc eugenolate) and as a component of mouth washes (1 to 5%), which are used for inflammatory changes in the oral and pharyngeal mucosa [31, 47]. Germany's Commission B9 (dentistry) of the Federal Institute for Drugs and Medical Devices (BfArM) has disallowed its use in root canal procedures due to possible penetration into periapical tissue thereby causing inflammation and possible sensitization [30].

In folk medicine, cloves are decocted or chewed for bad breath, and clove oil is used for dyspeptic complaints. Clove oil is also used for fighting nausea (single dose: 0.05 to 0.2 ml) [37]. It is applied locally, undiluted, for tooth pain (a cotton swab is soaked with a few drops of clove oil and stuck into the opened pulp cavity; the risk of pulp (sensitive tissue at center of tooth) degeneration must be taken into account). Ethanolic solutions are used for rheumatic complaints or muscle pains [37, Ü39], and ointments (10%) are used for preventing mosquito bites [45].

Clove-Nut-Gugelhupf

150 g ground hazelnuts, 300 g butter, 180 g confectioner's sugar, 1/2 teaspoon of ground clove, 6 egg yolks, 150 g flour, 1 teaspoon of baking powder, 50 g grated chocolate, egg white from 6 eggs, 120 g sugar, some butter and flour for the cake tin, confectioner's sugar for decoration.

Roast the hazelnuts very shortly in the oven at 160 °C and let them cool. Whip the butter with the confectioner's sugar and the ground cloves to a foamy consistency and add the egg yolk in small portions. Sift the flour and baking powder and mix with the ground hazelnuts and grated chocolate. Cream the egg white with the sugar and fold the mixture alternately with the foamy butter bit by bit into the flour mixture. Preheat the oven to 180 °C. Brush the Gugelhupf pan with melted butter and sprinkle with flour. Pour the batter into the cake pan and wipe even with a spatula. Bake in the preheated oven for about one hour. Let the Gugelhupf cool a bit and turn the cake pan around to release the cake from its form and sprinkle with confectioner's sugar [Ü90].

Literature

[1] Ahmad F. et al., Insect Sci. Its Appl. 16(3/4):391–393 (1995), ref. CA 128: 150622e.

[2] Anonym, Dtsch. Apoth. Ztg. 133(48): 4593 (1993).

[3] Bae E.A. et al., Biol. Pharm. Bull. 21(9): 990–992 (1998).

[4] Beuchat L.R., Food Preserv. 1994: 167–179 (1994).

[5] Brieskorn C.H. et al., Phytochemistry 14.2308–2309 (1975).

[6] Briozzo J. et al., J. Appl. Bacteriol. 66:69–75 (1989).

[7] Brodin P., Endod. Dent. Traumatol. 4:1–11 (1988).

[8] Brown S.A. et al., Blood Coagul. Fibrinol. 3:665–668 (1992).

[9] Bullerman L.B. et al., J. Food Sci. 42:1107–1109.

[10] Cai L., Ch.D. Wu, J. Nat. Prod. 59(10): 987–990 (1996).

[11] Chung Sh. et al., Biosci. Biotechnol. Biochem. 61(1):118–123 (1997).

[12] Debelmas A.M., J. Rochat, Plant Méd. Phytother. 1:23–27 (1967).

[13] Deininger R., Z. Phytother. 12(6): 205–212 (1991).

[14] Dewhirst F.E., Thesis, University of Rochester, N.Y. 1978, zit. nach Lit. 13

[15] Dirks U., K. Herrmann, Z. Lebensm. Unters. Forsch. 179:12–16 (1984).

[16] Dorman H.J., S.G. Deans, J. Appl. Microbiol. 88(2):308–316 (2000).

[17] Fischer I.U. et al., Xenobiotica 20:209–222 (1990).

[18] Gopalakrishnan M. et al., J. Sci. Food Agric. 50:111–117 (1990).

[19] Grade A.C., B.P.M. Martens, Dermatologica 178:217–220 (1989).

[20] Hartnoll G. et al., Arch. Dis. Childh. 69:392–393 (1993).

[21] Hitikoto H. et al., Appl. Environ. Microbiol. 39:818–822 (1980).

[22] Hollander F., Lauber F.U., Proc. Soc. Exp. Biol. Med. 87:34 (1948).

[23] Huneck S., Phytochemistry 11:3311–3312 (1972).

[24] Jamahara J. et al., J. Pharm. Dyn. 6: 281–286 (1983).

[25] Jayathilakan K., T.S. Vasundhara, K.V. Kumudavally, J. Food Sci. Technol. 34(2):128–131 (1997).

[26] Kim H.M. et al., J. Ethnopharmacol. 60(2):125–131 (1998).

[27] Koller W.D., Z. Lebensm. Unters. Forsch. 173:99–100 (1981).

[28] Koller W.D., Z. Lebensm. Unters. Forsch. 169:457–461 (1979).

[29] Koller W.D., Z. Lebensm. Unters. Forsch. 168:102–105 (1979).

[30] Kommission B9 beim BfArM, BAnz vom 24.09.1992, S. 7948.

[31] Kommission E beim BfArM, BAnz-Nr. 223 vom 30.11.1985

[32] Krikorian-Manoukian A., A.R. Ratsimamanga, CR Acad. Sci. 264:1350–1352 (1967), ref. CA 66:114288t.

[33] Kumari M.V.R., Cancer Lett. 60:291–294 (1991).

[34] Kurokawa M. et al., Antiviral Res. 27 (1/2):19–37 (1995).

[35] Lawrence B.M., Perfum. Flavorist 13:57–58 (1988).

[36] Lawrence B.M., Perfum. Flavorist 9:35–45 (1984).

[37] Leung A.Y., in: Encyclopedia of Common Natural Ingredients used in Food, Drugs and Cosmetics, John Wiley & Sons, Cichester, Brisbane, Toronto 1980, p. 37.

[38] Linde H., Arch. Pharmaz. 316:971–972 (1983).

[39] Mabrouk S.S. et al., Z. Lebensm. Unters. Forsch. 171:344–347 (1980).

[40] Masada Y., Analysis of Essential Oils by Gas Chromatography and Mass Spectrometry, John Wiley Sons, New York 1976.

[41] Menon A.N., C.S. Narayanan, Flav. Fragrance J. 7:130–132 (1992).

[42] Meyer J., in: H.D. Reuter et al. (Hrsg.), Wirksamkeitsnachweis pflanzlicher Analgetika. Phytotherapie, Grundlagen – Klinik – Praxis, Hippokrates Verlag, Stuttgart 1987.

[43] Oya T. et al., Biosc. Biotechnol. Biochem. 61(2):263–266 (1997).

[44] Perez C., Anesini C., Am. J. Clin. Med. 22(2):169–174 (1994).

[45] Perutz A. et al., Pharmakologie der Haut, Springer-Verlag, Berlin 1930.

[46] Reiter M., W. Brandt, Arzneim. Forsch. 35:408–414 (1985).

[47] Riethe P. et al., Arzneimitteltherapie in der Zahn-, Mund- und Kieferheilkunde, Thieme Verlag, Stuttgart 1980.

[48] Ruzicka L., K. Hofmann, Helv. Chim. Acta 19:114–128 (1936).

[49] Schröder R., Kaffee, Tee und Kardamom. Tropische Genussmittel und Gewürze. Geschichte, Verbreitung, Anbau, Ernte, Aufbereitung, Ulmer-Verlag, Stuttgart 1991.

[50] Schulz J.M., K. Herrmann, Z. Lebensm. Unters. Forsch. 171:193–199 (1980).

[51] Sensch O. et al., Planta Med. 59(7):A687 (1993).

[52] Shahidi F. et al., J. Food Lipids 2(3):145–153 (1995).

[53] Skarbane K., D. Powell, Substance P, Dublin, Boole Press 1983, ref. in Lit. 13, s.o.

[54] Srivastava K.C., Prostglandins, Leukot. Ess. Fatty Acids 48:363 (1992).

[55] Stahl E. (Hrsg.), Chromatographische und mikroskopische Analyse von Drogen, Fischer Verlag, Stuttgart, New York 1978.

[56] Thompson D.C. et al., Chem. Biol. Interact. 77:137–147 (1991).

[57] Toda S. et al., Planta Med. 60(3):282 (1994).

[58] Vösgen B., K. Herrmann, Lebensm. Unters. Forsch. 170:204–207 (1980).

[59] Wagner H. et al., Planta Med. 37:9–14 (1979).

[60] Wagner H., L. Sprinkmeyer, Dtsch. Apoth. Ztg. 113:1159–1166 (1973).

[61] Walter R.H., Phytochemistry 11:405–406 (1972).

[62] Yukawa T.A. et al., Antiviral Res. 32(2): 63–70 (1996).

[63] Zaidi S.H. et al., Ind. J. med. Res. 46:732–738 (1958).

[64] Zhang Y., Y. Chen, Phytochemistry 45(2): 401–403 (1997).

[65] Zheng G.Q. et al., J. Nat. Prod. 55(7): 999–1003 (1992).

Literature references identified by Ü can be found in the general listing of books and monographs at the back of this book.

Coriander

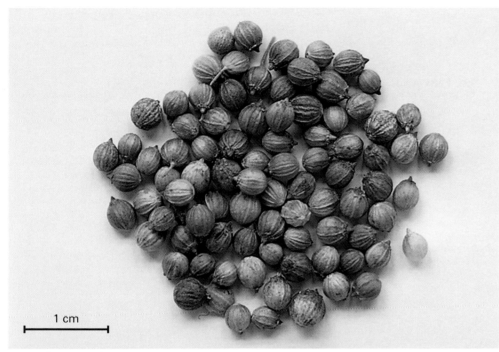

Fig. 1: Coriander fruits

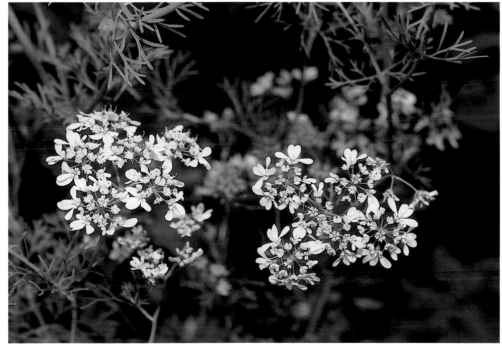

Fig. 2: Coriander (*Coriandrum sativum* L.)

Plant source: *Coriandrum sativum* L.

Taxonomic classification: *Coriandrum sativum* L. var. *vulgare* ALEF., fruit diameter 3 to 5 mm, *Coriandrum sativum* L. var. *microcarpum* DC., fruit diameter 1.5 to 3.0 mm.

Family: Umbelliferous plants (Apiaceae, synonym Umbelliferae).

Common names: Engl.: coriander (fruit), cilantro (leaf), Chinese parsley; Fr.: coriandre, Persil arabe; Ger.: Koriander, Gartenkoriander, Koliander, Schwindelkorn, Wanzenkraut, Wanzendill, Wanzenkümmel, Arabische Petersillie, Chinesische Petersilie.

Description: Annual herb, growing to a height of up to 0.8 m, having an unpleasant odor reminiscent of shield bugs, glabrous, with spindle-shaped tap root, round stem, finely grooved, branched in the upper part. Leaves are light green, glabrous, alternate, the lower ones with long petiole, entire-margined or crenate, readily falling off; the leaves that follow later are 1- to 3 times pinnatisect, the marginal leaf very enlarged, the upper and middle leaves sitting on a broad sheath with skin-like margin. The main stem axis and lateral branches each end in a terminal, flat umbel with 3 to 5 rays; involucre absent or consisting only of an inconspicuous leaf, small involucres consist of 3 filiform leaflets. Flowers radial, 5 sepals, the two outer ones significantly longer than the three inner ones, 5 petals, white or reddish, the outer unpaired ones of the radial, marginal flowers 2 to 4 mm long, with 2 deep clefts, the vicinal ones larger than the 2 inner ones, 5 anthers, 2 styles, ovary inferior, bilocular; the fruit is a double achene, composed of 2 mericarps which remain closed upon ripening and usually do not split into their mericarps, forming a spherical fruit. Flowering period is from June to August [37].

Native origin: Native to the eastern Mediterranean region, and introduced through cultivation in North Africa, South- and Central Europe, East Asia, North- and South America.

Main cultivation areas: Egypt, India, Russian Federation, Morocco and the USA, followed by, among others, Hungary, Poland, Czech Republic, Holland, France, Italy, Turkey, the Balkan countries, Germany, China, Iran, Central- and South America.

Main exporting countries: Bulgaria, Morocco, Hungary, Romania, Egypt, France, Italy, Turkey, Russian Federation, and other Eastern European countries.

Cultivation: Coriander prefers light, sandy, chalky soil in sunny or half-shaded dry places, but also thrives in damp, cool locations. Sowing takes place, depending on the weather, from the end of March until April spaced apart 25 to 30 cm. The seed should not be covered more than 1 cm deep. Harvest takes place in August or September, when the fruits in the center umbel are ripe [Ü41]. In Germany, small-grain varieties are cultivated such as 'Csillag', 'Hrubcicky', 'Jantar', 'Lozen 1', 'Sandra', and 'Thüringer' [Ü14, Ü21].

Culinary herb

Commercial forms: Coriander seeds: the dried, ripe fruits, large-grain (75 to 100 fruits/g, southern origins like Morocco and India) or small-grain (more than 130 fruits/g, East European origins), crushed or coarsely ground fruits, dried coriander leaf (cilantro), coriander essential oil and coriander oleoresin.

Production: Harvest takes place prior to the fruits becoming completely ripe, usually using a harvester-thresher, early in the damp morning hours, because after the dew dries the fruits fall off easily. Post-har-

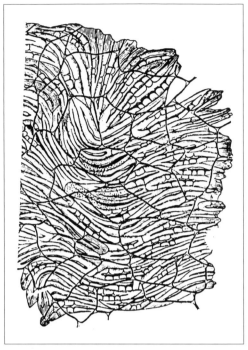

Fig. 3: Coriander. Fibrous layer of the mesocarp. From Ü25.

vest, the fruits are air dried in a storage space [Ü21].

Forms used: The whole, dried fruits, powdered fruit, roasted, crushed fruits, fresh herb (Chinese parsley, cilantro, Mexican parsley, kinsa).

Storage: The dried, whole fruits are stored in well-sealed metal- or glass containers, protected from light and moisture, and have a shelf life of several years. The fresh herb can be frozen in plastic bags; drying is not recommended.

Description. Whole fruit (Fig. 1): Yellowish-brown, smooth and spherical double achenes, consisting of mericarps which are firmly attached to each other, diameter 1.5 to 5 mm, more rarely up to 7 mm in fruits with oval shape, with 10 wavy, not very prominent main ribs and 8 to 10 straight and clearly protruding secondary ribs; remains of the calyx and style are recognizable.

Description. Powdered fruit: Brown colored powder; the chloral hydrate slide preparation shows fragments of the prominent, wavy-bent, fibrous layer, which is a characteristic feature of the mesocarp (see Fig. 3); also present are the numerous fragments of the endosperm with small oxalate druses, oil droplets (some free), aleuron grains and pieces of the exocarp with polygonal, thick-walled cells (containing oxalate crystals) and beneath, layers of transversal cells, "parquetry-cells" of the endocarp, fragments of vascular bundles and oil streaks. Starch must be absent [Ü25, Ü29, EB6, Ph Eur].

Odor: The fresh, unripe fruits and the fresh herb have a disagreeable odor, reminiscent of shield bugs; after drying or maturing, spicy-aromatic with sweetish note, **Taste:** Spicy, somewhat burning.

History: Coriander is one of the oldest spices. It was already mentioned in ancient Sanskrit texts, in the Old Testament ("Passah-spice") and in the Papyrus Ebers (about 1550 BCE). It has been known in China for about 2,000 years. The Romans and Greeks used coriander as a wine flavoring. With the Roman occupation, coriander was brought to Central Europe and England. In a local government decree by Karl the Great, "Capitulare de villis" (authored in about 795 CE, see footnote, Anise), its cultivation was called for. Introduced to the USA in the late 17th century [Ü73, Ü92, Ü97].

Constituents and Analysis

DIN- and ISO-Standards: ISO-Standard 2255 (Coriander).

Constituents of the fruits

- Essential oil: 0.1 to 2% (higher content in small fruit varieties, larger fruit varieties often contain only 0.1 to 0.3%), with the main component linalool (coriandrol, particularly the $(3S)$-(+)-enantiomer, 45 to 85%) and predominantly α-pinene (1 to 15%), limonene (0 to 4%), γ-terpinene (traces to 15%), *p*-cymene (0 to 15%), camphor (0 to 10%), geraniol (0 to 7%) and geranyl acetate (1 to 20%). The composition depends on the chemotype. Chemotypes from Arabian Peninsula and the Indian subcontinent do not contain limonene or camphor. The unripe fruits contain unsaturated aldehydes, which are also typical for the herb (see below) [3, 4, 5, 10, 15, 17, 22, 28–30, 33, Ü30].

- Fatty oil (13 to 21%), with a high proportion of bound petroselinic acid (about 38%) [Ü37].
- Hydroxycoumarins (very small amounts): Scopoletin, umbelliferone [20].
- Hydroxycinnamic acid derivatives: Caffeic acid, most likely occurring in the form of quinic acid derivatives, particularly chlorogenic acid, 4- and 5- caffeoylquinic acid, *p*-coumaroyl- and feruloylquinic acids [13, 34].
- Triterpenes: Coriandrinondiol [26].

Constituents of the herb

- Essential oil: The main components are unsaturated, aliphatic aldehydes (up to 83%, some of them with a shield-bug like odor), particularly (*E*)-dec-2-enal (about 46%, content decreasing during growth), (*E*)-dodec-2-enal (about 10%), (*E*)-tetra-dec-2-enal (about 6%), (*E*)-undec-2-enal (about 6%), (*E*)-tridec-2-enal and linalool (content increasing during growth), furthermore, among others, dec-2-enol (about 9%) and decanal (about 4%) [31]. Older publications refer to saturated aldehydes as the main components [24, 32, 33].
- Isocoumarins: Coriandrones A to E, coriandrin, dihydrocoriandrin [36].
- Flavonoids: Quercetin- and kaempferol-3-*O*-glycosides, as well as quercetin-3-*O*-glucuronide, rutin and isoquercitrin, among others [23].
- Alkylphthalides [16].

Tests for Identity: Organoleptic, macroscopic and microscopic analysis as well as TLC of the ground fruits, according to Ph Eur; the composition of the essential oil can be determined with GC or GC/MS respectively [3, 22, 29].

Quantitative analysis: The essential oil content of the fruits can be determined volumetrically using steam distillation of the freshly ground fruits, according to Ph Eur, with xylol in the graduated tube.

Adulterations, Misidentifications and Impurities are hardly possible, due to the characteristic appearance of the fruit.

Actions and Uses

Actions: Coriander fruit has a mild spasmolytic effect. Due to its salivation and bile secretion promoting effects it is appetizing and has digestive action. The essential oil and evaporation residues of coriander macerates have shown good antibacterial and antifungal activity [4, 25].

In rats, the addition of coriander fruits to a high fat diet with added cholesterol inhibits the increase of blood lipid content, and the level of LDL and VLDL decreased while that of HDL increased. The authors found indications that coriander stimulated cholesterol excretion via bile acids. The blood level of lipid peroxides decreased [8, 9]. Coriander fruits in feed (6.25%) delayed the onset of streptozotocin-induced diabetes in mice [28]. Aqueous extracts of coriander fruit lowered the progesterone concentration in serum and inhibited the implantation of fertilized egg cells in rats fed high doses (250 to 500 mg/kg body weight). Teratogenic effects did not occur at this dosage [1].

Toxicology: Based on existing data, there is no acute or chronic toxicity with the regular use of coriander as a spice. The sensitization potential is small; despite the often-detected antibodies, allergic reactions generally are rare and only observed in atopic patients and in cases of frequent occupational exposures. Allergic reactions are also possible in individuals who are allergic to other Apiaceae plants (e.g. celery, carrots, parsley, anise, fennel, caraway) or to Asteraceae plants like mugwort (celery-mugwort-spice-syndrome) [19, 27, 35, 38, Ü39].

Culinary use: Coriander is especially popular in India, China, Thailand, Vietnam, Iran, Russia, North Africa, Latin America, in the Middle East, and also in Northern Europe.

The whole fruits are usually added at the beginning of cooking. They can be, however, ground and sprinkled over a finished dish. The aroma impact can also be enhanced by lightly roasting the fruits before use. Crushed fruits rapidly lose their aroma, so they should be crushed shortly before use, e.g. in a spice mill. The leaves should be finely cut and added to the finished dish before serving.

Coriander fruits are used as a spice in the preparation of sauces, marinades, meat dishes (lamb, pork, goat, rabbit, game, fowl, ragouts, meat loaf), sausage products, fish, shellfish, vegetables (cauliflower, celery), mushrooms (especially champignons) and lentil dishes, in the baking of bread, whole grain rolls and spelt bread (usually combined with anise and caraway), but also of sweet baked goods, e.g. ginger spice bread, honey biscuits and spiced biscuits, as well as fruit compotes (e.g. pears, mangos, apple sauce) and plum jam. Likewise, they can serve as a spice for pickling cucumbers, red beets and mushrooms as well as in the preparation of sauerkraut (often together with caraway). In some countries (e.g. in Belgium) coriander fruits are added as a flavor component of top fermented beers [Ü13, Ü17, Ü45, Ü51, Ü55, Ü71, Ü74, U90, Ü107].

The fresh leaves serve, predominantly in India, Thailand, China and South America, usually combined with other spices, as a flavor component of salads, soups (e.g. fish soups) and meat dishes. It is an essential component of South American guacamole, a thick sauce made from avocadoes and tomatoes. In Central Europe, it is used as a spice in stir-fried vegetables, of fish or meat from the wok, of salads (rice-, noodle-, vegetable salads), chutneys, relishes and soups. The taste of meals that have been spiced with coriander leaves is an acquired taste. While many people completely reject it, some gourmets love it [Ü51, Ü53, Ü79, Ü90].

The essential oil is used, especially by the spirits industry, as a flavor component of aperitifs and liqueurs, e.g. Danziger Goldwasser, Boonekamp and Cordial Medoc. Furthermore it is used in the baked goods and confectionery industries.

Combines well with: (Coriander herb) basil, chilies, fresh mint, garden cress, garlic, onions, savory and watercress, (Coriander fruit) allspice, chilies, clove, cumin, fennel, garlic, lovage, mint and pepper [Ü55].

As a component of spice mixes and preparations: → Baharat, → Bread spice, → Cake spice, → Chili con carne spice, → Curry powder, → Dukkah, → English pudding spice, → Fish spice, → Garam masala, → Ginger bread spice, → Harissa, → Masala, → Mélange classique, → Parisian pepper, → Pickling spice, → Plum jam spice, → Poultry spice, → Salsa comum, → Sambal badjak, → Sambhar powder, → Sausage spice, → Seven seas spice, → Spiced biscuit spice, → Tabil, → Table mustard, → Tandoori, → Tika paste, → Zhug.

Other uses: The essential oil from coriander is used in the perfume industry and as a raw material for the production of linalool. The fatty oil of coriander serves as the starting material for the isolation of petroselinic acid, which is further processed to yield lauric acid and adipic acid.

Medicinal herb

Herbal drugs: Coriandri fructus, Coriander fruit, contains not less than 3 ml/kg of essential oil [Ph Eur], Coriandri fructus aetheroleum, Coriander oil [USP-NF], obtained by steam distillation from the dried, ripe fruit.

Indications: Coriander is used for dyspepsia and for loss of appetite. Coriander is used in the form of tea infusions of the crushed fruits (1 g/cup, daily dosage: 3 g), ethanolic extracts (e.g. coriander tincture) and the essential oil (internal: 1 to 3 drops with sugar or honey, 2 to 3 times daily, external: in a diluted form as an embrocation) [21, Ü106].
In India, coriander fruit is used for coughs, bladder problems, fever and dysentery, in the form of tea infusion applied locally for eye problems, and in Central- and South America, among other places, it is used for menstrual problems [2, 11, 12, 14, Ü92].

Baked Potatoes with Coriander
(Serves 4)
8 to 12 potatoes (about 1.6 kg). 1/2 l olive oil, salt, 1 teaspoon of crushed coriander fruits, 2 yolks, 2 teaspoons lemon juice, 2 garlic cloves, 1 teaspoon of table mustard, freshly ground white pepper, 4 tablespoons of whipped cream, chives, tomatoes, 1 lemon.

Wash the potatoes thoroughly and cut them in half. Brush the cut surface with oil and sprinkle with salt and some of the coriander. Place the cut potatoes face down on a baking sheet and bake them on the middle rack at 250 °C for 10 minutes; reduce the temperature to 150 °C and bake them for another 35 minutes. While the potatoes are in the oven, mix the yolks with salt, pressed garlic cloves, mustard and pepper, then incorporate the remaining oil bit by bit with a handmixer. The obtained mayonnaise is mixed with the whipped cream and seasoned to taste. Sprinkle the remaining coriander and chives on top of the mayonnaise and the potatoes. Serve with slices of tomatoes and lemons [Ü95].

Literature

[1] Al-Said M.S. et al., J. Ethnopharmacol. 21:165–173 (1987).

[2] Arseculeratne S.N. et al., J. Ethnopharmacol. 13:323–335 (1985).

[3] Bandoni A.L. et al., J. Ess. Oil Res. 10(5):581–584 (1998).

[4] Baratta Z.M. et al., J. Ess. Oil Res. 10:618–627 (1998).

[5] Borges P. et al., Nahrung 14:811–834 (1990).

[6] Cai Y.N. et al., Carcinogenesis 18(1): 215–222 (1997).

[7] Ceska O. et al., Phytochemistry 26(1): 165–169 (1987).

[8] Chitra V., S. Leelamma, Plants Foods Hum. Nutr. 51(2)167–172 (1997).

[9] Chitra V., S. Leelamma, Indian J. Biochem. Biophys. 36(1):59–61 (1999).

[10] Coleman W.M., B.M. Lawrence, J. Chromatogr. Sci. 30:396–398 (1992).

[11] De Montellano B.A., C.H. Browner, J. Ethnopharmacol. 13:57–88 (1985).

[12] Dimayuga R.E., J. Agundez, J. Ethnopharmacol. 17:183–193 (1986).

[13] Dirks U., K. Herrmann, Zeitschr. Lebensm. Unters. Forsch. 179:12–16 (1984).

[14] Fleurentin J., J.M. Pelt, J. Ethnopharmacol. 8:237–243 (1983).

[15] Formacék, V., K.H. Kubeczka, Essential Oils Analysis by Capillary Gas Chromatography and Carbon-13-NMR Spectroscopy, John Wiley & Sons, Chicester, New York, Brisbane, Toronto, Singapore 1982.

[16] Gijbels M.J.M. et al., Fitotherapia 53:17–20 (1982).

[17] Góra J. et al., Riv. Ital. EPPOS (Spec. Num., 15th Journees Internat. Huiles Essentielles, 1996:761-766 (1997).

[18] Jaspersen-Schib R., Dtsch. Apoth. Ztg. 132(13):621–625 (1992).

[19] Jensen-Jarolim E. et al., Clin. Exp. Allergy 27(11):1299–1306 (1997).

[20] Kartnig T., Fette Seifen Anstrichm. 68(2):131–134 (1966).

[21] Kommission E beim BfArM., BAnz-Nr. 173 vom 18.09.86.

[22] Krüger H. et al., Drogenreport 9(15):22–26 (1996).

[23] Kunzemann J., K. Herrmann, Z. Lebensm. Untersuch. Forsch. 164:194–200 (1977).

[24] Macleod A.J., J. Sci. Food Agric. 27:721–725 (1976).

[25] Maruzzella J.C., M. Freundlich, J. Am. Pharm. Assoc. 48(6):356–358 (1959).

[26] Naik C.G. et al., Curr. Sci. 52(12):598–599 (1983).

[27] Niinimäki A. et al., Allergy 44:60–65 (1989).

[28] Perineau F. et al., Parfum Cosmet. Aromes 98:79–84 (1991).

[29] Pino J. et al., Nahrung 37:119–122 (1993).

[30] Pino J.A. et al., J. Ess. Oil Res. 8:97–98 (1996).

[31] Potter Th.L., L.S. Fagerson, J. Agric. Food Chem. 38:2054–2056 (1990).

[32] Reisch J. et al., Planta Med. 14(3):326–336 (1966).

[33] Schratz E., S.M.J.S. Quadry, Planta Med. 14(3):310–325 (1966).

[34] Schulz J.M., K. Herrmann, Z. Lebensm. Unters. Forsch. 171:193–199 (1980).

[35] Stäger J. et al., Allergy 46:475–478 (1991).

[36] Tanaguchi M. et al., Phytochemistry 42(3): 843–846 (1996).

[37] Weymar H., Buch der Doldengewächse, Neumann Verlag, Radebeul 1959 (1959).

[38] Wüthrich B., T. Hofer, Dtsch. Med. Wschr. 109:981–986 (1984).

Literature references identified by Ü can be found in the general listing of books and monographs at the back of this book.

Cumin

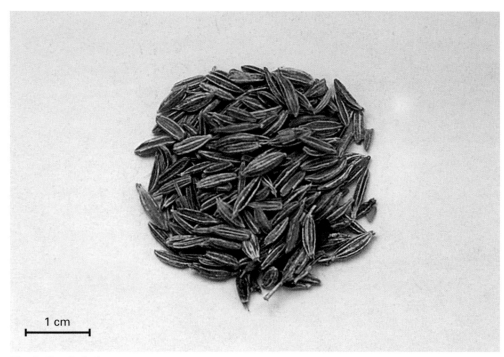

Fig. 1: Cumin fruits

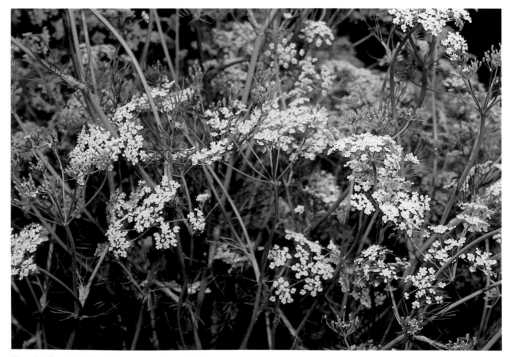

Fig. 2: Cumin (*Cuminum cyminum* L.)

Plant source: *Cuminum cyminum* L.

Synonym: *Cuminum odorum* SALISB.

Family: Umbelliferous plants (Apiaceae, synonym Umbelliferae).

Common names: Engl.: cumin, Roman caraway, Egyptian caraway; Fr.: cumin, cumin de prés; Ger.: Kreuzkümmel, Cumin, Kumin, Mutterkümmel, Römischer Kümmel, Italienischer Kümmel, Spanischer Kümmel, Türkischer Kümmel, Ägyptischer Kümmel, Welscher Kümmel, Polnischer Kümmel, Kala, Wanzen-Kümmel, Scharfer Kümmel.

Description: Annual herb, up to 0.5 m in height, glabrous (except the fruits), stem furcated. Tender leaves situated transversely on the leaf-sheaths, finely dissected, with lineal leaf-tips, the lower ones mostly twofold ternate; main axis and lateral branches with terminal, composite umbel having 3 to 5 rays, long involucre and long small involucres, mostly longer than the umbels and rays thereof. Radial flowers with 5 petals, white or pink, wide emarginated, with long retroflexed tips, 5 stamina, 2 styles, inferior ovary, 2-partite. The fruit is a 6 mm long and 1.5 mm wide, double achene that is crowned by subulate calyx tips, attached to a furcated carpophore; the individual mericarps do not easily separate. Flowering period is from June to August.

Native origin: Original occurrence is not entirely certain. Cumin is probably native to the Nile valley; since ancient times it has been widely distributed in northern Africa and southwestern Asia to India, now naturalized in southern Spain, southern France and Sicily.

Main cultivation areas: India and Iran followed by, among others, China, Sri Lanka, Pakistan, Turkey, Russian Federation, Central- and South America.

Main exporting countries: India and Iran. The supply in Germany comes from Turkey.

Cultivation: Cumin is grown in subtropical and tropical regions. It prefers deep, rich soil in sunny locations. For growing in one's own garden, cumin can be planted by seed (light dependent germination) in March in seed bowls indoors in a warm area, and then transplanted outside at the end of May [Ü2, Ü71].

Culinary herb

Commercial forms: Cumin: dried fruits, whole or ground, cumin essential oil and cumin oleoresin.

Production: About 40 days after sowing and shortly before the fruits are fully ripe, the plants are pulled out, dried, and thrashed in order to collect the fruits.

Forms used: Cumin: ground or crushed dried fruits, crushed roasted fruits. They should be crushed immediately before use.

Storage: The dried fruits can be stored for several years in well-closed metal- or glass containers, protected from light and moisture; ground cumin loses its aroma rapidly.

Description. Whole fruit (Fig. 1): Double achenes, mostly not separated into their mericarps, often with the remains of the pedicel; greenish gray to golden brown, 5 to 7 mm long and 1.0 to 1.5 mm wide, at the upper end with a roundish stylopodium with 2 short, bent styles; the mericarps have 5 yellowish main ribs and 4 less prominent, darker colored secondary ribs. Lens magnification reveals the multi-seriate, 120 to 200 µm long villiform trichomes with rounded tips [Ü37].
The **powdered fruit** is yellowish brown with characteristic fragments of the epidermis having thin, wavy-walled polygonal cells, irregularly striated cuticula, stomata and multi-celled, multi-seriate trichomes with rounded tips or remains thereof. Also present are groups of oblong stone cells from the sclerenchymatous layer of the mesocarp. Additionally, the powder contains numerous endosperm cells with oil droplets, aleuron grains and small calcium oxalate rosettes. Furthermore, groups of thick-walled transversal cells from the endocarp (Fig. 3), fragments of the mostly yellowish brown colored and very broad secretory canals and fragments of the vessels with sclerenchymatous fibers. Starch is absent [Ü48].

Odor: Peculiar aromatic, reminiscent of shield bugs, **Taste:** Aromatic and pungent, slightly bitter.

History: Cumin was already used during antiquity in Asia Minor and in the Mediterranean region. It was mentioned in the "Papyrus Ebers" (authored around 1550 BCE) and by Dioscorides (1st century CE). It was used as a pepper substitute in ancient Rome. The Old Testament of the Bible also mentions this spice. Since the 12th century, it has been cultivated in Spain [Ü2, Ü92].

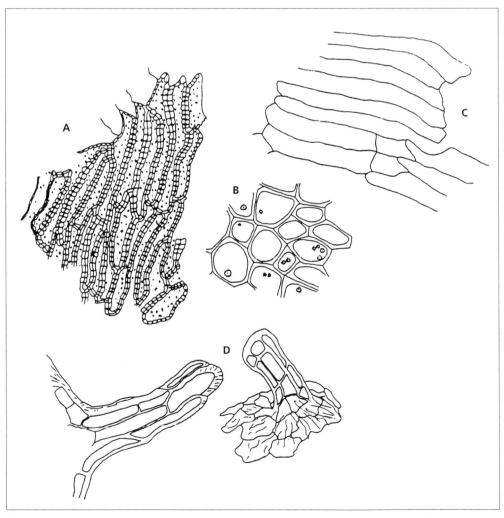

Fig. 3: Cumin. **A** Groups of oblong stone cells from the sclerenchymatous layer of the mesocarp, **B** Endosperm cells with small calcium oxalate rosettes **C** Groups of transversal cells from the endocarp **D** Fragments of the epidermis with multicellular, multiseriate trichomes with rounded tips. From Ü48.

p-Mentha-1,4-diene-7-al → Cuminaldehyde + p-Menth-3-ene-7-al

Constituents and Analysis

DIN- and ISO-Standards: ISO-Standard 6465 (Cumin).

Constituents

- Essential oil: 2.5 to 6.0%, the main component in fresh cumin is p-mentha-1,4-dienal; main components in the steam-distilled essential oil are cuminaldehyde (19 to 35%, some sources claim up to 72%), γ-terpinene (15 to 29%), β-pinene (10 to 22%), p-cymene (8 to 12%) and p-mentha-1,3-diene-7-al (about 16%), other monoterpenes occur proportionally below levels of 3%. Safrole has also been detected. The main odoriferous constituents include cuminaldehyde, p-mentha-1,4-diene-7-al and p-mentha-1,3-diene-7-al. Cuminaldehyde and p-menth-3-ene-7-al develop partially (or perhaps entirely) by disproportionation and isomerization from p-mentha-1,4-diene-7-al [4, 9, 16–18]. In the essential oil from fruits of Turkish origin, p-mentha-1,3-diene-7-al was absent; the main components were γ-terpinene (about 30%), p-cymene (about 25%), β-pinene (about 20%) and cuminaldehyde (about 18%) [2].
- Flavonoids (0.05 to 0.1%), the components are race-specific, with luteolin- and apigenin-7-O-glucoside (and 7-O-glucuronosylglucoside, respectively) as well as apigenin-7-O-apiosylglucoside and apigenin-5-O-glucoside [7, 8, 13].
- Fatty oil (10 to 15%) with a high content of bound petroselinic acid.

Tests for Identity: Macroscopic and microscopic analysis, as well as TLC of the extract; cuminaldehyde serves as the reference substance [Ü37].

Quantitative analysis: The content of essential oil can be determined volumetrically with steam distillation and xylol in the graduated tube [Ph Eur].

Adulterations, Misidentifications and Impurities have been described, particularly with → Caraway or Black cumin (see below). Admixtures of caraway fruits are easily detected due to the absence of trichomes. Black cumin is smaller than cumin and has a sweet taste. Synthetic colorants (to improve appearance) have also been detected in the whole and powdered fruits [Ü37].

Actions and Uses

Actions: Cumin stimulates salivation, secretion of gastric juice, excretion of bile and intestinal motility, and therefore improves digestion. Rats that were fed cumin (1.25% in feed) for 8 weeks showed elevated activity of pancreas amylase, of trypsin and chymotrypsin. Single doses had no effect [6].
Cumin extracts inhibited the growth of mycotoxins from mycotoxigenic molds [7, 10]. In animal experiments (rats), cumin extracts have shown estrogenic activity [11]. Cumin fed to healthy rabbits increased glucose tolerance. The possibility that cumin and other herbs with similar activity may help control and prevent diabetes mellitus is under discussion [13]. Cumin inhibited the induction of tumors induced by carcinogenic substances in rats [1].

Toxicology: Based on existing data, there is no acute or chronic toxicity with the normal use of cumin as a spice.
In the AMES-test, a mutagenic effect from the polar fractions of the extract and from the urine of rats, after eating feed that contained the fraction, was observed [14].
Cumin has a moderate sensitization potential. Allergic reactions are possible, however, in individuals who are allergic to other Apiaceae plants (e.g. anise, caraway, carrots, celery, fennel, parsley) or to Asteraceae plants like mugwort (celery-mugwort-spice-syndrome) [15, 19, Ü39].

Culinary use: Cumin is used especially in northern Africa, India, Indonesia, Thailand, Malaysia, Mexico, southern USA, Turkey, Spain and Portugal. In northern Africa, cumin is an important component of couscous (steamed wheat groats with meat, vegetables, chickpeas and raisins), Merguez (lamb) sausage, in Indonesia of mutton dishes, in Thailand and Malaysia of fish- and poultry curry and in Mexico and Texas of chilli con carne. In India it is an essential component of a few spice mixtures (see below). In European cooking, it is used relatively rarely. In Holland and in Switzerland it is an important spice for some varieties of cheese (Edam) and in France for pastry specialties. In Russia, it serves as a flavor component of beer and kvass. In a few countries, cumin is also used as a bread spice in the same way as caraway.
It is recommended that cumin should be lightly roasted in the pan without fat prior to use. Due to its strange, penetrating taste, which is unusual for westerners, it should be measured carefully.
In Central Europe cumin is used, but only rarely, as a spice in meat dishes, soups (potato-, pea-, onion soup), sauces (especially tomato-based, but also garlic sauces for fish dishes), chutneys (e.g. mango chutney), cabbage dishes, salads (e.g. tomato salad) and pickles [Ü20, Ü55, Ü71, Ü90, Ü92, Ü95].
Cumin essential oil is used in the liqueur industry as an aromatic component of herbal liqueurs and in the food industry in the production of spice essences.

Combines well with: Bay leaf, cardamom, chillies, cinnamon, clove, garlic, ginger, and nutmeg.

As a component of spice mixes and preparations: → Baharat, → Bomboe sajoer lodeh, → Cajun spice, → Chat masala, → Curry powder, → Dukkah, → Garam masala, → Panch phoron, → Ras el hanout, → Sambhar powder, → Seven seas spice, → Tandoori.

Other uses: The essential oil of cumin is used in the perfume industry.

Medicinal herb

Herbal drugs: Cumini fructus, Cumin, Cumini aetheroleum, Cumin essential oil.

Indications: Cumin is used similarly as caraway for digestive complaints, especially for cramp-like stomach- and intestinal problems, flatulence and diarrhea. Today it is used primarily in veterinary medicine. In some countries it also serves as a remedy for relief of menstrual pains and is misused as an abortive [5, 12, 18].

Similar Spices

Black cumin (zira), *Bunium persicum* (BOISS.) FEDCH. (Apiaceae), also incorrectly referred to as → Black cumin (black caraway, black zira), occurs in Iran, the Russian Federation (Central Asia), Afghanistan, and Pakistan, and is cultivated especially in India. The fruits and the essential oil are used as spice ingredients, and the tubers serve as a vegetable [Ü61, Ü92, Ü98].

Great pignut (earth chestnut, great earthnut), *Bunium bulbocastanum* L. (Apiaceae), is native to the Balearic Islands, and western Central Europe to northwestern Yugoslavia. The fruits serve as a spice and the leaves and tubers are used as vegetables [Ü61, Ü98].

Literature

[1] Aruna K., V.M. Sivaramakrishnan, Food Chem. Toxicol. 30(11):953–956 (1992).
[2] Borges P., Pino J., Nahrung 37:123–126 (1993).
[3] Ceska O. et al., Phytochemistry 26(1): 165–169 (1987).
[4] Farag S.E.A., M. Abo-Zeid, Nahrung 41(6):359–361 (1997).
[5] Farnsworth N.R. et al., J. Pharm. Sci. 64:535–598 (1975).
[6] Górna-Binkul A. et al., J. Chromatogr. A., 734(2):297–302 (1996).
[7] Halim A.F., S.A. Ross, Egypt. J. Pharm. Sci. 18:245–252 (1977).
[8] Khafagy S.M. et al., Pharmazie 33(5): 296–297 (1978).
[9] Lawrence B.R., Perfumer Flavorist 5:6–16 (1980).
[10] Mabrouk S.S. et al., Z. Lebensm. Unters. Forsch. 171:344–347 (1980).
[11] Malini T., G. Vanithakumari, Indian J. Exp. Biol. 25:442–444 (1987).
[12] Middelkoop T.B., R.P. Labadie, J. Ethnopharmacol. 8:313–320 (1983).
[13] Roman-Ramos R. et al., J. Ethnopharmacol. 48(1):25–32 (1995).
[14] Shashikanth K.N., Akiyoshi Hosono, Agric. Biol. Chem. 50:2947–2948 (1986).
[15] Stäger J. et al., Allergy 46:475–478 (1991).
[16] Tassan C.G., G.F. Russel, J. Food Sci. 40:1185–1188 (1975).
[17] Varo P.T., D.E. Heinz, J. Agric. Food Chem. 18:234–238, 239–242 (1970).
[18] Verghese J., Perfumer Flavorist 16:61–64 (1991).
[19] Wüthrich B., T. Hofer, Dtsch. Med. Wschr. 109:981–986 (1984).

Literature references identified by Ü can be found in the general listing of books and monographs at the back of this book.

Dill

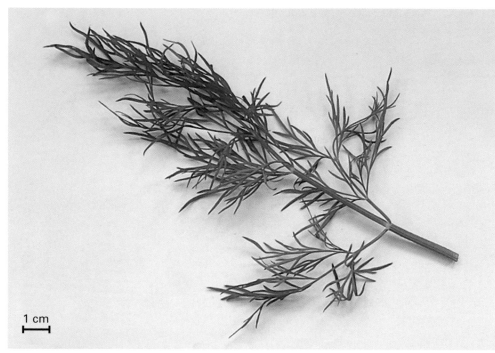

Fig. 1: Dill leaf

Plant source: *Anethum graveolens* L.

Taxonomic classification: The species is subdivided as follows:
Anethum graveolens L. var. *graveolens* (field dill), which grows wild in Southern- and Southwestern Asia,
Anethum graveolens var. *hortorum* ALEF. (garden dill), which is only known as a cultivated plant.
Only garden dill is used as a culinary spice. Some authors have also classified the species *Anethum sowa* ROXB. as *Anethum graveolens* L. ssp. *sowa* (ROXB. ex FLEMING) GUPTA (See below: Similar culinary spices).

Family: Umbelliferous plants (Apiaceae, synonym Umbelliferae).

Common names: Engl.: dill; Fr.: aneth odorant; Ger: Dill, Dille, Däll, Dillfenchel, Gurkenkraut, Gurkenkümmel, Blähkraut, Kapernkraut, Bergkümmel, Tille.

Description: Annual herb, growing to a height of 1.5 m. Stem round, finely grooved, with white and green striations, glabrous, dark green, bluish pruinose on the upper part, with a spindle-shaped tap root. Leaves alternate, the lower ones stalked, 2 to 3 times pinnate, lobes lineal and filiform, with a short leaf sheath with a white margin and an auriculate tip. The main axis and the side branches bear a terminal, composite umbel, each up to 20 cm in diameter, with numerous rays; involucres are absent. The flowers are radial, with 5 yellow petals, 5 stamina, 2 styles, ovary inferior and bilocular. The fruits are double achenes (cremocarps) being suspended on a bifurcate carpophore and remaining closed. Flowering period is from June to September.

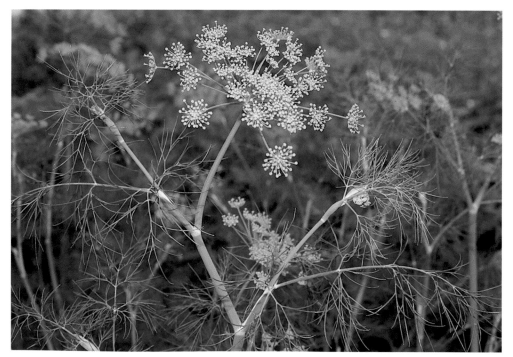

Fig. 2: Dill (*Anethum graveolens* L.)

Native origin: Dill probably originates from the region between the Caucasus and India, although other authors believe that it is native to the Mediterranean region. Today, garden dill is not found in the wild.

Main cultivation areas: Europe, especially Holland, Romania, Bulgaria and Poland, as well as Northern Africa, USA, Chile, Caribbean Islands, Argentina, Paraguay, and China.

Main exporting countries: Dill fruits come mainly from Central- and Eastern-Europe, especially Hungary, Holland, and the Balkan countries.

Cultivation: The soil requirements for dill are minor. The soil should be fine and crumbly, but not too sandy. Dill does not tolerate stagnant moisture. Because the stalk breaks easily, it is advisable to cultivate dill in a location protected from wind. Dry or damp soil is suitable for cultivation of dill plants for production of dill herb, and dry locations are best for dill seed. For the production of dill seed, sowing should take place starting in April in rows of 20 to 30 cm apart, and the seeds should only be lightly covered. In order to have a continuous supply of dill herb, small areas can be seeded in 14-day intervals from April to July [Ü14]. Varieties with an especially high leaf yield include 'Aros', 'Blattreicher/St. Wagner', 'Bouquet', 'Diwa', 'Dukat', 'Elefant', 'Gewöhnlicher', 'Herkules', 'Pikant', 'Sari', 'Tetra', and 'Vierling'. 'Gewöhnlicher' can be used for production of dill seed [Ü14, Ü21].

Culinary herb

Commercial forms: Dill tips: dried, fine-cut, usually freeze-dried young shoots and leaves, Dill weed: herb with flowers or unripe fruits, Dill seed: dried fruits. Fresh dill herb is sold in the vegetable market, and the essential oil of the fruits (dill seed oil) or herb (dill weed oil) is also available.

Production: Dill tips can be harvested after 6 to 8 weeks. Fresh herb that is used

for pickling is cut by hand or mechanically at the start of the flowering period. The fruits are harvested just before they are completely ripe, and as they are beginning to turn brown. Mowing should take place in the morning or in cloudy weather with sufficiently high humidity in order to keep the fruits from dropping off. The harvested herb is swathed and field dried, and after drying it is taken from the field and threshed [Ü14, Ü21].

Forms used: Fresh, non-flowering or flowering herb, usually without the lower part of the stem, the dried, threadlike parts of the pinnate leaflets, and the fresh or dried fruits.

Storage: The fresh herb can be stored wrapped in plastic bags in the refrigerator for a few days. It can also be stored, finely chopped, in plastic containers or in ice trays deep-frozen with water for about 8 to 10 months. Drying of dill herb is not optimal due to the considerable loss of aroma. The dried herb and fruits can be stored for several years in well-sealed metal- or glass containers, protected from light and moisture.

Description. Fruits (Fig. 3): The achenes are mostly separated from each other, reddish-yellow to yellowish-brown, smooth, glabrous, 4 to 5 mm long, 2 to 3 mm wide, lentil-shaped, compressed, outlines oval to ovate, with 5 filiform and light-colored ribs, which are broadly winged at the margins [Ü29, Ü48]

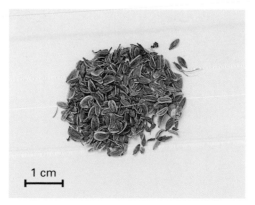

1 cm

Fig. 3: Dill fruits

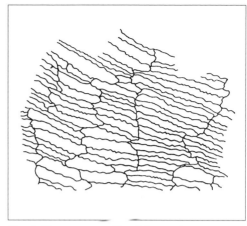

Fig. 4: Transverse cells of the endocarp. From Ü48

Herb: For the fresh herb, see description of the plant. The dried herb (dill tips, Fig. 1) of commerce is cut, dark green, consisting only of short filiform, about 0.5 mm wide and about 1 cm long leaf tips.

Powdered fruits: Characteristic are the transverse cells of the endocarp (Fig. 4), the wide, dark secretory ducts, the fibrous bundles and the sclerenchyma cells of the outer ribs as well as the numerous endosperm cells with very small oxalate rosettes, spherical oil droplets and aleuron grains [Ü29].

Odor, Taste. Ripe fruits: Odor very faint, fennel-like. The taste is mild at first, then pungent, somewhat acrid, caraway-like, **Herb:** Odor and taste reminiscent of parsley.

History: Dill was already used during antiquity. In the "Papyrus Ebers", it was mentioned as a medicinal plant. Its use in old Palestine has been documented in the New Testament. Arabs, Romans and Greeks also used dill. In Neolithic lake dwellings along the shores of Swiss lakes in the subalpine zone, dill has also been found. A local government decree by Karl the Great, "Capitulare de villis" (authored in about 795 CE, see footnote under → Anise), called for the cultivation of dill. In the 9th and 10th century, it was introduced to England [23].

Constituents and Analysis

Constituents of the fruits

- Essential oil: 2.5 to 5% (rarely up to 8%); the composition is race-specific; the main components are (S)-(+)-carvone (D-carvone, 18 to 81%), dihydrocarvone (0.1 to 62%) and (R)-(+)-limonene (10 to 50%), furthermore α- and β-phellandrene, dill ether ((+)-(3R, 8S, 9R)-3,9-epoxy-p-menth-1-ene, contributing to the aroma), among others, and dillapiol (trace amounts to 5%, in samples of Egyptian origin up 27%, possibly A. g. var. sowa, see below) [2, 6, 9–12, 18, 19, 21, 22, 24, 26, Ü43].
- Flavonoids: The main component is kaempferol-3-β-D-glucoside as well as vicenin, among others [7, 25].
- Coumarin derivatives: Bergaptene, umbelliferone and xanthotoxin (very small amounts) [1].
- Fatty oil (10 to 20%) [Ü43].

Constituents of the herb

- Essential oil: 0.2 to 2.3% (0.05 to 0.75%, calculated with reference to the fresh herb); the main components are (S)-(+)-α-phellandrene (26 to 65%, high content before development of the flower buds) and dill ether (5 to 32%, high content during flowering), both constituents are responsible for the typical odor of dill; also (+)-limonene (3 to 55%), β-phellandrene (up to 10%), p-cymene (up to 4%), D-carvone (content depends on the developmental stage of the plant, increasing with age, the variety and the way the essential oil is obtained; herb from Reunion contained 0.4%, from Finland 0 to 2.5%, from Germany 12 to 29%, from the USA 0 to 40%, from India 25 to 42% and from Hungary 25 to 50%); furthermore β-phellandrene, p-cymene, p-menth-2-ene-1,6-diol, 8-hydroxygeraniol, 2-methylbutyric acid methyl ester and piperitone [2, 4–6, 9, 13, 22, 27].
- Flavonoids: The main components are quercetin-3-O-β-D-glucuronide and isorhamnetin, furthermore quercetin- and isorhamnetin-3-O-glucoside, -3-galactoside, 3-rhamnoglucoside and vicenin [25, Ü43].
- Coumarin derivatives: Scopoletin, anethum-coumarin [1].

Tests for Identity: Organoleptic examination of the herb or fruits, as well as macroscopic and microscopic analyses or GC, GC/MS and GC/IRMS assays [3, 5, 6, 8, 11, 19, 27].

Quantitative assay: The content of essential oil can be determined with steam distillation, following the Ph Eur procedure with xylol in the graduated tube.

Adulterations, Misidentifications and Impurities: Indian dill is a possible adulterant. Its distinction is based on the relatively high content of dillapiol in its fruits.

Actions and Uses

Actions: For dill fruits, stimulation of salivation and gastric juice secretion is presumed. Due to the high carvone content, dill fruits have good spasmolytic activity (→ Caraway). Like all essential oils, dill oil also has antimicrobial effects [14, 16, 20]. Fresh dill herb has a similar effect on salivation and gastric juice secretion as dill fruit. The intensity of the spasmolytic action, which is dependent, predominantly, on the carvone content (see above), is probably variable depending on the variety. Dried dill herb has little effect due to its low essential oil content.

Toxicology: Based on existing data, there is no acute or chronic toxicity with the regular use of this herb as a spice [16]. The sensitization potential is low [Ü39].

Culinary use: Dill is indispensable in Nordic cooking. In Sweden it is a universal spice. It is also well liked in North- and Central America.

Dill should not be cooked or only very briefly due to very rapid volatilization of the essential oil.

The whole herb with nearly ripe fruits serves as a spice for pickling cucumbers (dill pickles, pickled gherkins), red beets, onions, tomatoes and white cabbage (sauerkraut) and, as well as the fresh or dried dill tops, to spice meat- (e.g. chicken) and fish dishes (especially salmon, fresh eel, carp, young herring), crabs, lobster, egg dishes (e.g. hard boiled eggs), ground meat, mushroom dishes, light sauces (dill sauce, e.g. for lamb, chicken or veal), dips, broths, clear soups, leaf salads, potato salads, herb vinegar (dill vinegar), herb butter, quark, fresh cheese, mayonnaise and remoulade [Ü2, Ü13, Ü79, Ü86, Ü90].

Dried dill fruits are used, especially in Northern Europe, in the same way as caraway, e.g. in bread, in France they are strewn over cake, and are also used for the spicing of fish and vegetable dishes (cauli-

Carvone   Dihydrocarvone   Limonene   α-Phellandrene

β-Phellandrene   Dill ether   Dillapiol

flower, sauerkraut, carrots, zucchini), grilled lamb or pork, or stews. It is also added to vegetable juices (e.g. tomato juice) [Ü2].

The essential oil of dill seeds is used as a flavor component of various liqueurs. Dill herb oil and dill essence are used in the food industry for the production of flavor ingredients.

Combines well with: Borage, garlic, onions, and shallots. While compatible with many other spice herbs, it is best used, however, alone.

As a component of spice mixes and preparations: → Bologna spice mix, → Chat masala, → Cocktail sauce, → Fish spice, → Frankfurter green sauce, → Herb butter, → Mixed pickles spice, → Pickle spice, → Poultry spice, → Quark spice, → Salad spice, → Soup spice, → Table mustard, → Vegetable spice.

Other uses: S-(+)-Carvone can be used to inhibit potato germination [26].

Medicinal herb

Herbal drug: Anethi fructus, Dill fruit, contains not less than 2.5% essential oil [EB 6].

Indications: Dried dill fruit is used for indigestions, especially for mild cramping pain of stomach and enterospasms, bloating and epigastric fullness. Dill fruit can be prepared in the form of a tea infusion (2 g freshly crushed or ground dill fruits per cup; adult daily dose: 2 to 6 g). The infusion is also used in folk medicine, similarly to that of caraway fruit, as a lactation promoting remedy (lactagogue). Germany's Commission E issued a negative monograph for dill herb because its activity has not been proven [15].

Similar culinary spices

Indian dill, *Anethum sowa* ROXB., fruits are used as a spice in India, Japan, Malacca Peninsula, and in Java, e.g. in lentil stews, but are also chewed after meals. The main component in the essential oil of the fruits is dillapiol. D-Carvone and limonene are also present [11, Ü93].

Kalakeitto (Finnish Fish Soup)
250 g of potatoes, 750 g fish (for example pike, mackerel, eel, cod, sea salmon, 2 tablespoons of flower, 1/2 l of milk, 3 teaspoons of chopped dill, condiment, table salt.

Peel and wash the potatoes; dice them into small cubes, add salt and boil them until half-done. Clean the fish, remove the fish bones and cut it into bite-sized pieces; place the fish pieces on top of the potatoes and cook them slowly, on low heat, until done. Mix in flour and milk and bring to a boil; simmer the soup for 8 min. Add the chopped dill, salt and condiment. Serve with dark bread and butter [Ü23].

Literature

[1] Aplin R.T., C.B. Page, J. Chem. Soc. 23:Soc. 2593 (1967).

[2] Bauermann U. et al., Drogenreport 6(10): 24–30 (1993).

[3] Betts T.J., J. Pharm. Pharmacol. 21(4): 259–262 (1969).

[4] Bonnlander W., P. Winterhalter, J. Agric. Food Chem. 48(10):4821–4825 (2000).

[5] Brunke E.J. et al., J. Ess. Oil Res. 3:257–267 (1991).

[6] Charles D.J. et al., J. Ess. Oil Res. 7:11–20 (1995).

[7] Dranik L.I., Khim. Prir. Soedin. (2):268 (1970).

[8] Faber B. et al., Fragrance J. 12(5):305–314 (1997).

[9] Göckeritz D. et al., Pharmazie 34(7): 426–429 (1979).

[10] Hälvä S. et al., J. Agric. Science in Finland 60(2):93–100 (1988).

[11] Hammer K., H. Krüger, Drogenreport 8(13):20–23 (1995).

[12] Huopalathi R., R. Lathinen, Flavour Fragrance 3:121–125 (1988).

[13] Huopalathi R., R.R. Linko, J. Agric. Food Chem. 31:331–333 (1983).

[14] Kellner W., W. Kober, Arzneim. Forsch. 4:319 (1954).

[15] Kommission E bei BfArM, BAnz-Nr. 193 vom 15.10.87 (1987).

[16] Kommission E beim BfArM, BAnz-Nr. 193 vom 15.10.1987.

[17] Kozawa M. et al., Chem. Pharm. Bull. 24:220 (1976).

[18] Krüger H., K. Hammer, J. Ess. Oil Res. 8(2):205–206 (1996).

[19] Mahran G.H. et al., Int. J. Pharmacog. 30:139–144 (1992).

[20] Maruzella J.C., A. Sicurella, J. Am. pharmac. Assoc. 49:692 –694 (1960).

[21] Poggendorf A. et al., Pharmazie 32(10): 607–613 (1977).

[22] Püst U., Untersuchungen über die ätherischen Öle in der Wurzel, Kraut und Früchten verschiedener Seselinae, Dissertation Hamburg 1976.

[23] Scholz H., Natürlich 17(6):32–36 (1997).

[24] Schreier P. et al., Lebensm. Wiss. Technol. 14:150–152 (1981).

[25] Teuber H. et al., Z. Lebensm. Unters. Forsch. 167(2):101–104 (1978).

[26] Van Der Mheen H., Beitr. Züchtungsforsch. 2(1):162 166 (1996).

[27] Van Der Mheen H., Beitr. Züchtungsforsch. 2(1):226–227 (1996).

[28] Vera R.R., J. Chane-Ming, J. Ess. Oil Res. 10:539–542 (1998).

Literature references identified by Ü can be found in the general listing of books and monographs at the back of this book.

Fennel

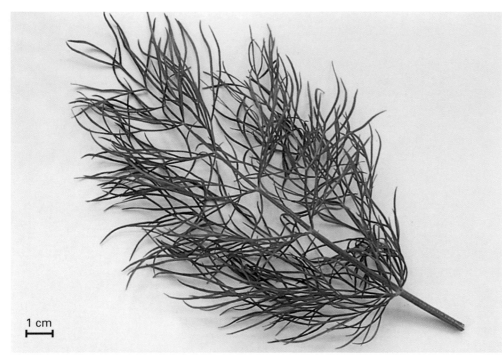

Fig. 1: Fennel leaf

1 cm

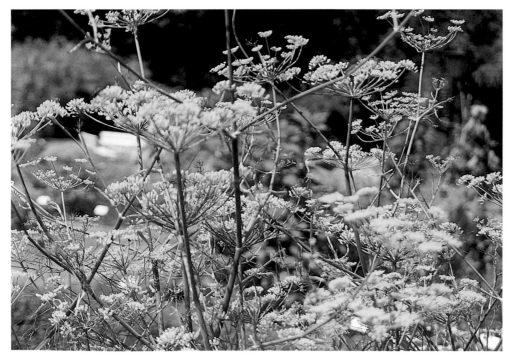

Fig. 2: Fennel (*Foeniculum vulgare* MILL.)

Plant source: *Foeniculum vulgare* MILL.

Synonyms: *Foeniculum capillaceum* GILIB., *Foeniculum officinale* ALL., *Anethum foeniculum* L.

Taxonomic classification: The species is differentiated by the following subspecies and varieties:
- *F. v.* MILL. ssp. *piperitum* (UCRIA) COUT., pepper fennel,
- *F. v.* MILL. ssp. *vulgare* (Syn.: ssp. *capillaceum* (GILIB.) HOLMBOE), garden fennel,
- - *F. v.* MILL. ssp. *vulgare* var. *azoricum* (MILL.) THELL., Florence fennel, finocchio,
- - *F. v.* MILL. ssp. *vulgare* var. *dulce* (MILL.) BATT. et TRAB., sweet fennel,
- - *F. v.* MILL. ssp. *vulgare* var. *vulgare*, bitter fennel, wild fennel.
The borderline between the varieties *F. v.* ssp. *vulgare* var. *vulgare* and *F. v.* ssp. *vulgare* var. *dulce* is not fixed, so a precise separation between the two is almost impossible to make. *F. v.* MILL. spp. *piperitum* and *F. v.* ssp. *vulgare* var. *azoricum* are cultivated as vegetables [10].

Family: Umbelliferous plants (Apiaceae, synonym Umbelliferae)

Common names: Engl.: fennel, sweet fennel; Fr.: fenouil, aneth doux (sweet fennel); Ger: Fenchel, Brotsamen, Brotwürzkörner, Brotanis, Frauenfenchel, Fenicht, Kinderfenchel.

Description: Annual to perennial herb, up to 2.5 m high, with beet-like root. Leaves alternate, the lower ones have petioles with a leaf sheath at the bottom; the upper leaves are sessile, glabrous, 3- to 4 times pinnatisect with awl-shaped tip. The primary and secondary stems bear each a single composite umbel with 4 to 25 unevenly long rays, without involucre or involucre.

The flowers are radial with 5 petals, deep yellow, 5 stamina, 2 styles, inferior ovary, bilocular. The fruit is a double achene with two mericarps, which remain closed and attached to a bifurcate carpophore (in some varieties they are detached). Flowering period is from July to September.
F. v. ssp. *vulgare* var. *vulgare* is triennial to quadrennial and rarely exceeds a height of 1.25 m; this variety has a hard and pithy stem. *F. v.* ssp. *vulgare* var. *dulce* is annual or biennial, with a soft tubular stem, growing to a height of 1.25 to 2.5 m.

Native origin: South- and Southwestern Europe, today widely distributed in almost all of Europe (with the exception of Northern Europe), Northern Africa, Asia Minor, Caucasus Region, Iran and Central Asia, and naturalized in North America, Eastern Asia, Malaysia, Indonesia, New Zealand, and South Africa, among other countries.

Main cultivation areas: Bitter fennel: Eastern Europe, especially Bulgaria, Czech Republic, Slovakia, Poland, Hungary, Romania, and Germany (Thuringia, Saxony), Sweet fennel: France, as well as Egypt, Bulgaria, China, India, Japan, Yugoslavia, and Turkey, among other countries.

Main exporting countries: Egypt and Turkey, followed by Spain, France, Czech Republic, Russian Federation, China, Japan, and India.

Cultivation: Fennel is not very demanding on soil quality, other than it does not thrive in too alkaline or too dry soil. Bitter fennel, grown as an annual, can be sown already by mid-March in row widths of about 30 to 50 cm. Varieties for annual cultivation include, among others, 'Berfena', 'Chumen' and 'Magnafena', and for biennial cultivation varieties include 'Großfrüchtiger', 'Romanesc' and 'Soroksári' [Ü14, Ü21].

Culinary herb

Commercial forms: Fennel seed: ripe, dried whole fruits, ground or broken, essential oil of sweet fennel, oleoresin of sweet fennel.

Production: Harvest is carried out at the end of October to the beginning of November, usually with a threshing machine, when the upper umbels take on a grayish-green color [Ü21]. For personal use, one can snip off the almost ripe multiple fruits and hang them up inside a paper bag to dry and further ripen. Leaves and stalks should be harvested prior to flowering. If only the leaves and stalks are desired, it is best to trim the plant back in order to prevent flowering.

Forms used: Dried fruits, fresh or dried leaves and stalks harvested before the flowering period, essential oil; due to the bitter taste of essential oil distilled from bitter fennel, the food industry uses the oil of sweet fennel and its oleoresin almost exclusively.

Storage: The fresh leaves can be stored in plastic bags in the refrigerator for a few days, chopped and frozen in the freezer, or preserved in olive oil or vinegar, as well as kept in dried form. The dried fruits are stored in well-sealed porcelain, glass or metal containers, protected from light, heat and moisture.

Description. Whole fruits (Fig. 3): They consist of the whole, cylindrical, 3 to 12

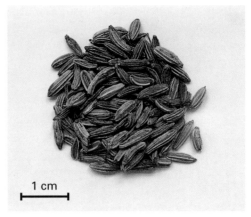

1 cm

Fig. 3: Fennel fruit

mm long and 4 mm wide fruits, with broadly rounded lower surface and a narrower, yellowish-green to yellow-brown upper part; the double achenes, sometimes separated into their mericarps. The individual achenes bear 5 distinct, somewhat curved ridges. Under magnification, the cross section reveals on the back 4 and on the front 2 secretory canals [Ü49].
For a description of fennel leaves (Fig. 1), see: Description.

Powdered fruits: Powder of bitter fennel is greenish-yellow, and that of sweet fennel is gray-brown to gray-yellow. Microscopic examination reveals the prominent parenchyma cells with reticulate thickenings of the wall (reticulate parenchyma, cells with large window-like oval or rounded pits) and "parquetry" cells of the endocarp (Fig. 4). Also present are the fragments of the thick-walled exocarp with few stomata, the secretory ducts with thin-

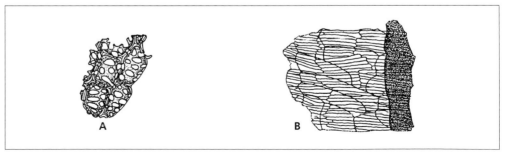

Fig. 4: Fennel. **A** Parenchyma cells of the endocarp with reticulate thickenings of the walls **B** "Parquetry" cells from the inner epidermis of the endocarp, beneath these cells parenchymatic tissue, to the right the remains of an oil duct. From Ü49.

walled, yellowish-brown remains of the epithelial tissue and the thick-walled endosperm as well as aleuron grains, oil droplets, oxalate microrosettes and fragments of the vascular bundles with lignified fibers. Starch must be absent [Ü49].

Odor: Aromatic (Bitter fennel), mildly sweet (Sweet fennel), **Taste:** First sweetish then somewhat bitter and burning (Bitter fennel), spicy and anise-like (Sweet fennel).

History: Fennel was already used by the Babylonians in 3000 BCE. The Egyptians used fennel as well, and it was often mentioned by Greek authors. Plinius the Elder (23–79 CE), in his "Naturalis Historia", praised its attributes as a good spice and medicine. The Arabs and Chinese also used this herb. In a local government decree by Karl the Great, "Capitulare de villis" (authored in about 795 CE, see footnote, → Anise) and in medieval herb books, fennel is also mentioned [for details see Lit. 14].

Constituents and Analysis

Constituents of the fruits
■ **Essential oil:**
Bitter fennel fruits: 3 to 8.5%, with the main components *trans*-anethole (50 to 75%, besides traces of *cis*-anethole), (+)-fenchone (15 to 30%, bitter tasting) and 2 to 6% estragole (methyl chavicol, with a sweetish taste).
Sweet fennel fruits: 0.8 to 3.0%, with the main components *trans*-anethole (80 to 95%), fenchone (less than 10%, mostly less than 1%), and estragole (0.8 to 6%).
Both subspecies contain, among these constituents, anise alcohol, anisaldehyde and monoterpenes, e.g. (*R*)-limonene, α-pinene, camphene, *p*-cymene, myrcene, α- and β-phellandrene, sabinene, γ-terpinene, *cis*-β-ocimene and terpinolene. Glycosides of a few of these compounds occur in the fruits [1, 10, 20, 29, 34, 36, 44, 47, 61, 62, 65].

Fruits of other chemical races:
There are chemical races which cannot be assigned to these subspecies based on the composition of the essential oil: for example those which contain less than 50% *trans*-anethole (0.3 to 39%), more than 30% fenchone or more than 30% methyl chavicol (30 to 84%), respectively [7, 8, 23, 24, 27, 34, 41].
■ Phenylacrylic acids, phenylallyl alcohols, phenolcarboxylic acids: These include, among others, *p*-hydroxycinnamic acid, caffeic acid, most likely occurs in the form of quinic acid derivatives, particularly chlorogenic acid, 4- and 5-caffeoylquinic acid, *p*-coumaroyl- and feruloyl quinic acids, 4-*O*-β-D-glucosylsinapyl alcohol, 4,9-di-*O*-β-D-glucosylsinapyl alcohol and 4-β-D-glucosyloxybenzoic acid [17, 42, 63, 64].
■ Hydroxycoumarins (traces): Osthenol, scoparin and umbelliferone, among others [Ü 37].
■ Furanocoumarins (traces): Bergaptene, imperatorin and psoralene, among others [13, Ü37].
■ Flavonoids (very little): Kaempferol-3-*O*-glucoronide, quercetin-3-*O*-glucoronide, and in some races isoquercitrin (quercetin-3-*O*-glucoside), kaempferol-3-*O*-arabinoside, foenicularin (quercetin-3-*O*-arabinoside) and rutin [25, 26, 35].
■ Trimeric stilbene derivatives and their glycosides: Foeniculosides I to V, miyabenol C, *cis*-miyabenol C, zizybeoside I and icaviside A₄ [44–46].
■ Fatty oil (9 to 21%): With a 45 to 60% petroselinic acid component in the triacylglycerols [60].
■ Proteins (20 to 30%).

Constituents of the herb
Content of essential oil in the leaves is 0.7 to 1%; about the same qualitative composition as in the fruits, but in addition to *trans*-anethole, the lower leaves also contain high concentrations of monoterpenes (in *F. v.* var. *vulgare*, up to 37% α-pinene, up to 42% α-phellandrene, and in var. *dulce*, up to 75% limonene) [51, 62]. In chemical races of Spanish origin, the main components were found to be α-phellandrene (9 to 27%), limonene (18 to 25%), fenchone (18 to 19%) and estragole (about 12%) [23].

Tests for Identity: Organoleptic examination, in addition to macroscopic and microscopic analysis, as well as TLC of the extract [59, Ph Eur] or the essential oil [6, 22, 31, Ü101]. Sweet fennel is identified by the absence or only a faint zone of fenchone. A differentiation of bitter fennel from sweet fennel (and their essential oils) can be achieved by GC [9, 11, 19, 22, 24, 33, Ph Eur, DAB].

Quantitative assay: The content of essential oil can be determined volumetrically with steam distillation, xylol in the graduated tube [Ph Eur]. The content of anethole, fenchone and estragole can be determined with GC [Ph Eur, DAB].

Adulterations, Misidentifications and Impurities: It is possible that sweet fennel is confused with bitter fennel. Sweet fennel is usually lighter colored and has a sweetish taste with no bitter aftertaste; the mericarps of sweet fennel are more rarely separated from each other, although a certain distinction based on morphological

trans-Anethole   Estragole   Fenchone

and anatomical differences is not possible [48]. The estragole content of bitter fennel must be below 6%, and that of sweet fennel below 10%. These specifications rule out the use of fennel from a few geographical origins (such as Czech Republic, Slovakia, Spain, and India); these can contain up to 80% estragole [57].

Actions and Uses

Actions: Fennel promotes digestion and has carminative action. Fennel has been shown to increase gastrointestinal motility and secretion [53, 54]. In rabbits, it has been shown that fennel (24 mg/kg body weight, orally) stimulated gastrointestinal motility and also reduced the inhibition of motility caused by sodium pentobarbitone (25 mg/kg body weight, intravenously) [43]. In low concentrations, fennel oil (5 to 25 ml fennel water via catheter through intestinal fistula of dog in situ) [49] or anethole (10 to 25 mg/l fluid bath, small intestine of mouse in vitro) stimulated gastrointestinal motility, and in high concentrations (above 50 mg/l fluid bath) had a relaxing effect [28].

Due to its spasmolytic activity, fennel relieves intestinal colics. Aqueous-ethanolic extracts of fennel (1:3.5 (w/v), ethanol 31%, 2.5 and 10 ml/l fluid bath) have shown in vitro atropine-like inhibition of spasms induced by acetylcholine and carbachol in guinea pig ileum. Aqueous extracts of fennel (2 to 3 g/kg body weight) have shown similar effects in cat small intestine in situ and in isolated guinea pig ileum. The tonus increasing effects of acetylcholine, pilocarpine, physostigmine or barium chloride are also antagonized by fennel oil (10 mg/l fluid bath) in vitro in the small intestine of various test animals [21, 43, 52, 55].

Fennel extracts have expectorant activity. In isolated bronchial mucosa of frog, it could be shown that a fennel infusion promoted the transport of particles through the ciliary beats [55]. Inhalation of anethole or fenchone has shown secretolytic action in rabbits [12].

A blood pressure lowering effect of fennel fruits has been reported [45].

In animal experiments, estrogenic effects were observed in female ovarectomized rats after administration of the residues on evaporation of an acetone extract of sweet fennel (0.5 to 2.5 mg/kg body weight) such as increased libido and increased weight of the mammary glands and uterus. In male rats, it caused a decrease in the protein concentrations in the testicles and vas deference, and in normal female rats it led to an increase in mammary gland weight, among other effects [3, 4, 38, 68, overview in Lit. 2].

Similar to all essential oils, fennel oil has antimicrobial action [1, 37–39, 43, 50].

Extracts of fennel fruit provide good antioxidative protection for fatty oils [42, 46].

Toxicology: Based on existing data, there is no acute or chronic toxicity with the normal use of fennel fruits or herb.

The sensitization potential is low. Allergic reactions such as rhinitis, conjunctivitis and asthma are possible, in particular, if there is an existing allergy towards other apiaceous foods (e.g. celery, carrot, parsley) or mugwort. Cross-reactions with paprika and pepper, due to antibodies towards two antigens of fennel with molecular masses of 67 to 75 KD, have been observed [30, 56, 58, 67].

During pregnancy, the consumption of preparations with high amounts of fennel essential oils should be avoided because of estrogenic effects, but the use of fennel as a spice does not pose a risk.

Medicinal products with a high estragole content (>10%) should be not be used due to a possible hepatocarcinogenic effect of estragole [16, 18, 40, 66], which, however, has only been documented in animal tests.

Culinary use: Fennel is especially revered in French and Italian cooking. It is also widely used in the countries of Southeastern Asia.

Fennel fruits should be crushed immediately before use (e.g. with a pestle and mortar), filled into a tea ball or a gauze sack and placed in the food to steep prior

to cooking, and removed just before serving. Due to its strong flavor, it should be used sparingly. For sprinkling on bread and other baked goods, whole fennel fruits are used.

Fennel fruits, usually sweet fennel, are used similarly as caraway, for example as a spice for breads (fennel bread) and pastries, sauces for cooked fish or pork, crustaceans or spaghetti, marinades, soups (e.g. cabbage-, leek-, potato soups, Provençal fish soup, bouillabaisse), meat dishes, fish dishes (e.g. mackerel, trout, sardines, sea grayling), red cabbage, red beets, mushrooms, compotes, cheeses, salad dressings and mayonnaise. Fennel fruits are also used as a preservative, e.g. for preserves of pickles, pumpkins, carrots as well as sauerkraut, and for inlaying with herring. Fennel fruits can also be used for preparing strawberry marmalade and apple- and quince jelly.

Florentine salami (finochiona) spiced with fennel is especially enjoyed in Italy. Fennel fruits also serve as a spice for grilled or baked meat in Italy. On the street corners in central Italy, slices of porchetta (a sucking pig) coated with fennel, garlic and rosemary are sold.

In India, candied fennel fruits are chewed after meals to promote good digestion. And for spicing Indian dishes, they are briefly roasted.

Chopped fresh fennel leaves or young shoots serve as a garnish and appetizer for mayonnaises, remoulade, sauces, vinaigrettes, soups, vegetable dishes, meat- and fish dishes, seafoods, peas and beans, quark, yogurt and green salads (e.g. Italian Cartucci). One can also prepare a spicy salad by adding fennel sprouts.

The dried stalks are an important component of Provençal cooking [Ü10, Ü17, Ü19, Ü55, Ü71, Ü73, Ü93, Ü95].

Combines well with: Chilies, dill, garlic, oregano, parsley, sage or thyme.

As a component of spice mixes and preparations: → Bread spice, → Curry powder, → Five-spice mix, → Herb mixtures for grilling and smoking, → Herb vinegar, → Panch phoron, → Tofu spice.

Other uses: Fennel tea is recommended for facial compresses, especially for fatty skin, for eye rinses and oral care remedies. Fennel powder, blended with warm milk, is used for skin smoothing masks. The essential oil is used as an aromatic component of oral care products as well as occasionally in the perfume industry [Ü24]. Bitter fennel oil is used to produce anethole for the liqueur industry, which uses it, for example, to make the French Pastis and Fenouilette or the Greek Ouzo.

Similar culinary spices: → Anise.

Medicinal herb

Herbal drugs: Foeniculi amari fructus, Bitter fennel (contains not less than 40 ml/kg of essential oil, of which not less than 60% is anethole, not less than 15% is fenchone, and not more than 5% is estragole) [Ph Eur], Foeniculi dulcis fructus, Sweet fennel (contains not less than 20 ml/kg of essential oil, of which not less than 80% is anethole, not more than 10% is estragole, and not more than 7.5% is fenchone) [Ph Eur], Foeniculi amari fructus aetheroleum, Bitter-fennel fruit oil (contains 12 to 25% fenchone, 55 to 75% *trans*-anethole, 1 to 10% *alpha*-pinene, 0.9 to 5.0% limonene, not more than 6% estragole, not more than 0.5% *cis*-anethole, and not more than 2% anisaldehyde) [Ph Eur].

Indications: Fennel fruits are applied for digestive complaints such as mild, cramp-like gastrointestinal pains, bloating and flatulence, as well as for catarrhs of the upper respiratory tract. Fennel fruits are used in the form of tea infusion or tincture. Especially in pediatric medicine fennel honey or fennel syrup are used for loss of appetite or catarrhs of the respiratory tract. The daily dosage is 5 to 7 g of dried fennel fruit or equivalent preparations (for children from 4 to 10 years 4 to 6 g, 1 to 4 years 3 to 5 g, and under 1 year 2 to 4 g) [1, 5, 15, 32]. In folk medicine, it is also used for amenorrhea (emmenagogue), to promote lactation (lactagogue) and for obesity [2, 41]. Externally, fennel water or fennel tea infusion is used for conjunctivitis [41].

Broiled Herring with Fennel Filling

4 whole, deboned herrings, 2 teaspoons of chopped fennel leaves, 1/2 teaspoon of chopped parsley, 30 g of butter, salt, 1 teaspoon of lemon juice.

Wash the herrings and make three diagonal incisions on each side. Combine the fennel, parsley and salt, and place the mixture into the incisions and the body cavity. Melt the butter with the lemon juice in a broiling pan. Place the fish in the pan and turn them over immediately so that they are covered with the butter sauce. Place the pan under the electric grill and broil each side of the fish on high heat for 4 to 5 minutes [Ü79].

Literature

[1] Afzal H., MS. Aktar, J. Pak. Med. Assoc. 31:230–232 (1981).
[2] Albert-Puleo M, J. Ethnopharmacol. 2(4): 337 (1980).
[3] Annusuya S. et al., Indian J. Physiol. Pharmacol. 29:21–26 (1988).
[4] Annusuya S. et al., Indian J. Med. Res. 87:364–367 (1988).
[5] Anonym, ESCOP-Monographs, Foeniculi fructus, Fennel (1996).
[6] Ballarini C., J. Ballarini, Pharmazie (8): 544 (1972).
[7] Barazani O. et al., Planta Med. 65(5): 486–489 (1999).
[8] Bernáth J. et al., J. Ess. Oil Res. 8:247–253 (1996).
[9] Betts T.J., J. Pharm. Pharmacol. 20: 61S–64S (1968).
[10] Betts T.J., J. Pharm. Pharmacol. 20(6): 469–472 (1968).
[11] Betts T.J., J. Chromatogr. 626(2):294–300 (1992).
[12] Boyd E.M., E.P. Sheppard, Pharmacology 6:65–80 (1971).
[13] Ceska O. et al., Phytochemistry 26(1): 165–169 (1987).
[14] Czygan F.C., Z. Phytother. 8:82–85 (1987).
[15] De Smet P.A.G.M. et al. (Eds.), in: Adverse Effects of Herbal Drugs, Springer Verlag Berlin, Heidelberg, New York 1992, Bd. 1, p. 91–95.
[16] De Vincenzi M. et al., Fitoterapia 71(6):725–729 (2000).
[17] Dirks U., K. Herrmann, Zeitschr. Lebensm. Unters. Forsch. 179:12–16 (1984).
[18] Drinkwater N.R. et al., J. Nat. Cancer Inst. 57:1323–1331 (1976).
[19] Fehr D., Pharm. Ztg. 127(46):2520–2522 (1982).
[20] Fehr D., Pharm. Ztg. 125:1300–1303 (1980).
[21] Forster H., Z. Allgemeinmed. 59:1327–13331 (1983).
[22] Gabrio Th. et al., Pharm. Zentralhalle 125(8):459–462 (1986).
[23] Garcia-Jiménez N. et al., J. Ess. Oil Res. 12:159–162 (2000).
[24] Guillen M.D., M.J. Manzanos, Chem. Mikrobiol. Technol. Lebensm. 16(5/6): 141–145 (1994).
[25] Harborne J.B., N.A.M. Saleh, Phytochemistry 10:399–400 (1971).
[26] Herrmann J., J. Kunzemann, Dtsch. Apoth. Ztg. 117:918–920 (1977).
[27] Hethelyi I., Olaj, Szappan, Kozmet 44(2): 64–67 (1995), ref. CA 123: 312503t.
[28] Imaseki I., Y. Kitabatake, Yakugaku Zasshi 82:1326–1328 (1962).
[29] Ishikawa T. et al., Chem. Pharm. Bull. 47(6):805–808 (1999).
[30] Jensen Jarolim E. et al., Clinical experim. Allergy 27(11):1299–13011 (1997).
[31] Karlsen J. et al., Planta Med. 17:281–293 (1969).
[32] Kommission E beim BfArM, BAnz Nr. 74 vom 19.04.1991.
[33] Kraus A., F.J. Hammerschmidt, Dragoco Report 27:31–40 (1980).
[34] Krüger H., K. Hammer, J. Ess. Oil Res. 11:79–82 (1999).
[35] Kunzemann J., K. Herrmann, Z. Lebensm. Untersuch. Forsch. 164: 194–200 (1977).
[36] Lawrence B.M., Performer and Flavorist 9(1984): 49–60, 14(1989): 47–49, 17(1992): 44–46 (1992).
[37] Lord C.F., W.J. Husa, J. Am. Pharm. Assoc. 43:438–440 (1954).

[38] Malini T. et al., Indian J. Physiol. Pharmacol. 29:21–26 (1985).

[39] Maruzzella J.C., M. Freundlich, J. Am. Pharm. Assoc. 48(6):356–358 (1959).

[40] Miller E.C. et al., Cancer Res. 43:1124–1134 (1983).

[41] Mills S. et al. (Eds.), Principles and Practice of Phytotherapie, Churchill Livingstone, Edinburgh 2000, p. 374–378

[42] Nakayama R. et al., Nippon Kasei Gakkaishi 47(12):1193–1199 (1996), ref. CA 126:182498u.

[43] Niiho Y. et al., Japan. J. Pharmacol. 27:177–179 (1976).

[44] Ono M. et al., Chem. Pharm. Bull. 44: 337–342 (1996).

[45] Ono M. et al., Chem. Pharm. Bull. 43: 868–871 (1995).

[46] Ono M. et al., Food Sci. Technol. Int., Tokyo 3(1):53–55 (1997), ref. CA 127: 064843a.

[47] Opdyke D.J.L., Food Cosmet. Toxicol. 14:309 (1976).

[48] Parzinger R., Dtsch. Apoth. Ztg. 136(7): 529–530 (1996).

[49] Plant O.H., G.H. Miller, J. Exp. Pharmacol. Ther. 27:149–164 (1926).

[50] Ramadan F.M. et al., Chem. Mikrobiol. Technol. Lebensm. 2:51–55 (1972).

[51] Ravid U. et al., J. Nat. Prod. 46:848–851 (1983).

[52] Reiter M., W. Brandt, Arzneim. Forsch. 35:408–414 (1985).

[53] Schilcher H., Therapiewoche 36: 1100–1112 (1986).

[54] Schilcher H., Dtsch. Apoth. Ztg. 124(29): 1433–1442 (1984).

[55] Schuster K.P., Wirkungsstärke und Wirkungsverluste spasmolytisch wirksamer Arzneidrogen, galenischer Zubereitungen und Arzneifertigwaren, geprüft am isolierten Darm des Meerschweinchens und am Darm der Katze in situ, Dissertation Ludwig-Maximilian-Universität 1971.

[56] Schwartz H.J. et al., Ann. Allergy Asthma Immunol. 78(1):37–40 (1997).

[57] Shah C.S. et al., Planta Med. 18:285–295 (1970).

[58] Stäger J. et al., Allergy 46:475–478 (1991).

[59] Stahl E. (Hrsg.), Chromatographische und mikroskopische Analyse von Drogen, Fischer Verlag Stuttgart, New York 1978.

[60] Stepanenko G.A. et al., Khim Prir. Soedin (6):827–828 (1980).

[61] Tóth L., Planta Med. 15:371–389 (1967).

[62] Tóth L., Planta Med. 15:157–172 (1967).

[63] Trenkle K., Pharmazie 27:319–324 (1972).

[64] Trenkle K., Planta Med. 20(4):289–301 (1971).

[65] Venskutonis P.R. et al., J. Ess. Oil Res. 8:211–213 (1996).

[66] Wiseman R.W. et al., Cancer Res. 47: 2275–2283 (1987).

[67] Wüthrich B., T. Hofer, Dtsch. Med. Wschr. 109.981–986 (1984).

[68] Zava D.T. et al., Proc. Soc. Exp. Biol. Med. 217(3):369–378 (1998).

Literature references identified by Ü can be found in the general listing of books and monographs at the back of this book.

Fenugreek

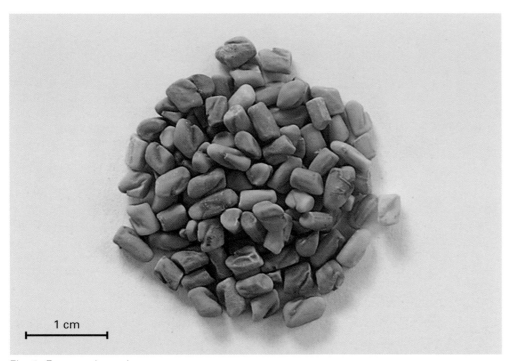

Fig. 1: Fenugreek seeds

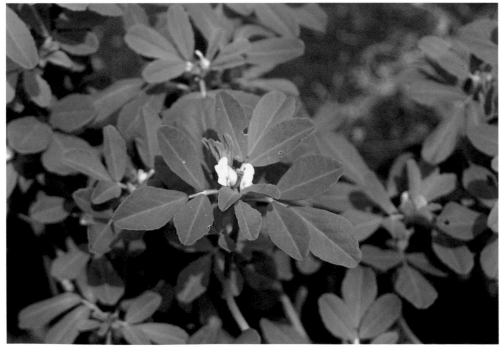

Fig. 2: Fenugreek (*Trigonella foenum-graecum* L.)

Plant source: *Trigonella foenum-graecum* L.

Taxonomic classification: The habitus of this species is quite variable. An infraspecific classification has been described, but it is rarely applied [50, Ü42].

Family: Pea family (Fabaceae, synonym: Papilionaceae; some authors also place it with Caesalpiniaceae and Mimosaceae in the legume family, Leguminosae).

Common names: Engl.: fenugreek, amber fenugreek, fenugrec; Fr.: fénugrec, senegré, trigonelle; Ger.: Bockshornklee, Griechischer Heu, Kuhhornklee.

Description: Annual herb, up to 60 cm tall. Leaves trifoliate, leaf stalks 0.5 to 2 cm and leaflets 1 to 3 cm long, obovate to oblong-lanceolate, dentate, with membrane-like stipules. The flowers are single or in pairs situated in the leaf axils 0.8 to 1.8 cm long, calyx tubular and membranaceus, corolla pale yellow, light-violet at the base and twice as long as the sepals; wings (alae) half as long as the flag (vexillum), the keel (carina) is obtuse. The pods are 2.5 to 15 cm long, 0.5 to 1 cm wide, erect, with a 2 to 3 cm long beak-like projection and containing 4 to 20 seeds. Flowering period is from June to July [Ü42].

Native origin: China, India, Iraq, northwestern India, and Ethiopia (naturally occurring or possibly escaped from cultivation?).

Main cultivation areas: Mediterranean countries (Egypt, Turkey, Morocco, Syria, Greece, southern France), Sudan, western- and central Asia, Arabian countries, India, China, Japan, North America (California), and Argentina.

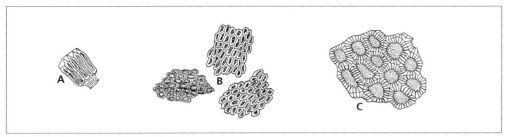

Fig. 3: Fenugreek, components of the testa. **A** Palisade layer with an adjacent cell of the hypodermal stratum (side view), **B** Cross sections of the palisade layer at different heights, **C** Hypodermal stratum (top view). From Ü49

Main exporting countries: India, Pakistan, China, Morocco, Turkey, France, and Argentina.

Cultivation: Fenugreek prefers nutrient-rich, slightly calcareous, not too light soil in warm, sunny locations. Propagation by sowing occurs at the start of April, set in rows about 25 cm apart. The seeds should not be planted any deeper than 3 cm [Ü21, Ü45].

Culinary herb

Commercial forms: Fenugreek seed (India and Pakistan: Methi): the ripe, dried, whole or ground seeds and fenugreek oleoresin.

Production: The herb can be harvested when a growth height of about 20 cm is attained. The seed harvest is carried out, usually by combine, when the lower pods begin to dry up and split. In small-scale cultivation or in developing countries, the whole plant is pulled out, dried, threshed, winnowed and cleaned [Ü21].

Forms used: Dried fenugreek seeds (whole or ground), roasted ground seeds, fresh (rarely dried) herb, and young pods.

Storage: The freshly cut leaves or shoots can be stored in plastic bags for a few days in the refrigerator. The seeds are stored in airtight porcelain-, glass- or suitable metal containers, protected from light and moisture. The dried seeds have a long shelf life.

Description. Whole seed (Fig. 1): For the morphology of the leaves, see description of the whole plant. The seeds are very hard, flattened, yellowish-brown to reddish-brown, more or less rhomboidal with rounded edges, about 3 to 5 mm long and 1.5 to 2 mm thick. The larger side shows a diagonal groove, which divides the seeds into two unequal parts.

Powdered seed: The seed powder is yellowish-brown, and the chloral hydrate slide preparation shows the characteristic fragments of the epidermal layer and the hypodermal stratum. The lumen of the palisade-like epidermal cells is bottle-shaped; view from the top reveals the "bottlenecks" as finely punctate cells. The cells of the hypodermal stratum have radially arranged thickenings, which, when viewed from the top, resemble stone cells (Fig. 3). Furthermore, mucilage cells of the endosperm, among others, are present. Starch, fibers and oxalate crystals must be absent [Ü49].

Odor: The seeds have a strongly aromatic and characteristic odor reminiscent of celery or lovage. The spicy odor of the leaves becomes stronger during drying, **Taste:** The seeds are mucilaginous when chewed, and faintly bitter. The leaves taste somewhat pungent and slightly bitter.

History: Fenugreek is one of the oldest medicinal- and cultivated plants. In India, the Near East and Egypt, it has been cultivated for millennia. A government decree by Karl the Great ("Capitulare de villis", authored in about 795 CE), which regulated agricultural practices, called for the cultivation of fenugreek (see footnote, → Anise) [Ü61].

4,5-Dimethyl-3-hydroxy-2(5H)-furanone (sotolone)

4-Methyl-3-hydroxy-2(5H)-furanone

Trigonelline

Trigofoenoside A

Constituents and Analysis

DIN- and ISO-Standards: ISO-Standard 6575 (Fenugreek).

Constituents of the seeds

- Essential oil: 0.01 to 0.02%, containing 3-hydroxy-4,5-dimethyl-2(5H)-furanone (sotolone) and 3-hydroxy-4-methyl-2(5H)-furanone, among others (both responsible for the characteristic odor). Furthermore, the steam distillate contains, among others, dihydroactinidindiolide, dihydrobenzofuran and n-hexanol. β-Elemene and ε-muurolene, among others, as well as aliphatic hydrocarbons have been detected in headspace analyses [11, 18, 19, Ü83].
- Trigonelline (coffearine, *N*-methylbetaine of nicotinic acid): 0.2 to 0.4% [29].
- Saponins: 1.2 to 3%; in the intact, ripe seeds 3,26-bisglycosides with Δ^4-furostene-, Δ^5-furostene- or 5α-furostane skeletons; they taste bitter and include, among others, trigofoenosides A to G, which, after hydrolytic cleavage of their glucose moiety at C-26, convert to spirostanol glycosides of which 12 aglycones are known; mainly diosgenin (about 10%), yamogenin (16%, the mixture is also known as trigonellagenin) and gitogenin (12%) [19, 21, 27, 52]. In fenugreek of Indian origin, trigofoenoside A and glycoside D, as well as trigoneosides Ia, IIa, IIb, IIIa, IIIb, IVa, Va, Vb, VI, VIIb, VIIIb and IX have been isolated [60]; in material of Egyptian origin, glycoside D, trigonelloside C, compound C and the trigoneosides Ia, Ib, Va, Xa, Xb, XIb, XIIa, XIIb, and XIIIa were detected [34, 59].
- Peptide esters of diosgenin: Foenugraecine [17, 59].
- Flavonoids: Particularly glycosyl flavones such as vitexin, isovitexin, vicenin-1, vicenin-2, orientin- und isoorientin as well as saponaretin [4, 55].
- Isoflavonoids: 0.3% rotenoids (in the fruits) [24].
- Mucilage: 20 to 45%, β-(1→4)-mannans, substituted with α-(1→6) galactosyl moieties [13, 14, 16].
- Lipids: 6 to 10%, triacylglycerols, phospholipids and glycolipids [22].
- Sterols: The main components are β-sitosterol and cholesterol [8].
- Proteins: 23 to 30% (rich in L-lysine and L-tryptophan) [16].
- Proteinase inhibitors: Bowman-Birk protease inhibitors, which are polypeptides inhibiting trypsin and chymotrypsin [57, 58].

Constituents of the leaves

- Saponins: Steroid glycosides, with diosgenin as aglycone, such as graecunins A, B, C, D, E, F and G [54].
- Flavonoids: Kaempferol- and quercetin-3-*O*- and 3,7-*O*-glycosides [54].
- Isoflavonoids: Formononetin and rotenoids [24, 54].
- Coumarin derivatives: Trigoforin (3,4,7-trimethylcoumarin), 4-methyl-7-acetoxycoumarin and scopoletin [54, 56].
- Lignans: γ-Schisandrin [56].

Tests for Identity: Macroscopic and microscopic examinations as well as TLC analysis, according to Ph Eur.

Quantitative assay: TLC of the sapogenins [15] or GC of its trifluoracetyl derivatives [27]. Evaluation of the mucilage content based on the swelling index [Ph Eur].

Adulterations, Misidentifications and Impurities have not been observed.

Actions and Uses

Actions: On the basis of its aromatic, slightly bitter taste, fenugreek has appetizing and digestion promoting effects. With ingestion of large amounts of the crushed seeds, e.g. as a roborant, digestive disturbances are conceivable due to its content of proteinase inhibitors. Whether the proteinase inhibitors are destroyed upon cooking, or not, has yet to be investigated. As an appetite stimulant, administration in rats of a protein-free and defatted fenugreek seed extract (containing 12.5% steroidal saponins and 0.002% 4,5-dimethyl-3-hydroxy-2(5H)-furanone; 10 or 100 mg/300 g body weight per day, mixed in feed for 14 days) caused a 20% increase in food consumption [35]. Isolated saponins (12.5 mg/300 g body weight) had the same effect [38]. Administration of fenugreek seed powder in rats (50 or 200 mg per animal, orally) increased bile flow by about 29% and 35%, respectively [9]. Fenugreek seed has anti-ulcerogenic activity. With the administration of aqueous extracts in rats, healing of gastric ulcers was enhanced [33].

In animal experiments [1, 6, 7, 26, 30, 40, 41, 53] and in humans [23, 31, 32, 42, 44, 47, 48], administration of fenugreek seeds lowered blood-glucose levels. As one example, non-insulin-dependent diabetics lowered their blood-glucose levels by 25% with the addition of 15 g fenugreek seed powder to meals [31], and insulin-dependent diabetics lowered their blood-glucose levels by 20% by taking 50 g of fenugreek seed powder, twice daily [42]. Similar to other mucilage-containing herbs, fenugreek increases the viscosity of the intestinal contents, and consequently it retards absorption by reducing the diffusion speed of food components. Thereby, the occurrence of glucose concentration peaks in the blood is prevented following the ingestion of food. In this regard, the mucilage-rich endosperm fraction of the seed is the most active part. The proteins and saponins do not contribute to this activity. Ethanolic extracts (mucilage-free) have no effect [1, 7, 31, 40].

In animal tests [9, 41, 43, 49, 51, 53] and in humans [12, 44–46, 48], fenugreek seeds lowered both the lipid- and cholesterol levels in the blood. Isolated saponins (12.5 mg/300 g body weight/day, orally) also lowered the blood cholesterol level in rats [38]. It is probably the saponins, through a complex formation with cholesterol, that inhibit its absorption, and through their interactions with bile salts inhibit the reabsorption [51]. At a daily dosage of 50 g powdered fenugreek, twice daily, diabetic and hyperlipidemic nondiabetic subjects attained an approximate 25% reduction of total serum cholesterol after 10 to 20 days. The LDL- and VLDL- levels were lowered by about 30% and the triglyceride level dropped 18 and 38%, respectively, while the HDL level remained unchanged [45, 46].

In diabetic rats, by comparison to normal rats, supplementation with fenugreek seeds in the diet lowered elevated lipid peroxidation in the blood, and there was an increase in the concentration of circulating antioxidants in the blood [39].

In rats, the addition of 3% glycolic acid to the diet produced oxalate urolithiasis, with concomitant administration of fenugreek seeds (500 mg/kg body weight, for 4 weeks) reduced the quantity of calcium oxalate deposited in the kidneys [5].

Saponins from fenugreek and foenugraecine have antiphlogistic activity [10, 17].

Toxicology: Based on existing data, there is no acute or chronic toxicity with the regular use of fenugreek seed or herb as a spice [2, 35].

The sensitization potential is small. However, there are two literature cases of serious allergic reactions caused by inhalation of fenugreek seed powder or after external application of a mucilaginous fenugreek seed preparation for dandruff [36]. Administration of a crude fenugreek saponin extract to male rats (saponin content 0.6%, 100 mg/animal per day, for 60 days) led to sterility of the test animals [25].

Culinary use: Fenugreek seeds are especially enjoyed in India, Sri Lanka, northeastern Africa, China and southern Europe, and to a lesser extent in the USA. In India, fenugreek is a component of curry dishes and chutneys. In Egypt and Ethiopia, it is used as a spice for fish- and meat dishes, but also for stews and vegetable dishes. In northern Africa, porridge-like meals are spiced with powdered fenugreek seed. In Russia, it serves as a component in baked goods and in onion-, potato-, and mushroom soups.

In Iran, the fresh leaves are a component of herb stews or, dried, of spice mixes for meat. In Egypt and India, in particular, the fresh leaves are enjoyed as a vegetable or they are cooked together with spinach and other green vegetables, or with starch-containing tuberous vegetables (e.g. potatoes, yams). The roasted, crushed seeds are used in some countries (Turkey, India, China, Arabian countries) as a coffee substitute or coffee admix and also as a component of oriental types of halva (see: → Sesame).

Fenugreek seeds are used in whole, ground or crushed forms. Often, they are very briefly (!) roasted (dry, without fat) in order to reduce their bitterness. The very hard seeds can be soaked in water overnight in order to make them easier to crush. The powder should be used sparingly because they have a strong spice impact. The whole seeds are used to spice roast lamb, roast beef and roast pork, and also to sprinkle on breads, cookies or biscuits [Ü13, Ü17, Ü71, Ü98].

Fenugreek seed powder adds a special character to fish soups, gourd vegetables, onion vegetables, eggplant, potatoes, meat loaf and flat breads [Ü71]. In the alpine countries, it is used as a spice in herb cheeses [Ü92]. It also serves as an ingredient for pickling of vegetables in vinegar and for sprinkling over roasted dishes or fish dishes [Ü55, Ü68].

A meal can be prepared by cooking the soaked seeds together with lentils [Ü55].

Fresh or dried leaves are especially suited for seasoning in onion soups, omclets and herb sauces [Ü55, Ü71, Ü74, Ü98].

Fresh, young, tender leaves can be mixed in with salads. The slightly bitter-tasting sprouts are a vitamin-rich addition to soups, salads or omelets, and they complement sandwiches made with tomatoes or cheese [Ü13, Ü17, Ü55, Ü68, Ü96].

Fenugreek extract is also used as a flavor component in mango chutney and artificial maple syrup [Ü68].

As a component of spice mixes and preparations: → Chemen, → Curry powder, → Panch phoron, → Sambhar powder.

Other uses: The powdered seed is used by the fellah class (in Arab countries) together with corn meal (1:2) as bread flour. It also serves as an aromatic component mixed with tobacco. The seeds can be used as a source material for obtaining diosgenin, which is of value as the raw material for semi-synthesis of steroid hormones.

Medicinal herb

Herbal drug: Trigonellae foenugraeci semen, Fenugreek, the swelling index is not less than 6 [Ph Eur].

Indications: Internally for loss of appetite (daily dose of 6 g crushed dried seed or in galenical preparations), and externally as a poultice for local inflammations (cook 50 g in 250 ml water for 5 minutes and apply as a warm poultice) [28].

In folk medicine, it is taken orally as mucilage for catarrh of the upper respiratory tract, for promotion of milk production in mammary glands, for lowering the blood-glucose level in diabetics, as well as taken by the tablespoonful several times daily, as a roborant [Ü106].

In Arabian folk medicine, fenugreek seed diet is used for preventing kidney stones [5].

Similar spice herbs

Sweet trefoil (blue fenugreek), *Trigonella caerulea* (L.) SER. var. *caerulea* (Synonym: *T. melilotus-caerulea* (L.) A. et GR., Fabaceae), occurs in the wild in the Caucasia region and in the Crimea (possibly as an escape from cultivation), and is cultivated in Alpine countries and northern Africa. The dried, powdered herb is a component of green herb cheeses (whey-cheese, Schabziger) and serves as a bread spice (South Tyrolean Vintschgerl). The seeds are also used as a condiment [Ü61, Ü98].

Kasuri methi, *Trigonella corniculata* (L.) L. (Fabaceae), is native to the Mediterranean region and western Asia, and cultivated in India, where the seeds and herb are used as a spice and cooked as a vegetable [Ü61].

Literature

[1] Abdel-Barry J.A. et al., J. Ethnopharmacol. 58(3):149–155 (1997).

[2] Abdel-Barry J.A., M.H. Al-Hakiem, J. Ethnopharmacol. 70(1):65–68 (2000).

[3] Abdo M.S., A.A. Al-Kafawi, Planta Med. 17(1):14 (1969).

[4] Adamska M., J. Lutomski, Planta Med. 20:224–229 (1971).

[5] Ahsan S.K. et al., J. Ethnopharmacol. 26:249–254 (1989).

[6] Ajabnoor M.A., A.K. Tilmisany, J. Ethnopharmacol. 22:45–49 (1988).

[7] Ali L. et al., Planta Med. 61(4):358–360 (1995).

[8] Artaud J. et al., Rev. Fr. Corps Gras 35:435–440 (1988).

[9] Bhat B.G. et al., Nutr. Rep. Int. 32:1145 (1985).

[10] Bhattacharya S.K. et al., Rheumatism 6:1 (1971).

[11] Blank I. et al., ACS Symp. Ser. 1997, 660 (Spices):12–28 (1997).

[12] Bordia A. et al., Prostaglandines, Leukotrienes, Essent. Fatty Acids 56(5):379–384 (1997).

[13] Chatterjee B.P. et al., Carbohydrat Res. 104:348–353 (1982).

[14] Clermont S. et al., Phytochemistry 21: 1951–1954 (1982).

[15] Dawidar A.M., M.B.E. Fayez, Z. Anal. Chemie 259(4):283 (1972).

[16] Elmafda I., Nahrung 19:683–686 (1975).

[17] Ghosal S. et al., Phytochemistry 13:2247–2251 (1974).

[18] Girardon P. et al., Planta Med. 51:533–534 (1985).

[19] Girardon P. et al., Lebensm. Wiss. Technol. 19:44–46 (1986).

[20] Gupta R.K. et al., Phytochemistry 25: 2205–2207 (1986).

[21] Gupta R.K. et al., Phytochemistry 24: 2399 (1986).

[22] Hemavathy J., J.V. Prabhakar, Food Chem. 31:1–7 (1989).

[23] Hillaire-Buys D. et al., Diabetologia 36 (Suppl. 1):A119 (1993).

[24] Kamal R. et al., J. Med. Aromat. Plant Sci. 19(4):988–993 (1998).

[25] Kamal R. et al., Phytother. Res. 7:134 (1993).

[26] Khosla P. et al., Indian J. Physiol Pharmacol. 39(2):173–174 (1995).

[27] Knight J.C., J. Chromatogr. 133:222–225 (1977).

[28] Kommission E beim BfArM, BAnz-Nr. 22a vom 01.02.1990.

[29] Kuhn A., H. Gerhard, Arch. Pharmaz. 281:378–379 (1943).

[30] Madar Z., Nutr. Rep. Int. 29:1267–1272 (1984).

[31] Madar Z. et al., Eur. J. Clin. Nutr. 42: 51–54 (1988).

[32] Madar Z., J. Arad, Nutr. Res. 9:691 (1989).

[33] Meshal I.A. et al., Fitoterapia 56:236 (1985).

[34] Murakami T. et al., Chem. Pharm. Bull. 48(7):994–1000 (2000).

[35] Muralidhara et al., Food Chem. Toxical. 37(8):831–838 (1999).

[36] Patil S.P. et al., Ann. Allergy Asthmam. Immunol. 78(3):297–300 (1997).

[37] Petit P. et al., Pharmacol. Biochem. Behav. 45(2):369–374 (1993).

[38] Petit P.R. et al., Steroids 60(10):674–680 (1995).

[39] Ravikumar P., C.V. Anuradha, Phytother. Res. 13(3):197–201 (1999).

[40] Ribes G. et al., Proc. Soc. Exp. Biol. Med. 182:159–166 (1986).

[41] Riyad M.A. et al., Planta Med. 54:286–290 (1988).

[42] Sharma R.D., Nutr. Res. 6:1353–1364 (1986).

[43] Sharma R.D., Nutr. Rep. Int. 33:669–677 (1986).

[44] Sharma R.D. et al., Eur. Clin. Nutr. 44(4):301–306 (1990).

[45] Sharma R.D. et al., Phytother. Res. 5:145 (1991).

[46] Sharma R.D. et al., Eur. J. Clin. Nutr. 44(4):301–306 (1990).

[47] Sharma R.D. et al., Phytotherapy Res. 10:332–334 (1996).

[48] Sharma R.D., T.C. Raghuram, Nutr. Res. 10:731–739 (1990).

[49] Singhal P.C. et al., Current Sci. 51(3):136 (1982).

[50] Sinskaja E.N., Kulturnaja Flora SSSR 13(1), Moskva, Leningrad: 503–516 (1950).

[51] Stark A., Z. Madar, Br. J. Nutr. 69(1): 277–287 (1993).

[52] Taylor W. et al., J. Agric. Food Chem. 45(3):753–759 (1996).

[53] Valette G. et al., Atherosclerosis 50:105–111 (1984).

[54] Varshney I.P. et al., J. Nat. Prod. 47:44–46 (1984).

[55] Wagner H. et al., Phytochemistry 12:2548 (1973).

[56] Wang D. et al., Chung Kuo Chung Yao Tsa Chih 22(8):486–487 (1997), ref.: Medline.

[57] Weder J.K., K. Haußner, Z. Lebensm. Untersuch. Forsch. 193(4):242–246 und 321 (1991).

[58] Weder J.K.P., K. Haußner, Z. Lebensm. Untersuch. Forsch. 192:455–459 und 535–540 (1991).

[59] Yoshikava M. et al., Heterocycles 47(1): 397–405 (1998).

[60] Yoshikawa M. et al., Chem. Pharm. Bull. 45(1):81–87 (1997).

Literature references identified by Ü can be found in the general listing of books and monographs at the back of this book.

Garden cress

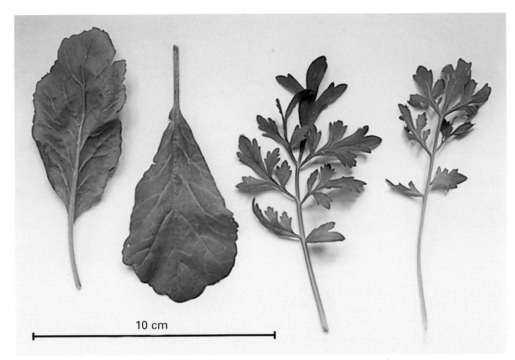

Fig. 1: Garden cress leaf, single basal leaves, pinnately dissect leaves of the stem.

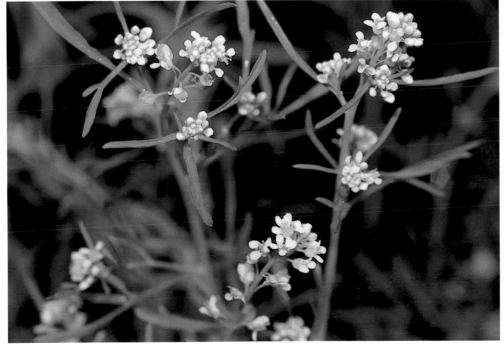

Fig. 2: Garden cress (*Lepidium sativum* L. ssp. *sativum*)

Plant source: *Lepidium sativum* L. ssp. *sativum*.

Synonym: *Lepidium hortense* FORSSK.

Taxonomic classification: Aside from the wild form, *L. s.* ssp. *spinescens* (DC.) THELL., there are numerous cultivated relatives with different leaf-shapes and seed colors.

Family: Mustard family (Brassicaceae, synonym Cruciferae).

Common names: Engl.: garden cress, pepperwort; Fr.: cresson alénois, cressonette, nasitort; Ger.: Gartenkresse, Gresich, Pfefferkraut, Tellerkresse.

Description: Annual herb, stalks up to 50 cm tall, mostly branched in the upper part, bluish pruinose. Leaves short petiolate, the lower ones are pinnatipartite, the upper ones undivided, lineal, glabrous, sometimes grayish pruinose (there are other cultivars with split, smooth or curly leaves, which have broad single basal leaves). The flowers are arranged in terminal- and axillary racemes and have 4 sepals, 4 petals, white or reddish, indistinctly unguiculate, 2 short and 4 long stamina, anthers often purple, superior ovary. The fruit is a 5 to 6 mm long, 3 to 4 mm wide, roundish-ovoid silicule, broadly winged towards the top, containing nearly smooth, reddish-brown, ovate seeds. Flowering period is from May to July [11, Ü37].

Native origin: Northeastern Africa, Egypt, the Near East, and naturalized in Europe.

Main cultivation areas: Cultivated almost exclusively as a garden plant in temperate to warm-temperate zones, for example in Europe, Northern Africa, Ethiopia, the Near East, Transcaucasia, India, China, Japan, and North America.

Main exporting countries: Only traded locally.

Cultivation: The plant prefers humus, loosely packed, slightly damp soil in sunny or partially shaded locations. The seeds germinate within two days and grow very quickly. Therefore, in order to have a constant supply of fresh, young leaves, they should be planted from March to September in intervals of 14 days in row widths of about 10 cm. Keep in mind that plants sown in high summer will have a low leaf yield because they flower more rapidly. In the winter months, garden cress can be grown without a problem in the windowsill in soil, sand or on a sieve in hydroponics, or to obtain sprouts, they can be grown on damp cellulose or baking paper. Cultivated varieties include, among others, 'Glattblättrige', 'Extra Krause', 'Großblättrige Neuheit' and 'Einfache' (the latter is especially suitable for growing indoors) [10, Ü33, Ü96].

Culinary herb

Commercial forms: Sprouted seeds in a damp substrate, the plant tops, and rarely the fresh leaves.

Production: A harvest is already possible 12 to 20 days after planting, as long as the plants are about 5 to 7 cm tall [Ü96].

Forms used: Fresh, young leaves, and sprouted seeds.

Storage: This herb must be used fresh; preservation is not recommended.

Description. Whole herb (Fig. 1): Fresh leaves: See description of the plant.

Odor: Spicy, **Taste:** Pungent and bitter-sweet when chewed.

History: It was already cultivated in Rome and Greece during antiquity; the Romans introduced it to extramediterranean parts of Europe [Ü61].

Constituents and Analysis

Constituents

- Glucosinolates: In the fresh leaves, 0.1 to 0.2% (about 0.6% with reference to the dried herb), the main components are glucotropaeolin, small amounts of gluconasturtiin and other glucosinolates (See → Garden nasturtium, Fig.). Due to the presence of myrosinase and other enzymes, which further convert the mustard oils (alkyl- and alkarylisothiocyanates, see → General Chapter 2, Fig. 12), decomposition products of glucotropaeolin are formed after tissue damage, that are, besides small amounts of benzylisothiocyanate, particularly phenylacetonitrile (benzyl cyanide, about 50%), and in the germinated seeds benzylthiocyanate. Other cleavage products include, among others, hex-5-enonitrile, pent-4-enonitrile, pent-4-enylisothiocyanate, but-3-enylisothiocyanate, 3-phenylpropionitrile, 2-phenylethylthiocyanate, 2-phenylethanol, benzaldehyde and benzylalcohol. Odor and taste are largely determined by the isothiocyanates [3–6, 8, 9].
- Vitamin C: 40 to 60 mg/100 g (calculated with reference to the fresh drug) [Ü98].
- Hydroxycinnamic acid esters: Such as quinic acid, among others.

Tests for Identity: Tests can be carried out with sensory and macroscopic analysis, as well as by detection of the glucosinolates and desulfoglucosinolates with TLC or HPLC [for literature see → Watercress].

Quantitative assay: The glucosinolate content can be determined with RP-HPLC [for literature see → Watercress].

Adulterations, Misidentifications and Impurities can be excluded since the leaves originate exclusively from cultivated sources.

Actions and Uses

Actions: Due to its pungent taste, it has appetite stimulating and digestion promoting action.
Fresh garden cress is a urinary antiseptic. The volatile components of urine from test subjects, who consumed 50 g of garden cress salad, inhibited the growth of *Bacillus subtilis*, *Escherichia coli* and *Staphylococcus aureus* [12]. Likewise, benzyl mustard oil has good antibacterial activity even in very weak dilutions. Antiviral properties have also been observed in mice [7].

Benzylisothiocyanate

Benzylthiocyanate

Phenylacetonitrile

3-Phenylpropionitrile

Pent-4-enylisothyocyanate

Hex-5-enonitrile

But-3-enylisothyocyanate

Pent-4-enonitrile

Toxicology: Based on existing data, there is no acute or chronic toxicity with the regular use of the leaves as a salad or as a salad ingredient. Inhibition of iodine-accumulation in the thyroid gland and the occurrence of goiter (due to iodine deficiency) caused by the rhodanides, which are present as enzymatic decomposition products in all glucosinolate containing plants, occurs only with chronic consumption of very high amounts; such high amounts cannot be reached by normal consumption of the leaves [Ü100]. Due to the irritating effects of mustard oils, this herb should not be consumed by patients with stomach and intestinal ulcers and by children under the age of four.

Culinary use: Under no circumstances should garden cress be heated. Also, due to the high volatility of its mustard oil, chopping the leaves leads to loss of aroma. Washing the leaves should be kept to a minimum, unless absolutely necessary.

The fresh, young leaves are used as a spice and garnish for pan-fried meats, quark, fresh cheese, herb mayonnaise, dips, remoulade, chutneys, sauces (cress sauce, e.g. for chicken, turkey, fish), potato salad, clear soups, cold cream sauces, egg dishes and salads (tomato salad, egg salad, mixed salads) as well as side dishes for soups and cold plates. Garden cress is also very well suited as a salad, for preparation of herb butter or to sprinkle on sandwiches [Ü1, Ü13, Ü30, Ü45, Ü46, Ü55, Ü56, Ü79].

The sprouted seeds are used as a garnish or they are eaten fresh [Ü55].

Garden cress is mostly used solo and rarely in combination with other spring herbs.

Other uses: In Ethiopia, the seeds are used to produce edible oil [Ü61].

Medicinal herb

Herbal drug: Lepidii sativi herba, Garden cress herb (obsolete).

Indications: Formerly used as an antiscurvy remedy, as a "blood purifier", as an expectorant and for urinary tract infections, among other uses. The medicinal use of garden cress is no longer practiced. In Northern Africa, it has also been used for gonorrhea [Ü37].

Similar glucosinolate-containing herbs used in salads

Common winter cress (Brown water cress is also designated as winter cress, see → Watercress): *Barbarea vulgaris* R. BR. ssp. *vulgaris* (Brassicaceae, Engl.: common winter cress, yellow rocket, bitter cress; Fr.: herbe de Sainte Barbe; Ger.: Barbarakraut), native to Europe, Northern Africa, Asia, and naturalized in North America and New Zealand. Important constituents include its glucosinolates, of which the main components are gluconasturtiin (2-phenylethylglucosinolate), (*2R*)- and (*2S*)-glucobarbarine (1-hydroxy-2-phenyl-ethylglucosinolate), and following enzymatic cleavage, 2-phenylethylisothiocyanate, 3-phenylpropionitrile and 1-hydroxy-2-phenylethylisothiocyanate are formed. The leaves are used as a salad or as salad ingredients [13, Ü98].

Land cress (American cress, *B. verna* (MILL.) ASCHERS.), only very rarely cultivated in gardens in Europe, e.g. in France and England, and in North America, is used in the same way as common winter cress.

Common scurvy grass, *Cochlearia officinalis* L. (Brassicaceae, Engl.: scurvy grass, spoonwort; Fr. cranson; Ger.: Löffelkraut, Löffelkresse), is native to the Atlantic coasts, the North Sea and the Baltic Sea and, today, is also cultivated, but only on a small scale. Its important constituents are the glucosinolates, of which the main component is glucocochlearine (converting to butyl mustard oil = butylisothiocyanate, after enzymatic cleavage) [2], as well as numerous tropane alkaloids including, among others, cochlearine (3α-3-hydroxybenzoyl)-tropine) [1], and vitamin C (80 to 200 mg/100 g). Scurvy grass was formerly used as an important anti-scurvy remedy by sailors. Today, especially in the Nordic countries, is serves as a spice for herb butter, herb cheese and bread spreads. It is used raw as a salad herb and cooked as a vegetable. In Germany, scurvy grass is a protected endangered plant. In England, English scurvy grass (*C. anglica* L.) is also cultivated, and it is used as a salad side dish [Ü92, Ü98]. See also → Black mustard, → Garden nasturtium, → Hoary cress, → Persian mustard, → Sarepta mustard, → Watercress, → White mustard.

Literature

[1] Bachmann P. et al., 45th Ann. Congr. Soc. Med. Plant Res. (Abstracts) C03 (1997).

[2] Cole R.A., Phytochemistry 15:759–762 (1976).

[3] Gil V., A.J. MacLeod, Phytochemistry 19:1365–1368, 1369–1374, 2071–2076 (1980).

[4] Gmelin R., A.I. Virtanen, Acta chem. Scand. 13:1474–1475 (1959).

[5] Hasapis X., A.J. Mac Leod, Phytochemistry 21:291–296, 1009–1013 (1982).

[6] Hrncirik K., J. Velisek, Potravin Vedy 15(3):161–172 (1997).

[7] Klesse P., P. Lukoschek, Arzneim. Forsch. 5:505–507 (1955).

[8] MacLeod A.J., R. Islam, J. Sci. Food Agric. 27:909–212 (1976).

[9] Saaivirta M., Planta Med. 24:112–119 (1973).

[10] Schmidt L., Drogenreport 6(9):39–40 (1993).

[11] Weymar H., Buch der Kreuzblütler, Neumann Verlag, Leipzig-Radebeul 1988.

[12] Winter A.G., L. Willeke, Naturwissenschaften 40:167–168 (1953).

[13] Zrybko C. et al., J. Chromatogr. A767 (1/2):43–52 (1997).

Literature references identified by Ü can be found in the general listing of books and monographs at the back of this book.

Garden nasturtium

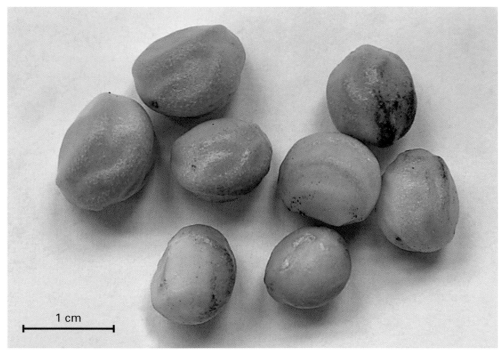

Fig. 1: Garden nasturtium, unripe fruits

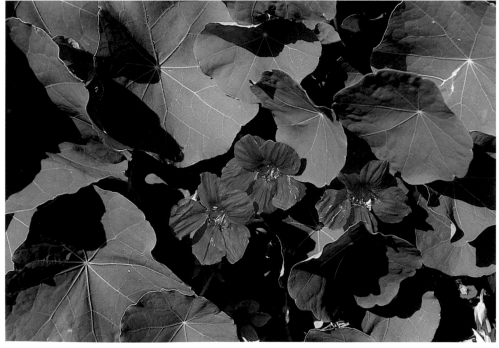

Fig. 2: Garden nasturtium (*Tropaeolum majus* L.)

Plant source: *Tropaeolum majus* L.

Taxonomic classification: The species can be subdivided into the climbing form, *Tropaeolum majus* L. var. *altum* Voss, and the bush form, *Tropaeolum majus* L. var. *nanum* Voss.

Family: Nasturtium family (Tropaeolaceae).

Common names: Engl.: garden nasturtium, nasturtium; Fr.: capucine grande, cresse du Pérou; Ger.: Kapuzinerkresse, Große Blumenkresse, Salatkresse, Salatblume, Großindische Kresse.

Description: Perennial, frost sensitive in Central Europe and therefore only cultivated as an annual in those regions; herbaceous, with underground stolons, bushy, 25 to 30 cm high, or creeping or climbing, respectively, tendrils up to 3 m long. Leaves dark green, glabrous, shield-like, 3 to 5 cm wide and long, with eccentrically arranged petioles. The dorsiventral flowers emerge from the leaf axils, having 5 sepals, 2 of them forming a lower lip and the other 3 fused as an upper lip, extending into a 3 cm long, bent spur, 5 petals, free, yellow to red, alternating with the sepals, 8 stamina, superior ovary, dehiscent, 3-partite fruit; individual fruits wrinkled, able to float in water. Flowering period is from July until the first frost [Ü37].

Native origin: Warmer regions of South America, especially Ecuador, Peru, Colombia, and grows wild in many subtropical and tropical areas.

Main cultivation areas: There is no cultivation for commercial purposes.

Cultivation: The plant prefers moderately nutrient-rich, loamy-sand soil in sunny to half-shade locations. It does not tolerate temperatures below 4 °C. In soil with high nitrogen content and with not enough sun, the plant will favor the production of more foliage and less flowering. In April cultivation, 3 to 4 mericarps per pot can be started indoors at 18 °C. In mid-May, they can be transplanted outdoors at 20 cm lines × 25 cm apart. After mid-May, it is also possible to plant by direct seeding. They can also be grown in pots or window boxes [Ü33, Ü96].

Culinary herb

Commercial forms: Not commercially traded.

Production: The shoot tips, leaves or flowers can be freshly picked any time. The fruits can be harvested any time as long as they are still green.

Forms used: Fresh leaves, shoots, flowers, flower buds and unripe fruits.

Storage: Leaves, shoot tips, flowers and flower buds should be consumed fresh; flower buds and unripe fruits pickled in vinegar have a shelf-life of about 6 months.

Description. Whole unripe fruits (Fig. 1): For leaves and fruits, see description of the whole plant; the flower buds are light green, 8 to 22 mm long, with a spurred calyx.

Odor: Acrid when crushed, **Taste:** Pungent when chewed.

History: In Peru and Bolivia, garden nasturtium was already used in pre-Columbian times as a spice and salad ingredient. In 1682, it was introduced from Peru to Central Europe by the Spaniards, where it was first cultivated in cloister gardens [21, Ü92].

Constituents and Analysis

Constituents

- Glucosinolates: About 0.1% (with reference to the fresh herb), in the seeds about 1%, with the main component glucotropaeolin (benzyl glucosinolate), in addition to 4-hydroxy- and 4-methoxybenzyl glucosinolate. Catalyzed by the enzyme myrosinase, which is stored in myrosine cells, mustard oils are formed by cleavage of the glucosinolates after tissue damage (Fig. 12, General Section). Glucotropaeolin is cleaved to benzyl mustard oil (benzylisothiocyanate, pungent taste, volatile) [8].
- Vitamin C: 300 to 320 mg/100 g (calculated with reference to the fresh leaves), and in the flowers, about 130 mg/100 g [17].
- Flavonoids: The main component is quercetin triglucoside [4].
- Caffeic acid derivatives: Chlorogenic acid, among others [4].
- Cucurbitacins: In the unripe fruits, cucurbitacin B, D and E [20].
- Xyloglucans (amyloids): Serving as energy storage of the seeds instead of starch [2, 7].
- Carotenoids, particularly in the flowers lutein and zeaxanthin [7].

Tests for Identity: Sensoric and macroscopic analysis. For the analysis of the glucosinolates, and the tests for identity with chemical or physico-chemical methods, see → Watercress.

Quantitative assay with RP-HPLC of the glucosinolates directly [1, 16] or in the form of desulfoglucosinolates with HPLC and GLC [9].

Actions and Uses

Actions: Due to the pungent taste, garden nasturtium has appetizing and digestion promoting action. The high antimicrobial activity (inhibitory concentration ca. 30 µg/ml) is dependent on the content of benzyl mustard oil in the chopped fresh plant (ca. 30 mg/100 mg, with reference to the fresh weight) [3, 5, 6, 10, 13, 18, 19]. Garden nasturtium has a urinary disinfectant action following oral ingestion, due to its content of benzyl mustard oil. This compound absorbs well and is excreted in the urine predominantly in the form of the metabolite N-acetyl-S-(N-benzylthiocarbamoyl)-L-cysteine that breaks down to N-acetyl-L-cysteine and benzyl mustard oil at pH 5 [15]. The exhalation of free benzyl mustard oil following oral ingestion has also been postulated [11]. The therapeutic use of benzyl mustard oil is not approved due to the lack of clinical studies to support efficacy [11].

Toxicology: Based on existing data, there is no chronic or acute toxicity in healthy individuals with the normal use of garden nasturtium as a spice or salad ingredient. Due to the skin and mucous membrane irritating effects of benzyl mustard oil, irritation of the kidneys can occur in patients with preexisting kidney disease. In case of overdose, albuminuria can occur also in healthy individuals, possibly due to damage of the glomeruli and tubuli. After the intake of large amounts, gastrointestinal disturbances are also possible [12].
The occurrence of an urticaria-like exanthema after the intake of garden nasturtium has been observed. Plant parts or benzyl mustard oil have the potential for contact allergenic activity [11, 12, 14, Ü39].

Culinary use: The young, freshly plucked leaves and shoots, and rarely the flowers, serve as salad side dishes, e.g. of cucumber

Glucotropaeolin   Benzyl mustard oil

salad. The leaves are also eaten alone as a salad. Due to the strong mucous membrane irritating benzyl mustard oil, not more than 15 g per meal and not more than 30 g per day should be eaten.

The young leaves picked to pieces are also used as a component of fillings for meat- and fish dishes as well as to spice soljanka, cream-, vegetable-, fish- and poultry soups, mushroom rice, scrambled eggs, omelets, quark, cream cheese as well as from mustard sauces and vinaigrettes to artichokes. Due to the volatility of the aromatic compound benzyl mustard oil, garden nasturtium should be added only shortly before completion of the dish. They can also be used to sprinkle on sandwiches and on cooked potatoes or mixed under risotto [Ü13, Ü55, Ü66, Ü74, Ü98, Ü107].

Stirring them into homemade strawberry-, peach-, apricot- and sour cherry marmalades immediately before bottling is recommended [Ü71].

The flower buds and unripe fruits are pickled in vinegar, similar to → Capers. They are soaked in salt water for 24 hours, strained, and then cooked with wine vinegar.

The flowers can be used alone or together with some white pepper corns for the preparation of herb vinegar, which takes on a striking orange tone. They are also suitable for the preparation of nasturtium butter (30 g chopped flowers mixed with 90 g soft butter and lemon juice to taste) [Ü47, Ü74]. The use of candied flowers as cake decorations has also been described [Ü108].

Combines well with: Chives, parsley, table mustard, and tarragon.

As a component of spice mixes and preparations: → Herb vinegar.

Medicinal herb

Herbal drug: Tropaeolum-majus fresh plant, essential oil of the fresh plant, obtained by steam distillation of the crushed, fermented plant material.

Indications: Taken internally as supportive treatment of urinary tract infections, catarrhs of the respiratory tract as well as externally for mild muscle pains. It is used in the form of preparations, e.g. fresh pressed plant juice, for which the daily dose corresponds to about 3×15 mg benzyl mustard oil. It should not be used in cases of stomach- or intestinal ulcers as well as bladder diseases, and should also not be dispensed to infants or toddlers [12].

Garden Nasturtium Drink à la Lechthaler

3 to 4 twigs of garden nasturtium (flowers and leaves), 140 ml milk, 3 teaspoons of natural yogurt, 10 ml mango syrup.

Mix the ingredients with 2 ice cubes in a blender and pour the mixture into a cold glass. For decoration, place a nasturtium flower on top of the drink [Ü57].

Literature

[1] Björnquist B., A. Hase, J. Chromatogr. 435:501–507 (1988).
[2] Courtois J.E. et al., Carbohydr. Res. 49: 439–449 (1976).
[3] Dannenberg H. et al., Hoppe-Seylers Z. Physiol. Chem. 303:248–256 (1956).
[4] Delaveau P., Physiol. Veg. 5:357–390 (1967).
[5] Ebbinghaus K.D., Med. Welt 1327–1329 (1962).
[6] Ebbinghaus K.D., Med. Welt 58–61 (1966).
[7] Franz G., Z. Phytother. 17(4):255–622 (1996).
[8] Gadamer J., Arch. Pharmaz. 237: 111–120 (1899).
[9] Hrncirik K. et al., Z. Lebensm. Unters. Forsch. A 206:103–107 (1997).
[10] Kienholz M. et al., Zbl. Bakt., I. Abt., Orig. 167:610–614 (1957).
[11] Kommission B6 beim BfArM., BAnz.-Nr. 52 vom 17.02.1993.
[12] Kommission E beim BfArM., BAnz-Nr. 162 vom 29.08.92
[13] Massier J., Med. Welt 2390–2393 (1964).
[14] Maurice P.D., Br. J. Dermatol. 137(4):661 (1997).
[15] Mennicke W.H. et al., Xenobiotica 18: 441–447 (1988).
[16] Minchington I. et al., J. Chromatogr. 247:141–148 (1982).
[17] Scheunert A., E. Theile, Pharmazie 7:776–780 (1952).
[18] Wechselberg K., Z. Hyg. 145:380–394 (1958).
[19] Winter A.G., Naturwissenschaften 41: 337–338 (1954).
[20] Wojciechowska B., L. Wizner, Herba Pol. 29(2):97–101 (1983).
[21] Wolters B., Dtsch. Apoth. Ztg. 138(45): 4340–4351 (1998).

Literature references identified by Ü can be found in the general listing of books and monographs at the back of this book.

Garlic

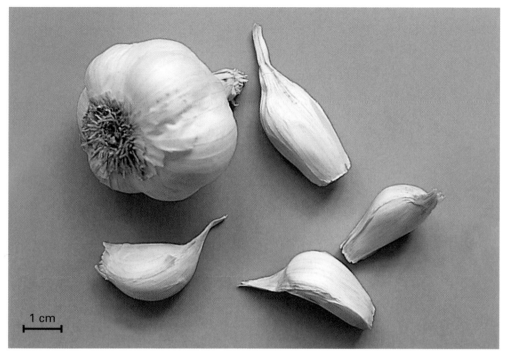

Fig. 1: Garlic bulb and cloves of garlic

Plant source: *Allium sativum* L. var. *sativum.*

Taxonomic classification: The species *Allium sativum* L. can be subdivided into the following varieties:
Allium sativum L. var. *sativum,* common garlic,
Allium sativum L. var. *ophioscordum* (also *ophioscorodon*) (LINK) DÖLL, serpent garlic, rocambole (see below: Similar culinary herbs),
Allium sativum L. var. *pekinense* (PROKH.) MAEKAWA apud MAKINO, Peking garlic (see below: Similar culinary herbs).

Family: Allium plants (Alliaceae; in older literature this species was placed in the lily family, Liliaceae).

Common names: Engl.: garlic, common garlic; Fr.: ail, ail blanc; Ger.: Knoblauch, Knobl, Knoblich, Knofel, Kofel, Knufloch, Windwurzel, Weingartenknoblauch.

Description: Perennial herb, 25 cm to 90 cm in height, with mostly composite bulbs, offset bulbs (cloves) oblong-ovoid (*A. s.* var. *sativum*) or roundish ovoid (*A. s.* var. *ophioscordum*), enclosed by a thin, skin-like membrane which is white, greenish, pink, purple or violet. Leaves are gray-green to bluish gray, flat, broadly linear, acuminate, with a keel below, somewhat grooved, with a rough margin (in *A. s.* var. *ophioscordum* not grooved, with a more or less smooth margin), up to 2 cm wide (in *A. s.* var. *pekinense* more than 2 cm wide). Stalk with inflorescence round, bearing leaves up to the mid-section. Sheath monophyllous with a long beak-like projection; inflorescence is a pseudoumbel with few flowers but bearing numerous, ovoid brood bulbs, up to 1 cm in diameter.

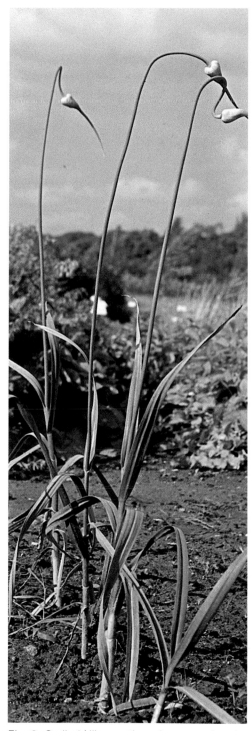

Fig. 2: Garlic (*Allium sativum* L. var. *sativum*)

Flowers with 6 perigone leaves, reddish-white or greenish and 6 stamina, shorter than the perigone, the inner ones with a short, blunt, tooth-like appendix on each side; sterile (only a few Asian cultivars produce viable seeds). Flowering period is July to August [Ü42].

Native origin: Probably native to central Asia, secondarily the central Mediterranean region, and from there it has spread through cultivation almost worldwide. Today, garlic is not known in the wild.

Main cultivation areas: China, India, Thailand, Egypt, South Korea Spain, Turkey, USA (California), Republics of the former Yugoslavia, Italy, and France.

Main exporting countries: Italy, Spain, Hungary, Czech Republic, the Balkan countries, Russian Federation, and Egypt. China is the main exporter of dried garlic.

Cultivation: Garlic prefers loamy-humus, deep, nutrient-rich soil in sunny locations. It is winter hardy. Due to its self-incompatibility, garlic or other Allium species should not be planted again in the same location for at least 5 years. Propagation is carried out vegetatively by planting cloves (separated from the bulb) or brood bulbs (secondary cloves formed in the umbel) in September until mid October, spaced at about 25×8 cm, at a depth of 3.5 to 5.0 cm. Garlic that is grown from brood bulbs will produce in the first year rounds (small bulbs without cloves) which can be used for planting in the autumn [Ü21, Ü96]. Cultivars include, among others, 'Stamm' (high allicin content), 'Thüringer' (without brood bulbs, it does not produce shoots), 'Burgenland', 'Mako' and 'Ungarisher' (Hungarian) [22, Ü21].

Culinary Herb

Commercial forms: Garlic: whole, fresh bulbs, loose, or the tops tied in bundles or woven into braids (garlic braids), summer garlic products (unripe bulbs with green,

whole or shortened leaves), dried or freeze-dried flakes, slices, granulated or powdered bulb, garlic juice, puréed garlic, garlic dry extract (spray-dried onto a carrier), garlic salt (mixture of 40% powdered garlic and 60% common salt), garlic essential oil (obtained by steam distillation), and garlic oleoresin. Smoked garlic bulbs are also commercially traded, which, due to the loss of their ability to germinate, have a longer shelf life than non-smoked bulbs. Garlic that is cultivated in southern latitudes is more aromatic than garlic grown in Central Europe.

Production: The ripe bulbs are harvested when the upper third of the of leaves have withered and the cloves begin to fill the skins (beginning of July to beginning of August). If harvested later than this, the bulbs begin to disintegrate in the cloves. In industrial farming, garlic is harvested using bulb diggers, digger-shakers, or other mechanical garlic harvesters (scooping, uprooting, stalk cutting), or plowshares with attached loaders. After field drying, the tops should be cut at 1 cm, the outer skin should be removed and the bulbs should then be cured in a well-ventilated room. In the retail trade, garlic is offered by small producers bundled or with the leaves woven into braids [Ü21]. Powdered- or granulated garlic is produced by cutting the cloves into slices and dehydrating in a tunnel dryer. Lyophilization is also practiced. By adding calcium stearate (flow agent), the free-flowability of powdered- or granulated garlic is improved [Ü93].

Forms used: Fresh garlic cloves, dried or freeze-dried preparations made from garlic cloves (powder, granules, flakes, garlic salt), and garlic purée.

Storage: The bulbs with a dried surface can be stored in a well-ventilated, dry location between 0 and 2 °C (also in attics; stored garlic is frost-resistant). Winter garlic (planted in fall, harvested in July) can be stored until February. Spring garlic (planted in spring, harvested in August) can be stored until May. In order to prevent the

bulb from drying out, the producers sometimes coat the bulbs with paraffin.

Description. Whole bulb (Fig. 1): Spherical to ovoid, composite bulb, diameter about 4 cm. The bulb consists of a hard, flattened base with root fibers on the lower end, and situated on top, a longish main bulb, surrounded by 8 to 20 longish and bent, somewhat angular secondary bulbs (cloves). The main and secondary bulbs are each enclosed by white to reddish, paper-like membranes. The entire bulb-aggregate is covered by several, dry whitish skins [EB 6].

Cut dried pieces: Horn-like, transparent, strongly hygroscopic disks or fragments.

Powdered garlic: Light yellow to light ochre-colored powder; microscopic examination of the chloral hydrate slide preparation reveals the numerous parenchyma fragments as well as groups of spiral and annular vessels, closely associated with thin-walled parenchyma. Numerous oxalate crystals in form of prisms are also present. Negative reaction for starch with iodine-solution [87, Ph Eur].

Odor: Fresh, uncut bulbs odorless, characteristic garlic odor when cut or crushed; the powder has only a faint, garlic odor.

Taste: Pungent, burning, and characteristic.

History: The origin of garlic cultivation was probably in southwestern Asia, about 6,000 years ago; it is one of the oldest cultivated plants. Since about 2000 BCE, garlic has been cultivated in Egypt. It is common knowledge that garlic played a significant role in promoting the health of slaves working on the great pyramids. Due to its antiseptic effects, garlic was used as a component for filling the body cavities of mummies. Garlic is also an important plant in the mythology of many cultures and peoples [48, Ü92].

Constituents and Analysis

DIN- and ISO-Standards: DIN-Standard 5560 (Dried garlic, trade specification), ISO-Standard 6663 (Garlic, cold storage).

Constituents

- Alliins (*S*-alk(ene)ylcysteine sulfoxides): 0.5 to 1.3% in the fresh bulbs, less in the leaves: (+)-*S*-Allyl-L-cysteine sulfoxide (alliin, about 1%), *trans*-(+)-*S*-(prop-1-enyl)-L-cysteine sulfoxide, (+)-*S*-ethylcysteine sulfoxide and (+)-*S*-methyl-L-cysteine sulfoxide [71, 108].
- Alliaceous oils: The non-volatile alliins come into contact with the enzyme allinase after tissue damage and are then transformed to the volatile alk(ene)-sulfenic acids, which spontaneously convert to compounds with characteristic garlic aroma, the alk(en)yl-alkane/-alkenethiosulfinates (Figs. 10 and 11,

General Part 2.3.4). 10 Dialkylthiosulfinates (0.5 to 1.0%) have been detected including, among others, allicin (allyl-prop-2-ene-thiosulfinate), methyl-prop-2-enethiosulfinate and prop-1-enyl-prop-2-enethiosulfinate [20, 44, 65, 77, 88].

- As decomposition products of the thiosulfinates arising during steam distillation, boiling or frying of garlic: Dialk(ene)oligosulfides, including diallyl-, methylallyl- as well as dimethyl-sulfides and –oligosulfides; they include compounds with 1 (3%), 2 (40%), 3 (37%), 4 (20%), 5 or 6 sulfur atoms, particularly diallyl trisulfide, diallyl disulfide, methylallyl trisulfide and diallyl sulfide, in addition to sulfur-free constituents such as propene and acetaldehyde, which quickly evaporate [1, 54, 112, 123, Ü83]. After steam distillation, a number of hydrophilic constituents have been isolated from the water phase, e.g. 3,5-diethyl-1,2,4-trithiolan, prop-2-ene-1-ol and 2,4-dimethylfuran [123].

- If comminuted garlic is processed in non-polar solvents, for example during oil maceration, the thiosulfinates with allyl functionality are converted to vinyldithiins (about 70%, 2-vinyl-[4H]-1,3-dithiin and 3-vinyl-[4H]-1,2-dithiin) and ajoene (12% *cis*- and *trans*-ajoene); dialkyldi- and –trisulfides have also been detected. Extraction with alcohol mostly yields diallyl-trisulfides, methylallyl-trisulfide and ajoene [77].

- The human organism metabolizes the thiosulfinates to the corresponding alk(ene)yl mercaptans (allyl mercaptan, methyl mercaptan) and metabolized into allylmethyl sulfide and diallyl sulfide. These compounds are partially eliminated through respiration or via the skin and mucous membranes. They are finally metabolized to sulfates and CO_2 [78, 84, 110, for a review of pharmacokinetics, see Lit. 62]. Alliins can also be transformed to alk(en)yl disulfides by intestinal flora [113].

- γ-Glutamylpeptides (about 1.6%, precursors of alliins, in the bulbs only): γ-Glutamyl-*S*-allylcysteine (0.24 to 0.56%), γ-glutamyl-*S*-*trans*-1-propenyl-cysteine (0.35 to 0.47%), γ-glutamyl-*S*-methylcysteine (0.06 to 0.2%) and γ-glutamylmethionine [42, 82, 108].

- Allithiamine (adduct of thiamin and allicin with full vitamin B_1 activity) [18].
- Adenosine: about 0.05% [83].
- Polysaccharides, oligosaccharides and monosaccharides: Particularly fructans (about 50%, neokestose-type), saccharose, scorodose, glucose, and fructose [15, 64, 82].
- Steroid saponins, triterpene saponins: Including, among others, sativoside-B1, -R1, -R2, protoeruboside B, F-gitonin [63].
- Flavonoids (traces): Quercetin- and kaempferol glycosides [42].
- Trace elements: Selenium [66], tellurium [74].

Tests for Identity: TLC, according to [97, Ü102, Ph Eur].

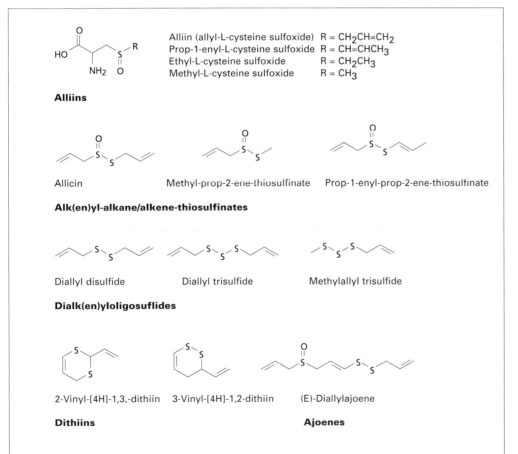

Alliin (allyl-L-cysteine sulfoxide) R = CH₂CH=CH₂
Prop-1-enyl-L-cysteine sulfoxide R = CH=CHCH₃
Ethyl-L-cysteine sulfoxide R = CH₂CH₃
Methyl-L-cysteine sulfoxide R = CH₃

Alliins

Allicin   Methyl-prop-2-ene-thiosulfinate   Prop-1-enyl-prop-2-ene-thiosulfinate

Alk(en)yl-alkane/alkene-thiosulfinates

Diallyl disulfide   Diallyl trisulfide   Methylallyl trisulfide

Dialk(en)yloligosuflides

2-Vinyl-[4H]-1,3,-dithiin   3-Vinyl-[4H]-1,2-dithiin   (E)-Diallylajoene

Dithiins   **Ajoenes**

Quantitative assay: The content of alliin and allicin can be determined with TLC [56, 87]; alliin levels can be evaluated with HPLC [86–88] or, after derivatization, with GC [71]. Another method for alliin quantification is the detection of ammonia, which develops after cleavage with immobilized alliinase [57, 70], and the HPLC determination of the allicin and other thiosulfinates after fermentation of garlic biomass [86–88, 115, 119, Ph Eur], as well as GC [86, 87] or headspace-GC analyses [46, 67]. The alk(en)ylsulfides and thiosulfinates are assayed with HPLC [78]; the former can also be detected in steam-distilled garlic oil by GC/MS or GC/FTIR [54, 123]. The sulfur content is determined according to [20], the steam-volatile constituents are quantified volumetrically [DAB], and the proteins are assessable via SDS-PAGE [85].

Adulterations, Misidentifications and Impurities can be excluded due to the typical appearance, taste and odor of garlic.

Actions and Uses

Actions: Garlic not only has appetite stimulant and digestion promoting effects, but also antilipidemic, antiatherosclerotic and antihypertonic action, thrombocyte aggregation inhibiting effects, and it stimulates fibrinolysis, in this way preventing infarction. Furthermore, it increases blood circulation in peripheral vessels, reduces the risk of tumor formation, activates thyroid gland activity, and has antihepatotoxic activity. Almost all of these effects can be attributed to the antioxidative effect of alliaceous oils. Additionally, garlic has also shown, among other activities, antimicrobial, anthelmintic, insecticidal and immune stimulant activity. The number of publications that have reported on the pharmacological actions of garlic is so great, that in the following section, there is only room for an overview of the exemplary literature. For the most part, results from in vitro studies have been left out.

Lowering of lipid levels in the blood: Garlic has been observed to show a lipid-lowering effect in numerous clinical studies [for an overview of studies up until 1989 see Lit. 75; additional findings reported in Lit. 24, 27, 51, 52, 81, 98, 104, 116]. Daily oral ingestion of 5 g fresh garlic for three weeks as part of a controlled standard diet led to a lowering of total cholesterol by 13% and triglycerides by 25% in healthy volunteers [52]. In a 16-week double blind, placebo-controlled study with hypercholesterolemic patients, a daily dose of 600 mg garlic powder tablets (standardized to 1.3% alliin) led to a 12% reduction of cholesterol concentration in serum in the experimental group and a 17% reduction of triglycerides concentration. [81]. In a randomized, double-blind, placebo-controlled study involving patients with primary hypercholesterolemia, given 0.9 g garlic powder/day (standardized to 1.3% alliin) for 4 months, a decrease of cholesterol level of 21% occurred [27]. In another study involving patients with primary hypercholesterolemia, after six months total cholesterol levels dropped by an average of 14%, triglyceride levels dropped by an average of 20%, LDL-values dropped by about 19% and HDL-values increased by about 18% following daily administration of an enteric coated garlic oil preparation (5 mg oil bound to beta-cyclodextrin, b.i.d.; main constituents diallyl disulfide and diallyl trisulfide) [98]. A meta-analysis of 16 studies found that one-month garlic powder therapy (600 to 900 mg daily) resulted in a lowering of total cholesterol levels by about 12%, which persisted for a minimum of 6 months. Lowered triglyceride levels were also observed [104]. A subsequent meta-analysis confirmed a "modest" lowering of total cholesterol levels (5.8%) due to the influence of dietary supplementation with garlic, however the authors doubt that this small lipid-lowering effect has clinical significance [107]. An anti-hypercholesterolemic effect has also been observed in animal experiments wherein garlic powder was added to feed with concomitant ingestion of a cholesterol rich diet [6, 50].
These observations stand in contrast to other study results [16, 17, 49, 80, 89, 105]. In a randomized, double-blind, placebo-controlled study involving patients with hyperlipoproteinemia, no significant changes in total serum cholesterol, HDL or LDL were observed following ingestion of 198 mg or 450 mg garlic, t.i.d. [80]. Likewise, no effect was attained in similarly designed studies with dried garlic powder in enteric-coated tablets at a dosage of 300 mg, t.i.d., for 12 weeks [49, 105]. Also, the application of garlic essential oil (5 mg oil bound to beta-cyclodextrin, b.i.d.) in a randomized, placebo-controlled study had no influence on serum lipoproteins, cholesterol absorption, or cholesterol synthesis [16].

Antiatherosclerotic effect: Garlic has demonstrated antiatherosclerotic effects in animal- and human studies. Ingestion of garlic powder (300 mg/d, 2 years) in seniors resulted in the maintenance of the arterial elasticity (measured by pulse wave velocity) [26]. In a randomized, double blind, placebo-controlled study, enteric-coated garlic powder tablets were administered to patients with advanced atherosclerotic plaque (300 mg, t.i.d.). In the garlic group, the reduction of the increase of atherosclerotic plaque volume in carotid and femoral artery (assessed by high-resolution ultrasound) ranged from 5 to 18% within the observation period of 48 months, and in a few cases there was even a decrease in plaque volume [69].
The antiatherosclerotic effect of garlic appears not only to be dependent upon the antilipidemic action, but rather it probably takes place, mainly due to a protection of blood lipids, especially LDL (see Chapter 4.8), from oxidative changes. Evidence for that theory is found in a study of mice fed a high-cholesterol diet supplemented with allicin solution (9 mg/kg body weight) for 15 weeks. The allicin-treated group had significantly lower atherosclerotic changes in the aortic sinus compared to the control group that was fed only a high-cholesterol diet. There were no significant differences between blood lipid profiles of either group [2]. Similar results have been attained in studies with rabbits [92]. In an ex-vivo study, LDL isolated from patients who took an aged garlic extract (2.4 g/day) for 7 days was significantly resistant to Cu2+-mediated oxidation [89].

Antihypertensive effect: Blood pressure lowering effects of 5 to 10% following ingestion of garlic have been observed in a few studies [for an overview of studies up until 1989 see Lit. 75; additional findings in Lit. 14, 58, 75, 81]. An antihypertensive effect has also been determined in animal studies [4, 6]. It has been deduced from rat studies that garlic exhibits a vasodilatative effect by modulation of the production and function of relaxing- and contracting factors of endothelial cells [59].

Inhibition of thrombocyte aggregation: This effect has been demonstrated in clinical studies [for an overview of studies up until 1989 see Lit. 75; additional findings in Lit. 5, 7, 47, 58, 94, 116]. In a double blind, placebo-controlled study involving subjects with elevated spontaneous thrombocyte platelet aggregation, after 4 weeks administration of 800 mg garlic powder (400 mg, t.i.d.; standardized to 1.3% alliin), decrease of circulating platelet aggregates in the blood, of thrombocyte aggregation tendency and of plasma viscosity was observed [58, 116]. Oral administration of one garlic clove per day (about 3 g) for 26 weeks reduced thromboxane B_2 levels in serum [58]. An ex-vivo study in humans showed that the administration of 5 ml of an aged garlic extract for 13 weeks delayed the ADP-induced platelet aggregation and diminished the total percentage of platelet aggregates in the blood though without significant changes in plasma level of thromboxane B_2 [94]. In rats, thromboxane B_2 levels in serum were significantly decreased by administration of an aqueous extract of garlic. Boiling the extract diminished its activity [25].

Enhancement of fibrinolytic activity: [For an overview of studies up until 1989, see Lit. 75; additional findings in Lit. 23, 32, 52]. Daily ingestion of 5 g fresh garlic by healthy volunteers for 3 weeks led to an increase of fibrinolytic activity from 77 units to 94.5 units (measurement of euglobulin lysis time) [52]. In a group of 50 patients with myocardial ischemia, fibrinolytic activity increased 6 hours after ingesting a dose of 500 mg fresh or baked garlic by 63% or 72%. After ingestion of the same daily dose for 4 weeks, at the end of the study period activity increased by 85% or 72% [32].

Lowering the risk of infarction: As proof of the speculation that antiatherosclerotic, antilipidemic and antihypertensive effects of garlic contribute to lowering the risk of infarction, a study involving 432 patients after cardiac infarction was carried out. They were treated with encapsulated garlic essential oil (0.1 mg/day) or placebo. After 3 years, blood pressure and blood cholesterol levels in the verum group were significantly lower than those in the placebo group and the number of re-infarctions in the verum group was reduced about 50% [23].

Antimicrobial action: In the agar diffusion test, fresh pressed juice of garlic inhibited the growth of both gram-negative and gram-positive bacteria and was also active against some antibiotic-resistant strains. 20 mg of the pressed garlic juice had the same effect as 10 μg of ampicillin [100]. Garlic powder, garlic oil, allicin or diallyl trisulfide have shown antibiotic effects against, among other species, *Helicobacter pylori* [30, 90, 106], *Staphylococcus aureus*, *Escherichia coli*, *Listeria monocytogenes* [72], *Staphylococcus epidermidis*, *Salmonella thyphi*, yeasts [12, 33], *Cryptococcus neoformans* [34] and *Giardia intestinalis* [8, 10, 12, 19, 29, 30, 33, 34, 72, 95, 100, 101, 106, 116, 120-122]. In vivo, the number of streptococcal bacteria and total coliforms in the intestinal flora of rats was reduced by garlic extract (1 g/rat for 3 days, activity equivalence with 8 mg tetracycline hydrochloride) to 1% of the original count, and lactobacillus to 10% [101].

A Chinese epidemiological study indicated that garlic consumption may protect against *Helicobacter pylori* infection and therefore may also protect against stomach ulcers and gastric cancer [122]. The same opinion is also shared by other authors [106].

The growth of pathogenic dermatophytes has also been strongly inhibited in the agar diffusion test or by topical application on rabbit skin (but not with oral administration) [8].

An antimicrobial effect in the blood and urine has also been demonstrated following ingestion of garlic [29].

Immune stimulating action: Garlic stimulates the production of cytokines (IL-2, TNF, and interferon-gamma) and the proliferation of macrophages, NK-cells and T-cells [73, 76].

Prevention against the induction of malignant tumors: There are numerous indications that garlic may prevent malignant tumors. Epidemiological studies in Japan and China have shown that increased consumption of garlic (as well as, among others, onion and Chinese leek) decreased the risk of occurrence of stomach- or esophagus cancer [19, 45]. In epidemiological studies in France, it was demonstrated that the probability of women getting breast cancer decreased with an increased consumption of garlic or onions (as well as fiber from cereals) [31]. An earlier, extensive study in Holland does not corroborate these results [39]. A meta-analysis of epidemiological studies carried out up to year 2000 showed, however, that for persons who regularly take garlic, the risk of intestinal cancer lowered from 1 to 0.69, and for stomach cancer from 1 to 0.53 [96]. Similar results are found in another meta-analysis [43].

Indications of the tumor preventing action of garlic arose also from experiments with animals. It has been shown that tumors induced by carcinogens (e.g. benzopyrene, 7,12-dimethyl benzanthracene, *N*-methyl-*N*-nitrosourea, dimethylhydrazine, nitrosomethylbenzylamine, diethylnitrosamine) can be inhibited by preparations made from raw garlic or some by its genuine isolated constituents (e.g. *S*-allyl cysteine) [for an overview of studies up until 1989, see Lit. 109, up to 1996, Lit. 117].

Administration of an aqueous garlic extract (250 mg/kg body weight, orally) effectively suppressed 7,12-dimethylbenzanthracene(DMBA)-induced carcinogenesis in the buccal pouches of male Syrian hamsters [14]. Garlic powder (1 to 4% in feed) prevented DMBA-induced breast cancer in rats [79], and the incidence of mammary tumorigenesis induced by *N*-methyl-*N*-nitrosourea in female rats was reduced by supplementation with garlic powder (20 g/kg body weight, a very high dose), S-allyl cysteine (57 μmol/kg body weight) or diallyl disulfide (57 μmol/kg body weight) by 76, 33 or 53%, respectively [97]. The incidence of colorectal adenocarcinoma in mice induced by 1,2-dimethylhydrazine was strongly reduced by gavage administration of diallyl sulfide [118].

The formation of carcinogenic substances by chemical reaction can also be inhibited by constituents of garlic and their degradation products. Diallyl disulfide inhibited the formation of carcinogenic heterocyclic aromatic amines in boiled pork juice [111], and S-allyl cysteine inhibited the formation of carcinogenic nitrosamines in the stomach [37].

In Mexico, in some Central- and South-American countries, and in Spain and India, garlic is used as an oxytocic agent, for dysmenorrhea and as an abortive. In animal experiments, estrogenic and ACTH-like effects have been shown [35, 36, 60].

Toxicology: Based on existing data, there is no acute or chronic toxicity in healthy people with the regular use of garlic as a spice or herbal remedy. Particularly in sensitive individuals, high doses of raw garlic, garlic powder, garlic juice or garlic oil can lead to stomach complaints, heart burn, nausea, vomiting, bloating, colic, diarrhea, micturition, cystitis and even fever. Raw garlic is contraindicated in stomach and duodenal ulcers. Since the alliaceous oils pass into breast milk, they can cause bloating in babies and hence, nursing mothers should avoid garlic or preparations thereof. With external use of garlic or garlic oil, skin irritation with blistering can occur, especially in children [36, 61, 75, 93, 103, Ü58].

In animals (rats, cats, dogs), which were fed high doses of garlic juice over a few weeks time, reduced body weight was observed, as well as damage to the gastric mucosa or anemia; at levels of 5 ml/kg body weight, a few laboratory rats died. The LD_{50} for garlic extracts is at 0.5 up to or exceeding 30 ml/kg body weight [21, 36, 41, 102].

The sensitization potential is moderate. The main allergen is diallyl sulfide but

antibodies against a macromolecular antigen (12 kDa) from garlic have also been detected. Eczema of the hands and more rarely conjunctivitis, runny nose or asthma (particularly with contact of airborne garlic dust) have been observed, particularly in kitchen personnel, vegetable venders and housewives as well in workers of the pharmaceutical industry. Cross reactions with onions are possible [9, 13, 28, 36, 40, 53, 61, 65, 91, Ü39].

Culinary use: The culinary use of garlic is highest in eastern and southeastern Asia, followed by the Mediterranean countries and South America. But also in Europe, following the end of the 2nd world war, it became more and more integrated partly from the adoption of exotic dishes and cooking traditions.

Sometimes it is just used to produce a delicate aroma of garlic, e.g. for salads and in some vegetable dishes (spinach, chard, zucchini, vegetable fennel) that are served in a bowl that has been rubbed with cut pieces of fresh garlic or with cloves of garlic that have been lightly browned in oil. Rubbing garlic over roasted meat is also practiced. If one desires a strong garlic taste, it is best to use the fresh cloves with the paper-like skin removed, chopped, in thin slices or cut into spikes (for larding), chopped in a garlic dicer or in a mortar (best with some salt) or squeezed through a garlic press. For garlic bulbs that have already begun to sprout, the green shoots should be removed. The serving size for Central European eating habits is 1 to 2 cloves, but in southern Europe up to 40 cloves are used for a meal that serves 4 persons. Flavor intensity can be varied depending on the point at which garlic is added to the meal, at the beginning or at the end of cooking. Adding it to hot oil destroys its aroma. Fresh garlic is preferable over dried products or other prepared forms [Ü2, Ü55, Ü91].

Garlic serves as a spice in meat dishes (roasted with, especially mutton, lamb, pork, calf, rabbit, chicken, goose), of sausages (salami, garlic sausage, ringed garlic sausage, garlic sausage for heating in water), fish dishes (e.g. zarzuela, a Spanish

seafood casserole), rice dishes, fried potatoes (one should avoid over browning of roasted garlic), egg dishes (e.g. omelets), salads (e.g. tomato salad, tsatsiki, mushroom salad, and garlic honey in fruit salads), of sauces, mayonnaises or dips (e.g. aioli sauce, a Provençal garlic mayonnaise, and skordalia, a Greek garlic mayonnaise) for noodles, fish, sea foods, poultry, game or vegetables, for salad dressings (e.g. as a component of garlic honey), quark, soups (e.g. potato soup) and vegetables [Ü2, Ü13, Ü23, Ü53, Ü55, Ü65, Ü74, Ü79, Ü91, Ü95]. Steamed in butter, garlic can be eaten as a vegetable [48].

Garlic is also popular as a bread topping. For this, one rubs peeled garlic cloves onto toasted white bread and then spreads butter over it. In the English literature, the preparation of garlic baguettes (garlic bread) is described. To prepare, the baguette is cut in two, lengthwise, and a mixture of about 80 g butter and 1 to 2 peeled, crushed garlic cloves (sometimes also with chopped parsley) is spread on the baguette pieces, which are then wrapped in aluminum foil and baked at about 180 °C for 10 to 15 minutes. It is served hot [Ü65, Ü79].

Garlic plants that have not formed bulbs, or fresh garlic herb can be used, chopped, like chives, as a bread and butter topping. Garlic butter is an essential addition to escargot, shellfish, and fish filets [Ü68].

Garlic herb oil can be added to soups and pot roast dishes. It is made by pickling the whole, peeled cloves of 4 to 8 garlic bulbs for 1 to 2 months in 600 ml olive oil along with thyme- and rosemary branches as well as a few bay leaves. Prior to pickling the garlic cloves, they are brushed with olive oil, wrapped in aluminum foil, and baked in the oven at 190 °C for about 15 minutes [Ü47].

Peeled, garlic cloves, pickled in vinegar, are used as a side dish for noodle dishes, baked chicken or cold meats [Ü55]. In Russian cooking, garlic is also used in the pickling of mushrooms and vegetables [Ü81].

Likewise, garlic can be used as a flavor component of alcoholic beverages (e.g. garlic vodka, garlic punch).

Combines well with: Basil, chillies, coriander, fresh ginger, lemongrass, onion, paprika, parsley, pepper, and watercress.

As a component of spice mixes and preparations: → A.1. Sauce, → Barbecue spice, → Bomboe, → Café de Paris spice mix, → Cajun spice, → Chemen, → Chili con carne spice, → Chili powder, → Fish spice, → Garlic salt (40% garlic powder + 60% cooking salt), → Green masala, → Gremolata, → Hamburger meat spice, → Harissa, → Herb butter, → Herb vinegar, → Lemon pepper, → Masala, → Meat spice, › Nam prik, → Persillade, → Pesto, → Pizza spice, → Quark spice, → Sambal badjak, → Sauce spice, → Soup spice, → Tai-ping China, → Tandoor, → Tika paste, → Tomato ketchup, → Tunisian spice blend, → Venison spice, → Zhug.

Other uses: In the rearing of young pigs, garlic was successfully employed to reduce the frequency of diarrhea thus increasing the growth performance [55].

Medicinal herb

Herbal drugs: Allii sativi bulbi pulvis, Garlic Powder [Ph Eur] contains not less than 0.45% allicin or Powdered Garlic [USP-NF] contains not less than 0.3% alliin and not less than 0.1% γ-glutamyl-(S)-allyl-L-cysteine), Powdered Garlic Extract [USP-NF] contains not less than 4.0% alliin, Garlic Fluidextract [USP-NF], Allii sativi aetheroleum, Distilled Garlic Oil (obtained by steam distillation of cut fresh, fermented garlic bulbs).

Indications: As adjunctive therapy to dietetic measures for hyperlipidemia and for prevention of age-related vascular changes. The recommended daily dose according to Germany's Commission E monograph (1988) is 4 g fresh garlic bulb (corresponding to about 1.3 g garlic powder) or equivalent preparations [68]. More recently, lower dosage levels have been shown to be sufficient [103].
In folk medicine, garlic is used for gastrointestinal disorders, among other conditions,

especially for flatulence and colic, as a cholagogue, for high blood pressure, as an antiatherosclerotic remedy, for bronchitis, menopausal conditions and as an anthelmintic. Dosage forms include fresh garlic, fresh pressed juice, dried powder, oily macerate of fresh homogenized garlic (usually in soft-gel capsules or in β-cyclodextrin coated dragées), garlic oil, obtained by steam distillation, and also rarely in the form of garlic tincture and garlic dry extract. Garlic juice, crushed garlic cloves or garlic slices are used applied externally for treatment of wounds, warts, corns, muscle pains, neuralgia and rheumatic diseases [3, Ü37, Ü60].
It should not be underestimated that garlic also plays a large role in the prevention of intestinal infections, especially in warmer climates.
There are some pharmaceuticals that release an insufficient quantity of allicin [11], so it is advisable to take preparations of garlic with sufficient allicin-forming potential, fresh garlic or garlic oil.

Similar culinary herbs

Serpent garlic (rocambole, sand leek, → Pearl onion, see: → Onion; Similar Allium species), *Allium sativum* L. var. *ophioscordum* (LINK) DÖLL, is cultivated nearly worldwide, and its bulbs and bulbils are used the same as garlic or also pickled in vinegar similar to pearl onions [Ü61, U74].

Peking garlic, *Allium sativum* L. var. *pekinense* (PROKH.) MAEKAWA apud MAKINO, is grown in gardens, predominantly in China and Japan. The bulbils are used as a spice [Ü61].

Twisted leaf garlic, *Allium obliquum* L., is cultivated in North- and Central Asia, Romania, and Siberia, and is used in the same way as garlic [Ü98].

Long-stamen onion, *Allium macrostemon* BUNGE, is native to Mongolia, China, Japan, Korea, and the eastern part of the Russian Federation, is cultivated and wild collected in Southeastern Asia, and used

in the same manner as garlic, especially in China and in the Republic of Georgia [Ü85].

Long-pointed leek, *Allium longicuspis* REGEL, is native to Central Asia, cultivated in Kazakhstan, and is used in the same way as garlic [Ü61].

Garlic Spread
1 small can of anchovies, 30 peeled garlic cloves, 1 bunch of parsley, 2 tablespoons of soft butter, 5 tablespoons of olive oil, some olive oil for roasting.

Drain the anchovies, rinse and mash them with a fork. Squeeze 15 garlic cloves in a garlic press, remove the parsley leaves from the thick leaf stalks and mince very finely. Mix the ingredients and process the mixture to obtain a paste. Dice the remaining garlic cloves, fry the pieces with a bit of olive oil until golden-brown and mix them with the paste [Ü53].

Literature

[1] Abraham K.O. et al., Lebensm. Wiss. Technol. 9(4):193–200 (1976).
[2] Abramovitz D. et al., Coron. Artery Dis. 10(7):515–519 (1999).
[3] Agarwal K.C., Med. Res. Rev. 16(1): 111–124 (1996).
[4] Al-Qattan K.K., A.M. Alnaqeeb, J. Ethnopharmacol. 66(2):217–222 (1999).
[5] Ali M. et al., Prostaglandins Leukot. Ess. Fatty Acids 60(1):43–47 (1999).
[6] Ali M. et al., Prostaglandins Leukot. Ess. Fatty Acids 62(4):253–259 (2000).
[7] Ali M., M. Thomson, Prostaglandins Leukot. Ess. Fatty Acids 53(3):211–222 (1995).
[8] Amer M. et al., Int. J. Dermatol. 19: 285–287 (1980).
[9] Anibarro B. et al., J. Allergy Clin. Immunol. 100(6 Pt):734–738 (1997).
[10] Ankri S., D. Mirelman, Microbes. Infect. 1(2):125–129 (1999).
[11] Anonym, Dtsch. Apoth. Ztg. 132(13): 643 (1992).

[12] Arora D.S., J. Kaur, Int. J. Antimicrob. Agents 12(3):257–262 (1999).

[13] Asero R. et al., J. Allergy Clin. Immunol. 101(3):427–428 (1998).

[14] Balasenthil S. et al., Cancer Detect. Prev. 23(6): 534–538 (1999).

[15] Baumgartner S. et al., Carbohydr. Res. 328(2):177–183 (2000).

[16] Berthold H.K. et al., J.A.M.A 279(23): 1900–1902 (1998).

[17] Berthold H.K., T. Sudhop, Curr. Opin. Lipidol. 9(6):565–569 (1998).

[18] Bitsch R., I. Bitsch, Dtsch. Apoth. Ztg. 129:65–68 (1989).

[19] Block E., Angew. Chem. 104:1158–1203 (1992).

[20] Block E., Dtsch. Apoth. Ztg. 129 (Suppl. 15):3–4 (1989).

[21] Bogin E. et al., J. Food Protection 47:100–101 (1984).

[22] Bomme U. et al., Arznei- und Gewürzpflanzen 1(2):55–60 (1996).

[23] Bordia A., Dtsch. Apoth. Ztg. (Suppl. 15):16–17 (1989).

[24] Bordia A., Am. J. Clin. Nutr. 34: 2100–2103 (1981).

[25] Bordia T. et al., Prostglandins Leukotrienes Fatty Acids 54(3):183–186 (1996).

[26] Breithaupt-Grögler K. et al., Circulation 96:2649–2655 (1997).

[27] Brosche T., D. Platt, Fortschr. Med. 108:703–706 (1990).

[28] Burden A.D. et al., Contact Dermatitis 30(5):299–300 (1994).

[29] Caporaso N. et al., Antimicrob. Agents Chemother. 23:700–702 (1983).

[30] Cellini L. et al., FEMS Immunol. Med. Microbiol. 13(4):273–277 (1996).

[31] Challier B. et al., Eur. J. Epidemiol. 14(8):737–747 (1998).

[32] Chutani B.K., A. Bordia, Atherosclerosis 38:417–421 (1981).

[33] Dankert J. et al., Zentralbl. Bakteriol. (Orig. A) 245(1/2):229–239 (1979).

[34] Davis L.E. et al., Planta Med. 60(6): 546–549 (1994).

[35] De Montellano B.A., C.H. Browner, J. Ethnopharmacol. 13:57–88 (1985).

[36] De Smet P.A.G.M. et al. (Eds.), in: Adverse Effects of Herbal Drugs, Springer Verlag Berlin, Heidelberg, New York 1992, Bd. 1, p. 91–95.

[37] Dion M.E. et al., Nutr. Cancer 28(1):1–6 (1997).

[38] Dorant E. et al., Gastroenterology 110(1): 12–20 (1996).

[39] Dorant E. et al., Breast Cancer Res. Treat 33(2):163–170 (1995).

[40] Eming S.A. et al., Br. J. Dermatol. 141(2):391–392 (1999).

[41] Farkas M.C., J.N. Farkas, J. Am. Anim. Hosp. Ass. 10:65 (1974).

[42] Fenwick G.R. et al., CRC Crit. Rev. Food Sci. Nutr. 22:199–377 (1985).

[43] Fleischauer A.T. et al., Am. J. Clin. Nutr. 72(4):1047–1052 (2000).

[44] Freeman G.G., R.J. Whenham., J. Sci. Food Agric. 26:1869 (1975).

[45] Gao C.M. et al., Jpn. J. Cancer Res. 90(6):614–621 (1999).

[46] Graham D.Y. et al., Am. J. Gastroenterol. 94(5) :1200–1202 (1999).

[47] Grünwald J., Dtsch. Apoth. Ztg. 131 (Suppl. 24):16–20 (1991).

[48] Hale S.: Knoblauchküche, Könemann Verlagsges mbH Köln, Lizenzausgabe einer engl. Ausgabe (Quintet Publishing Limited, London) 1995.

[49] Isaacsohn J.L. et al., Arch. Intern. Med. 158(11):1189–1194 (1998).

[50] Ismail M.F. et al., Pharmacol. Res. 39(2): 157–166 (1999).

[51] Jain A.K., Am. J. Med. 94:632–635 (1993).

[52] Jain R.C., Am. J. Clin. Nutr. 30:1380–1381 (1977).

[53] Jappe U. et al., Am. J. Contact Dermatitis 10(1):37–39 (1999).

[54] Jinovetz L. et al., Z. Lebensm. Unters. Forsch. 194:363–365 (1992).

[55] Jost M., Agrarforschung 3:479–481 (1996).

[56] Kappenberg F.J., H. Glasl, Pharm. Ztg.-Wissensch. 135(5):189–193 (1990).

[57] Keusgen M., Planta Med. 64(8):736–740 (1998).

[58] Kiesewetter H. et al., Clin. Pharm. Ther. Toxicol. 29:151–155 (1991).

[59] Kim-Park S., D.D. Ku, Clin. Exp. Pharmacol. Physiol. 27(10):780–786 (2000).

[60] Koch H.P., Z. Phytother. 13(6):177–188 (1992).

[61] Koch H.P., Dtsch. Apoth. Ztg. 132(27): 1419–1428 (1992).

[62] Koch H.P., Z. Phytother. 13(3):83, (1992).

[63] Koch H.P., Dtsch. Apoth. Ztg. 133(41): 3733–3743 (1993).

[64] Koch H.P. et al., Phytother. Res. 7:387–389 (1993).

[65] Koch H.P., G. Hahn: Knoblauch – Grundlagen der therapeutischen Anwendung von Allium sativum L., Urban & Schwarzenberg, München 1988.

[66] Koch H.P., W. Jäger, Dtsch. Apoth. Ztg. 128:993–995 (1988).

[67] Koch J. et al., Planta Med. 55:327–331 (1989).

[68] Kommission E beim BfArM., BAnz. 122 vom 06.07.88.

[69] Koscielny J. et al., Atherosclerosis 144(1): 237–249 (1999).

[70] Krest I., P. Milka, M. Keusgen, Pharm. Pharmacol. Lett. 7(4):145–147 (1997).

[71] Kubec R. et al., J. Chromatogr. A 862(1):85–94 (1999).

[72] Kumar M., J.S. Berwal, J. Appl. Microbiol. 84(2):213–215 (1998).

[73] Lamm D.L., D.R. Riggs, Urol. Clin. North Am. 27(1):157–162 (2000).

[74] Larner A.J., Med. Hypothesis 44(4): 295–297 (1995).

[75] Lau B.H.S.: New Protective Roles for Selected Nutrients, Allan R. Liss, Inc. 1989, p. 295–325.

[76] Lau B.H.S. et al., Mol. Biother. 3(2): 103–107 (1991).

[77] Lawson L.D., Dtsch. Apoth. Ztg. 131 (Suppl. 24):10–12 (1999).

[78] Lawson L.D. et al., Planta Med. 57(4): 363–370 (1991).

[79] Liu L. et al., Carcinogenesis 13(10): 1847–1851 (1992).

[80] Luley C. et al., Arzneim. Forsch. 36:766–768 (1986).

[81] Mader F.H., Arzneim. Forsch. 40:1111–1116 (1990).

[82] Matsuura H. et al., Planta Med. 62(1): 70–71 (1997).

[83] Michahelles E., Über neue Wirkstoffe aus Knoblauch (Allium sativum L.) und Küchenzwiebel (Allium cepa L.), Dissertation Ludwig-Maximilians-Universität München 1974 (1974).

[84] Minami T. et al., J. Food Sci. 54:763–765 (1989).

[85] Mochizuki E. et al., J. Assoc. Off. Anal. Chem. Int. 79(6):1466–1470 (1996).

[86] Müller B., R.D. Aye, Dtsch. Apoth. Ztg. 131 (Suppl 24):8–10 (1991).

[87] Müller B., A. Ruhnke, Dtsch. Apoth. Ztg. 133(24):2177–2187 (1993).

[88] Müller B.H., Beitrag zur Charakterisierung und Analytik von Alliin und Allicin in Knoblauch und seinen Zubereitungen, Dissertation Universität Erlangen-Nürnberg 1991.

[89] Munday J.S. et al., Atherosclerosis 143(2):399–404 (1999).

[90] O'Gara E.A. et al., Appl. Environ. Microbiol. 66(5):2269–2273 (2000).

[91] Peret-Pimiento A.J. et al., Allergy 54(6): 626–629 (1999).

[92] Prasad K. et al., J. Cardiovasc. Pharmacol. Ther. 2(4):309–320 (1997).

[93] Rafaat M., A.K. Leung, Pedriat. Dermatol. 17(2):475–476 (2000).

[94] Rahman K., D. Billington, J. Nutr. 130(11):2662–2665 (2000).

[95] Ross Z.M. et al., Appl. Environ. Microbiol. 67(1):475–480 (2001).

[96] Samaranayake M.D. et al., Phytother. Res. 14(7):564–567 (2000).

[97] Schaffer E.M. et al., Cancer Letters 102(1/2):199–204 (1996).

[98] Schiewe F.P., T. Hein, Z. Phytother. 16(6):343–348 (1995).

[99] Sendl A. et al., Planta Med. 58(1):1–7 (1992).

[100] Sharma V.D. et al., Indian J. Exp. Biol. 15:466–468 (1977).

[101] Shashikanth K.N. et al., Food Microbiol. 29:348–352 (1984).

[102] Shashikanth K.N. et al., Nutr. Rep. Int. 33:313–319 (1986).

[103] Siegers C.P., Dtsch. Apoth. Ztg. 129 (Suppl. 15):13–15 (1989).

[104] Silagy C., A. Neil, J.R. Coll. Physicians Lond. 28(1):39–45 (1994).

[105] Simons L.A. et al., Atherosclerosis 113(2):219–295 (1995).

[106] Sivam G.P. et al., Nutr. Cancer 27(2):118–121 (1997).

[107] Stevinson C. et al., Ann. Intern. Med. 133(6):420–429 (2000).

[108] Sticher O., Dtsch. Apoth. Ztg. 131 (Suppl. 24):3–4 (1999).

[109] Sumiyoshi H., M.J. Wargovich, Asia Pacific J. Pharmacol. 4:133–140 (1989).

[110] Tamaki T., S. Sonoki, J. Nutr. Sci. Vitaminol. (Tokyo) 45(2):213–222 (1999).

[111] Tsai Sh-J. et al., Mutagenesis 11(3):235–240 (1996).

[112] Velisek J. et al., Spec. Publ-R. Soc. Chem. 197 (Flavour Science):258–261 (1996), ref. CA: 126:237607m.

[113] Virtanen A.I., Phytochemistry 4:207–228 (1965).

[114] Vorberg G., B. Schneider, Natur Ganzh. Med. 3:62–66 (1990).

[115] Wagner H. , A. Sendl, Dtsch. Apoth. Ztg. 130(33):1809–1815 (1990).

[116] Walper A., Dtsch. Apoth. Ztg. 131 (Suppl. 24):20–25 (1991).

[117] Wargovich M.J., Biochem. Soc. Trans. 24(3):811–814 (1996).

[118] Wargovich M.J., Carcinogenesis 8(3):487–488 (1987).

[119] Winkler G. et al., Dtsch. Apoth. Ztg. 132(43):2312–2317 (1992).

[120] Yin M.C., W.S. Cheng, J. Food Prot. 61(1):123–125 (1998).

[121] Yin M.C., S.M. Tsao, Int. J. Food Microbiol. 49(1/2):49–56 (1999).

[122] You W.C. et al., Int. J. Epidemol. 27(6):941–944 (1998).

[123] Yu T.H. et al., J. Agric. Food Chem. 37(3):725–730 (1989).

Literature references identified by Ü can be found in the general listing of books and monographs at the back of this book.

Ginger

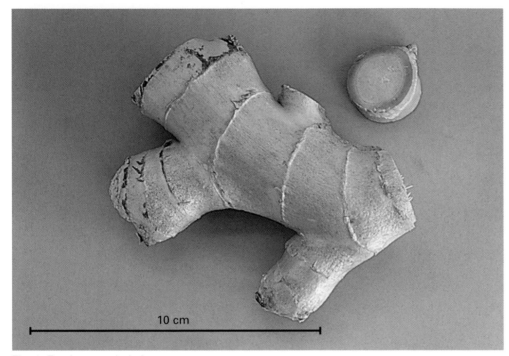

Fig. 1: Fresh, unpeeled ginger

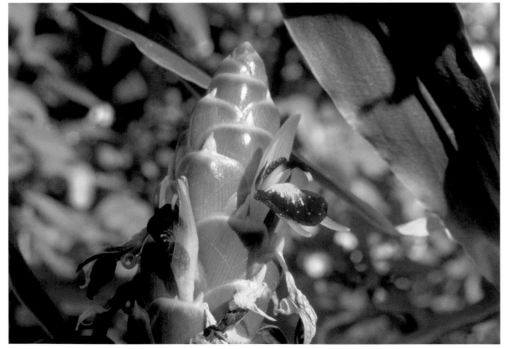

Fig. 2: Ginger (*Zingiber officinale* L.)

Plant source: *Zingiber officinale* L.

Synonym: *Amomum zingiber* L.

Family: Ginger family (Zingiberaceae).

Common names: Engl.: ginger, common ginger; Fr.: gingembre; Ger.: Ingwer, Echter Ingwer, Ingber, Immerwurzel, Schnapswurzel.

Description: Rhizomatous perennial with horizontal creeping rhizome, antler-like branched and bulbous thickened, somewhat flattened, with annular leaf scars and filiform roots. The up to 1 m high pseudostems are formed from the long sheaths of the reed-like leaves with longish-lanceolate, entire-margined lamina. The flowering stalks are growing up to 30 cm in length, bearing densely arranged sheathlike leaves. The inflorescences are spicular, ovoid, with about 5 cm long, single flowers situated in the axils of the bracts. The calyx is whitish, corolla yellow, with 3 clefts. The 3 stamina of the outer whorl form a petallike, purple colored, yellowish punctate lip, within the inner whorl only 1 stamen is fertile. Inferior ovary, 3-chambered, developing into a fleshy, berry-like capsule. Flowers and seeds are rare.

Native origin: Ginger is not known to occur in the wild, and it probably originated in India.

Main cultivation areas: Cultivated in many tropical countries, especially in India (over 20 varieties), Southern China, Malaysia, Nigeria and Sierra Leone, followed by, among others, Taiwan, Japan, Thailand, Sri Lanka, Vietnam, Jamaica, Hawaii, Indonesia, Australia (Queensland), and Brazil.

Main exporting countries: Predominantly China and Brazil, followed by Nigeria, Indonesia, Singapore, and West Malaysia.

Cultivation: The cultivation of ginger requires a tropical climate with high humidity and without large fluctuations in temperature as well as light but humus, sufficiently damp soil in half-shaded locations. Propagation is carried out vegetatively with pieces of rhizome [Ü89]. For growing ginger in pots, they must overwinter completely dry and not be exposed to temperatures below 10 °C [Ü56].

Culinary herb

Commercial forms: Ginger (ginger root): fresh, unpeeled rhizome (Fig. 1, green ginger), unpeeled or partially peeled only on the flattened sides (unpeeled ginger, coated ginger, black ginger), decorticated and dried (white ginger, peeled ginger, uncoated ginger), whole, cut ("sliced"), covered in sugar syrup or candied (Chylon ginger) or ground, dried and rarely unpeeled, treated with lime and/or sulfurized. In China and Japan, slices of the rhizome are preserved by pickling in brine, rice wine or rice vinegar (due to the pink color, which is often strengthened by synthetic food coloring substances, also described as red ginger, pickled in sweet vinegar as beni shoga [30].

Ginger is also described according to its origin: **Jamaican ginger** (light, pale yellow, peeled, fracture fibrous, pieces up to 12 cm long and up to 2 cm wide, very good quality, aromatic-pungent, with a citrus-like flavor, corresponds to the requirements of the German pharmacopoeia, top product "peeled bold", never treated with lime or bleached, **Indian ginger** (Bengal-, Cochin-, Calicut-, Malabar-ginger, bleached or unbleached, decorticated or partially peeled only on the flattened sides, Bengal-ginger, fine-aromatic, best Indian variety, Cochin-ginger is light brown to yellowish, burning-pungent, good quality Calicut-ginger is reddish-brown, moderately pungent, and smells lemony), **Chinese ginger** (unpeeled, pale brown, mild, often in slices, mostly traded in crystallized candied form or in a sugar solution), **Australian ginger** (light brown, peeled or unpeeled, moderately pungent, citrus-like aroma, mostly traded in preserved or crystallized form), **West African ginger** (very dark, usually unpeeled, with wrinkled cork tissues, sometimes also unpeeled or longitudinally split, very pungent, camphoraceous odor, inferior quality, usually only used in the meat processing industry and for the manufacture of oleoresins or essential oils), **Brazilian ginger** (unpeeled, giant variety, very large rhizome, usually traded fresh, plus chaipira variety).

Also commercially traded are **ginger essential oil** (ginger oil) and **ginger oleoresin** (golden brown, highly viscous oil, main components are essential oil (20 to 40%), pungent compounds (25 to 30%), in addition to, among others, triacylglycerols and waxes) [Ü37, Ü92, Ü98].

Production: For the production of dried ginger, the rhizomes are harvested about 8 to 10 months after planting, after the aerial parts of the plant have wilted. To obtain a less fibrous rhizome, e.g. for the fresh ginger market or for the production of candied ginger for ginger confectionery, the rhizomes are harvested earlier, after about 5 to 6 months. The washed rhizome, sometimes soaked over night in water, also often immersed briefly in hot water or hot water is poured over it, is broken into suitable sized pieces, freed from the roots and cork by scraping, rarely peeled with a bamboo knife (using a metal knife would spoil the taste), and dried. The removal of the cork layer must be done very carefully, because the secretion cells are situated, in part, directly below the cork layer. The rhizome may be coated with lime, especially in some parts of India (Kerala). For this purpose the rhizome is soaked and cleaned several times, in baskets submerged in lime milk, then dried. The process can be repeated several times. In addition, the rhizome is sometimes sulfurized. Decorticated ginger can also be treated in this way (bleached ginger). Lime and sulfurizing serve to beautify the product and protect it against infestations by insects or microorganisms. Rarely the rhizome is dried unpeeled, with only the cork of flanks removed or longitudinally split. In Australia, the fresh rhizome is dried in cut slices. Ginger is usually packed in jute sacks [35, Ü37].

To produce candied ginger, the rhizome is washed, hot water is poured over it and then soft-boiled. It remains in cold water for up to 3 days, and then boiling, concentrated sugar syrup is poured over it. After draining, the procedure is repeated, followed by drying (candied ginger) or coating in sugar syrup (Chylon, cut into plum-shaped pieces = plum ginger). Sometimes it is brightened up with rice flour.

Ginger can also be cut into thin slices and pickled (beni shoga).

Forms used: The fresh rhizome, decorticated and scraped or finely chopped, the peeled or unpeeled dried, ground rhizome, the candied, peeled rhizome, ginger essential oil, and ginger oleoresin.

Storage: The fresh rhizome can be preserved for several weeks in the refrigerator wrapped with paper towels and tightly packed in a plastic bag. Ginger can also be stored in the deep freezer and, upon demand, peeled and sliced while still frozen. It is also used pickled with vinegar, rice wine, salt brine or candied and coated with syrup, respectively; after opening, these products need to be refrigerated as well. The dried rhizomes are stored in well-closed containers protected from light, heat, moisture and insect infestation. During storage, the gingerols are slowly converted to shogaols. Elevated shogaol levels indicate excessive storage or thermal stress.

Description. Whole rhizome (Fig. 3): Antler-like (sympodial), planar branched, somewhat flattened, up to 12 cm long, up to 4 cm wide pieces; unpeeled ginger is light to red-brown, yellowish-gray pieces if peeled ("claw" or "hand", for the colors of different varieties, see: Commercial forms) [DAB].

Cut rhizome consists of whitish to light-yellow slices or cubiform pieces. The cross

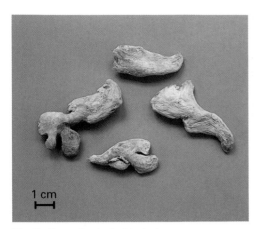

Fig. 3: Decorticated, dried ginger

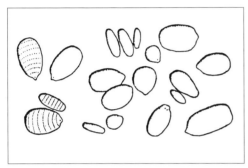

Fig 4: Starch grains from ginger [Ü37]

section shows, below the periderm, a narrow, somewhat dark parenchyma of the cortex, which is separated by a circular endodermis from the rather large and oval central stele. Numerous vascular bundles are scattered in the cortex and central stele. Cork or fragments thereof can be present [DAB].

Powdered rhizome: Light-yellow to yellowish-brown. Microscopic examination shows predominantly the characteristic, single, ovate to drop-shaped, flat, indistinctly layered, 20 to 25 µm long and 18 to 20 µm wide starch grains (Fig. 4) as well as the colorless fragments of parenchyma with partially intact oil cells with yellow content and tiny crystals. Also present are scalariform and reticulate vessels and non-ligneous, lightly thickened fibers, which, if viewed from the side, are on one side lobed in an arch-like fashion. In the unpeeled or partially peeled material, cork shreds with thick-walled cork cells are present [11, Ü37, Ü49].

Taste: Aromatic, more or less pungent and slightly bitter, **Odor:** Aromatic; in Indian, Chinese and Australian ginger with a lemon-like note.

History: Cultivation and use were already described in the oldest Chinese and early Indian (Sanskrit) texts. Ginger was introduced to Mediterranean regions by the Arabs and was used by the Greeks and Romans. Dioscorides (second half of the 1st century) and Plinius the Elder (23–79 CE) described its aromatic properties. The Roman cookbook "De re coquinaria" (10 volumes), which appeared under the name of Apicius in the 3rd century, mentions ginger as a valuable spice for meat and poultry sauces (see: Asafetida, footnote). Its application in Central Europe as a culinary spice was first mentioned in the 11th century. At that time, the monastery Hirschau already documented ginger as a common spice. Its use as a valuable aphrodisiac has also been noted. In the 13th century, the Arabs brought it to East Africa. In the 16th century, ginger was introduced to Western Africa by the Portuguese and to the West Indies during the Spanish conquests. In Australia, it has been cultivated since about 1940. In the 18th century, ginger almost disappeared from European cuisine, but today, with the new trend in East Asian cooking, it has found its way back as a popular kitchen spice [30, Ü92].

Constituents and Analysis

DIN- and ISO-Standards: DIN-Standard 10201 (Ginger, technical specifications), ISO-Standard 13 685 (Ginger and its oleoresins: Determination of the most pungent components: gingerols and shogaols).

Constituents
■ Essential oil: 1 to 4.3%, 160 components have been identified to date; the composition strongly depends on the origin. Usually, the main components are sesquiterpenes, including, among others:
– Sesquiterpene hydrocarbons (−)-zingiberene (7 to 50%), (−)-β-sesquiphel-landrene (2 to 12%, both components decline during storage), *ar*-curcumene (0.2 to 19%, increases during storage), (−)-β-bisabolene and (*E*)-α-farnesene,
– Sesquiterpene alcohols such as sesquiphellandrol and zingiberol (isomeric mixture of *cis*- and *trans*-β-eudesmol, which significantly contributes to the odor,
– Monoterpenes, including, among others, 1,8-cineole (traces to 13%), *p*-cymene (0.2 to 11%), nerolidol, (traces to 9%), α-pinene (1.8 to 4.2%), linalool (1.0 to 5.5%), furthermore, borneol, β-pinene, camphene, geraniol, citral (a high content causes a lemon-like aroma),
– Aliphatics, among others, nonanol (2 to 8%), propanal, (0.1 to 3.1%) [5, 10, 14, 17, 29, Ü37].
In a ginger variety of Indian origin, the main components were found to be *ar*-curcumene (about 19%), β-sesquiphellandrene (about 12%); the content of zingiberene was only at 7% [10]. The dried rhizome of another variety from Sri Lanka ("Sidda") contained mostly β-bisabolene (about 45%) and *ar*-curcumene (about 27%) [31]. Australian ginger contains mostly monoterpenes, particularly camphene (about 14%) and β-phellandrene (about 12%), in addition to 1,8-cineole (about 7%) and citral (geranial about 5% + neral about 4%) [10]. Ginger rhizomes from Madagascar also contained predominantly monoterpenes, including camphene (about 31%), γ-terpinene (about 12%) and geranial (about 10%), as well as, among others, α-pinene (about 7%), β-phellandrene (about 6%), 1,8-cineole (about 5%) and neral (about 4%), with only 2% zingiberene [33].
■ Monoterpene glycosides: (+)-Angelicoidenol-2-*O*-β-D-glucoside [53].
■ Phenylethyl-*n*-alkyl-ketones (phenylalkanones) and their derivatives:
– Gingerols (phenylalkanones), about 25% of the oleoresin, particularly [6]-gingerol (pungent tasting), furthermore [3]-, [4]-, [5]-, [8]-, [10]-, [12]-gingerol ([n] = amount of C-atoms from the fatty acid residues which biosynthetically are linked with a cinnamic acid derivative),

methyl gingerols (methylation at the asymmetrical C-atom or at the phenolic OH-group),

- Shogaols (5-desoxy-4,5-dehydro-gingerols), which are artifacts from the drying process and storage, developing from the gingerols by dehydration, especially [6]-shogaol (more pungent than [6]-gingerol, thus the pungency of the rhizomes is increasing during storage), as well as methylshogaols,
- Paradols (5-deoxy-gingerols): [6]-Paradol (only in traces),
- Gingerdiones, 1- and 5-dehydro-gingerdiones: particularly [6]-dehydrogingerdione,
- 6-Gingesulfonic acid,
- Zingerone (phenylethyl-methyl-ketone-derivatives, arising from the gingerols during storage; elevated levels are indicative of inferior quality) [6, 9, 14, 53].
- Gingerdiols (3-deoxy-3,5-dihydroxy-gingerols), particularly [6]-gingerdiol, its glycosides, as well as [6]-methylgingerdiol, [6]-gingerdioldiacetate and [6]-methylgingerdioldiacetate [4, 21, 22, 42].
- 1,7-Diarylheptanoids (curcuminoids) including, among others, hexahydro-curcumin (diarylheptandione), diarylheptanones (e.g. gingerenones A, B and C, isogingerenone B), diarylheptanonols, diarylheptanediols, cyclic diarylheptanoids and their acetates and diacetates [9, 21, 23, 24].
- Diterpenes: Galanolactone, (E)-8-β,17-epoxylabd-12-ene-15,16-dial; only present in the Japanese ginger variety "Kintoki", from Z. officinale ROSCOE var. rubens MAKINO, [18]).
- Ginger glycolipids A, B, C (monoacyldigalactosylglycerols) [53].
- Starch (about 50%).

Tests for Identity: With organoleptic, macroscopic and microscopic analysis as well as TLC, according to Ph Eur or USP-NF (see also Lit. [13]; for identity tests using micro-TLC, see Lit. [50]).

Quantitative assay: The content of essential oil can be determined volumetrically with steam distillation and xylol in the

Zingiberene

Sesquiphellandrene (R = H)
Sesquiphellandrol (R = OH)

ar-Curcumene

β Eudesmol

Gingerols (n = 1, 2, 3, 4, 6, 8, 10)
[6]-Gingerol (n = 4)

Shogaols (n = 1, 2, 3, 4, 6, 8, 10)

Zingerone

Gingerenone A (R = H)
Gingerenone B (R = OCH₃)

graduated tube [Ph Eur]. HPLC determination of the gingerols and total pungent compounds according to USP-NF or [39].

Adulterations, Misidentifications and Impurities: Japanese ginger (see below) can be recognized by its different aroma (reminiscent of bergamot oil) as well as by the occurrence of composite aleuron grains and oxalate druses. The rhizomes of other types of ginger are considerably larger. Addition of lime to improve appearance can be detected with acetic acid (bubbling due to the presence of $CaCO_3$).

Actions and Uses

Actions: Ginger rhizome, essential oil and oleoresin, due to their aromatic odor and aromatic-pungent taste, stimulate the flow of saliva, the secretion of gastric juices and intestinal motility, and therefore they have appetite stimulating and digestion promoting action. In animal experiments, after several weeks administration increased activity of various digestive enzymes was shown, e.g. intestinal lipase-, saccharase-, maltase-, trypsin- and chymotrypsin activity [11, 28, 36, 37, Ü37]. Ginger also stimulates choleresis. [6]-Gingerol has been shown to be the most active choleretic substance of ginger [52].

Ginger has anti-ulcerogenic activity. Aqueous dry extracts, that probably contain no essential oil, have caused a reduction in gastric juice production in animal tests. The extracts protect against ulcerogenic noxa (hydrochloric acid, indomethacin, acetylsalicylic acid, among others). As anti-ulcerogenic substances, [6]-gingerol, [6]-gingesulfonic acid, [6]-shogaol and zingiberene have been isolated [14, 21, 38, 51, 53, Ü37].

Ginger has antiemetic action, which has been demonstrated in animal studies and in numerous clinical studies [overviews found in Lit. 8, 11, 14, 19, Ü37]. Some constituents of ginger probably have a 5-HT$_3$-antagonistic action [46].

Ginger has antihyperlipidemic activity. In cholesterol fed rabbits, an ethanolic extract of ginger (200 mg/kg body weight, p.o.) significantly reduced elevated levels of serum cholesterol, triglycerides, lipoproteins and phospholipids. The severity of atherosclerotic lesions in the animals receiving ginger extract was also much lower [2]. In animal experiments, elevated cholesterol excretion and a lowering of serum cholesterol levels after administration of ginger oleoresin have been observed [14, 15, 43]. In mutant apolipoprotein E- deficient (E(0)) mice, ginger extract (250 µg/day, p.o., 10 weeks) led to a reduction of aortic atherosclerotic lesion areas by 44%, plasma triglycerides by 27% and plasma cholesterol by 29%. There was a 76% reduction of the cellular cholesterol biosynthesis rate in peritoneal macrophages and the capacity to oxidize LDL was reduced by 60%. The macrophages had a lower capacity to take up oxidized LDL (by 47%) [12].

In humans, ginger inhibits thrombocyte aggregation at high doses (10 g powder as single-dose) [3].

Ginger has antitumorigenic activity. Ginger extracts, in vitro in non-cytotoxic doses, inhibited Epstein-Barr-virus activation in Raji cells induced by 12-O-tetradecanoyl phorbol-13-acetate (TPA) [48] and pre-application of a ginger extract protected against skin tumors in mice after topical application of cocarcinogen TPA together with 7,12-dimethylbenz(a)anthracene [20]. In animal tests, [6]-gingerol and [6]-paradol showed antitumor promotional and antiproliferative effects [47].

Ginger potentiates the antioxidative defense system of the organism. In rats, ginger (1% in the feed) significantly lowered lipid peroxidation and significantly increased the blood glutathione content [1].

Dry extracts of ginger have antimicrobial, nematocide, molluscicidal and antischisto-somal action [16, Ü37]. Components of the essential oil, especially β-sesquiphellandrene and zingiberene, inhibit the replication of rhinoviruses [7].

Ginger extracts and the polar constituents of ginger rhizome, especially [6]-gingerol and shogaol, have antiphlogistic and antiedematic action [20]. In clinical studies, improvements of rheumatic complaints have been shown following oral administration [46]. The antiphlogistic effect occurs possibly through inhibition of cyclooxygenase and lipoxygenase [25].

In the Ayurvedic system of medicine, ginger is used for treatment of migraine headaches. Studies have shown a preventive effect with the addition of uncooked ginger with meals (decrease in frequency of episodes), and a symptomatic effect with migraine attacks 30 minutes after ginger is taken orally (500 to 600 mg powder in water). Additional doses are taken every 4 hours for 3 to 4 days [34].

A detailed overview of pharmacological actions and clinical studies on ginger can be found in Lit. 8 and 14.

Toxicology: Based on existing data, there is no acute or chronic toxicity with regular use of ginger as a spice [8]. At higher doses (single dose above 4 to 6 g), ginger can irritate the mucosa of the stomach. Contact allergies can occur in sensitive people [13].

Culinary use: In Indian and oriental cooking, ginger is combined mainly with fish. In Indonesian, Japanese and Chinese cooking, it is often used in combination with soy sauce and garlic, as a seasoning in meat-, fowl-, fish- and vegetable dishes. Chinese specialties prepared in a wok are hardly imaginable without ginger. Ginger is also very popular in Russian cooking. In Russia, and in other countries, ginger is a component of refreshing beverages (sbiten) with kvass and honey.

Due to the pleasant aroma, fresh ginger is preferred over dried ginger. In cooked dishes, ginger should be added about 20 minutes before the end of cooking time, and in sweet dishes as well as sauces about 1 to 5 minutes before finishing and for pastry it is mixed with the other ingredients.

Due to its strong spice intensity, it should be measured carefully.

Fresh ginger, with its cork layer scraped off, in grated form or in the form of juice made by squeezing grated or diced ginger through a garlic press is used as an ingredient in fruit desserts, salads (fruit salads, especially those that contain apples and/or bananas, and sweet-sour salads, e.g. carrot-, cucumber- or rice salad), sauces (e.g. tomato sauce), marinades, chutneys or pickles. Ginger is often used for canning pears and pickling cucumbers or pumpkins. As a spice for meat dishes (especially beef), vegetable dishes (e.g. red cabbage, celery puree), fish dishes (e.g. red bass) and rice dishes as well as crabs and prawns, fresh, peeled ginger, and ginger cut in slices or strips can be added to the dish and removed after finished cooking [26, Ü2, Ü13, Ü55, Ü59, Ü73, Ü95].

Dried, ground ginger is used especially as an ingredient in sweet baked goods (ginger biscuits, ginger cakes, ginger bread, ginger buns) and in puddings, and less often as a spice in soups, sauces, fish, meat, especially fowl dishes, and fruit salads as well as compotes. It is an integral component of many spice mixes (see below). In tropical countries (e.g. Saudi Arabia, Yemen), ginger is added to coffee (gahwa) or tea (Ü13, Ü55, Ü73).

Ginger syrup serves primarily as a component of fruit desserts, marmalades, sauces or chutneys. Candied ginger is used the same as fresh ginger in the bread- and confectionery industries (e.g. for the production of ginger chocolate, ginger jelly). Ginger confectionery, with chocolate-coated bars of candied ginger, is a popular sweet. Ginger jam with orange peels ("chow-chow") is very popular not only in China, but also in England [Ü55, Ü59, Ü73, Ü95]. Ginger oleoresin and ginger essential oil are used especially in the beverage industry, e.g. in bitter liqueurs such as angostura and Boonekamp, but also in the confectionery industry.

Ginger beer and ginger ale are well known and popular, mainly in the Anglo-Saxon countries. Ginger beer is a top-fermented beer with a high content of extract, for which commercially available industrially manufactured ginger extracts are used. Non-brewed ginger beer (Gingerade) can be made in a bottling factory by diluting commercial ginger beer concentrate with carbonated water. Its alcohol content is adjusted to 2%. Ginger lemonade (Ginger Ale) is alcohol-free and is produced from ginger concentrates mixed with lemon- and other fruit juices, capsicum extracts as well as frothing agents [Ü93].

English ginger bread is prepared with shredded wheat, butter and eggs and spiced with ginger, cinnamon and clove as well as honey [49].

Combines well: In salty dishes with black pepper, chillies, clove, coriander, cumin, garlic, onions, paprika, and soy sauce, and in sweet dishes with cardamom, cinnamon, and citrus fruits.

As a component of spice mixes and preparations: → Chat masala, → Chilli sauce, → Curry powder, → Fish spice, → Five-spice-mix, → Gingerbread spice, → Green masala, → La kama, → Masala, → Pastry spice, → Pickling spice, → Plum jam spice, → Poultry spice, → Quatre épices, → Ras el hanout, → Salsa comum, → Sausage spice, → Scappis spice mix, → Stollen spice, → Tandoori, → Tika paste, → Tomato ketchup, → Tridschataka.

Other uses: Ginger oil is used in the perfume industry as a component of heavy, oriental perfumes, and as a bath additive [30].

Medicinal herb

Herbal drug: Zingiberis rhizoma, Ginger rhizome, contains not less than 15 ml/kg of essential oil [Ph Eur].

Indications: Ginger is used for digestive problems, loss of appetite, nausea, symptoms of motion sickness, nausea following minor surgical procedures and Roemheld's syndrome. The single dose is 0.3 to 1.5 g, and daily dose is 2 to 4 g dried rhizome or equivalent preparations. Preferred dosage forms are powdered rhizome, ginger tincture (20 to 30 drops in some water, one half-hour before meals) or fluidextracts as a component of prepared medicines [8, 27]. For treatment of symptoms of motion sickness, 0.5 to 2 g of powdered ginger is taken 30 minutes before departure time and then every 4 hours another 0.5 to 2 g. Ginger is recommended for nausea and vomiting during the clinical course of cyto-static-therapy [44]. The essential oil can be incorporated in cough ointments.

In folk medicine, ginger tea is used for soothing stomachaches, dysmenorrhea and blood circulation problems. Ginger tincture is applied externally for treatment of rheumatic complaints and for pulled muscles. The essential oil, added to a fatty base (e.g. butter; 5 drops/100 g), is used as an external rub for coughs. Ginger mulled wine (5 slices fresh ginger rhizome, juice of half a lemon, a shot of red wine, honey and hot water) is a home remedy for treatment of influenza infections with moderate fever [49].

Similar culinary spices

Japanese ginger (myoga ginger), *Zingiber mioga* (THUNB.) ROSCOE (Zingiberaceae), native to Japan and China, cultivated in Japan, China and Hawaii, the material of commerce is usually peeled and treated with lime, more pungent than Jamaican ginger, the young leaves and shoots are also used [Ü61].

Martinique ginger (zerumbet ginger, wild ginger), *Zingiber zerumbet* (L.) ROSCOE (Zingiberaceae), is not known in the wild and is cultivated in Sri Lanka, India and Thailand. The essential oil in the rhizome has a race-specific composition with the main components being either zerumbone (ca. 36%, sesquiterpene), α-caryophyllene (humulene, ca. 17%) and camphene (ca. 16%) or α-terpineol (ca. 45%), myrcene (ca. 22%) and γ–terpinene (ca. 10%) [Ü43]. The rhizome is used the same as ginger, especially as a spice in unsweetened rice dishes as well as in fowl- and meat dishes. The leaves are eaten as a vegetable. The essential oil is used in the cosmetics industry [40, 41, Ü61].

Yellow zitwer (also known as Indian ginger or Bengal ginger), *Zingiber cassumunar* ROXB. (*Z. purpureum* ROSCOE, Zingiberaceae), is probably native to India, and is cultivated in many parts of tropical Asia. The main components of the essential oil in the rhizome are sabinene and ter-pinenol-4, and furthermore, among others, α- and β-pinene, myrcene, α-terpinene, limonene, terpinolene and *p*-cymene [32, Ü43]. The rhizome is used the same as ginger [Ü61, Ü92].

Mango ginger, *Curcuma amada* ROXB. (Zingiberaceae), is native to India, and cultivated in India and Pakistan. The rhizome is used similar to ginger and contains ca. 1 to 3% essential oil composed mainly of *ar*-curcumene (ca. 28%), camphor (ca. 11%), β-curcumene (ca. 11%), curzerenone (ca. 7%) and 1,8-cineole (ca. 6%) [45, Ü61].

Ginger Cake Slices
(For the Christmas Holiday season)
250 g butter, 250 g sugar, 6 eggs, 250 g ground hazelnuts, 250 g rubbed bittersweet chocolate, 100 g flour, 100 g finely diced, candied ginger, 250 g confectioner's sugar, juice of one lemon.

Preheat the oven to 180 °C. In a large bowl, mix the butter, sugar and eggs until foamy and continuously add the hazelnuts, bittersweet chocolate and flour; at the end, fold in the ginger. Butter a baking tin with a high rim and spread the cake mixture about 2 cm thick onto it. Bake for 25 min. Before removing from the oven, check with a tooth pick if the cake is done. Cut the cake while still hot into squares or triangular pieces and let them cool. Spread the frosting made from confectioner's sugar and lemon juice evenly over the slices. Before eating, store the ginger cake slices for 1 to 2 weeks in a well-closed tin-box [30].

Literature

[1] Ahmed R.S. et al., Indian J. Exp. Biol. 38(6):604–608 (2000).

[2] Bhandari U. et al., J. Ethnopharmacol. 61(2):167–171 (1998).

[3] Bordia A. et al., Prostaglandins Leukot. Ess. Fatty Acids 56(5):379–384 (1997).

[4] Charles R. et al., Fitoterapia 71(6): 716–718 (2000).

[5] Chen Ch.Ch., Ch.T. Ho, J. Agric. Food Chem. 36:322–328 (1988).

[6] Connell W.D., M.D. Sutherland, Austr. J. Chem. 22:1033–1043 (1969).

[7] Denyer C.V. et al., J. Nat. Prod. 57:658–662 (1994).

[8] ESCOP, ESCOP Monographs Zingiberis rhizoma, Ginger (1996).

[9] Endo K. et al., Phytochemistry 29(3): 797–799 (1990).

[10] Erler I. et al., Z. Lebensm. Unters. Forsch. 186:231–234 (1988).

[11] Falch B. et al., Dtsch. Apoth. Ztg. 137: 4267–4278 (1997).

[12] Fuhrman B. et al., J. Nutr. 130(5):1124–1131 (2000).

[13] Futrell J.M., R.L. Rietschel, Cutis 52(5): 288–290 (1993).

[14] Germer S., G. Franz, Dtsch. Apoth. Ztg. 137:4260–4266 (1997).

[15] Gujral S. et al., Nutr. Rep. Int. 17:183–189 (1978).

[16] Habsah M. et al., J. Ethnopharmacol. 72(3):403–410 (2000).

[17] Harvey D.J., J. Chromatogr. 212:75 (1981).

[18] Huang Q. et al., Chem. Pharm. Bull. 39:397–399 (1991).

[19] Jaspersen-Schib R., Dtsch. Apoth. Ztg. 132(13):621–625 (1992).

[20] Katiyar S.K. et al., Cancer Res. 56(5): 1023–1030 (1996).

[21] Kikuzaki H. et al., Phytochemistry 30(11): 3647–3651 (1991).

[22] Kikuzaki H. et al., Phytochemistry 31(5): 1783–1786 (1992).

[23] Kikuzaki H. et al., Chem. Pharm. Bull. 39(1):120–122 (1991).

[24] Kikuzaki H., N. Nakatani, Phytochemistry 43(1):273–277 (1996).

[25] Kiuchi F. et al., Chem. Pharm. Bull. 40: 387–391 (1992).

[26] Knieriemen H., Natürlich 16(3):39–43 (1996).

[27] Kommission E beim BfArM, BAnz-Nr. 85 vom 05.05.88, Berichtigung am 13.03.90 und am 01.09.90.

[28] Langner E. et al., Balance 1:5–16 (1997).

[29] Lawrence B.M., Perfumer and Flavorist 9:1–40 (1984).

[30] Lorenz B.: Leckere Gerichte mit Ingwer, Mary Hahn Verlag in der FA Herbig Verlagsbuchhandlung, München 1998.

[31] MacLeod A.J., N.M. Pieris, Phytochemistry 23:353–359 (1983).

[32] Masuda T., A. Jitoe, Phytochemistry 39(2):459–461 (1995).

[33] Möllenbeck S. et al., Flavour Fragrance J.12(2):63–69 (1997).

[34] Mustafa T., K.C. Srivastava, J. Ethnopharmacol. 29:267 (1990).

[35] Nair M.K. et al. (Eds.): Processings of the National Seminar on Ginger and Turmeric, Central Plantation Crops Research Institute, Kasaragod, India, 1980, p. 253.

[36] Platel K., K. Srinivasan, Int. J. Food Sci. Nutr. 47(1):55–59 (1996).

[37] Platel K., K. Srinivasan, Nahrung 44(1): 42–46 (2000).

[38] Sakai K. et al., Chem. Pharm. Bull. 37: 215–217 (1989).

[39] Sane R.T. et al., Indian Drugs 35(1):37–44 (1998).

[40] Seidemann J., Drogenreport 13(23):65–68 (2000).

[41] Seidemann J., Dtsch. Lebensm. Rdsch. 89:117–120 (1993).

[42] Sekiwa Y. et al., J. Agric. Food Chem. 48(2):373–377 (2000).

[43] Sharm I. et al., Phytotherapy Res. 10:517–518 (1996).

[44] Sharma S.S. et al., J. Ethnopharmacol. 57(2):93–96 (1997).

[45] Srivastava A.K. et al., J. Ess. Oil Res. 13:63–64 (2001).

[46] Srivastava K.C.T., T. Mustafa, Med. Hypotheses 39:342–348 (1992).

[47] Surh Y., Mutat. Res. 428(1/2):305–327 (1999).

[48] Vimala S. et al., Br. J. Cancer 80(1/2): 110–106 (1999).

[49] Vonarburg B., Natürlich 17(6):61–63 (1997).

[50] Wolf J., Pharm. Ztg. 140:4142 (1995).

[51] Yamahara J. et al., J. Ethnopharmacol. 23:299–304 (1988).

[52] Yamahara J. et al., J. Ethnopharmacol. 13:217–225 (1985).

[53] Yoshikawa M. et al., Chem. Pharm. Bull. 42:1226–1230 (1994).

Literature references identified by Ü can be found in the general listing of books and monographs at the back of this book.

Grains-of-paradise

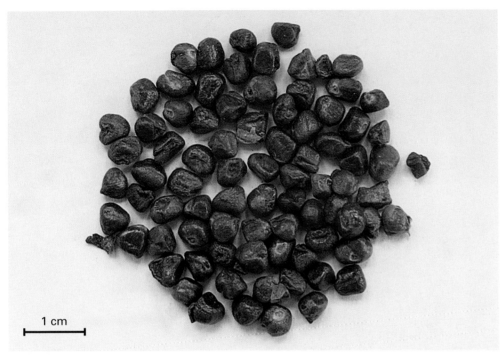

1 cm

Fig. 1: Grains-of-paradise

Plant source: *Aframomum melegueta* (ROSC.) K. SCHUM.

Synonym: *Amomum melegueta* ROSC.

Family: Ginger family (Zingiberaceae).

Common names: Engl.: grains-of-paradise, Guinea pepper, melegueta pepper, alligator pepper; Fr.: maniguette, semance de paradis, graine de maniguette ou de paradis; Ger.: Paradieskörner, Melaguetapfeffer, Meleguetapfeffer, Malaguetapfeffer, Guineakörner, Guinea-Kardamomen, Aligatorpfeffer, and Guinea-pfeffer.

Description: Rhizomatous perennial herb, up to 2 m high, bushy, leaves lanceolate, forming false stems with leaf-sheaths, flowers with large, mauve labellum having a bright yellow fleck, fruit a pear-shaped, large berry with 20 to 25 (possibly up to 100) seeds [2, Ü92].

Native origin: Tropical West Africa (Sierra Leone to Angola).

Main cultivation areas: Ghana, Guinea, Ivory Coast, and Sierra Leone, also frequently cultivated in tropical home gardens.

Main producing countries: Ghana. It is produced only for the local market and is of little importance for world trade.

Cultivation: The plant requires a humid climate and temperatures of at least 15 to 18 °C. It is propagated by rhizome cuttings [5, 6].

Culinary herb

Commercial forms: Grains-of-paradise, dried seeds.

Production: The fruits are collected shortly before ripening; the seeds are removed from the white, bitter fruit flesh and dried.

Forms used: Seeds.

Storage: Protected from light, moisture and insect infestation, in a cool place, in tightly closed glass-, porcelain- or metal containers.

Description: The whole seeds are 2 to 4 mm long, 2 to 3 mm wide, cacao-brown, light brown at the lower end, with small protuberances, hard and shiny; they may have a somewhat turbinate, angled shape due to the pressure in the fruit, and are mostly conically tapered at the stalk of the ovule (funiculus). The cross section is white [Ü60].

Taste: Pepper like, **Odor:** Aromatic, reminiscent of cardamom.

History: Grains-of-paradise was already in use by the ancient Romans. In Central Europe, it was employed as a pepper substitute and for flavoring of wine and beer. Under Elisabeth I, this spice played an important role as a seasoning for foods, wine and beer. Later, it was forgotten in Europe but experienced a renaissance during the World Wars as a pepper substitute (Ger.: "Appetitweizen"). Derived from the German name "Guinea-pfeffer", the Gulf of Guinea is called "Pfefferküste", meaning pepper-coast [1, Ü2].

Constituents and Analysis

Constituents

■ Phenylethyl-*n*-alkyl-ketones (phenylalkanones):
- Gingerols, particularly [6]-gingerol (pungent taste), and [8]-gingerol,
- Shogaols (5-desoxy-4,5-dehydro-gingerols), mostly [6]-shogaol (pungent taste), likely artifacts of the gingerols that arise during storage,
- Paradols (5-desoxy-gingerols): Including [6]-paradol and [8]-paradol, with pungent taste,
- Gingerdiones: [6]-Gingerdione (1-(4´-hydroxy-3´-methoxyphenyl)deca-3,5-dione) [4, Ü43],
- Zingerone (gingerone, see chemical structures → Ginger, artifact of the gingerols) [4].

■ Essential oil: 0.3 to 0.75%, the main components are α- and β-caryophyllene and their epoxides [8].

■ Tannins, starch, fatty oil [Ü60].

Tests for Identity: → Ginger.

Quantitative assay: The volumetric determination of the essential oil content is based on the Ph Eur procedure, using steam distillation and xylol in the graduated tube [Ph Eur].

Actions and Uses

Actions: Due to its essential oil and bitter substances content, it can be taken to promote the secretion of gastric juices and bile and therefore good digestion.
[6]-Paradol and [6]-shogaol, isolated from the dried seeds, have shown good antibiotic activity against various mycobacterium and Candida-species, while zingerone was shown to be inactive. Gram-negative bacteria were not influenced [4]. Extracts of the seeds and especially [6]-gingerol as well as [6]-shogaol have strong antifeedant activity against termites [3].

[6]-Gingerol

[6]-Shogaol

[6]-Paradol

[6]-Gingerdione

Toxicology: A single dose of 0.35 g seeds led to temporary visual impairment (double and blurred vision) in healthy volunteers [7].

Culinary use: Grains-of-paradise are used especially in Moroccan and Tunisian cooking. It is used in a similar manner as pepper, among others, as a seasoning for eggplant fruits, potatoes, braised lamb and fish, furthermore, especially in the UK and the USA, as a flavoring component of beer, wine, strongly aromatic liqueurs, whisky, brandy and of mulled wine [Ü2, Ü55, Ü73, Ü81].

As a component of spice mixes and preparations: → Ras el hanout.

Other uses: It is sometimes used in the perfume industry [Ü60].

Medicinal herb

Herbal drug: Paradisi semen, Grains-of-paradise.

Indications: Used in West African folk medicine as a carminative and diuretic, for the treatment of migraines and rheumatic diseases as well as an aphrodisiac [1].

Other Aframomum-species used as culinary herbs

Grains-of-paradise (alligator pepper), *Aframomum exscapum* (SIMS) HEPPER, native to and grown in tropical Africa, and used in the same way as *Aframomum melegueta* [Ü61].

Cameroon cardamom, see → Cardamom.

Korarima cardamom, see → Cardamom.

Madagascar cardamom, see → Cardamom.

Literature

[1] Anonym, Z. Phytother. 16(5):296 (1995).
[2] Engler A., Die Pflanzenwelt Afrikas, Bd. 2, Verlag von Wilhelm Engelmann, Leipzig; Bd. II, p. 386–387 (1908).
[3] Escoubas P. et al., Phytochemistry 40(4): 1097–1099 (1995).
[4] Galal A.M., Int. J. Pharmacogn. 34(1):64–69 (1996).
[5] Hall J.B., D.K. Abbiw, Econ. Bot. 31:321–330 (1977).
[6] Harten van A.M., Econ. Bot. 24:208–216 (1970).
[7] Igwe S.A. et al., J. Ethnopharmacol. 65(3): 203–206 (1999).
[8] Menut C. et al., Flavour Fragrance 6:183–186 (1991).

Literature references identified by Ü can be found in the general listing of books and monographs at the back of this book.

Hops

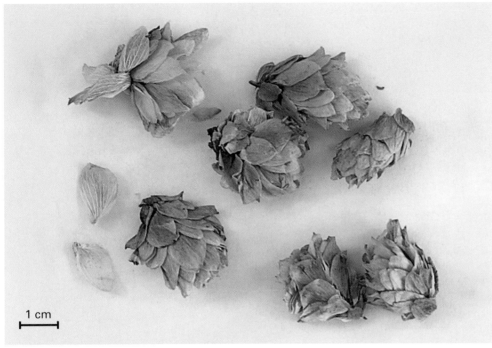

Fig. 1: Hop strobiles

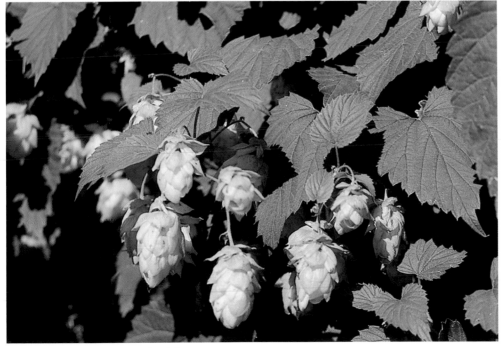

Fig. 2: Hops (*Humulus lupulus* L.)

Plant source: *Humulus lupulus* L.

Taxonomic classification: The species can be subdivided into numerous varieties. These subdivisions, however, are unimportant for the use of hops.

Family: Hemp family (Cannabaceae, synonymous with Cannabinaceae or Cannabidaceae. In older literature, it was assigned to the mulberry family, Moraceae).

Common names: Engl.: hops, hop; Fr. houblon; Ger.: Hopfen, Gemeiner Hopfen.

Description: Hardy, perennial vine, 3 to 6 m (rarely 12 m) long, dioecious, with a deep and robust rhizome from which grow numerous shoots; the rough stalk, is twining to the right, due to numerous hooked hairs. The long-stalked, broadly ovate, mucronate-dentate, opposite arranged leaves are 10 to 15 cm wide, mostly with 3 to 5 (sometimes up to 7) lobes. The male inflorescences are arranged in loose, axillary panicles, with rather inconspicuous flowers, about 3 mm long, with 5 whitish-green perigone leaves and 5 stamina; the female flowers are arranged in dense, spike-like inflorescences on short, side or terminal branches, later developing into characteristic, hanging, ovoid cones (strobiles) in which the flowers are arranged mostly in groups of 4, united in compound cincinni in the axils of a usually absent bract, with cordate stipules, fused forming an up to 2 cm long ovuliferous scale, which during the ripening period turns yellow-brown and becomes covered with glands; the ovary is enclosed in a bowl-like fashion by a prophyll, styles are absent, 2 stigmata, filiform. Flowering period is from July to August.

Native origin: Its origin is unknown (possibly Mongolia), but occurs in the wild as an escape from cultivation in Europe, Central- and Eastern Asia, Australia, and North America.

Main cultivation areas: Cultivated worldwide between the 25th and 55th latitudes, in Germany (especially in Hallertau, as well as Tettnang, Spalt, Hersbruck, Jura, the Elbe-Saale area, Baden/Bitburg/Rheinpfalz), as well as the Czech Republic (Saaz), France (Elsass-Lothringen), Slovakia, Poland, Austria, Belgium, Portugal, Spain, Ukraine, UK, USA, Canada, Chile, India, China, Japan, Australia, New Zealand, and South Africa.

Main exporting countries: Germany (especially Bavaria), the Czech Republic, Slovakia, China, and the USA.

Cultivation: Hops prefer slightly warming sandy-loam or loamy-sand, up to 2 m root permeable soil in an open, south facing position. Only female plants are grown in so-called hop gardens. Propagation is carried out using cuttings from female plants (10 to 18 cm long piece of a shoot from the previous year with 4 to 5 dormant buds, rhizome pieces with several buds or with root pieces). To facilitate climbing, a 6 to 7 m high trellis with wood- or concrete poles connected by wire and cables is used. In March, the hop rhizomes are removed and trimmed. After sprouting, the number of shoots (20 to 100) is reduced to 3 and these are trained to climb the twine. The plant reaches the trestle height during the flowering period at the end of June to the beginning of July. A hop plant is productive for 15 to 20 years [4, Ü21].

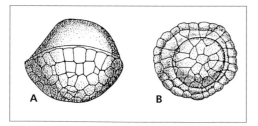

Fig. 3: Hops, glandular trichomes: **A** View from the side, **B** View from the top. From Ü49.

In Germany, aroma cultivars (A-hops) are cultivated, among others, including 'Hallertauer Medium Early', 'Hallertauer Tradition', 'Hersbrucker Late', 'Spalter', 'Tettnanger' and bittering cultivars (B-hops) 'Magnum', 'Northern Brewer', and 'Brewers Gold'. Other cultivars include, among others, the Czech variety 'Saazer', the Slovakian variety 'Savinja Golding', the Polish variety 'Lublin', the Austrian varieties 'Steirischer (Sanntaler)' and 'Malling', the English variety 'Fuggle' and the US variety 'Perle' [4, Ü21].

Culinary herb

Commercial forms: As a spice the dried inflorescences of female plants (hop strobiles) are used. Forms used for medicinal purposes are: hop strobiles, hop glands (hop grains, lupulinic glands, glandular hairs, obtained from hop strobiles by sieving, hop dust, lupulin, and lupulinum) and dry extracts, obtained by extracting hop strobiles or pellets (see below) with methanol or ethanol (30 to 70%) or with supercritical CO_2. For the brewing industry, baled cone hops (bale hops, moderately pressed), "Canned" hops (strongly compressed), powdered hops, and hop pellets (pulverized hop strobiles, often packed under vacuum with bentonite clay added at 20% prior to pelleting), each described according to their content of hop bitter substances (3 to 7% α-acids, 2.5 to 4% β-acids) as A-Hops (aroma hops) and B-Hops (bittering hops), hop soft extract (dark green, viscous consistency, extracted using supercritical CO_2, less often with ethanol, contains ca. 50% α-acids, 7% essential oil, graded according to bitter value), powdered hop extract (30 to 40% silica as carrier), isomerized hop extract (α-acids converted to iso-α-acids) and hop oil (obtained through steam distillation) [4, 15, 28].

Production: Hop strobiles are harvested about 5 weeks after flowering. The vines are cut about 1 to 2 meters above the ground using a so-called bottom cutter, and then the vines are fed into stationary

hop picking machines. The hops are then dried in a hop kiln for 5 to 6 hours at 65 °C with a stream of hot air passing through. After brief (cool) storage, they are packed into pressed bales [4, Ü21, Ü92].

Forms used: Dried inflorescence (hop strobiles), sieved glands (hop grains), and hop extracts which are preferred in the brewing industry.

Storage: In the brewing industry, not longer than 1 year below 10 °C, protected from light and moisture, in well-closed porcelain-, glass- or suitable metal containers. Hop extracts, if sealed properly, have a longer shelf life than the hop strobiles or glands.

Description. Hop strobile (Fig. 1): The ovoid, acuminate hop strobile is 2 to 5 cm long, stalked, consisting of numerous ovate, greenish-yellow, imbricate and scaly stipules and prophylls. The stipules are flattened and symmetrical, the prophylls are asymmetrical due to a furrow at the base of the leaf-like structure. The bases of the stipules and prophylls are covered with small orange-yellow glands [Ph Eur].

Hop glands: An orange-yellow, somewhat sticky powder obtained from hop strobiles by sieving.

Powdered hops: The hop glands are 150 to 250 µm wide, bowl-shaped, consisting of a monolayer of polygonal secretory cells, from which the cuticula is separating, thus forming a blister (Fig. 3). The resinous secretion is soluble in ethanol, ether or chloralhydrate [ÖAB]. In the greenish-yellow powder obtained from the strobile, fragments of the stipules and prophylls with wavy lobed epidermal cells are present, as well as single, cone-shaped covering trichomes with small oxalate druses.

Odor: Agreeable, aromatic, **Taste:** Spicy, weakly bitter, hop glands more intensely bitter; intense odor of isovalerianic acid indicates that the material has been stored for too long.

History: During Greek and Roman antiquity, the young shoots were eaten raw as salads. In the 8th and 9th century, its use as a beer flavoring was first reported in Central Europe. Cultivation since the 11th century near Spaet (Bavaria) and in Bohemia, since the 14th century in Sweden, since the 16th century in England and since the 18th century in North America. The large scale use of hops as a beer flavoring had been established by the beginning of the 19th century [9, Ü61].

Constituents and Analysis

Constituents
- Hop bitter substances (hop resin): 10 to 30% of the hop strobile, and 50 to 80% of the hop glands (methanol and ether extractable). They can be fractionated into:
  - Soft resin (soluble in hexane) consisting of hop bitter acids (α-acids and β-acids) and their breakdown products (e.g. iso-α-acids, lupoxes, lupdoxes) and:
  - Hard resin (insoluble in hexane) consisting of the oxidation products of hop bitter acids (δ acids) and lipophilic flavonoids.

During storage, the proportion of the content of soft resin decreases due to transformation into hard resin. Material that has been stored for longer than 1 year only contains 30 to 50% of the original bitter substances.

The bitter acids from hops are monoacylphloroglucinols with 2 dimethylallyl side chains (α-acids, humulone, 3 to 13% in the strobile) or with 3 dimethylallyl side chains (β-acids, lupulone, 3 to 8%), which differ from each other by the side chain at position 2. The α-acids humulone, cohumulone and adhumulone are intensely bitter, the β-acids lupulone, colupulone and adlupolone are hardly bitter. The hop bitter acids are easily transformed and auto-oxidized to form hexane-insoluble compounds. Upon heating of hop strobiles or extracts thereof (for example during the brewing process), through reduction of the rings of the α-acids cyclopentatrione compounds (iso-α-acids, intensely bitter) arose; the transformation of the β-acids leads to dihydrofuran derivatives, mostly with intact 6-carbon ring (including lupoxes A and B, lupdoxes A, bitter) [17, 22, 28, 34, 59, Ü37].

- Essential oil (hop oil): 0.05 to 1.7% in the strobiles (the monograph Lupuli strobulus of the German commission E requires not less than 0.35%) [33], 1 to 3% in the hop glands; the content strongly depends on the variety, length of storage and storage conditions. The main components are myrcene (25 to 62%), α-caryophyllene (humulene, 3.5 to 42%, high content in aromatic varieties), β-caryophyllene (2.7 to 17%), farnesene (0.1 to 21%) and undecan-2-one (2 to 17%), furthermore, among others, linalool, *trans*-4,5-epoxy-(*E*)-dec-2-enal, 2-methyl-but-3-ene-2-ol, fatty acid (such as acetic, propionic, isobutyric and isovalerianic) esters of aliphatic alcohols, alkenones, cyclic ethers, spiroketals, peroxides, epoxides, peroxy acids and organosulfur compounds, probably to a large extent auto-oxidation products [6, 20, 29, 34, 40, 66]. The content of the main essential oil components can be used to determine

Humulone   (R = – CH$_2$ – CH (CH$_3$)$_2$)
Cohumulone   (R = – CH (CH$_3$)$_2$)
Adhumulone   (R = – CH (CH$_3$) – CH$_2$ CH$_3$)

α-Acids

Lupulone   (R = – CH$_2$ – CH (CH$_3$)$_2$)
Colupulone   (R = – CH (CH$_3$)$_2$)
Adlupulone   (R = – CH (CH$_3$) – CH$_2$ CH$_3$)

β-Acids

Iso-α-acids

Lupoxes A

Xanthohumol   R = OCH$_3$
Desmethylxanthohumol   R = OH

Isoxanthohumol   R = OCH$_3$
8-Prenylnaringenin   R = OH

2-Methyl-3-butene-2-ol

the hop variety [39]. In a German hop variety ("Spalter"), the main odor components were myrcene, linalool and *trans*-4,5-epoxy-(*E*)-dec-2-enal [55]. 2-Methyl-but-3-ene-2-ol, a potentially active constituent, is a decomposition product of the α-acids. It is volatile and remains due to its solubility in water in the water phase after steam distillation. Fresh hops only contain traces (0.02%). Its content increases during storage (after 1 year 0.69%, after 2 years 0.75% and 3 years 0.76%), and later decreases (after 4 years, 0.49%) [20, 21, 28, 48, 70].

- Tannins: In the strobile 2 to 4% oligomeric proanthocyanidins [28].
- Chalcones: Xanthohumol (3´-prenyl-6´-*O*-methylchalconaringenin, at least 0.25%, decreasing upon storage) and desmethylxanthohumol (Fig. 31); race specific are, among others, xanthogalenol, 4´-*O*-methylxanthohumol, 3´-geranylchalconaringenin, α,β-dihydroxyxanthohumol, and iso-dehydrocycloxanthohumolhydrate. The chalcones easily convert (for example during drying, storage or brewing) to the corresponding flavanones, e.g. isoxanthohumol, prenylnaringenins and geranylnaringenins [56].
- Flavonol glycosides: Including astragalin, isoquercitrin, quercitrin, and rutin, among others [12, 54, 57–59].
- Phenylacrylic acids, phenylcarboxylic acids: Such as ferulic acid, caffeic acid, and its esters (chlorogenic acid, neochlorogenic acid), gallic acid and vanillinic acid [59].
- Polysaccharides [35].

Tests for Identity: Based on organoleptic, macroscopic and microscopic examination as well as on TLC [Ü77, Ü102, Ü106, Ph Eur]. Analysis of the flavonoids by TLC [23, PF X], of the essential oil by GC [11, PF X] or SFC-FTIR [2], and of the bitter substances by LC and MEKC [67].

Quantitative assay: Determination of the total resin content by extraction with 70% ethanol [Ph Eur]. The content of bitter substances can be evaluated with TLC [23], HPLC [5, 10, 18, 22, 26, 44] or micro-

LC as well as MEKC [67], and the xanthohumol content with HPLC [22]. Essential oil determination with steam distillation and xylol in the graduated tube [PF X]; qualitative analysis of its components with GC or GC/MS [11, 40]. For a GC-assay of 2-methyl-but-3-ene-2-ol, see [20].

Adulterations, Misidentifications and Impurities: Possible with hop strobiles from wild collection, which are recognizable by their lower content of extractives. Seeds must be absent; they indicate that the material originated from the wild.

Actions and Uses

Actions: Due to the bitter-aromatic taste, hops are appetite stimulating and digestion promoting. Hops stimulate the secretion of gastric juice [62].

In isolated rabbit- and guinea pig intestines and in rat uterus, an ethanolic hop extract (1 g hop strobiles/10 ml 70% ethanol, 0.001 ml/ml organ bath) produced a strong spasmolytic effect [7].

For the sedative effect of hops, there are positive results from animal experiments [68]. Intraperitoneal administration of 250 or 500 mg/kg body weight of a commercially available extract of hop strobile (extraction solvent and drug-to-extract ratio not declared), 30 minutes before each test, dose-dependently reduced motor activity of mice in the trailing wheel by 59% and 65%, respectively. The time to onset of convulsion, caused by administration of pentylenetetrazole (100 mg/kg body weight, i.p.), was significantly lengthened. The sleeping time after administration of pentobarbital (35 mg/kg body weight, i.p.) was dose-dependently increased. The authors postulated that hops have sedative and hypnotic action. Additionally, there were indications that hops have anticonvulsant, antinociceptive and hypothermic properties [37]. Ethanolic extracts of hop strobile have shown motility inhibiting action in mice, however aqueous extracts and hop oil (1 mg/kg body weight, i.p.) have not [38]. In a randomized, double blind, placebo-controlled

clinical study, a sleep-promoting and sedative effect of hop baths (hop extract 1%, 100 ml thereof in 100 liter warm bath water) was demonstrated [49]. 2-Methyl-3-butene-2-ol (0.8 g/kg body weight, i.p.), isolated from the volatile fraction of hop strobile, produced narcosis in mice for about 8 hours [21, 70, 71]. In rats, this substance (ca. 0.2 g/kg body weight, i.p.) had a motility-depressant effect of about 50%, which after 3 hours reached its maximum and after 9 hours subsided [69-71]. Because the dosage levels of 2-methyl-3-butene-2-ol that are necessary to produce a sedative effect in animal tests are so high, and because hop strobiles contain only a small amount of this compound, it alone cannot explain the sedative effect of hops. It is conceivable, however, that humans are more sensitive to the agent than mice and/or that lupulone metabolizes into 2-methyl-3-butene-2-ol in the human body after oral ingestion of hops [69].

In contrast to the above-mentioned results, no sedative effect was observed in humans following oral administration of hop glands (5×250 mg), α-acids (50 mg), β-acids (40 mg), hop oil (8 mg) or bitter substances isolated from beer (60 mg) [60]. Also, ethanolic hop extracts or lupulone (10 to 100 mg/kg body weight), applied orally by gavage in rats and mice, had no influence on motor activity and did not potentiate the activity of barbiturates [24]. Hop strobiles presumably have estrogenic activity [32, 46]. In the receptor-binding test, hops were bound to the calf uterine cytoplasmatic receptor. High binding activity was observed especially in cases where the hops were harvested at the end of the growth period (September) [24, 27]. Flavonoid-containing extracts of hop strobile elevated specifically the activity of estrogen-dependent alkaline phosphatase of a human endometrium adenocarcinoma line. Through activity-guided fractionation, 8-prenylnaringenin was found to have a high binding affinity to estrogen receptors from rat uteri [41]. The other prenyl- or the geranyl- naringenin derivatives, the chalcones and hop acids had no activity [31, 42]. The concentration of active constituents with estrogenic activity in hops (1.5 to 4.8 ng/g estradiol-β17-equivalent) is so low that no estrogenic effect can be expected from taking hops within the therapeutic dosage range or by drinking beer. In order to achieve an estrogenic effect comparable to the effective oral daily dose of about 2 mg estradiol-β17, one would have to consume about 400 kg of hop strobiles or 1,000 liters of beer [50]. Some other authors have found no estrogenic activity in hops [13].

Humulone has antiphlogistic action in the ear edema in mouse test. It inhibited activity against 12-O-tetradecanoylphorbol-13-acetate (TPA)-induced inflammation and arachidonic acid- induced inflammation, and the tumor-promoting effect of TPA on skin (1 µg/mouse) [72].

Hop extracts, hop oil or other isolated components (especially *trans*-isohumulone) have shown antimicrobial activity against gram-positive bacteria and some fungi, but not against yeast [8, 36, 51-53, 63].

Up to this point, there are only in vitro data available showing that xanthohumol inhibits osteoclasts and through it bone resorption [65], its cytotoxic effect on tumor cells [43, 64], its inhibitory effect on the induction of enzymes which activate carcinogens [25] and on the activity of diacylglycerol-acyltransferase [61].

Toxicology: Based on existing data, there is no acute or chronic toxicity with the normal use of hops by healthy individuals [1]. The LD_{50} value in animal tests (3.5 g ethanolic hop extract/kg body weight mouse, p.o.) is many times higher than the usual dose humans are exposed to when consuming hops as a flavoring or herbal remedy [24]. The ingestion of large amounts of hop glands or hop extracts can lead to symptoms such as headache, loss of appetite and bradycardia. Even staying in hop storage facilities can lead to symptoms of hop exposure. Intense contact with the fresh (!) strobile can lead to "hop picker's syndrome", which is characterized by headache, somnolence, conjunctivitis, blistering of the skin and joint aches (possibly due to percutaneous absorption of lipophilic hop constituents and inhalation

of the essential oil). Eye contact with hop constituents can lead to conjunctivitis.

The sensitization potential is moderate. Symptoms of an allergic reaction are particularly contact dermatitis, sometimes with blisters. Case reports in [30, 41, 45, 47, Ü58].

Culinary use: The volatile compounds of hops serve as flavor components of cheese (hop cheese, matured between layers of hops: Nieheimer cheese, Lüdger cheese, Westphalia herb cheese) [Ü98].

The young shoot tips and leaves of hops are eaten raw in salads or blanched in soups or as a vegetable, especially in Belgium and France. The secondary shoots (see below) that are thinned out in the hop gardens from March to April are consumed similar to green asparagus salad, rounded off with hollandaise sauce, vinaigrette or mayonnaise. As a delicacy, the shoots are baked in beer batter or filled in pancakes [Ü1, Ü45, Ü98].

Its primary area of use is in the brewery industry. Hops give beer a pleasant, aromatic taste, extend the shelf life (antibacterial action, precipitation of the protein) and increase its foaming stability. Today, brewers mostly use standardized hop extracts, obtained by high-pressure extraction with supercritical CO_2 (although not permitted for German Pilsner Special and strong light beer (Märzen)).

Other uses: Hop extracts are used in skin cosmetics and bath products due to their postulated "skin-stretching" effects [Ü24]. The odor compounds of hops are also employed in the perfume industry. The fibers of the shoots can be used as a raw material for crude textiles and ropes.

Medicinal herb

Herbal drugs: Lupuli flos, Hop strobile, contains minimum 25% matter extractable by alcohol (70 per cent V/V) [Ph Eur], Lupuli glandula, Hop glands, contain minimum 70% matter extractable by ether [ÖAB].

Indications: For health disorders such as nervousness, restlessness and states of anxiety as well as difficulty falling asleep. Single-dose for oral administration is 0.5 g of hop strobile. Hops are taken in the form of powdered strobiles, tea infusions (1 to 2 teaspoonfuls hop strobile in 150 ml hot water, 2 to 4 times daily) or aqueous-ethanolic extracts (1 to 2 ml tincture, 1:5, 60% ethanol, 1 to 3 times daily). Although there are no data available on the safety during pregnancy, according to the usual practices its use should be avoided by pregnant women [1, 33]. Dry extracts, produced with methanol, ethanol or water, and usually at high temperatures, do not contain all of the typical hop constituents. The efficacy of these extracts has not been substantiated. Therefore therapeutic use of supercritical CO_2 extracts should be preferred [15]. Additionally, the tea infusion of the dried strobiles is used to stimulate the appetite and to increase the secretion of gastric juice due to its bitter action [Ü106]. Hop pillows and baths (with the addition of hop extracts) are used to promote sleep (volatility of 2-methyl-3-butene-2-ol, possibly via percutaneous absorption?). Hops have been prescribed for sexual neuroses in men (possible estrogenic effects?) [14, 16].

Hop glands are used mainly in the form of a 30% ointment for the treatment of poorly healing wounds and ulcers.

Literature

[1] Anonym, ESCOP Monographs: Lupuli flos, Hop. Strobile (1997).

[2] Auerbach R.H. et al., J. Assoc. Off. Anal. Chem. Int. 83(3):621–626 (2000).

[3] Bravo L. et al., Boll. Chim. Farm. 113(5): 310–305 (1974).

[4] Breitner G., Z. Phytother. 13(5):151–154 (1992).

[5] Buckee G.K., C.D. Baker, J. Inst. Brew. 93:468–471 (1987).

[6] Buttery R.G., Chem. and Ind.: 1225–1226 (1966).

[7] Caujolle F. et al., Agressologie 10:405–409 (1969).

[8] Cookson J.S., A. Lawton, Brit. med. J. 2:376–379 (1953).

[9] Czygan F.C., Z. Phytother. 13(5):141–150 (1992).

[10] Daud I.S., S. Kusinski, J. Inst. Brew. 92:559–567 (1986).

[11] Eri S. et al., J. Agric. Food Chem. 48(4):1140–1149 (2000).

[12] Etteldorf et al., Z. Naturforsch. C 54(7/8):610–612 (1999).

[13] Fenselau C., P. Talalayl, Cosmet. Toxicol. 11:597–603 (1973).

[14] Fintelmann V., Z. Phytother. 13(5):165–168 (1992).

[15] Forster A., Z. Phytother. 13(5):162 (1992).

[16] Ganzer B.M., Pharm. Ztg. 137(38):2894–2898 (1992).

[17] Giedraityte G. et al., Biologija 1996(1):69–73 (1996), ref. CA 126:198729f.

[18] Hann J.T., Chromatographia 24:510–512 (1987).

[19] Hänsel R. et al., Planta Med. 45:224–228 (1982).

[20] Hänsel R. et al., Z. Naturforsch. 35c:224–228 (1980).

[21] Hänsel R. et al., Z. Naturforsch. 35c:1096–1097 (1980).

[22] Hänsel R., J. Schulz, Dtsch. Apoth. Ztg. 126:2033–2037 (1986).

[23] Hänsel R., J. Schulz, Dtsch. Apoth. Ztg. 126:2347–2348 (1986).

[24] Hänsel R., H.H. Wagener, Arzneim. Forsch. 17:79–81 (1967).

[25] Henderson M.C. et al., Xenobiotica 30(3): 235–251 (2000).

[26] Hermans-Lokkerbol A.C.J., R. Verpoorte, J. Chromatogr. A 669:65–73 (1994).

[27] Hesse R. et al., Zbl. Vet. Med. A 28:442–454 (1981).

[28] Hölzl J., Z. Phytother. 13(5):155–161 (1992).

[29] Jahnsen V.J., J. Inst. Brew. 69:460 (1963).

[30] Jirasek L. et al., Acta Univ. Carol. Med. Suppl. 10:539 (1960).

[31] Keukeleire De D. et al., Pharm. Pharmacol. Lett. 7(2/3):83–86 (1997).

[32] Koch W., G. Heim, Münch. Med. Wschr. 95:845 (1953).

[33] Kommission E beim BfArM, BAnz 228 vom 05.12.1984, Berichtigung 13.03. 1990.

[34] Krofta K. et al., Kvasny Prum. 42(7–8):237–240 (1996), ref. CA 125:326932k.

[35] Kumai A., R. Okamoto, Toxicol. Lett. 21:203–207 (1984).

[36] Langezaal C.R. et al., Pharm. Weekbl. Sci. 14(6):353–356 (1992).

[37] Lee K.M. et al., Planta Med. 59(7, Suppl): A691 (1993).

[38] Löffelholz K., ZYMA-Symposium, München, Symposiumsbericht ZYMA GmbH, München, S. 63-72 (1978).

[39] Maier J., Hopfen-Rundschau 278 (1978).

[40] Malizia R.A. et al., J. Ess. Oil Res. 11:13–15 (1999).

[41] Milligan S.R. et al., J. Clin. Endocrinol. Metab. 84(6):2249–2252 (1999).

[42] Milligan S.R. et al., J. Clin. Endocrinol. Metab. 85(12):4912–4915 (2000).

[43] Miranda C.L. et al., Food Chem. Toxicol. 37(4):152–158 (1999).

[44] Narziss L., L. Scheller, Monatsschr. Brauwiss. 37:496–504 (1984).

[45] Newmark F.M., Ann. Allergy 41:311–312 (1978).

[46] Okamoto R., A. Kumai, Acta Endocrinol. 127:371–377 (1992).

[47] Raith L., K. Jäger, Contact Dermatitis 11:53 (1984).

[48] Rode J. et al., 46th Ann. Congress of the Soc. for Med. Plant Res. 1998 Vienna, Abstracts, D04.

[49] Rosen van M. et al., Z. Phytother. 16(5, Suppl.):26.

[50] Sauerwein H., Meyer H.H.D., Monatsschr. Brauwiss. 50(7/8):142–146 (1997).

[51] Schmalreck A.F., M. Teuber, Can. J. Microbiol. 21:205–212 (1974).

[52] Simpson W.J., A.R.W. Smith, J. Appl. Bacteriol. 72:327–334 (1992).

[53] Smith N.A., P. Smith, J. Inst. Brew. 99:43 (1993).

[54] Song-San S. et al., Phytochemistry 28(6):1776 (1989).

[55] Steinhaus M., P. Schieberle, Food Chem. 48(5):1776–1783 (2000).

[56] Stevens J.F. et al., J. Agric. Food Chem. 47(6):2421–2428 (1999).

[57] Stevens J.F. et al., Phytochemistry 53(7):759–775 (2000).

[58] Stevens J.F. et al., Phytochemistry 44(8):1575–1585 (1997).

[59] Stevens R., Chem. Rev. 67:19–71 (1967).

[60] Stocker H., Schweiz Brau. Rundsch. 78:80 (1967).

[61] Tabata N. et al., Phytochemistry 46(4):683–687 (1997).

[62] Tamasdan S. et al., Farmacia (Bucharest) 29:71–75 (1981).

[63] Teuber M., Applied Microbiology 19:871 (1970).

[64] Tobe H. et al., Biosc. Biotechnol. Biochem. 61:1027–1029 (1997).

[65] Tobe H. et al., Biosc. Biotechnol. Biochem. 61(1):158–159 (1997).

[66] Tressl R. et al., Agric. Food Chemistry 26:1426–1430 (1978).

[67] Verschuere M. et al., J. Chromatogr. Sci. 30(10):388–391 (1992).

[68] Wohlfahrt R., Beiträge zum Nachweis sedativhypnotischer Wirkstoffe in *Humulus lupulus* L., Dissertation FU Berlin 1982.

[69] Wohlfahrt R. et al., Monatsschr. Brauwiss. 34:430, 432 (1981).

[70] Wohlfahrt R. et al., Arch. Pharm. 315:132–137 (1982).

[71] Wohlfart R. et al., Planta Med. 48:120–123 (1983).

[72] Yasukawa K. et al., Oncology 52:156–158 (1995).

Literature references identified by Ü can be found in the general listing of books and monographs at the back of this book.

Horseradish

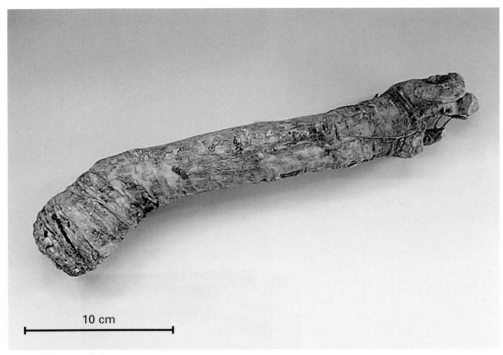

Fig. 1: Horseradish root

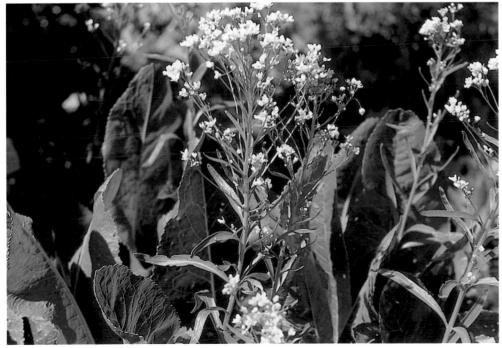

Fig. 2: Horseradish (*Armoracia rusticana* Ph. Gaertn., B. Mey. et Scherb.)

Plant source: *Armoracia rusticana* Ph. Gaertn., B. Mey. et Scherb.

Synonyms: *Armoracia lapathifolia* Usteri, *Cochlearia armoracia* L.

Family: Mustard family (Brassicaceae, synonym Cruciferae).

Common names: Engl.: horseradish; Fr.: cran, mérédic, cranson, raifort sauvage; Ger.: Meerrettich, Kren, Chren, Krien, Koren, Pfefferwurzel, Pferderettich, Bauernsenf.

Description: Perennial herb with a thick, cylindrical and fleshy, up to 60 cm long root bearing multiple, enlarged root crowns and underground stolons. In the first year, the plant produces only basal rosette-leaves, 30 to 100 cm in length, with a long petiole, leaf blade slightly wavy, oblong-ovate, cordate at the base, with an unevenly crenate margin; in the second year, several, up to 1.5 m high, hollow, angular and furrowed, glabrous stalks emerge, branched in the upper part. The leaves on the stalks are lanceolate, short-petiolate or sessile, broadly crenate to pectinate-pinnatifid. The multiflorous inflorescences are composed of numerous racemes. The 4 erect, patulous sepals are 2.5 to 3 mm long, the white petals are 4.5 to 7 mm long; 2 short and 4 long stamina are present, the ovary is superior, and the small fruit is a 4 to 6 mm long silicule. The smooth seeds are usually sterile. Flowering period is from May to July [19, Ü37].

Native origin: Probably native to southern Russia and eastern Ukraine, today it is growing wild throughout most of Europe, and has been naturalized in other continents.

Main cultivation areas: Cultivated in almost all temperate zones, mostly on a small-scale. In Germany it is grown in Upper Franconia, Thuringia, and Spreewald.

Main exporting countries: Austria, Poland, and the Russian Federation.

Cultivation: Horseradish is usually cultivated as an annual and needs deep, humus, and medium-heavy soil with a good water supply. Propagation is carried out from the beginning of April through the beginning of May with lateral roots (root cuttings) obtained from the previous year's cultivation, which must be at least 1 cm in size and 20 to 30 cm long (planted at intervals of about 70×15 cm). In June or July, the roots are uncovered again and the new side roots and side shoots that have formed are rubbed off to minimize branching. When growing horseradish for personal use, take note when purchasing root cuttings that they have been cut with a slanting cut on the lower end and a straight cut on the top. Once planted in the garden, it is nearly ineradicable. In order to prevent the plant from spreading, horseradish should be planted in a buried, open-bottom container with a diameter of 60 to 80 cm and about 1 m deep. There are no cultivars in existence. The individual growing regions have their own selections, e.g. Bavarian, Austrian, Styrian choice, Edelkofener and Nederlinger [2, Ü21, Ü96].

Culinary herb

Commercial forms: Horseradish: the fresh roots (rods, often shrink wrapped), furthermore conserves with various preparations of the grated, fresh roots, marinated roots, root juice, the ground and dried roots, furthermore essential oil of horseradish.

Production: Horseradish is harvested in the autumn after the leaves die off or in the following spring with a specialized plow (horseradish plow) or a shaker sieve digger. Then the small roots are cut off and

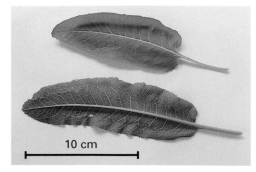

Fig. 3: Horseradish leaves

the main root cleaned by hand. For the production of grated horseradish root, the small roots can also be used [2, Ü21].

Forms used: The grated fresh root, the powder or dried root, pasty conserves of the grated root, and the fresh young leaves.

Storage: Horseradish roots harvested in late fall (October/November) can be stored at –2 °C wrapped in foil for up to 2 years. Roots that have been harvested earlier or were stored above 0 °C lose their pungent taste rapidly. In the past, the roots were covered with wet sand and stored in a cool cellar for later consumption. They can also be sliced and pickled in wine vinegar or grated before storage in the deep freezer.

Description. Whole root (Fig. 1): Up to 60 cm long and up to 6 cm thick, cylindrical roots, mostly with transverse striations and multiple root crowns at the top; gray-yellow outer surface and, visible in the cross section, a broad, white cortex enclosing a yellowish xylem. For a description of the leaves (Fig. 3), see plant description.

Odor: Pungent upon rubbing, **Taste:** Extremely pungent and burning when chewed.

History: Horseradish was probably first cultivated during antiquity. The cultivation in Central Europe has been documented since the 12th century. Since the 16th century, horseradish has been extensively grown in gardens [Ü92].

Constituents and Analysis

Constituents

▪ Glucosinolates (slightly bitter tasting): 0.2 to 0.6%, the main compounds are sinigrin (about 0.15%) and gluconasturtiin (about 0.1%). Other glucosinolates, occurring in smaller amounts include, among others, glucobrassicanapin (4-pentenylglucosinolate) and the 3-indolylmethylglucosinolates glucobrassicin, 4-methoxyglucobrassicin and 4-hydroxybrassicin. Upon tissue damage, the glucosinolates come into contact with the enzyme myrosinase that is located in the myrosine-cells, and thereby, the alkyl- or alkarylisothiocyanates (mustard oil) are formed (see Fig. 12 in the General Section 2.3.2). From sinigrin, the readily volatile, pungent smelling and hot tasting allylisothiocyanate (allyl mustard oil, 21 to 55%, with lacrimatory action) is formed; gluconasturtein transforms into 2-phenylethylisothiocyanate (2-phenylethylmustard oil, 15 to 40%) and glucobrassicanapin into 4-pentenylisothiocyanate. The glucobrassicins do not yield stable isothiocyanates; later ones transform

N=C=S Allylisothiocyanate

H₃C—N=C=S Methylisothiocyanate

N=C=S Ethylisothiocyanate

N=C=S 2-Phenylethylisothiocyanate

N=C=S Isopropylisothiocyanate

N=C=S Pent-4-enylisothiocyanate

N=C=S sec.-Butylisothiocyanate

into the corresponding 3-hydroxy-methylindole derivatives and rhodanide. Other isothiocyanates, which have been detected at lower levels, are methyl-, ethyl-, isopropyl-, and sec.-butylisothiocyanate (2-butylisothiocyanate). Based on older references, allyl mustard oil in horseradish can react, probably enzymatically catalyzed, with water to form diallylthiouric acid and the strongly active antibiotic compound carbonyl sulfide [6, 9, 11, 18, Ü100]. The leaves of the horseradish plant only contain low amounts of glucosinolates.

- Ascorbic acid (Vitamin C): About 0.6% [Ü37].
- Flavonoids: Including, among others, quercetin, kaempferol and 3-O-[2-O-(β-D-xylopyranosyl)-β-galactopyranosyl)] derivatives of these aglycones [10, 15, Ü43].

Tests for Identity: Sensoric, macroscopic and microscopic analysis as well as TLC of the glucosinolates and, after fermentation, of the steam-distilled mustard oils [Ü101].

Quantitative assay: The content of glucosinolates can be determined with HPLC [1], or, in form of desulfoglucosinolates, with HPLC or GLC [9]; the mustard oils, obtained after fermentation, are assayed with GC [7, 13].

Actions and Uses

Actions: Due to its pungent taste, horseradish causes a reflex action that stimulates the secretion of saliva, gastric juice and bile fluid, and therefore is an appetite and digestion promotion stimulant. Extracts of horseradish have shown spasmolytic action in animal experiments [17]. The volatile constituents have antimicrobial action [8, 12]. Following oral administration of 10 to 25 g of grated horseradish, substances excreted in the urine inhibited the growth of *Bacillus subtilis*, *Escherichia coli* and *Staphylococcus aureus* [20]. Due to its skin irritant effect, grated horseradish, when applied externally, led to an increase of skin blood circulation.

Toxicology: Based on existing data, there is no chronic or acute toxicity in healthy individuals with the normal use of the roots. Due to the skin- and mucous membrane-irritating effects of the mustard oils, the intake of higher doses can lead to irritation of the stomach, kidneys and urinary tract in sensitive individuals. Therefore, horseradish should not be used in cases of gastric and intestinal ulcers and inflammatory kidney disease. Intense skin contact can lead to irritations, and to inflammation with prolonged exposure. Workers in the horseradish processing industry showed symptoms such as lacrimation, headaches, coughing, exhaustion and symptoms of irritation of the mucous membranes [Ü58, Ü100].

Culinary use: In Germany, and abroad, horseradish serves as a typical German cooking spice. It reached France through the Alsatian population ("moutarde des allemands"). It is used predominantly in southern Germany and Austria, and also to a lesser extent in the cooking of many other European regions.

Used are the fresh, peeled roots, which have been grated or preferably, cut in a blender (to protect against eye irritation), as well as pasty horseradish root preparations or the dry powder. Upon grating of the horseradish root, not only the glucosinolates are split moreover the phenolic compounds come into contact with peroxidases and oxidation- and polymerization reactions result in the formation of brown products. The discoloration can be slowed down by slight acidification with lemon juice or vinegar. Due to the rapid volatility of the mustard oil, one should grate horseradish shortly before use and then add it to the dish, when it is table ready and cooled down. One can also place grated horseradish on the table, mixed with sweet cream and some lemon juice (or sweet vinegar) for self-service. Dry horseradish products must be soaked in luke-warm (fermentation!) water prior to use. Grated horseradish is used, often as a side dish, slightly acidified with lemon juice and its taste is softened by the addition of cream, sour cream, quark, yogurt and/or grated apples.

Horseradish root serves as a spice in meat dishes, especially of roast beef, soured boiled rump, mutton, marinated beef, game and tongue, of fish dishes, e.g. carp, mackerel, tuna fish or tench, of smoked fish, e.g. trout or salmon, of oysters, ham, cold cuts, cold meats, hard boiled eggs, small sausages, mashed potatoes, Thuringian dumplings, potatoes baked in aluminum foil, of piquant sauces or dips for fish, poultry or vegetables, of chicken-, red beet-, tomato- and potato salads, mayonnaise, quark, fresh- or cottage cheese as well as a filling for avocados. In Scandinavia, people make a cranberry-horseradish cream as an extender for game [Ü20, Ü23, Ü30, Ü47, Ü56, Ü59, Ü63, Ü66, Ü68, Ü79, Ü92, Ü97, Ü107, Ü108].

Commercially available, table-ready, grated horseradish usually also contains table salt, sugar, vinegar, citric acid, cream and spices [Ü98].

Horseradish cut into slices serves as an added ingredient for pickling cucumbers, red beets and mixed pickles.

Young horseradish leaves can be added to salads. In Russia they are also added to pickled mushrooms or pickled cucumbers and tomatoes [Ü81].

Combines well with: Bay leaf, chives, clove, garlic, mint, onions, and pepper.

As a component of spice mixes and preparations: → Horseradish mustard, → Horseradish vinegar, → Meat spice, → Moscow Horseradish (made from horseradish, red beets, salt, vinegar, sugar, and spices), → Pickling spice, → Table mustard.

Medicinal herb

Herbal drug: Amoraciae rusticanae radix, Horseradish root, fresh or dried.

Indications: Horseradish is taken internally for catarrhs of the respiratory tract and for supportive therapy for infections of the lower urinary tract (average daily dose is 20 g for the fresh root, or equivalent preparations, e.g. fresh pressed plant juice). Externally, it is applied for catarrhs of the respiratory tract and as a hyperemic treatment for mild muscle pains (preparations containing maximum 2% mustard oils). Horseradish should not be used by patients with gastric- and intestinal ulcers and inflammations of the kidneys, nor by children under 4 years of age [14].

Similar spice herbs

Meadow horseradish, *Armoracia sisymbrioides* (DC.) CAJAND., native to western and eastern Siberia to Sakhalin Island, where it is cultivated in gardens and used in the same way as horseradish [Ü61].

Wasabi (Japanese horseradish), *Wasabia japonica* (MIQ.) MATSUM. (*Eutrema wasabi* (SIEB.) MAXIM., Brassicaceae) is native to and cultivated in Japan (especially in Honshu). From the glucosinolates that it contains, 10 volatile mustard oils can be formed, of which the main component is allyl mustard oil [13]. The rhizomes have an apple green flesh. They are grated raw or used in dry powdered form as a spice in traditional Japanese dishes, especially meals prepared with raw fish (sashimi, sushi). The dry powder is stirred in luke-warm (!) water and the resulting mash is left to stand for about 10 minutes (fermentation). The paste can be used not only for sushi and sashimi, but also as a component of grill sauces or salad marinades in a mayonnaise base and as a spice of fish- and meat dishes (added after cooking is finished) [Ü55, Ü61].

Horseradish tree, *Moringa oleifera* LAM. (*M. pterygosperma* GAERTN., Moringaceae), an up to 10 m high tree, native to northern India, cultivated especially in subtropical countries of Asia and Africa, but also in Central America. The main constituents of the root are glucosinolates: Glucotropaeolin, which, following damage to tissue, forms benzyl mustard oil (0.05% benzylisothiocyanate), and 4-[(4'-α-rhamnosyloxy)benzyl]glucosinolate is formed from 4[(α-L-rhamnosyloxy)benzyl]-isothiocyanate. The latter glucosinolate is also found in the seeds (0.9%, up to 9% in the defatted seeds). The leaves contain the glycosides 4-[(4'-O-acetyl-α-rhamnosyloxy)benzyl]isothiocyanate, niaziminine A and niaziminine B, furthermore the nitrilglycosides niazirine, niazirinine and niazidine, the thiocarbamates niazine A, niazine B and niazimicine, nitrile esters, carbamates and polysulfide sulfinates [3–5, 16, Ü43]. Primarily the roots are used as a spice in the same way as horseradish. The fruits, which are up to 45 cm long and up to 2.5 cm thick, with up to 20 triangular, pea-sized, black- to gray brown seeds with 3 paper thin, white wings, are eaten in the form of salads and curries. The seeds are the source of the so-called oil of ben (fatty oil). The leaves, flowers and young fruits are also used as vegetables [Ü61, Ü92].

> **Baked potatoes in aluminum foil with horseradish butter**
> (Serves 6).
> 6 large potatoes, salt, 50 g fresh horseradish, 1 to 2 teaspoons lemon juice, 1 bundle of dill, 150 g butter, freshly ground pepper, Worcestershire sauce.
>
> Wash the potatoes thoroughly by scrubbing them with a brush under running tap water and parboil them unpeeled in salt water for 20 minutes. Finely grate the horseradish and add a few drops of lemon juice. Chop the dill and mix one teaspoon with the horseradish and butter; season with salt, pepper and Worcestershire sauce. In aluminum foil, form the butter into a roll and place it for 15 minutes in the deep freezer. Wrap the potatoes individually in aluminum foil and bake them in the pre-heated oven at 200 °C for 20 to 25 minutes. Take the butter out of the foil, roll it in the remaining dill and cut it into 12 slices. Open the foil of the potatoes a bit and make a criss-cross incision, then slightly squeeze them. Serve them with 2 butter slices for each potato [Ü95].

Literature

[1] Betz J.M., S.W. Page, Planta Med. 56: 590–591 (1990).
[2] Bomme U., Kulturanleitung für Meerrettich, Heil- und Gewürzpflanzen 44, Merkblätter für Pflanzenbau, LBP Freising (1988).
[3] Faizi S. et al., J. Nat. Prod. 57(9): 1256–1261 (1994).
[4] Faizi S. et al., Planta Med. 64(3):225–228 (1998).
[5] Faizi Sh. et al., J. Nat. Prod. 60(12): 1317–1321 (1997).
[6] Gilbert J., H.E. Nursten, J. Sci. Food Agric. 23:527–539 (1972).
[7] Grob K., P. Matile, Phytochemistry 19: 1778–1789, 1789–1793 (1980).
[8] Halbeisen T., Arzneim. Forsch. 7:321–324 (1957).
[9] Hrncirik K., J. Velisek, Potravin. Vedy 15(3):161–172 (1997), ref. CA 127: 217829c.
[10] Hrncirik K. et al., Z. Lebensm. Unters. Forsch. A 206:103–107 (1997).
[11] Isaac O., E. Kohlstaedt, Arch. Pharmaz. 295:165–173 (1962).
[12] Kienholz M., Arzneim. Forsch. 13:768–771, 920–926, 980–986, 1109–1116 (1963).
[13] Kojima M. et al., J. Pharm. Soc. Japan. 93:453–459 (1973).
[14] Kommission E beim BfArM, BAnz-Nr. 85 vom 05.05.1988.
[15] Melchior Larsen L, et al., Phytochemistry 21:1029–1033 (1982).
[16] Murakami A. et al., Planta Med. 64(4): 319–323 (1998).
[17] Peichev P. et al., Eksperim. Med. Morfol. 5:47–5 (1966), zit. bei Ü37.
[18] Schildknecht H., G. Rauch, Naturforsch. B 17:800–803 (1962).
[19] Weymar H., Buch der Kreuzblütler, Neumann Verlag, Leipzig-Radebeul 1988.
[20] Winter A., M. Hornbostel, Naturwissenschaften 40:489–490 (1953).

Literature references identified by Ü can be found in the general listing of books and monographs at the back of this book.

Hyssop

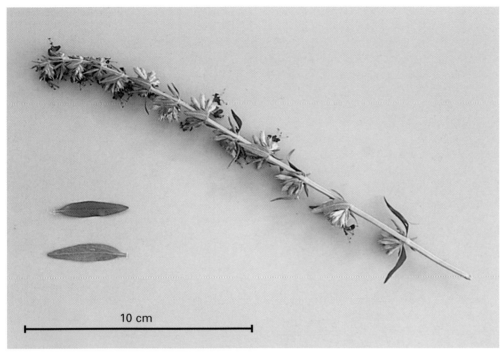

Fig. 1: Hyssop shoot tips and hyssop leaves

Plant source: *Hyssopus officinalis* L.

Taxonomic classification: *Hyssopus officinalis* L. ssp. *officinalis* is the main cultivated subspecies with the following varieties:
Hyssopus officinalis L. ssp. *officinalis* var. *angustifolius* (BIEB.) BENTH.,
Hyssopus officinalis L. ssp. *officinalis* var. *vulgaris* BENTH.,
Hyssopus officinalis L. ssp. *officinalis* var. *decussatus* PERS.
Furthermore, the following subspecies occur, among others:
Hyssopus officinalis L. ssp. *canescens* (DC.) BRIQ. (France, Spain),
Hyssopus officinalis L. ssp. *montanus* (JORDAN et FOURR.) BRIQ. (France),
Hyssopus officinalis L. ssp *aristatus* (GODR.) BRIQ. (France, Spain, Balkan countries).

Family: Mint family (Lamiaceae, synonym Labiatae).

Common names: Engl.: hyssop; Fr.: hysope; Ger.: Ysop, Isop, Eisop, Josefskraut, Joseph.

Description: Subshrub with strong, multi-headed taproot and tetragonal branches, up to 60 cm high. The foliage leaves are opposite arranged, linear-lanceolate, entire-margined, nearly sessile, 1 to 3.5 cm long, 2 to 6 mm wide, bearing glandular scales on both sides. The flowers are arranged in dense, secund, up to 10 cm long false spikes, which are connected to cymes. The flowers are 8 to 12 mm long, the tubulate calyx has 5 uniform teeth, the bilabiate, dark-blue perianth has 4 stamina surpassing it, the stylus is longer than the

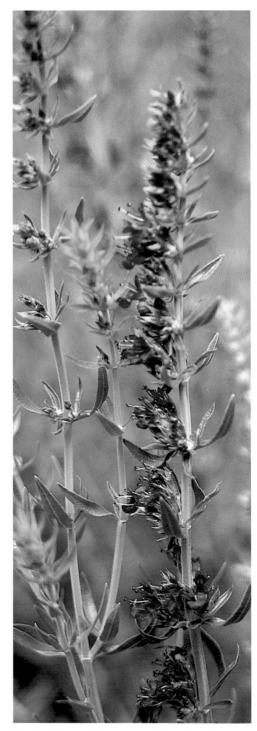

Fig. 2: Hyssop (*Hyssopus officinalis* L.)

stamina, the superior ovary is divided in 4 locules. Flowering period is June until September [25, Ü 37].

Native origin: Southern- and Southeastern Europe, Morocco, Algeria, Caucasus region, Iran to Southern Siberia, in the Middle Ages it was introduced in Western- and Central Europe.

Main cultivation areas: Southern France, Italy, former Yugoslavia, Bulgaria, Hungary, Germany, Czech Republic, Russian Federation, the USA, and India.

Main exporting countries: France, Italy, Hungary, and the Czech Republic.

Cultivation: Hyssop prefers loose, calcareous soil in sunny locations. Hyssop is planted in March in trays or seed flats, in May it must be pricked out and planted outside in row widths of 40 to 60 cm. It is also possible to propagate in the spring or early summer with cuttings or stock divisions. The plant is productive for 3 to 5 years. Varieties include 'Blankyt', 'Kekviragu' and 'Perlay' [Ü17, Ü21].

Culinary herb

Commercial forms: Hyssop: dried herb with flowers, dried branch tips, dried rubbed herb, and hyssop essential oil.

Production: In the first year after the beginning of the bloom, and in the second year in June and September it is harvested either with a sickle or with a cutter-loader. For production of the leaf material, after drying, it is rubbed by hand or industrially rubbed with a sheller. For production of the essential oil, the fresh herb is chopped and immediately distilled. The leaves and shoot tips can be harvested fresh continuously as required.

Forms used: Fresh leaves and shoot tips, dried, rubbed herb.

Storage: The fresh herb can be stored in sealed plastic bags in the refrigerator for a few weeks. Drying leads to considerable aroma loss. The dried leaves are stored in well-closed metal- or glass containers, protected from light and moisture.

Description. Whole herb (Fig. 1): See description of the plant.

Cut herb: Characterized by the violet-blue pruinose calyces, which only project the stamina and the style, the light-green, narrow, rolled-up leaf pieces, with glandular scales on both sides, as well as the tetragonal, pubescent stem fragments [Ü37]. Microscopic examination of the chloral hydrate preparation shows the epidermis with strongly refractive sphaero-crystals and diacytic stomata, capitate trichomes and few short dentiform trichomes, along the leaf venation, as well as multicellular articulate trichomes with thickened basal cell (Fig. 3), labiate glandular scales with 8 secretory cells and finely ribbed pollen grains with 6 pores [Ü48].

Odor: Spicy, camphoraceous, **Taste:** Spicy, mint-like, and somewhat bitter.

History: Hyssop was already known as a medicinal- and aromatic plant in ancient times. The bible also mentions it several times. It was valued in ancient Greece and

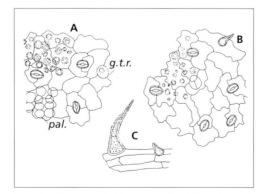

Fig. 3: Hyssop. **A** Upper leaf epidermis with stomata, sphaero-crystals, capitate trichome (g.t.r.) and part of the transparent palisade parenchyma (pal.), **B** Lower leaf epidermis with stomata, sphaero-crystals, capitate trichome and dentiform covering trichome, **C** Epidermis of the fragments from the leaf venation with dentiform covering trichome and multicellular, articulate trichome. From Ü48.

Rome as well as by Arab tribes. In the 12th century, the Benedictine monks spread its cultivation in Central Europe [Ü55, Ü56, Ü92].

Constituents and Analysis

Constituents

- Essential oil: 0.3 to 1% (in the fresh herb 0.03 to 0.16% of fresh weight). The main components are strongly dependent on the subspecies, variety, race and also on climate conditions, developmental stage of the plant, the method of obtaining the essential oil, and other factors.

In cultivated races, the dominant components are pinocamphone (*trans*-pinocamphone, up to 62%), isopinocamphone (*cis*-pinocamphone, up to 43%), β-pinene (up to 23%) and limonene (up to 12%); also present are, among others, pinocarvone, germacrene D, α- and β-phellandrene, β-caryophyllene, sabinene, myrcene and β-bourbonene. ISO-Standard 9841 (1991 E) requires a pinocamphone content of 5.5 to 17.5%, for isopinocamphone 34.5 to 50% and for β-pinene 13.6 to 23% [8, 11, 15, 19, 20, 22].

From not closely defined varieties of wild-growing species (from India), the main components isopinocarvone (about 38%) and pinocarvone (about 23%) have been identified [21].

In Spanish provenances (*H. o.* ssp. *aristatus?*), 1,8-cineole (40 to 53%), β-pinene (about 17%) and isopinocamphone (3 to 30%) were found, as well as α-pinene and sabinene, among others. Methyleugenol (eugenol methyl ether, about 38%), limonene (37%), origin Montenegro (*H. O.* ssp. *aristatus?*) [5].

In *H. o.* ssp. *aristatus*, the main components of the essential oil were methyleugenol + limonene + 1,8-cineole (44 + 16 + 12%), myrtenol + β-pinene + isopinocamphone (33 + 19 + 10%), β-pinene + 1,8-cineole (25 + 23%) or 1,8-cineole + isocamphone + β-pinene (40 to 48 + 28 to 16 + 9 to 11%) [13, 22].

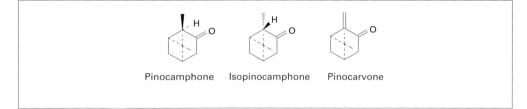

Pinocamphone   Isopinocamphone   Pinocarvone

In *H. o. L. var. decumbens* the following constituents have been detected; linalool (about 50%), 1,8-cineole (about 13 to 15%) and limonene (about 5%), among others, as well as α- and β-pinene, β-caryophyllene [15–17].

- Hydroxycinnamic acid derivatives (known as "labiate tannins"): 2 to 8%, mainly rosmarinic acid and caffeic acid, isoferuloyl-D-glucoseester [10, 12, 24].
- Flavonoids: 3 to 6% diosmin (bitter!), 5 to 6% hesperidin(?) and vicenin-2, among others [7, 12].
- Diterpenes: Marrubiin [1].
- Triterpenes: Oleanolic acid, ursolic acid [Ü43].

Tests for Identity: The herb can be identified with sensoric examination, macroscopic and microscopic analysis as well as with TLC according to PF X [described in Lit. Ü37].

Quantitative assay: The content of essential oil can be determined volumetrically with steam distillation using a graduated tube prefilled with xylol, according to the European Pharmacopoeia [Ph Eur]; its composition is assayed with GC [5, 22] or GC/MS [13,17].

Adulterations, Misidentifications and Impurities are possible with different subspecies. The species can be differentiated based on their GC-profiles.

Actions and Uses

Actions: Due to its aromatic and bitter taste, hyssop is appetizing and digestion promoting.

Methanolic extracts of the dried herb have shown a weak antispasmodic action in vitro with carbachol-induced (0.1 μmol/l) contraction of guinea pig trachea preparation in organ bath [3].

Diosmin, which occurs in relatively high concentrations in the dried herb, is known for its blood vessel protective and antiphlogistic actions [13].

Chloroform extracts of the dried herb and hyssop essential oil inhibit the growth of various bacteria and the yeast *Candida albicans*. For this activity, the linalool-strain is significantly more active than the pinocarvone/isopinocarvone-strain [14, 15, 18]. The essential oil has also shown good antimicrobial activity against virulent strains of *Mycobacterium tuberculosis*. The antiviral action observed in vitro [4], which is dependent on the rosmarinic acid content, is only relevant with topical application.

In animal tests (chickens), hyssop oil (0.01 to 0.5 ml/kg body weight, p.o.) demonstrated a remarkable anthelmintic effect [6].

Toxicology: Based on existing data, there is no acute or chronic toxicity with the use of hyssop as a spice and for tea infusions at normal doses.

The essential oil at high doses may trigger cramps and epileptic attacks due to its pinocamphone content. In rats, 0.13 g of the essential oil per kg body weight, i.p., led to tonicoclonic spasms. The LD_{100} in rats, i.p, is 1.6 ml essential oil/kg body weight. After the administration of 2 to 3 drops over several days to a 6-year old child, and 30 or 100 drops, respectively, to adults, spasms have been observed [9, Ü37, U58].

Allergic reactions have not been observed up to this point; such reactions, however, cannot be completely ruled out in cases of existing allergy against lamiaceous plants [2].

Culinary use: Hyssop is used predominantly in Southern European and Oriental cooking, e.g. for the seasoning of veal. Due to its intense taste, hyssop should be measured sparingly. It should not be cooked with the meal because of the rapid loss of aroma.

Freshly chopped leaves or shoot tips, and rarely the dried, rubbed herb, are used as a seasoning of soups, meat dishes (beef and mutton, ragouts, roulade, fillings), fatty fish dishes (eel), egg- and noodle dishes, poultry-, potato-, vegetable- and legume soups (peas, white, red or green beans), mushroom rice, cauliflower, salads (bean-, tomato-, cucumber-, celery-, lettuce), marinades, herb vinegars, herb butter, herb sauces, herb omelets, dips, quark as well as cream cheese. Hyssop herb preserved in sugar syrup can be used as a seasoning of fruit desserts [Ü1, Ü13, Ü51, Ü86, Ü91].

The flowers have low seasoning strength and can be used as a garnish of salads or sliced meat plates [Ü17, Ü51].

Fresh hyssop is suitable for the preparation of alcoholic herbal drinks, and dried hyssop for making herbal teas [Ü57, Ü71]. Frequent use, e.g. as a house tea, must be cautioned against because chronic toxicity has not been ruled out with certainty.

The essential oil is used for the manufacture of spice essences and liqueurs (Abtei, Altvater Benediktiner, Chartreuse, Kartäuser) [Ü55, Ü92].

Combines well with: Chervil, garlic, parsley, pepper, and onions.

As a component of spice mixes and preparations: → Fines Herbes, → Herbes de Provence.

Other uses: The essential oil is used in the perfume industry.

Medicinal herb

Herbal drug: Hyssopi herba, Hyssop herb, no longer found in more recent German-language pharmacopoeias, Hysope PF X (1988).

Indications: In folk medicine it is used for treatment of diseases of the respiratory tract, asthma, digestive problems, intestinal catarrhs, cardiac complaints, menstrual complaints and to stimulate blood circulation (2 to 4 g dried herb prepared in the form of tea infusions or 2 to 4 ml of tincture, t.i.d.), among other uses. Because efficacy for the above-listed indications for use are not substantiated, the German Commission E did not approve a therapeutic use for hyssop [9]. Extracts of the dried herb are also used as a gargle for pharyngitis.

Potato soup with hyssop

1 to 2 teaspoons butter, 1 onion (finely minced), 4 large potatoes, 3/8 l vegetable broth, some white wine, 1/2 cup cream, hyssop, pepper, cayenne pepper.

Heat the butter in a pot and sauté the onions until they sweat and become transparent. Peel and dice the potatoes and sauté them with the onions for a short time. Add white wine to the hot ingredients in the pan and add all the vegetable broth; let all the soup ingredients simmer for 8 to 10 minutes on medium heat. Season generously with salt, pepper, cayenne pepper and hyssop. The ingredients are puréed in a food processor or with a hand mixer. Before serving, mix in the cream and garnish with fried bacon crumbs, if desired [Ü1].

Literature

[1] Balansard J., Compt. Rend. Soc. Biol. 117: 1014 (1934).
[2] Benito M. et al., Ann. Allergy Asthma Immunol. 76(5):416–418 (1996).
[3] Bergendorf O. et al., Planta Med. 61(4): 370–371 (1995).
[4] Büechi S., Dtsch. Apoth. Ztg. 138(14): 1265–1274 (1998).
[5] Gorunovic M.S. et al., J. Ess. Oil Res. 7: 39–43 (1995).
[6] Hilal S.H. et al., Egypt. J. Pharm. Sci. 19:177–184 (1978).
[7] Husain S.Z., K.R. Markham, Phytochemistry 20:1171–1173 (1981).
[8] Kerrola K., B. Galambosi, H. Kallio, J. Agric. Food Chem. 42:776–781 (1994).
[9] Kommission E beim BfArM., BAnz.-Nr. 162 vom 29.08.1992.
[10] Lamaison J.L. et al., Ann. Pharm. Franc. 46:103–108 (1990).
[11] Lawrence B.M., Perfum. Flavorist 20(5):96–98 (1995).
[12] Marin F.R. et al., Planta Med. 64(2):181–182 (1998).
[13] Piccaglia R. et al., J. Ess. Oil Res. 11:693–699 (1999).
[14] Recio M.C. et al., Phytother. Res. 3:77–80 (1989).
[15] Renzini G. et al., J. Ess. Oil Res. 11:649–654 (1999).
[17] Salvatore G. et al., RIV Ital. EPPOS (Spec. Num., 15th Journees Internationales, Huiles Essentielles, 1996):673–681 (1997), ref. CA 127:351016p.
[18] Salvatore G. et al., J. Ess. Oil Res. 10(5):563–567 (1998).
[19] Sattar A.A. et al., Pharmazie 50(1):62–65 (1995).
[20] Schultz G., F. Stahl-Biskup, Flavour Fragr. J. 6:69–74 (1991).
[21] Schütz G., Flavour and Fragrance 6:69–73 (1991).
[22] Shah N.C., Indian Perfum. 35:49–52 (1991), zit. Lit. 17 (s.o.).
[23] Tsankova E.T. et al., J. Ess. Oil Res. 5:609–611 (1993).
[24] Vallejo M.C.G. et al., J. Ess. Oil Res. 9(5):567–568 (1995).
[25] Varga E. et al., Acta Pharm. Hung. 68(3):183–188 (1998).
[26] Weymar H., Buch der Lippenblütler und Rauhblattgewächse, Neumann Verlag, Radebeul 1961.

Literature references identified by Ü can be found in the general listing of books and monographs at the back of this book.

Juniper

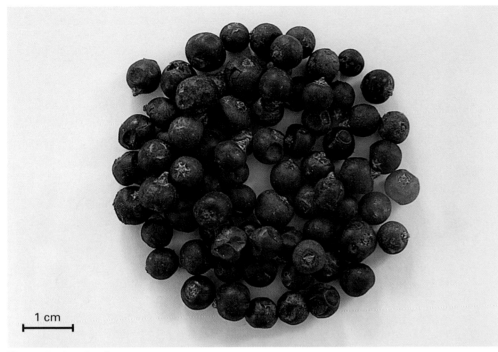

Fig. 1: Juniper berries

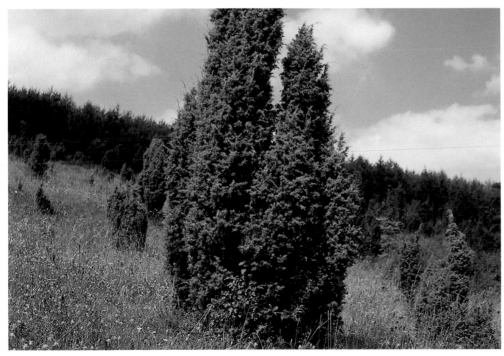

Fig. 2: Juniper (*Juniperus communis* L.)

Plant source: *Juniperus communis* L.

Taxonomic classification: The species can be classified in subspecies and/or varieties. Of the subspecies there exist numerous garden varieties (e.g. of *J. communis* the varieties 'Hibernica' (columnar growing, reaching up to 5 m high), 'Compressa', 'Hornibrookii' and 'Prostrata' (are only 30 to 75 cm high)). The galbulus (cone berry) that is used as a medicinal- and culinary herb originates almost exclusively from the subspecies *J. communis* L. ssp. *communis*.

Family: Cypress family (Cupressaceae).

Common names: Engl.: juniper, common juniper; Fr.: genévrier; Ger.: Wacholder, Gemeiner Wacholder, Machandel, Hageldorn, Kranawitt, Kronawitt, Kaddig, Reckolder, Recholder, Rankholder.

Description: Dioecious, evergreen shrub, up to 3 m tall (seldom up to 12 m) with rigid, acicular and very pointed leaves. Both male and female flowers are yellowish and inconspicuous. The female plants develop cone berries with a characteristic triradiate mark resulting from the fusion of the 3 hypsophylls at the top. The false berries are green in the first year after fertilization, ripening in the second or third year, becoming blue-black and bluish pruinose [Ü106].

Native origin: Europe, Northern Africa, North-, Central- and Western Asia, North America.

Main cultivation areas: Cultivation takes place worldwide, mainly as an ornamental shrub.

Main exporting countries: Croatia, Albania, Italy, Romania, Hungary, Southern

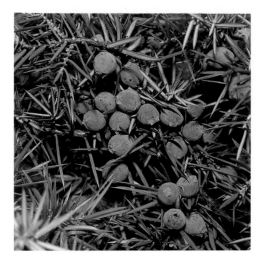
Fig. 3: Juniper twig with berries

France, Spain, Sweden, North America, and Northern Africa.

Cultivation: Juniper prefers sandy, permeable soil. Propagation from seeds is easily possible. For growing in the garden it is expedient to purchase young plants in a container [Ü45].

Culinary herb

Commercial forms: Juniper berries: the ripe whole or rough-chopped juniper berries, essential oil of juniper berries, and juniper berry oleoresin

Production: The cone berries are wild collected. Harvest of the ripe bluish-black berries takes place from the end of August until mid-September. They are dried at room temperature and separated from the leaf- and stem pieces by sieving. Even though juniper is protected under German conservation law, wild collection of the berries is permitted [Ü37].

Forms used: Fresh or dried juniper berries, in spice mixes the rough-chopped juniper berries.

Storage: In a cool place, protected from light and moisture in airtight porcelain-, glass- or suitable metal containers not

longer than 1 year. During storage of crushed or ground berries, the aroma quickly dissipates.

Description. Whole fruit (Fig. 1): Globose, berry-like fruits, diameter 6 to 10 mm, violet-brown to black-brown, often bluish pruinose, with triradiate, fused cleft and 3 indistinct protuberances at the apex, sometimes with the remains of the peduncle at the base; the inner part of the sticky yellow fruit pulp contains mostly 3, very hard, angular seeds [Ph Eur].

Powdered fruit: The powder contains polygonal, thick-walled, dotted epidermis cells with colorless walls and brown content; the loose, thin-walled parenchyma of the cotyledons shows the embedded large, yellow, ovate-elongated cells with ligneous walls, known as barrel-shaped cells, and the fragments of the stone cell layer of the testa with single calcium oxalate crystals (Fig. 4), collenchymatically thickened hypodermal cells, fragments of the above-mentioned cleft with papillose-dentate epidermis cells, fragments of the thin-walled endosperm and embryonic tissue with oil-droplets and aleuron grains; starch is absent [Ü25, Ph Eur].

Odor: After crushing, aromatic, turpentine-like, **Taste:** Sweet and aromatic-spicy, then slightly bitter.

History: Juniper was already described in the Papyrus Ebers (authored in about 1550 BCE) as a remedy against digestive and urinary complaints and dropsy. It was also used in the Middle Ages for the above-mentioned indications. Juniper plays an important role in mythology [18, 32, Ü92].

Constituents and Analysis

DIN- and ISO-Standards: ISO-Standard 7377 (Juniper berries).

Constituents
- Essential oil: 0.5 to 3.4%, the main components depend strongly on a variety of factors, including, among others, the

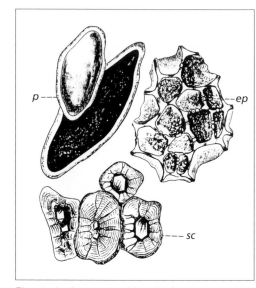
Fig. 4: Juniper, ep epidermis fragment, p barrel-shaped cells from the fruit pulp, sc stone cells of the testa with oxalate crystals. From Ü25.

country of origin (chemical races?), the elevation above sea-level where it occurs, the growth habit and the season of harvest: α-pinene (9 to 76%, high levels in low altitude growing conditions), sabinene (0.2 to 50%, high levels in mountainous conditions), β-myrcene (7 to 23%), limonene (1 to 11%), terpinenol-4 (0.3 to 17%), citronellol (5 to 13%), germacrene D (up to 10%), β-caryophyllene (1 to 8%), α-caryophyllene (humulene, 1 to 5%), β-pinene (2 to 6%), furthermore, among others, γ-muurolene, α-terpineol, borneol, geraniol, thujene, camphene, p-menthane, p-cymene, bornyl acetate, pyrazine, pyridine derivatives, in some origins also 1,8-cineole (up to 7%) [4, 6, 10, 14, 17, 23, 31, 35].
- Diterpenes: Junicedral, *cis*-communic acid, isocommunic acid, among others [5, 24].
- Invert sugar: About 30% [Ü43].
- Hydroxycoumarins: Umbelliferone, among others [19].
- Flavonoids: Rutin, quercitrin, isoquercitrin, 7-*O*-glycoside of hypolaetin, scutellarin, apigenin, luteolin and 7-hydroxy-4´5,6-methoxyflavone, 3-*O*-arabinosylglucoside of quercetin, 6-*O*-

xyloside of scutellarin and 6-hydroxyluteolin, kaempferol-3-*O*-rhamnoside, kaempferol-3-*O*-glucoside, the biflavonoids amentoflavone, cupressoflavone, robustaflavone, poducarpusflavone and hinokiflavone [9, 19].

- Proanthocyanidins and their monomeric precursors: (+)-Catechin, (−)-epicatechin, (+)-gallocatechin and (−)-epigallocatechin [8], among others.

The occurrence of lignans is disputed [6].

Tests for Identity: The berries are analyzed with TLC [34, Ph Eur], the essential oil of juniper berries with GC [2, 4, 31] or GC/MS [3, 4] or HPLC [Ph Eur].

Quantitative assay: The content of essential oil is determined volumetrically after steam distillation of the crushed berries with xylol in the graduated tube [Ph Eur], the compounds of the essential oil by HPLC [Ph Eur].

Adulterations, Misidentifications and Impurities with berries from other Juniperus-species are possible. They can be recognized microscopically by the branched barrel-cells of the fruits of other Juniperus-species [Ü106].

Actions and Uses

Actions: Due to the aromatic, slightly bitter taste, juniper berries are appetizing and digestion promoting. Extracts of the dried fruits are supposed to stimulate intestinal peristalsis and resolve intestinal spasms [13, 21]. Juniper berry oil in very high doses has shown choleretic action (rats, 250 to 500 mg/kg body weight, in olive oil, intraduodenal, increased biliary flow from 13 to 87%) [36].

In animal studies a diuretic effect could be shown at very high doses of juniper infusion (16 to 125 mg, p.o., per animal or per kg body weight?) [37] or of juniper berry oil (1 mg/kg body weight!) [11]. The diuretic effect has also been demonstrated in humans [18]. The diuretic effect is attributed mainly to terpinenol-4, which in contrast to the terpene hydrocarbons does not have nephrotoxic action [12]. Because the excretion of salts (saluresis) is not increased, the action is instead referred to as water diuresis (aquaresis) [6, 20, 28, 30, 32, 37].

An inflammation inhibiting, antiexudative action has been demonstrated with p.o. application of a dry extract (100 or 110 mg/kg body weight, suspended in water, p.o.) in Carrageenan-induced rat paw edema [22]. Decoctions of juniper berries (p.o. application, corresponding to 250 mg berries/kg body weight) had a blood sugar reducing effect in normoglycemic rats. In rats with streptozotocin-induced diabetes (corresponding to 125 mg berries/kg body weight), the blood sugar level was also reduced, loss of body weight was prevented and animal mortality was reduced [29].

Similar to all essential oils, the oil of juniper berries has antimicrobial action [6].

Toxicology: There is no acute or chronic toxicity with the occasional use of juniper berries as a spice or medicine at normal doses.

In older animal tests, kidney damage after the administration of large doses of essential oil of juniper berries has been observed [32]. In newer tests, this observation could not be confirmed. In rats with a daily intake of 100 to 1000 mg/kg body weight or terpinenol-4, respectively, at doses of 400 mg/kg body weight, p.o, dissolved in sesame oil, over a period of 28 days, no pathological changes in the function and morphology of the kidneys could be observed in these animals (yet there was no increase in diuresis). The concerns that long term use or overdoses of juniper berries could cause kidney damage are therefore no longer justified. However, until the potential risk has been clarified, juniper berries should not be taken for longer than 1 week without a doctor's prescription [16].

The dried extract obtained with 50% ethanol from the fruits at very high doses (300 mg or 500 mg/kg body weight, intragastral, day 1 to 7 after fertilization) had a fertilization-inhibiting effect in rats. The implantation rate was reduced by 50 or 80%, respectively, and the number of embryos was significantly reduced. Administration after implantation (days 14 to 16) led to abortion [1, 25, 26].

Contraindications for the external use of essential oil from juniper berries are skin damage, acute skin diseases, feverish- and infectious diseases, cardiac insufficiency and hypertension [15].

Culinary use: Juniper berries are used as a seasoning predominantly in Northern- and Western European cooking and somewhat also in Russian cooking.

Whole juniper berries are added before cooking or frying to dishes that require longer cooking time. For the preparation of marinades, dressings and sauces, they are crushed before use in order to make a rapid release of the essential oil possible. In many dishes it is a good idea to add the berries inside an herb sack or metal tea ball so that the juniper berries can be pulled out before serving or before the meal is consumed. It should be measured carefully (3 whole or 2 crushed berries for one portion).

Juniper berries serve mainly as an ingredient for marinades (for meat- and venison), fish brew, sauces (red wine sauce, buttermilk sauce) and fillings for game- and poultry dishes (venison, wild boar, pigeon, duck), as a seasoning of veal, lamb, mutton, pork and beef as well as of fish, as a seasoning for stews, e.g. for beef stew and white beans, for pastas, sauerkraut, red cabbage, white cabbage, sauces (e.g. juniper cream sauces), corned beef, smoked meats and sausage products [Ü30, Ü55, Ü78, Ü81, Ü93, Ü95].

Juniper berries are also used as a pickling spice for sauerkraut, vegetables, cucumbers, red beets, pearl onions and pumpkins. In combination with coriander they are used as pickling brine for meat [Ü1, Ü45, Ü53, Ü59, Ü71].

Juniper berries can also be used as a spice in jellies (especially apple jelly), marmalades, pomace, fruit cakes (especially apple cake) and English plum pudding [Ü68, Ü98].

Juniper berries play a large role in the production of alcoholic spirits. Juniper schnapps is made from neutral spirit or fine grain distillate with the addition of juniper distillate (pouring the neutral spirit over the juniper berries followed by distillation) or from juniper low wine (crude distillate of fermented juniper berries), e.g. Gin, Steinhäger, Genever, Doornkaat, Machandel, Borowiezka and Brinjewec. The addition of juniper essential oil in alcoholic beverages is forbidden in Germany [Ü30, Ü92, Ü98].

Combines well with: Bay, clove, fennel, garlic (crushed berries, garlic and salt rubbed onto wildfowl before roasting), marjoram, mints, parsley, and thyme, with allspice and pepper (as a seasoning of beef), with mugwort (for roasted wild boar), with allspice, bay leaves, clove, pepper, and white mustard (as a pickling spice).

As a component of spice mixes and preparations: → Fish spice, → Meat spice, → Pickling spice, → Vegetable spice, → Venison spice.

Other uses: Juniper berries are also used as an additive to smoking mixtures for sausages [Ü93].

Medicinal herb

Herbal drugs: Juniper pseudo-fructus, Juniper berries, contain minimum 10 ml/kg essential oil [Ph Eur], Juniperi aetheroleum, should contain 20 to 30% α-pinene, 1 to 12% β-pinene, 1 to 35% β-myrcene, 2 to 12% limonene and 0.5 to 10% terpinenol-4 [Ph Eur].

Indications: Used for dyspeptic complaints such as eructation, pyrosis and epigastric fullness, in the form of tea infusions and decoctions, alcoholic extracts and wine extracts (daily dose 2 to 10 g of the dried berries, corresponding to 20 to 100 mg essential oil, for infusions 150 ml boiled water poured over 2 g of the freshly crushed berries and steeped for 10 minutes) [16, Ü12, Ü106]. Juniper berries with low terpene hydrocarbon content essential oil (ratio of terpinenol-4 to monoterpene hydrocarbons of 1 : 3 to 1 : 5) are recommended for use as diuretics for irrigation therapy for inflammatory and bacterial diseases of the lower urinary tract and for prevention and treatment of gravel [7, 31]. The therapeutic use of juniper berries and their essential oil is contraindicated in cases of inflammatory renal diseases and during pregnancy and their culinary use should also be considered cautiously.

Moreover, in folk medicine, juniper berries are used for cystitis (without kidney inflammation), gout and for rheumatic complaints, among other conditions. Chewing on juniper berries is supposed to mask bad breath [6, Ü37].

Juniper oil is used externally in baths intended to induce hyperemia, in folk medicine in the form of juniper spirits (juniper berry oil : ethanol 90% in a ratio of 1 : 9) as an embrocation for rheumatic diseases, for acne, psoriasis, seborrhea as well as eczema, and also taken internally (5 to 10 drops/d juniper oil) for low urinary output, for irrigation therapy, prostate inflammations, rheumatism, flatulence and intestinal colic [6, 27, 33, Ü37].

Juniper Sauerkraut
1 finely minced onion, 1 crushed garlic clove, 1 finely chopped apple, 60 g margarine, 5 to 7 crushed juniper berries, 500 g sauerkraut, 1/2 l broth, 1 cup of yogurt or sour cream.

The minced onion, garlic and apple are sautéed in melted margarine on low heat until soft. Add the crushed juniper berries, broth and sauerkraut and cook on low heat for 2 to 3 minutes. Pour the mixture in a fireproof oven form and let it cook in the oven at 140 °C for 45 to 60 minutes. Shortly before serving, add yogurt or cream. Serve with grilled pork chops or small bratwursts [Ü109].

Literature

[1] Agrawal O.P. et al., Planta Med. Suppl. 98–101 (1980).

[2] Analytical Methods Committee, Analyst 109:1351–1352 (1984), zit. in Ü30.

[3] Caramiello R. et al., J. Ess. Oil Res. 7(2):133–145 (1995).

[4] Chatzopoulou P.S., S.T. Katsiotis, Planta Med. 59(6):554–556 (1993).

[5] De Pasqual Teresa J. et al., Am. Quim. 73(4):568–573 (1977).

[6] De Smet P.A.G.M. et al. (Eds.): Adverse Effects of Herbal Drugs, Springer Verlag Heidelberg 1993, Vol. 2, p. 217–229.

[7] ESCOP, ESCOP Monographs Juniperi fructus, Juniper berry (1997).

[8] Friedrich H., R. Engelshowe, Planta Med. 33(3):251–257 (1978).

[9] Hiermann A. et al., Sci. Pharm. 64(3/4): 437–444 (1996).

[10] Hoerster H. et al., Rev. Med. (Tirgu-Mures, Rom.) 20(2):215–218 (1974).

[11] Janku I. et al., Experientia 13:255–256 (1957).

[12] Janku I. et al., Arch. Exp. Path. Pharmakol. 238:112–113 (1960).

[13] Klare K., Med. Welt 1:1089–1090 (1927).

[14] Klein E., H. Farnow, dragoco Rep. 11(10):223–226 (1964).

[15] Kommission B8 beim BfArM., BAnz. Nr. 127 vom 12.07.1990.

[16] Kommission E beim BfArM., BAnz-Nr. 228 vom 05.12.84.

[17] Koukos P.K., K.I. Papadopoulou, J. Ess. Oil Res. 9(1):35–39 (1997).

[18] Kreitmair H., Pharmazie 8:187–192 (1953).

[19] Lamer-Zarawska E., Pol. J. Chem. 54(2):213–219 (1980).

[20] Lasheras B. et al., Plant Méd. Phytothér. 20:219–226 (1986).

[21] Leers H., Hippokrates 11:1117–1123 (1940).

[22] Mascolo N. et al., Phytother. Res. 1:28–31 (1987).

[23] Maurer B., Perfum. Flavorist 19:19–27 (1994).

[24] Pascual J. de et al., Phytochemistry 22: 300–301 (1983).

[25] Prakash A.O., Int. J. Crude Drug Res. 24:19–24 (1986).

[26] Prakash A.O. et al., Acta Eur. Fertilitatis 16:441–448 (1985).

[27] Reglin F., Praxis-telegramm 3–4 (1994).

[28] Roberts S., J. Pharm. Belg. 41:40–45 (1986).

[29] Sánchez de Medina F. et al., Planta Med. 60(3):197–200 (1994).

[30] Schilcher H., Dtsch. Apoth. Ztg. 124: 2429–2436 (1984).

[31] Schilcher H. et al., Pharm. Ztg-Wissensch. 138(3/4):85–91 (1993).

[32] Schilcher H., B.M. Heil, Z. Phytother. 15(4):205–213 (1994).

[33] Schmidt G.P., Heilpraxis Magazin 32–34 (1992).

[34] Stahl E. (Hrsg.): Chromatographische und mikroskopische Analyse von Drogen, Fischer Verlag Stuttgart, New York 1978.

[35] Vernin G. et al., Phytochemistry 27: 1061–1064 (1988).

[36] Vogel G., Arzneim. Forsch. 25: 1356–1365 (1975).

[37] Vollmer H., A. Giebel, Arch. Exp. Path. Pharmacol. 190:522–534 (1938).

Literature references identified by Ü can be found in the general listing of books and monographs at the back of this book.

Leek

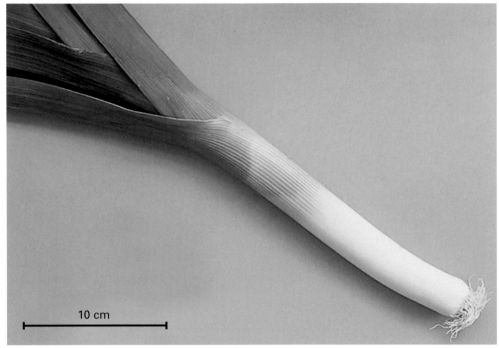

Fig. 1: Leek

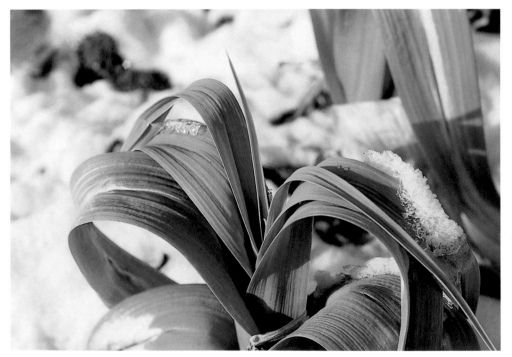

Fig. 2: Leek (*Allium porrum* L. var. *porrum*)

Plant source: *Allium porrum* L. var. *porrum*.

Synonym: *Allium ampeloprasum* var. *porrum* J. GAY.

Taxonomic classification: The species *Allium porrum* L. can be subdivided in the following varieties:
A. porrum L. var. *porrum*, leek, and *A. porrum* L. var. *sectivum* F.H.H. LUEDER, pearl onion, see below.

Family: Allium plants (Alliaceae; in older literature this species was placed in the lily family, Liliaceae).

Common names: Engl.: leek, common leek, purret; Fr.: poireau, porreau; Ger.: Porree, Lauch, Winterlauch, Breitlauch, Spanischer Lauch, Suppenlauch, Welschzwiebel.

Description: Perennial herb, 30 to 100 cm tall, flowering in the second year, cultivated for 1 year only. Foliage leaves are lanceolate, ribbon-like, parallel-veined, unifacial and up to 1 m long; the leaf bases are stem like arranged. The inflorescence is a multiflorous pseudoumbel with a unifoliate, bulging coat with a long tip. The flowers have 6 bright-purple perigone leafs, 6 stamina and a three chambered ovary. The fruit is a three-chambered capsule with 1 to 2 seeds. Flowering time is from June until August.

Native origin: Probably native to the Eastern Mediterranean region, not known in the wild, possibly originating from *A. ampeloprasum* L., wild leek.

Main cultivation areas: Leek is cultivated worldwide, in Germany especially in North Rhine-Westphalia; France is the essential growing region.

Main exporting countries: France.

Cultivation: Leek requires humus- and nutrient rich, deep, damp soil in sunny to half-shaded locations. Summer leek seeds are planted in pots in January, cultivated at 16 to 20 °C, seedlings are pricked out and transplanted outdoors in April, spaced at 15 × 40 cm, after April seeds can be sown directly in the field. Autumn leek is sown in March or April in pots and transplanted in May or June. Winter leek seeds can be sown outdoors at the end of May, usually left covered to overwinter in the plot. It is also possible to purchase planting stock. It is recommended to plant in mounds, thereby producing plants with a long, white scape [Ü96]. Numerous varieties exist. Cultivars of Summer leek suitable for cultivation include: e.g. 'Alma' and 'Ekkehard', for cultivation of Autumn leek: 'Bavaria', 'Blaugrüner Herbst (with numerous selections)', 'Genita', 'Janos', 'Kampus', 'Merkur' and 'Pancho', for cultivation of Winter leek: 'Blaugrüner Winter (with numerous selections)', 'Pollux' and 'Poros'. For industrial utilization, exclusively summer or autumn leek varieties are cultivated [Ü15].

Culinary Herb

Commercial forms: Leek: fresh, non-flowering plant, preferably with a long, strong scape of which a large portion is white, without noteworthy bulb formation, or dried scape, cut into pieces 1 to 1.5 cm long and 0.5 to 1 cm wide.

Production: Harvest of summer leek is carried out from the beginning of July to the end of August, of autumn leek from the beginning of September to December and of winter leek in the autumn or spring.

Forms used: Fresh or dried lower plant parts, cut into disks, seldom leaves also.

Storage: At 0° C and 95% relative humidity, fresh leek can be stored up to 3 months; at –1 to –2 °C, up to 5 months [Ü98]. For household use, leeks can be

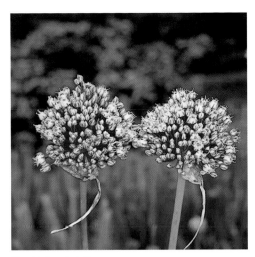

Fig. 3: Leek inflorescence

stored for a few weeks in plastic bags in the refrigerator; Winter leek, if not kept in the garden through the winter, can be covered with sand or soil and stored for several months in the basement.

Description. Whole herb (Fig. 1): For the non-flowering plant, see: Description.

Odor: Alliaceous upon bruising, **Taste:** Mild, onion-like.

History: Leek has been cultivated by the peoples of the Mediterranean since antiquity [Ü92].

Constituents and Analysis

Constituents

- Alliins (S-alk(ene)ylcysteine sulfoxides), in undamaged plant parts, the following substances have been detected: S-Methyl-L-cysteine sulfoxide and S-propyl-L-cysteine sulfoxide. Based on the decomposition products [2, 4, 11], it must be assumed that S-prop-enyl-L-cysteine sulfoxide (see chemical structures → Onion) also occurs.
- Alliaceous oils: Upon bruising of the plant, the non-volatile alliins come into contact with the enzyme alliinase and are converted to volatile alk(en)yl-sulfenic acids. The latter transform spontaneously into the characteristically smelling, alliaceous decomposition products of raw leek, the alk(en)yl-alkane/alkenethiosulfinates (Fig. 10, General Section). Also detected were, among other components, (E,Z)-prop-1-enyl-mehanethiosulfinate (29%), propyl-propanethiosulfinate (25%), (E)-methyl-prop-1-enthiosulfinate (21%), methyl-propanethiosulfinate (7%), propyl-methanethiosulfinate (6%), (E)-propyl-prop-1-enethiosulfinate (5%), allyl-prop-1-enethiosulfinate and zwiebelanes (about 10%, see chemical structures → Onion) [3].

Methyl-L-cysteine sulfoxide   R = CH₃
Propyl-L-cysteine sulfoxide   R = CH₂CH₂CH₃
Prop-1-enyl-L-cysteine sulfoxide   R = CH = CHCH₃

Prop-1-enyl-methane-thiosulfinate

Propyl-propane-thiosulfinate

Methyl-prop-1-ene-thiosulfinate

Methyl-propane-thiosulfinate

Methylpropyldisulfide   Dipropyldisulfide   Prop-1-enylpropyldisulfide   Prop-1-enylpropyltrisulfide

The sulfinates transform spontaneously into dialk(en)ylmono- and oligosulfides, mainly into methyl-propyl-disulfide and dipropyl-disulfide; this process is accelerated during cooking. 65 other compounds have also been identified in the steam distillate, including, among others, prop-1-enyl-propyl-disulfide, prop-1-enyl-propyl-trisulfide, allylalcohol, 2-methylpentanal, hex-3-ene-1-ol, 2,3-dihydro-2-*n*-hexyl-5-methylfuran-3-one, 2,3-dihydro-2-*n*-octyl-5-methylfuran-3-one and 3,4-dimethylthiophene [1, 9, 13, 15]. Responsible for the odor are the alk(en)yloligosulfides and also, among others, *n*-propanal, 2-methylpent-2-enal (both with weak lacrimatory action), hex-2-enal and propanethiol. The qualitative composition and the ratio of the individual constituents depend on the cultivar and origin [12, 13].

- Steroid saponins: Mono- and bisdesmosides with the aglycones porrigenins A, B and C, 12-ketoporrigenin, neoporrigenins A and B, agigenin, neoagigenin [5, 6, 7, 10].
- Flavonoids: Isoquercitrin (quercetin-3-glucoside) and astragalin (kaempferol-3-glucoside), among others [16].
- Dibenzofuran derivatives [7].
- Monosaccharides, oligosaccharides, polysaccharides, including, among others, saccharose (about 18%), water-soluble polysaccharides (10 to 15%), particularly mucilage-forming fructans, arabans and pectins [8, 14].
- Vitamin C: 15 to 30 mg/100 g (fresh weight) [Ü98].

Tests for Identity: → Asafetida, → Onion.

Quantitative assay: → Asafetida, → Onion.

Adulterations, Misidentifications and Impurities: Not known.

Actions and Uses

Actions: On the basis of the pungent taste of raw leeks as well as the slightly irritant action of their alliaceous oils on the gastric mucosa and due to the aromatic odor and taste of cooked leeks, they are appetizing and digestion promoting. The isolated saponins inhibit in vitro the growth of tumor cells [5]. Other studies of pharmacological action are not known.

Toxicology: Based on existing data, there is no chronic or acute toxicity in healthy individuals with the consumption of leek as a spice or vegetable. In sensitive persons, leek can cause colics and flatulence.

Culinary use: Leek is used worldwide. In Scotland it is used in cook-a-leekie soup, a national dish. Leek is used in the same manner as onions and cooked with the meal.

Cut, fresh leek is used as a seasoning of sauces, vegetable stews, meat soups, fish- and meat dishes as well as soufflés [Ü63, Ü81].

Fresh leek can be eaten raw as a salad or as an addition to a salad or cooked as a vegetable.

Combines well with: Pepper.

As a component of spice mixes and preparations: → Bouquet garni, → Soup greens.

Similar spice herbs: → Onion.

Medicinal herb

Herbal drug: Allium-Porrum, whole plant.

Indications: In folk medicine is it used for helminth and as a diuretic remedy [Ü60].

Literature

[1] Auger J., E. Thibout, Can. J. Zool. 57: 2223 (1979), ref. in Ü37.
[2] Block E., Angew. Chem. 104:1158–1203 (1992).
[3] Block E. et al., J. Agric. Food Chem. 40:2431–2438 (1992).
[4] Bonnet R. et al., CR Acad. Sci. Ser. D. 279:1919 (1974).
[5] Carotenuto A. et al., J. Nat. Prod. 60(10): 1003–1007 (1997).
[6] Carotenuto A. et al., Phytochemistry 51(8): 1077–1082 (1999).
[7] Carotenuto A. et al., Gazz. Chim. Ital. 127(9):523–536 (1998).
[8] Darbyshire B., R.J. Henry, New Phytol. 87:249 (1981), ref. in Ü37.
[9] Dembele S., P. Dubois, Ann. Techn. Agr. 22:121 (1973), ref. in Ü37.
[10] Fattorusso E. et al., J. Agric. Food Chem. 48(8):3455–3462 (2000).
[11] Fenwick G.R. et al., CRC Crit. Rev. Food Sci. Nutr. 22:199–377 (1985).
[12] Ferary S., J. Auger, J. Chromatogr. A. 750(1+2, 4th Intern Symp. on Hyphenated Techniques in Chromatography and Hyphenated Chromatographic Analyzers, 1996):63–74 (1996), ref. CA: 126: 059106n.
[13] Noleau I. et al., J. Ess. Oil Res. 3:241–256 (1991).
[14] Rubat de Mérac M.L.: Recherches sur le métabolisme glucidique du genre Allium et en particulier d'Allium ursinum L., Theses (Sci. nat.) Univ. Paris 1949, ref. in Ü43.
[15] Schreyen L. et al., J. Agric. Food Chem. 24(2):336–341 (1976).
[16] Starke H., K. Herrmann, Z. Lebensm. Unters. Forsch. 161:25 (1976).

Literature references identified by Ü can be found in the general listing of books and monographs at the back of this book.

Lemon balm

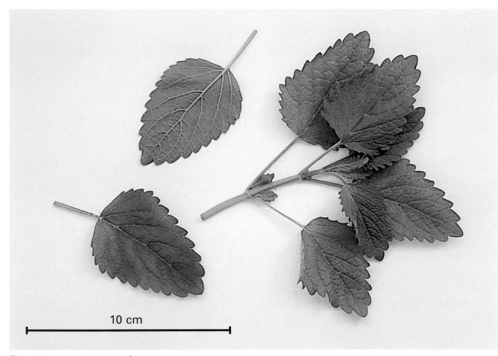

Fig. 1: Lemon balm leaf

10 cm

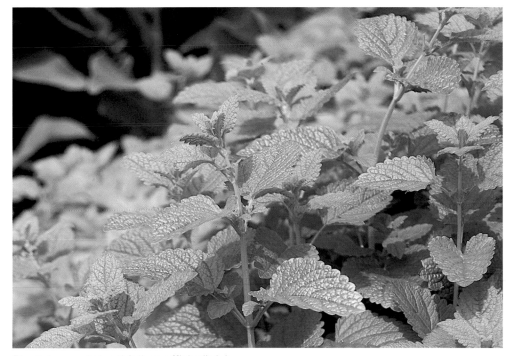

Fig. 2: Lemon balm (*Melissa officinalis* L.)

Plant source: *Melissa officinalis* L.

Taxonomic classification: The species is subdivided as follows:
Melissa officinalis L. ssp. *officinalis* (Synonym: *Melissa officinalis* f. *officinalis* (L.) Briq.),
Melissa officinalis L. ssp. *altissima* (Sibth. et Sm.) Arcang.,
Melissa officinalis L. ssp. *inodora* (Bornm.) Bornm.
The cultivated forms are derived from the first listed subspecies.

Family: Mint family (Lamiaceae, synonym Labiatae).

Common names: Engl.: lemon balm, melissa, bee balm; Fr.: mélisse, citronelle, citronade; Ger.: Melisse, Zitronen-Melisse, Citronelle, Bienenkraut, Honigblatt.

Description: Perennial herb with multi-headed rootstock, erect stem, quadrangular, branched, glabrous or sparsely hairy, up to 90 cm high. Leaves opposite, ovate to rhomboid, 2 to 6 cm long, up to 4 cm wide, upper surface pubescent or glabrous, lower surface glabrous or at most, with hairs along the veins, long petiolate, leaf margin with regular broadly crenate serration; occasionally, small shoots are present in the leaf axils. The 3 to 5 flowers occur in the leaf axils in whorl-like fashion; the calyx is tubular-campanulate with short teeth, 7 to 9 mm long, bilabiate, the upper lip is tridentate, the lower lip has 2 aristate, densely pubescent teeth bending upwards, tubular corolla, 8 to 15 mm long, bluish-white, pale-lilac or faintly yellowish-white, bilabiate, with domed 2-lobed upper lip, lower lip 3-lobed, the middle lobe is larger than the side lobes, 4 stamina, fused in the upper part, superior ovary, diphyllous, divided into 4 locules. The fruit separates into 4 one-seeded, chestnut brown-colored nutlets, about 2 mm long. The flowers mostly do not appear before the second year. Flowering period is from June to September [53, Ü21, Ü37].

Native origin: Eastern Mediterranean region to western Asia.

Main cultivation areas: Europe, Morocco, Algeria, Canada, USA, Mexico, Cuba, Peru, and temperate zones of Asia.

Main suppliers: Germany (Thuringia, Saxony-Anhalt, Franconia), Spain, Romania, Bulgaria, southern France, and the Russian Federation.

Cultivation: Lemon balm prefers sunny locations with not too dry, warm sandy soil or sandy loam soil with good supply of humus. Partial shade or shade are tolerated, but this diminishes the essential oil content. The plant is self-incompatible but should also not be grown subsequent to other mint family plants in the same place. Sowing can be done in March in the green house and transplanted outside in May, spaced 30 × 30 cm apart. Direct seeding is possible with a distance of 60 cm between the rows. With direct seeding, however, there is no harvest in the first year of cultivation. The populations can be used for 3 to 4 years. For growing lemon balm in an individual garden, it is advisable to buy the plants in herb pots or divide old plants. Cultivated are upright varieties (derived from the German variety 'Aufrechte Erfurter Melisse', which grows rapidly, with large leaves, but having a high stem part, somewhat frost sensitive, winterkilling is possible) or in the first season, low lying varieties (derived from the German variety 'Quedlinburger niederliegende Melisse', little growth in the 1st year, small leaves, frost resistant); cultivars grown additionally in Europe include, among others, 'Citronella', 'Citra', 'De Dobrotesti', 'Melisa 2', and 'Landor' [Ü21, Ü96, for an evaluation of other varieties see Lit. 47].

Culinary herb

Commercial forms: Lemon balm: dried leaves, cut or cut dried herb, in the vegetable trade the fresh herb or annual small plants in herb pots are also available, and lemon balm essential oil.

Production: On industrial farms, lemon balm is cut before flowering with a cutter bar mower or a loader combine harvester from June to mid-July and again in mid-September. In the 2nd growing season a 3rd cutting is also possible. Lemon balm is dried in a belt drier at 35 to 40 °C, the chopping and separating of stems and leaves is done through sieves or air separator. On small-scale farms, once to twice yearly the leaves are cut by hand before the flowering period, removed from the stems and dried. Fresh leaves for daily use can be harvested throughout the entire vegetation period [Ü21].

Forms used: For culinary use the fresh, rarely dried leaves, and lemon balm essential oil.

Storage: The fresh leaves can be stored in plastic bags in the refrigerator for a few days or in the ice compartment or deep freezer for a couple of months. The dried herb should be kept in well-closed metal-, glass- or porcelain containers, as cool as possible (cyclization of citronellal!), protected from light and moisture. Since the level of essential oil rapidly diminishes, lemon balm herb should not be stored longer than 1 year.

Description. Whole leaf (Fig. 1): See description of the whole plant (for details on the anatomy, see Lit. [57]).

Cut leaf: Thin, mostly folded, when dried somewhat brittle leaf fragments, upper surface distinctly darker than the lower surface, with prominent venation on the lower surface. Under lens magnification, bristly hairs are discernible on the upper surface, and on both surfaces, punctate lamiaceous glandular scales are visible.

Powdered leaf: Green leaf powder with numerous, uni- and bicellular, canine tooth-like conical trichomes, mostly multicellular bristles with thin, streak-like verrucate and cuticula, as well as typical, lamiaceous, glandular scales. Sclerenchymatic fibers occur very scarcely or are entirely absent [Ü49].

Odor and **Taste:** Aromatic and lemon-like when fresh. The essential oil content in the dried leaves dissipates rapidly; hence they are mostly taste- and odorless.

History: The use of lemon balm as a medicinal and culinary herb dates back to antiquity. It was already mentioned in the "Historia plantarum" by Theophrastus of Ephesos (372–287 BCE). Arab and Persian physicians (e.g. Avicenna, 980–1027 CE) praised it as a mood elevating and gastric secretion stimulating remedy. In the 10th century, the plant was introduced to Spain by the Arabs, and later was brought to Central Europe by Benedictine monks. In the compendium "Physica" by Hildegard von Bingen (1098–1179), the effects of lemon balm are documented. In the 16th century, it was already cultivated in several European countries. Since 1611, it has been used along with other medicinal plants in the manufacture of "Karmelitergeist" [22, Ü92].

Constituents and Analysis

Constituents

▪ Essential oil: 0.05 to 0.3% in the fresh leaves (calculated with reference to the dried leaves); in some cultivars grown in Mediterranean countries (e.g. Spain), up to 0.4%. The main components are citral (a mixture of geranial = citral a and neral = citral b, in lemon balm, the compositional ratio ranges from 4:3 to 5:3) and citronellal (about 98% (+)-enantiomer and 2% (–)-enantiomer, both are the main odoriferous constituents, together making up 50 to 97% of the essential oil). The ratio of these two components is highly variable. In the leaves of most provenances, the content of citral (10 to 90%, average about 50%) is higher than the content of citronellal (0.1 to 40%, average 8%). In some provenances, however, particularly in mature leaves during and after anthesis, the citronellal content can also be higher. Other components are, among others, β-caryophyllene (about 28% of the essential oil, converting to β-caryophyllene epoxides I and II during storage), germacrene D (up to 15%, sometimes absent), 6-methylhept-5-ene-2-one (up to 9%), geranyl acetate (up to 6%), α-copaene (up to 5%), nerol (up to 5%), methyl citronellate (up to 5%, sometimes absent) and geraniol [1, 8, 11, 13, 17, 18, 31, 32, 35, 39, 43–45, 50, 57, 58], as well as glycosides of the volatile constituents, e.g. glycosides of citronellol, phenyl ethanol, eugenol, benzyl alcohol and oct-1-ene-3-ol [5].

During drying and storage, citral and citronellal are rapidly lost. In the dried material of commerce, only very little or no citral and citronellal, respectively, are detectable; often, caryophyllene epoxides dominate [38].

In *M. o.* ssp. *inodora*, the main components are β-caryophyllene as well as β-cubebene (15% each) and citral (about 12%) [42]. *M. o.* ssp. *altissima* only contains traces of citral and citronellal, the main components in this subspecies are germacrene D (32 to 54%) and β-caryophyllene (7 to 22%) [9, 58].

- Hydroxycinnamic acid derivatives (labiate tannins): Up to 7%, including, among others, rosmarinic acid (about 5%), caffeic acid, chlorogenic acid, 2-(3′,4′-dihydroxyphenyl)-1,3-benzodioxol-5-aldehyde, "melitric" acids A and B (caffeic acid trimers) [2, 12, 19, 22, 28, 48].
- Hydroxycoumarin derivatives: Aesculetin [21].
- Flavonoids: 0.2 to 0.7%, glycosides of luteolin, apigenin, quercetin and kaempferol, including, among others, luteolin-3′-glucuronide, cynaroside (luteolin-7-*O*-glucoside), cosmosiin (apigenin-7-*O*-glucoside), furthermore rhamnazin (3,7-dimethoxykaempferol) and 7-methoxykaempferol [6, 14, 16, 21, 36, 40, 49].

- Triterpene acids: Particularly ursolic acid (about 0.3%) and oleanolic acid [6].

Tests for Identity: Sensoric, macroscopic and microscopic analysis, as well as TLC of leaf extracts [20, 43, 57, Ü77, Ü102, DAB, Ph Helv] or TLC of the essential oil obtained from the leaves [43, 57, Ph Eur]. For the analysis of essential oil in commerce, GC, GC-MS or GC-IRMS analysis is required [15, 45]. For the identification of subspecies, DNA-fingerprint analyses are now also used for medicinal and culinary herbs [54].

Quantitative assay: The content of essential oil can be determined volumetrically with steam-distillation, using a prefilled graduated tube containing xylol, decalin or 1,2,3,4-tetramethylbenzene [57, Ph Eur]. The content of citral and citronellal can be determined with TLC [20, described in Lit. Ü37] or GC (see above); hydroxycinnamic acid derivatives are quantified colorimetrically, according to Ph Eur. The rosmarinic acid content can be determined with HPLC [12], or after silylation with GC [41].

Adulterations, Misidentifications and Impurities: Not to be expected since the material of commerce originates exclusively from cultivated sources. Possible adulteration with the non-official subspecies *M. officinalis* ssp. *altissima* can be recognized by the almost complete absence of citronellal and citral (neral + geranial), and based on morphological and anatomical characteristics [58]. A high content of stem parts (<10%) [Ph Eur] is considered an impurity.

Lemon balm essential oil is very expensive since it only occurs at low levels in the leaves. Adulterations and substitutions, for example, with the essential oil from → West Indian lemongrass or other Cymbopogon-species, lemon catnip (*Nepeta cataria* L. var. *citriodora* (BECK.) BALB, see below), as well as *Eucalyptus citriodora* HOOK. (Myrtaceae) and *Litsea cubeba* PERS. (Lauraceae) have been described [45].

Actions and Uses

Actions: Due to its aromatic taste, lemon balm causes a reflex action that stimulates the secretion of saliva, gastric juice and bile fluid, and therefore it has appetite stimulating and digestion promoting action.

In animal experiments (mice), application of lemon balm oil and some its constituents (among others, citral, citronellal, β-caryophyllene) by stomach tubes led to motility inhibition, explained as sedative activity, in a photoelectric barrier cage. The effect occurred at doses as low as 1 mg/kg body weight (β-caryophyllene, citral, citronellal or 3.1 mg/kg body weight lemon balm oil) [51]. Lemon balm oil or some of its constituents, especially β-caryophyllene and citral, also inhibited motility in mice when added to the breathing air [3].

In in-vitro studies using organ preparations from test animals (ileum, jejunum, trachea), the essential oil, citral or citronellal demonstrated antispasmodic effects. The EC_{50} for lemon balm oil in the guinea pig tracheal muscle preparations was 22 mg/liter, and 7.8 mg/liter in the electrically stimulated longitudinal muscle of the ileal myenteric plexus [4]. Spasmolytic effects were also observed with saturated aqueous solutions of lemon balm oil [10]. Whether these effects can be reproduced with oral administration of therapeutic doses in humans remains to be investigated. The same holds true for the sedative, sleep inducing and analgesic effects that have been observed in animal tests (mice) following intraperitoneal administration of lyophilized aqueous-ethanolic extracts of lemon balm leaf [46].

Lemon balm oil and citral have both shown a good antimicrobial effect [34]. Antiviral activity has been observed for aqueous extracts of lemon balm leaf in vitro and with parenteral application [7, 22, 24, 25, 29, 56], which is mainly due to the rosmarinic acid content, and probably only works with topical application.

Extracts of lemon balm leaf have good antioxidative activity. The main antioxidative active substances are rosmarinic acid and 2-(3′,4′-dihydroxyphenyl)-1,3-benzodioxol-5-aldehyde [27, 48].

Toxicology: Based on existing data, there is no acute or chronic toxicity with the normal use of lemon balm as a seasoning and in form of tea infusions. The sensitization potential is low. Case reports of allergic reactions are not known [Ü39].

Culinary use: The fresh, chopped leaves or shoot tips are used. The dried leaves are not suitable for use as a seasoning because most of their essential oil has evaporated. Due to the rapid loss of aroma when heated, the leaves should not be cooked with meals. Instead they should be added to the dish just shortly before serving. If allowed to infuse for a long time, they will turn brown. Due to their intense flavor, relatively small amounts are sufficient for seasoning.

Fresh chopped lemon balm leaves are suitable especially to enhance the flavor of cold dishes and beverages such as salads (e.g. of green salad, fruit salad, but also of cucumber-, potato-, egg- and fish salad), salad dressings, dips, raw fruit or vegetable dishes, refreshing beverages, punch (wine punch, strawberry punch), milk drinks, milk puddings, summer drinks, cold sweet soup or white wine punch, ice cream dishes, yogurt, quark, fresh cheese, creams, desserts, marmalades (strawberry-, peach-, apricot- and quince marmalades), as well as for pickling of cucumbers and tomatoes and as a component of herb vinegars, herb oils as well as herb butter. It is rarely used as a seasoning in warm dishes such as fruit soups, herb soups, chicken bouillon, sauces, omelets, meat dishes (rabbit, lamb, calf, mutton, game), poultry dishes (e.g. in fillings for roast chicken), vegetable dishes (e.g. of young vegetables, rutabaga and peas), fish dishes (e.g. trout) and mushroom dishes (e.g. champignons). Chopped lemon balm leaves sprinkled over buttered bread is a recommended delicacy. It is also suggested to place a twig of fresh lemon balm in the teapot with Earl Grey or Ceylon tea [Ü1, Ü2, Ü17, Ü47, Ü55, Ü59, Ü74, Ü79, Ü86, Ü92, Ü107].

Whole lemon balm leaves are also used as a garnish, e.g. for fish dishes, or candied as a cake garnish [Ü17].

Lemon balm oil is used as a flavor ingredient of herb liqueurs (Abtei, Alpenkräuter-likör, Aromatique, Cordialmedoc, Feinbitter, Chartreuse) as well as in the production of medicinal- and herbal spirits [Ü92].

Combines well with: Lemon, in green salads with borage, dill and tarragon, herb sauces with chervil, lovage and parsley, and as a spice for quark with fennel and hyssop [Ü59].

As a component of spice mixes and preparations: → Fish spice, → Frankfurter green sauce, → Herb vinegar (for preparation of lemon balm vinegar, place 2 to 3 fresh lemon balm branches in a bottle with wine vinegar and let it soak in a warm location for 2 weeks [Ü47]).

Other uses: The essential oil is used in the perfume industry. Due to its high price however, it is likely to have been replaced by distillates of Cymbopogon-species (→ West Indian lemongrass).

Medicinal herb

Herbal drugs: Melissae folium, Lemon balm leaf, contains not less than 4.0% of total hydroxycinnamic derivatives expressed as rosmarinic acid. Requirements for a specific essential oil content are not provided. The occurrence of essential oil obtained by steam distillation, however, is a prerequisite, since it serves as the test solution for the TLC identification [Ph Eur]. Melissae aetheroleum, Melissa oil, due to its high price is rarely used medicinally.

Indications: Lemon balm is used for nervous sleep disturbances and functional gastrointestinal complaints. The dosage is 1.5 to 4.5 g dried leaf per cup of tea infusion, several times daily [23]. Furthermore, other reported indications for use include states of restlessness, irritability, and digestive complaints such as minor spasms. The suggested dosage for oral administration is 2 to 3 g prepared as a tea infusion, 2 to 3 times daily, tincture (1 : 5 in 45% ethanol) 2 to 6 ml, t.i.d., or other preparations at equivalent dosage levels [4]. Additionally, lemon balm is used for psychovegetative cardiac disorders, biliary disorders, and dysmenorrhea. In psychiatric practice, it is used not only for treating sleep disturbances but is also used as an anxiolytic [55]. Extracts of lemon balm and the essential oil are used in the form of baths for skin inflammations and neurovegetative disturbances as well as in the form of poultices and ointments for skin infections (astringent action of the labiate tannins, antiviral action of rosmarinic acid), e.g. for Herpes labialis [4, 25, 26, 33, 52, Ü106].

Other culinary herbs with a lemon-like aroma

Lemon catnip, *Nepeta cataria* L. var. *citriodora* (BECK.) BALB. (Lamiaceae), is grown mainly for the production of essential oil in Europe, North America, India, and China. The leaves and flower buds are also used as spices. The essential oil contains citral (about 5 to 15%) as well as, among others, citronellol, elemol and nepetalactone [32]. It has cockroach repellent action [Ü61].

Moldavian dragonshead (Turkish lemon balm), *Dracocephalum moldavica* L. (Lamiaceae), is an annual plant, native to southern Siberia, and China, and cultivated in Romania, Bulgaria, and the Russian Federation, among other locations. The main components of the essential oil of the variety 'Arat' are geranyl acetate (about 60%) and citral (about 20%) [32]. It is used similarly to lemon balm [Ü61, Ü81].

Crested late-summer mint, *Elsholtzia ciliata* (THUNB.) HYL. (Lamiaceae), cultivated in eastern Asia, the main constituent of its essential oil is citral (about 20%) [32].

Mexican giant hyssop (lemon hyssop), *Agastache mexicana* (H.B.K.) LINT. et EPLING. (Lamiaceae), is native to northern Mexico, and cultivated in the USA. The main constituents of the essential oil obtained from the leaves are pulegone, menthone, isomenthol, limonene and citronellal (about 3.5%), which are jointly responsible for the aroma [32]. The leaves are used as a seasoning in salads, egg dishes, and for preparing beverage teas [30, Ü61, Ü81].

Lemon geranium (apple scented geranium), *Pelargonium odoratissimum* (L.) L'HERIT ex AIT. (Geraniaceae), is cultivated in France, Spain, and Brazil, among other countries, for the production of its essential oil, of which its main constituents are geraniol (about 65%) and citronellal (about 6%) [32].

Other culinary herbs with a lemon-like aroma include, among others, some types of ginger (→ Ginger), → West Indian lemongrass, muscatel sage (→ Sage), → Lemon, lemon basil (→ Basil), lemon thyme (→ Wild Thyme and Thyme) and lemon wormwood (→ Mugwort).

Lemon balm drink

4 to 5 lemon balm leaves, 2 thin cucumber slices, 10 ml lemon juice (freshly squeezed), 10 ml corn syrup or molasses, ginger ale (Schweppes).

Combine all the ingredients, except the Ginger Ale, in a glass with ice cubes. Fill up with ginger ale [Ü57].

Literature

[1] Adzet T. et al., Planta Med. 58:562–564 (1992).

[2] Agata I. et al., Chem. Pharm. Bull. 41: 1608–1611 (1992).

[3] Ammon H.P.T., Therapiewoche 39:117–127 (1989).

[4] Anonym, ESCOP Monographs: Melissae folium, Melissa leaf (1996).

[5] Baerheim Svendsen A., I.J.M. Merkx, Planta Med. 55:38–40 (1989).

[6] Brieskorn C.H., Arch. Pharmaz. 307:603–613 (1974).

[7] Büechi S. Dtsch. Apoth. Ztg. 138(14): 1265–1274 (1998).

[8] Carnat A.P. et al., Pharm. Acta Helv. 72(5):301–305 (1998).

[9] Dawson B.S.W. et al., Flavour Fragr. J. 3:167–170 (1988).

[10] Debelmas A.M., J. Rochat, Plant. Med. Phytother. 1(1):23–27 (1967).

[11] Enjalbert F. et al., Fitoterapia 54:59–65 (1983).

[12] Gracza L., P. Ruff, Arch. Pharmaz. 317: 339–345 (1984).

[13] Hefendehl F.W., Arch. Pharm. 303:345–357 (1970).

[14] Heitz A. et al., Fitoterapia 71(2):201–202 (2000).

[15] Hener U. et al., Pharmazie 50:60–62 (1995).

[16] Hodisan V., Clujul. Med. 70(2):280–286 (1997).

[17] Hollá M. et al., J. Ess. Oil Res. 9:481–484 (1997).

[18] Hose S. et al., Pharmazie 52:247–243 (1998).

[19] Janicsák G. et al., 46th Ann. Congress of the Soc. for Med. Plant Res. 1998 Vienna, Abstracts, B17 (1998).

[20] Kloeti F. et al., Fresenius' Z. Anal. Chem. 312:352–354 (1985).

[21] Koch-Heitzmann I., W. Schultze, Z. Phytother. 9(3):77–85 (1988).

[22] Koch-Heitzmann I., W. Schultze, Dtsch. Apoth. Ztg. 124(43):2137–2145 (1984).

[23] Kommission E beim BfArM, BAnz-Nr. 228 vom 05.12.84, Berichtigung 13.03.1990.

[24] König B, J.H. Dustmann, Naturwissenschaften 72:659–661 (1985).

[25] Koytchev R. et al., Phytomedicine 6(4): 225–230 (1999).

[26] Kümel G. et al., Dtsch. Apoth. Ztg. 131(30): 1609 (1991).

[27] Lamaison J.L. et al., Fitoterapia 62:166–171 (1991).

[28] Lamaison J.L. et al., Ann. Pharm. Franc 48:103–108 (1990).

[29] Louis S.K. et al., Proc. Soc. Exp. Biol. Med. 124:865–869 und 869–874 (1967).

[30] Manjarrez A., V. Mendoza, Perfumery Ess. Oil Record 57:561 (1966), zit. bei Ü43.

[31] Meyer W., G. Spiteller, Z. Naturforsch., C: Biosc. 51(9/10):651–656 (1996).

[32] Mikus B., J. Schaser, Drogenreport 8(13): 32–38 (1995).

[33] Mohrig A., Dtsch. Apoth. Ztg. 136(50): 4575–4580 (1996).

[34] Möse J.R., G. Lukas, Arzneim. Forsch. 7:687–692 (1957).

[35] Mulkens A., I. Kapetanidis, J. Nat. Prod. 51:496–498 (1988).

[36] Mulkens A., I. Kapetanidis, Pharm. Acta Helv. 62:19–22 (1987).

[37] Mulkens A., I. Kapetanidis, Pharm. Acta Helv. 63:266–270 (1988).

[38] Nykänen I., L. Nykänen, Lebensm. Wiss. Technol. 19:482–485 (1986).

[39] Pino J.A. et al., J. Ess. Oil Res. 11:363–364 (1999).

[40] Reiter M., W. Brandt, Arzneim. Forsch. 35:408–414 (1985).

[41] Reschke A., Z. Lebensm. Unters. Forsch. 176:116–119 (1983).

[42] Sarer E., G. Kökdil, Planta Med. 57: 89–90 (1991).

[43] Schultze W. et al., Dtsch. Apoth. Ztg. 129:155–163 (1989).

[44] Schultze W. et al., Planta Med. 55: 219–220 (1989).

[45] Schultze W. et al., Dtsch. Apoth. Ztg. 135(7):557–577 (1995).

[46] Soulimani R. et al., Planta Med. 57(2): 105–109 (1991).

[47] Stahn T., U. Bomme, Herba Germanica 2(2):78–90 (1994).

[48] Tagashira M., Y. Ohtake, Planta Med. 64(6):555–558 (1998).

[49] Thieme H., Pharmazie 28:69–70 (1973).

[50] Tittel G. et al., Planta Med. 46:91–98 (1982).

[51] Wagner H., L. Sprinkmeyer, Dtsch. Apoth. Ztg. 113:1159–1166 (1973).

[52] Walz A., Dtsch. Apoth. Ztg. 136(1):26 (1996).

[53] Weymar H., Buch der Lippenblütler und Rauhblattgewächse, Neumann Verlag, Radebeul 1961.

[54] Wolf H.Th. et al., Planta Med. 65(1):83–85 (1999).

[55] Wong A.H.C. et al., Arch. Gen. Psychiatry 55(11):1033–1044 (1998).

[56] Yamasaki K. et al., Biol. Pharm. Bull. 21(8):829–833 (1998).

[57] Zänglein A. et al., Dtsch. Apoth. Ztg. 135(50):4623–4639 (1995).

[58] van den Berg T. et al., Pharmazie 52(10): 802–807 (1997).

Literature references identified by Ü can be found in the general listing of books and monographs at the back of this book.

Lemon verbena

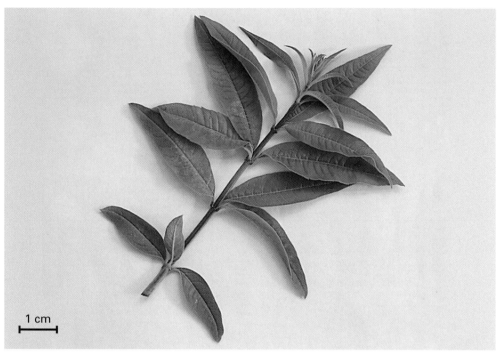

Fig. 1: Lemon verbena top

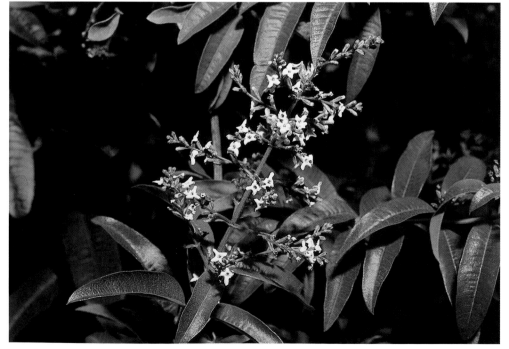

Fig. 2: Lemon verbena (*Aloysia triphylla* (L'HÉRIT.) BRITT.)

Plant source: *Aloysia triphylla* (L'HÉRIT.) BRITT.

Synonyms: *Lippia triphylla* (L'HÉRIT.) KUNTZE, *Aloysia citriodora* PALAU, *Lippia citriodora* (ORT. ex PERS.) H.B.K.

Taxonomic classification: The classification of this plant to different genera (Aloysia, Lippia, Verbena, Zapania) can easily lead to confusion.

Family: Vervain or verbena family (Verbenaceae).

Common names: Engl.: lemon verbena, vervaine; Fr.: verveine citronée, verveine odorante, citronelle; Ger: Zitronenstrauch, Aloysie, Echte Verbene, Zitronenverbene, Verbenenkraut, Mexikanischer Oregano.

Description: Shrub, 1 to 1.5 m (seldom up to 4.5 m) tall, deciduous. The foliage leaves are short stalked, long-acuminate, entire-margined, glanduliferous on the under-surface and verticillate arranged. The small numerous flowers are arranged in paniculate spikes, have a hairy tetrarch calyx, 4 white or bright-violet, at the bottom connate petals, 2 short and 2 longer stamina and a two-chambered ovary. The small dry fruit contains 2 monospermous stones. Flowering time is from June until September [Ü37, Ü42].

Native origin: Uruguay, Argentina, Chile, and Brazil.

Main cultivation areas: Mexico, Chile, Argentina, Brazil, Mediterranean region (especially Morocco, Algeria, Turkey, Southern France and Israel), South Africa, southern parts of the Russian Federation, and India.

Main exporting countries: Chile, Israel, and Morocco.

Cultivation: Lemon verbena prefers loose, well drained soil in sunny to half-shade positions in moist and warm climates. Propagation is carried out with cuttings or stolons. The plants do not tolerate temperatures below 4 °C. Lemon verbena is also a popular pot- or tub plant in temperate latitudes, especially in the USA. Tip cuttings from the lower part slightly ligneous, cut directly below a leaf node, can be easily grown underneath jars. Propagation from seeds is also possible; regular watering and fertilizing is necessary. In light quarters, they can overwinter at 5 to 10 °C, with less watering but not allowed to completely dry out. While overwintering the plants drop some of their leaves, which often are only replaced in the summer [Ü17, Ü32, Ü66].

Culinary herb

Commercial forms: Lemon verbena herb: dried leaves, whole herb ("feuille à feuille") or bulk commodity ("verveine standard", rubbed, dedicated for tea bags), verbena oil (oregano oil).

Production: After the second vegetation period the young lateral branches can be cut twice annually, usually before the blooming period in July and then once more in October. After rapid drying, usually by hanging up in bundles, the rolled up leaves are stripped off [Ü37].

Forms used: Fresh leaves (the dried leaves also for the preparation of tea), and verbena oil.

Storage: The fresh leaves can be stored in plastic bags in the refrigerator for a few days. Dried leaves are to be stored in tightly closed porcelain-, glass- or suitable metal containers, in a dark and cool place.

Description. Whole herb (Fig. 1): See plant description, the leaves are 8 to 12 cm long, 2 to 2.5 cm wide; in their dried state, they are strongly rolled up, revealing the lower surface on the outside, midrib strongly prominent on the lower surface from which leaf veins branch off perpendicularly. The upper leaf surface is whitish punctuate and rough due to cystolithic trichomes [PF X].

Powdered herb: Light green fragments of the upper epidermis with stout, cystolithic trichomes, which are surrounded by rosette-like cells, epidermis of the lower leaf surface with numerous anomocytic stomata and glandular trichomes [PF X].

Odor and **Taste:** Lemon-like.

History: The plant was introduced to Europe by the Spaniards in the 17th century, and was often grown in Mediterranean gardens.

Constituents and Analysis

Constituents

- Essential oil: 0.1 to 0.7% in the dried leaves, the main components are 20 to 40% carbonyl compounds: geranial (citral a, 15 to 25%), neral (citral b, about 15%), methylheptenone (about 2%), citronellal and photocitrals A, epi-A and B (significantly contributing to the odor, formed by photocyclisation of citral), furthermore (–)-limonene (10 to 20%), 1,8-cineole (3 to 6%), geraniol (about 6%), spathulenol (about 5%), camphor (about 4%), germacrene D (about 4%), bicyclogermacrene (about 4%), β-caryophyllene (about 2%), geraniol, geranyl acetate, nerol, neryl acetate [4, 5, 7]. In a chemotype from Argentina, the main components were myrcenone (about 36%), (–)-thujone (about 13%), lippifoli-1(6)-ene-5-one (about 9%) and limonene (about 7%) [7]; in a different material (grown in Thuringia, Germany), the main components were geraniol (24%), nerol (19%) and limonene (16%) [11].
- Flavonoids: Including, among others, luteolin-7-O-glucoside, luteolin-7-O-glucuronylglucoside, luteolin-7-O-glucoronosylglucuronoside, 7-O-glucosides of apigenin and diosmetin, free flavones, methoxylated flavones such as eupafolin, cirsimaritin, salvigenin and eupatorin [1, 15, 16].
- Iridoids: About 0.1%, verbenalin and geniposidic acid [10, 14].
- Hydroxycinnamic acid derivatives: 3 to 7% verbascoside, among others [10].

Tests for Identity of the leaf material with TLC [PF X], for verbena oil TLC [PF X] or capillary GC [4, 5].

Quantitative assay of the essential oil volumetrically, after steam distillation and addition 1% NaCl with xylol in the graduated tube [PF X], and of the carbonyl constituents in the essential oil, calculated as citral, with oximtitration [DAB, → Zitronenöl].

Adulterations, Misidentifications and Impurities: Due to the characteristic lemon-like odor of the leaves, misidentifications are unlikely. Adulteration of lemon verbena oil is conceivable due to its high price. Possible substitutes include the so-called "Spanish verbena oil" (from *Thymus hyemalis* LANGE, see below) or the "East-Indian verbena oil" (→ West Indian lemon grass).

Geranial (Citral a)   Neral (Citral b)   Photocitral A   epi-Photocitral A

Actions and Uses

Actions: Due to their aromatic taste, the leaves of lemon verbena are appetite stimulating and digestion promoting.

Valid studies of the pharmacological actions exist only for verbena oil. In the isolated guinea pig small intestine it showed spasmolytic action (2×10^{-4} ml/ml bath liquid). It counteracted histamine-induced contractions [17]. Verbena oil has antibacterial action (MHK 0.62 µg/ml for Streptococcus- and Lactobacillus-species) [12].

Toxicology: Based on existing data, there is no acute or chronic toxicity with the use of normal doses of lemon verbena leaves or lemon verbena oil. The sensitization potential of verbena oil is, depending on the batch tested, weak to moderate [6].

Culinary use: Finely chopped leaves in small quantities (!) are used as a flavoring of fruit- and vegetable salads, desserts (e.g. stewed pears in lemon verbena leaf flavored syrup), fruit pudding, pudding sauces, cakes, ice creams, fruit tortes as well as fresh fruit drinks and sorbets, mainly with peaches or strawberries, whole leaves, which are removed after stewing, for refining of sauces, rice dishes, for fillings of poultry and fish [Ü17, Ü55, Ü66, Ü74, Ü79].

Fresh, finely chopped or ground leaves mixed with butter are suitable as a basic spread for toast with fish or grilled meat [Ü79].

Dried leaves placed in a sugar jar, ensure fresh aroma of its content [Ü74].

Verbena oil is also used, albeit rarely, in the liqueur industry (Vervaine du Velay).

Combines well with: Lemon balm and lemon thyme.

Other uses: The fresh or dried leaves (lemon verbena tea, vervaine tea), alone or in combination with licorice or peppermint, serve as a house tea. The essential oil is also used in the perfume industry, due to its high price mostly for fine perfumes.

Medicinal herb

Herbal drugs: Lippiae triphyllae folium, Verbena herb (according to PF X minimum 0.4% essential oil), Lippiae triphyllae aetheroleum (Aloysiae citriodorae aetheroleum), Verbena oil.

Indications: In France it is used for digestive problems, nervousness and somnipathy (5 to 20 g of the dried leaf per 1 litre water as a tea infusion, 2 to 5 cups daily, 3 to 6 drops of verbena oil 2- to 3-times daily). The essential oil is also applied externally for poorly healing wounds in the form of cataplasms [Ü37].

Other Verbenaceae used as culinary herbs

Mexican oregano, American oregano, *Lippia graveolens* H.B.K. (Verbenaceae), native to tropical and subtropical America, cultivated in Central America, California, sweetish, somewhat fragrant like clove, contains 0.3 to 2.5% essential oil, of which the main components are carvacrol (comprising 0.5 to 41%) and thymol (0.2 to 57%), 1,8-cineole (2 to 14%) and *p*-cymene (8 to 28%) [2, 3, 7, 8, 13]. It is used as a seasoning of meat-, bean- and vegetable stews, the dried herb is also a component of Mexican seasonings such as chili powder or chili con carne seasoning [9].

Spanish thyme, *Lippia micromera* SCHAU., native to South America, cultivated in Trinidad and Tobago in gardens, the leaves are used in the same way as those of *Lippia graveolens* [see above] [Ü61].

Literature

[1] Carnat A. et al., Planta Med. 61(5):490 (1995).
[2] Compadre C.M. et al., Planta Med. 53: 495–497 (1987).
[3] Dominguez X.A., Planta Med. 55:208–209 (1989).
[4] Garnero J., Parfum Cosmet. Aromes 13: 29–39 (1977), zit. Ü37.
[5] Kaiser R., D. Lamparski, Helv. Chim. Acta 59:1797–1802 (1976).
[6] Kligman A.M., W. Epstein, Contact Dermatitis 1:123–239 (1975).
[7] Kustrak D., Farm. Glas. 52(9):221–231 (1996).
[8] Lagouri V. et al. Z. Lebensm. Unters. Forsch. 197:20–23 (1993).
[9] Melchior H., H. Kastner, Gewürze: Botanische und chemische Untersuchungen, Parey Verlag, Berlin 1974.
[10] Mende R., M. Wichtl, Dtsch. Apoth. Ztg. 138(31):2904–2910 (1998).
[11] Mikus B. et al., Drogenreport 10(18): 68–73 (1997).
[12] Pellecuer I. et al., Plant Med. Phytother. 14:83–98 (1980).
[13] Pino J. et al., Nahrung 33:289–295 (1989).
[14] Rimpler H., H. Sauerbier, Biochem. Syst. Ecol. 14:307–310 (1986).
[15] Skaltsa H., G. Shammas, Planta Med. 54: 265 (1988), zit. Ü37 (1988).
[16] Tomás-Barberán F.A. et al., Phytochemistry 26:2281–2284 (1987).
[17] Torrent Marti M.T., Rev. R. Acad. Farm. (Barcelona) 14:39–55 (1976), zit. Ü37.

Literature references identified by Ü can be found in the general listing of books and monographs at the back of this book.

Lesser Galangal

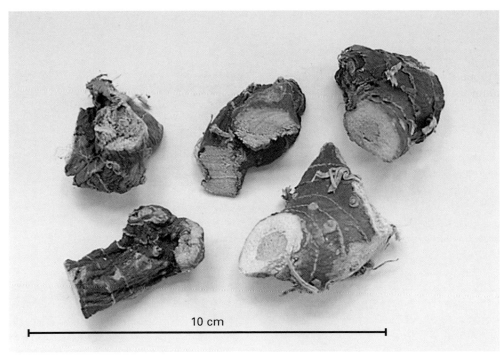

Fig. 1: Lesser galangal rhizome

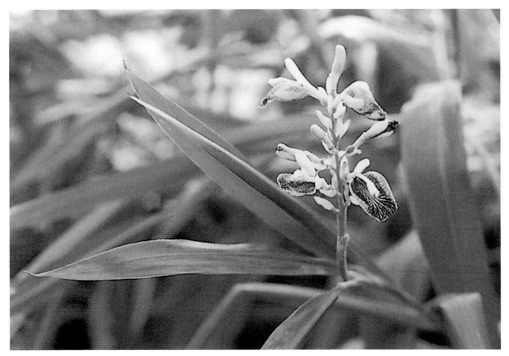

Fig. 2: Lesser galangal (*Alpinia officinarum* HANCE)

Plant source: *Alpinia officinarum* HANCE.

Synonyms: *Alpinia malaccensis* (BURM.) ROSCOE, *Languas officinarum* FARWELL.

Family: Ginger family (Zingiberaceae).

Common names: Engl.: lesser galangal, Chinese galangal, Chinese ginger, East Indian root; Fr.: galanga officinal, petit galanga, galanga de la Chine; Ger: Galgant, Echter Galgant, Kleiner Galgant, Kleine Galanga, Galant, Siam-Ingwer, Thai-Ingwer.

Description: Rhizomatous perennial herb, rhizome horizontal creeping, slender, cylindrical, smooth, with many branches, about 2 cm thick, up to 1 m long. The rhizome produces sterile pseudo-stems originating from the leaf-scars, as well as 0.6 to 1.5 m long flowering scapes. The non-flowering stems bear paired and lineal-lanceolate, entire-margined leaves (up to over 30 cm long), with a pointed tip and a somewhat prominent mid-rib. The scapes bear sheath-like leaves. The inflorescences form dense, terminal racemes. The corolla has a tubular base and is trilobate in the upper part, there are 6 stamina, their outer rim forms a perianth-like, white lip with red veins, and the inner rim contains one single fertile stamen, and the other two are filiform, situated just above the inferior, trilocular ovary. The red fruit is a quasi-spherical, pea-sized capsule [Ü45].

Native origin: South- and East coasts of the Chinese island of Hainan and the coastal areas just across on the mainland, as well as Thailand, Indonesia, Sri Lanka, Moluccas, Java, and Sumatra.

Main cultivation areas: Cultivated in Thailand, China (Hainan, Leitschou), Japan, India, Vietnam, Indonesia (Sumatra, Java,

Acetoxychavicol acetate

Dihydroyashabushiketol $R_1=R_2=H$

5-Hydroxy-7-(4''-hydroxy-3''-methoxyphenyl)
1-Phenyl-3-heptanone $R_1=OH$, $R_2=OCH_3$

Ages. In the 12th century, Hildegard von Bingen reported its use for stomach and intestinal complaints. In the 16th and 17th centuries, lesser galangal was imported to Central Europe via Russia (hence the German name "russische Wurzel"). It has been used since then not only as a medicine but also as a spice, similar to ginger [Ü81, Ü92].

Constituents and Analysis

Constituents

▪ Essential oil: 0.5 to 1.5%, the main component is 1,8-cineole (up to 50%), furthermore α- and β-pinene, myrcene and sabinene, among others, including small amounts of phenyl propane derivatives such as eugenol, chavicol and 1'-acetoxychavicol acetate [10, Ü106].

▪ Phenylethyl-n-alkyl-ketones (phenylalkanones): Gingerols, responsible for pungency (see Ginger) [Ü106].

▪ Diarylheptanoids: Complex mixture known as galangol or alpinol, diarylheptane-3-one, diarylheptane-3,5-dione, diarylheptane-3-ol-5-one, diarylhept-4-ene-3-one, diaryl-hept-1-ene-3-one and diarylheptane-3-hydroxy-methyl-5-one, among others, including dihydroyashabushiketol and 5-hydroxy-7-(4''-hydroxy-3''-methoxyphenyl)-1-phenyl-3-heptanone (with pungent taste), [5–7].

▪ Flavonoids: Quercetin-3-methyl-ether, isorhamnetin, "kämpferide" (3,5,7-trihydroxy-4'-methoxyflavone), galangine (3,5,7-trihydroxyflavone) and galangine-3-methyl ether [Ü60, Ü106].

▪ Starch (20 to 25%).

Tests for Identity with TLC [DAC 86, Ü106].

Quantitative assay: The content of essential oil can be determined volumetrically with steam distillation with xylol in the graduated tube [DAC 86].

Adulterations, Misidentifications and Impurities are possible with the rhizomes of *Kaempferia galanga* L. They are up to 4 cm thick and have a light-colored central

Moluccas), Sri Lanka, Malaysia, and the Antilles.

Main exporting countries: China, Thailand, Indonesia, Vietnam, and Sri Lanka.

Cultivation: The plant requires a tropical, humid climate. Propagation is done by rhizome cuttings. Rhizomes can be harvested at the earliest after 4 to 5 years [Ü89].

Culinary herb

Commercial forms: Lesser galangal: dried rhizome pieces often with the thin, brown skin removed, also cut or ground, fresh, unpeeled rhizome, and pickled rhizome.

Production: The approximately 1 m long rhizomes of 4 to 10 year old plants are washed after being dug up, cut into 5 to 10 cm long pieces, and dried [Ü89, Ü93].

Forms used: The fresh, rubbed rhizomes are best, but the dried rhizome is also used.

Storage: The fresh rhizome can be stored in the refrigerator wrapped in paper towels inside a plastic bag. The dried rhizomes are stored in glass-, porcelain- or metal containers protected from light, moisture, heat and insects.

Description. Whole rhizome (Fig. 1): Pieces of the rhizome, about 3 to 10 cm long, 1 to 2 cm thick, cylindrical, often knee-shaped bent, ramified; the cross sections is yellowish-brown on the inside and reddish-brown on the outside. The longitudinally striated surface bears small root-scars, which originate from the rhizome branches; also present are narrow, wavy, whitish fimbriate, nearly annular remains of the cataphyllary leaves, 0.5 to 1 cm apart. The fracture is fibrous and cinnamon-brown [Ü49, DAB 6].

Powdered rhizome: Contains a high amount of thick-walled, starchy parenchyma with scattered, brown and suberised secretory cells as well 25 to 80 μm wide, club-shaped, starch grains with prominent eccentric layering. Cork cells are absent. The epidermis is small-celled, brown and often multi-layered with some stomata. Also present are reticulate, scalariform and pitted vessels, abundant non-lignified, sclerenchymatic fibers, and surrounding the vascular tissue, small, elongated, non-suberised secretory cells [Ü49].

Odor: Agreeable and spicy, **Taste:** Aromatic, pungent and slightly bitter, reminiscent of ginger but not as pungent ("mild ginger").

History: Lesser galangal was already used in China during antiquity as a stomachic and spice. Plutarch (46–119 CE) mentioned this herb, and the Arabs have used it as well. Avicenna (980–1037 CE) praised its therapeutic attributes. Lesser galangal reached Central Europe during the Middle stele. Rhizomes from other *Alpinia* species have different TLC-profiles.

Actions and Uses

Actions: Due to its essential oil and bitter substances content, lesser galangal rhizome has a stimulant effect on the secretion of gastric- and biliary juices. 1´-Acetoxychavicolacetate has fungicidal, tumor- and phagocytosis inhibiting action. Presumably it slows down the activation of protein kinase C and the activation of the tumor triggering Epstein-Barr-Virus [13, 16]. The diarylheptanoids have been shown in vitro to be inhibitors of prostaglandin biosynthesis (IC_{50}: 2 to 170 µM) [7].

Culinary use: Lesser galangal is frequently used in Indonesian, Malaysian, Thai and Chinese cooking. Similarly to ginger, it is used to spice meat-, fish- and sweet dishes, but it is also added to salads and vegetables. The Indonesian rice dish, Nasi goreng, which is spiced with lesser galangal, is also known in Europe. Thus far, lesser galangal is used only rarely in Germany. As a spice, lesser galangal can be used in place of ginger. Rubbed, fresh lesser galangal or powdered lesser galangal serve as spices in meals made from fish- and sea foods (especially shrimps), lamb, braised chicken, exotic sauces, clear broths, stews, eggs, salads and vegetables [Ü13, Ü51, Ü55, Ü73].

Combines well with: Mugwort.

As a component of spice mixes and preparations: → Bomboe, → Curry powder, → Ras el hanout, → Sambal, → Stollen spice.

Other uses: Extracts of lesser galangal are used in liqueurs, especially digestive bitters (e.g. Boonekamp, Abtei, Stonsdorfer, among others), and in Scandinavia and Russia also in beer and kvass.

Medicinal herb

Herbal drug: Galangae rhizoma, Lesser galangal, contains not less than 0.5% essential oil [DAC, Ph Helv].

Indications: For digestive complaints and loss of appetite. The single dose is 0.5 to 1.5 g dried rhizome or equivalent preparations, and the daily dose is 2 to 4 g. Usually it is taken as a tincture [EB 6], daily dose: 2 to 4 g [8].

Similar culinary spices

Greater galangal (Siamese galanga, Java galanga, Thai ginger, Siam ginger), *Alpinia galanga* (L.) WILLD. (Synonym: *Languas galanga* (L.) STUNTZ, Zingiberaceae) occurs in Southeastern Asia, and is cultivated in Java and in the Philippines. The main components of the essential oil from its rhizomes are β-santalene, 1,8-cineole, β-bisabolene, *trans*-β-farnesene, α-bergamottene, terpinenol-4 and α-pinene, in addition to, among others, 1´-acetoxychavicol (galangal acetate, pungent tasting), chavicol acetate, chavicol, linalool, geranyl acetate, eugenol, bornyl acetate, citronellyl acetate, 2-acetoxy-1,8-cineole, 3-acetoxy-1,8-cineole and methyleugenol (eugenol methyl ester) [2, 3, 9, 11, 18]. Greater galangal rhizome serves as a spice in rice dishes, baked goods and alcoholic beverages especially in Thailand, Malaysia and Java. Outside of this region, it is rarely used. In these countries, the fruits are used similarly [1, 14, Ü61].

Light galangal, *Alpinia speciosa* (WENDL.) K. SCHUM. (Synonym: *A. zerumbet* (PERS.) BURTT et R.M. SM.), shell ginger, porcelain lily, Zingiberaceae), occurs in Northeast India and Myanmar, and is cultivated in India, Myanmar and Malaysia. The essential oil isolated from the fresh rhizomes contains, among other compounds, 1,8-cineole, methylcinnamate, α- and β-pinene, nerolidol, α-caryophyllene epoxide and β-eudesmol. Additionally, the rhizomes contain dihydro-5,6-dehydrokawain and 5,6-dehydrokawain. The rhizome is used similarly to lesser galangal and/or ginger, and the aromatic leaves serve as a wrap for cooked rice [4, 12, Ü43, Ü61].

Kaempferia galanga, *Kaempferia galanga* L. resurrection lily (Zingiberaceae), occurs in India, and is cultivated in Java, the Philippines and in the Sudan. The rhizomes contain 2.4 to 4.0% essential oil, of which the main components are cinnamic acid ethyl ester (about 25%) and *p*-methoxy cinnamic acid methyl ester (ca. 30%), and furthermore, borneol, camphor and Δ^3-carene. The rhizomes, but also the leaves, are used in India and Java for spicing unsweetened rice dishes, poultry- and meat dishes [15, 17, Ü61, Ü92, Ü93].

Southeast Asian Style Chicken
(Serves 2 to 4)
8 Chicken drumsticks, 6 crushed garlic cloves, 1 tablespoon black pepper (freshly ground), 2 tablespoons lesser galangal (ground), 1/2 teaspoon salt, oil.

Mix the garlic, pepper, lesser galangal and salt. Rub the drumsticks with the spice mixture and put them, covered, for 3 to 4 hours in the refrigerator. Then, pour oil into a frying pan up to height of 5 cm and place it on the hot burner. The oil should be hot but not smoke. Fry the drumsticks until they are golden-brown and done inside. Hold the chicken pieces over a paper towel to drip off excess oil and serve with rice [Ü55].

Literature

[1] Burkhil I.H., A Dictionary of Economic Products of the Malay Penninsula, Vol. 1 and 2, Ministry of Agriculture and Co-operatives, Kuala Lumpur, Malaysia 1966, ref. in Ü82.

[2] Chana J.S., Forum Aromather. Aromapflege 10:52–55 (1996).

[3] De Pooter H.L. et al., Phytochemistry 24:93–96 (1985).

[4] Hsu S.Y. et al., Planta Med. 60(1):88–90 (1994).

[5] Inoue T. et al., J. Pharm. Soc. Japan. 98:1255 (1978) , zit. in Ü43.

[6] Itokawa H. et al., Chem. Pharm. Bull. 29:2383–2385 (1981).

[7] Kiuchi F. et al., Chem. Pharm. Bull. 30:2279–2282 (1982).

[8] Kommission E beim BfArM, BAnz-Nr. 173 vom 18.09.86, Berichtigung am 13.03.90.

[9] Kubota K. et al., Agric. Food Chem. 47(2):685–689 (1999).

[10] Lawrence B.M. et al., Perfum Ess. Oil Rec. 60:89–96 (1969).

[11] Mori H. et al., Nippon Shokuhin Kagaku Kogaku Kaishi 42(12):989–995 (1995), ref. CA 124:115734p.

[12] Morita M. et al., Pharm. Bull. 44:1603–1606 (1996).

[13] Murakami A. et al., J. Agric. Food Chem. 48(5):1518–1523 (2000).

[14] Perry L.M., Medicinal Plants of East and Southeast Asia: Attributed Properties and Use, MTI Press, Cambridge, Massachusetts 1980

[15] Seidemann J., Pharmazie 47(8):636–639 (1992).

[16] Watanabe N. et al., Biosc. Biotechnol. Biochem. 59(8):1566–1567 (1995).

[17] Wong K.C. et al., Flavour Fragr. 7:263–266 (1992).

[18] Yang X., Eilerman R.G., J. Agric. Food Chem. 47(4):1657–1662 (1999).

Literature references identified by Ü can be found in the general listing of books and monographs at the back of this book.

Lovage

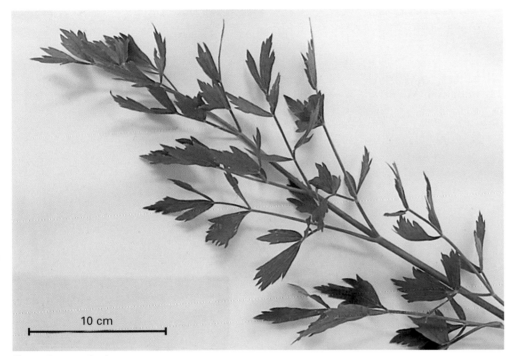

Fig. 1: Lovage leaf

Plant source: *Levisticum officinale* W.D.J. KOCH.

Synonym: *Ligusticum levisticum* L.

Family: Umbelliferous plants (Apiaceae, synonym Umbelliferae).

Common names: Engl.: lovage, garden lovage, bladder seed; Fr.: livèche; Ger: Liebstöckel, Maggikraut, Suppenlob, Liebstock, Bergliebstock, Lusch, Großer Eppich, Stecklaub, Lüppsteckel.

Description: Perennial herb, flowering in the 2nd year, 1 to 2 m high, taproot carrot-like thickened, furrowed, branched, with multiple headed and long, finger-thick roots. Cylindrical hollow stem, glabrous, pruinose, grooved and branched in the upper part. The main leaves are dark green, shiny, the lower ones bipinnate, the upper ones singly pinnate or entire-margined, lamina triangular-rhomboid, the lower leaves up to 70 cm long, leaflets broadly ovate, cuneiform at the base, three-lobed or broadly serrate. The flowers are arranged in terminal, composite umbels, up to 12 cm wide, with 12 to 20 rays, involucre and small involucres are numerous, with marginally ciliate-papillose serration, the upper surface is rough due to pointed papillae. The radial flowers have 5 pale yellow petals, with an inwardly bent tip, 5 stamina, 2 styles and an inferior bilocular ovary. The fruit is an almost circular double achene, separated into mericarps, which are still attached to a bifurcate carpophore; the mericarps are frequently curved. Flowering period is July to August [30].

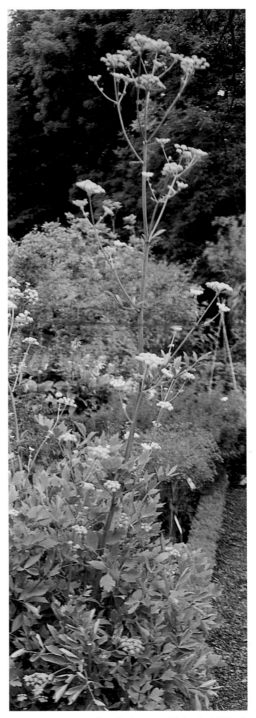

Fig. 2: Lovage (*Levisticum officinale* W.D.J. KOCH)

Native origin: Iran and Afghanistan, and introduced to Europe and the USA. The wild form is possibly *Levisticum persicum* FREYN et BORNM.

Main cultivation areas: Germany (Thuringia), Poland, Czech Republic, Switzerland, the Netherlands, the Balkan States, and the USA.

Main exporting countries: Germany (Thuringia), Poland, the Netherlands, and the Balkan States.

Cultivation: Lovage prefers deep, humus- and nutrient rich, moist soil in full sun to part-shade locations. Direct seeding can take place in August or April in rows of 40 to 65 cm apart. There are no bred varieties. In the seed trade a 'medium coarse leafy' variety (with much foliage and stout roots) is available. Propagation by root division is possible in the spring [Ü2, Ü21]. For a single household, one plant is sufficient, and can be up to 10 to 15 years old [Ü86].

Culinary herb

Commercial forms: Lovage leaf: dried leaves, cut or ground, lovage root: dried rhizome with roots, lovage seed: dried fruits, furthermore the fresh bundled herb, fresh plants in herb pots, lovage essential oil and lovage oleoresin both obtained from the fruits, and rarely from the herb and roots.

Production: The herb harvest can take place in the first year in July, and during early September and October, in the second year after June using a bar mower, cutting loader, grass harvester, or similar equipment. In the autumn of the plant's last productive year, the roots can be dug up. After washing, they are cut into 10 to 15 cm long pieces. The fruits are harvested by combine or thresher [Ü21]. Leaves for personal use can be plucked year round.

Forms used: Fresh, chopped leaves, dried, cut or ground leaves, the fresh or dried roots, and the whole broken fruits.

Storage: The fresh leaves can be stored for a few days, with the cut stalks immersed in water, or wrapped in plastic in the refrigerator (at temperatures between -1 and +2 °C, the shelf-life is 8 weeks), The whole leaves can be stored frozen in a freezer bag, or also finely cut, with water in the ice-tray. Drying leads to loss of aroma. The dried leaves, roots and seeds are kept in well-closed metal- or glass containers, protected from light and moisture. Especially the dried roots are prone to insect-infestation.

Description. Leaf (Fig. 1): See description of the whole plant. Microscopic examination reveals the sinuate-polygonal cells on both sides, with striated cuticula; trichomes and calcium oxalate crystals are absent [Ü37].

Fruit (Fig. 3): Elliptic, 5 to 7 mm long and half as wide, yellow to brown, after separation of the double achene, curved or crescent-shaped, with 5 ribs that are winged at the margin [Ü37].

Root: Short rhizome, up to 5 mm thick, often split longitudinally, light gray-brown to yellowish brown, often with transverse girdling, with up to 25 cm long and 1.5 cm thick roots; the fracture is mostly smooth and shows a wide, yellowish-white cortex and a narrow, brown-yellow xylem [Ph Eur].

Odor: Strongly aromatic, reminiscent of soup seasoning, **Taste:** Sweetish then pungent, slightly bitter.

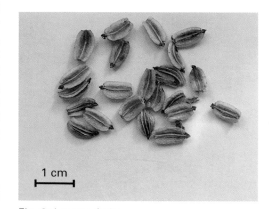

1 cm

Fig. 3: Lovage fruits

History: Lovage was already used medicinally in ancient Greece as a stomachic, carminative and spasmolytic. Via Italy it was introduced to Central Europe by Benedictine monks, where it has been cultivated as a medicinal and spice plant since the 8th century. In antiquity and during the Middle Ages, the fruits and roots were already not only considered good remedies against gastric complaints, loss of appetite, flatulence, retention of urine and hoarseness, but they were also recommended for the topical treatment of snake-, scorpion- and dog bites. In the imperial decree of Karl the Great "Capitulare de villis" (see footnote in → Anise monograph), the cultivation of lovage was called for [24, 28].

Constituents and Analysis

Constituents of the herb
- Essential oil: 0.8 to 1.7% (0.08 to 0.39%, calculated with reference to the fresh herb), with the main components α-terpinylacetate (35 to 48%), β-phellandrene (about 25%), phthalides (about 12%, mostly ligustilide) [3, 9, 26].
- Coumarins: About 0.1% [9,12].
- Furanocoumarins: About 0.3%, including bergaptene, among others [21, Ü100].
- Hydroxycoumarins: Umbelliferone [1].
- Flavonoids: 0.25%, particularly rutin [21].
- Unusual amino acids: 2-Aminoadipic acid, saccharopin [28].
- Vitamin C: 254 to 407 mg / 100 g (in the leaflets, calculated with reference to the fresh herb) [23].

Constituents of the fruit
- Essential oil: 0.8 to 1.1%, with the main components β-phellandrene (up to 60%), phthalides, especially ligustilide [9,26].
- Furanocoumarins: Imperatorin, bergaptene, psoralene, traces of xanthotoxin [5, 20].

Constituents of the root:
- Essential oil: About 0.4 to 1.7% (with 50 to 70% phthalides as the main com-

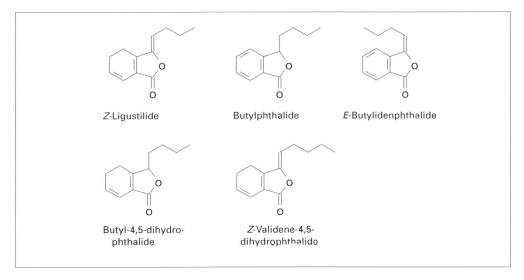

Z-Ligustilide   Butylphthalide   E-Butylidenphthalide

Butyl-4,5-dihydro-phthalide   Z-Validene-4,5-dihydrophthalide

ponents); with Z-ligustilide (3-n-butylidene-4,5-dihydrophthalide) dominating (83 to 93%), furthermore, Z-butylidenphthalide (ligusticum lactone, 3 to 7%), E-ligustilide (2 to 5%), Z-3-n-validene-4,5-dihydrophthalide (1 to 5%), 3-n-butyl-4,5-dihydrophthalide (senkyunolide), 3-butylphthalide and dimeric phthalides, among others; also present are β-phellandrene (about 17%), citronellal (13%), limonene (about 9%), cis-β-ocimene (about 5%), α- and β-pinene, as well as pentylcyclohexadiene [7–9, 13, 26, 27].

- Coumarin and coumarin derivatives: Coumarin and umbelliferone [1, 10, 18].
- Furanocoumarins: About 0.4%, with bergaptene and psoralene, among others [Ü100].
- Polyines: (+)-Falcarindiol [7].
- Sterols: β-sitosterol-β-glucoside [29].

Tests for Identity: Organoleptic, macroscopic and microscopic examination, as well as TLC analysis [25, Ü102, Ph Eur, Ph Helv, DAC 86]. The determination of the essential oil composition can be carried out with GC/MS and GC/FTIR [8]; the phthalide components can be identified with GLC, GC/MS or TLC [13].

Quantitative assay: The essential oil content is determined with steam-distillation, according to Ph Eur, with xylol in the graduated tube.

Adulterations, Misidentifications and Impurities: Due to their similar odor, celery leaves and fruits might be mistaken for lovage. The leaves from lovage are, in contrast to celery, bipinnate; the fruits are significantly larger than celery fruits (which are only up to 1.5 mm long). Accidental adulterations with roots from → Angelica, parsnip and → Salad burnet can be recognized with TLC [11, Ü102, Ph Eur].

Actions and Uses

Actions: Due to their aromatic, slightly pungent and slightly bitter taste, all plant parts have a reflex action which stimulates salivation, secretion of gastric juices, bile excretion and intestinal motility, and therefore they stimulate appetite and digestion.

In animal tests, extracts of the root slightly increased the quantity of urine and/or the excretion of chloride or urea [29]. Similar results have been confirmed in humans [6]. In rats, an estrogenic effect has been observed [22]. This author is not aware of any studies on the activity of the leaves and fruits, but similar effects must be supposed.

The phthalides have shown a mild sedative effect in animal tests in high doses (100 mg/kg body weight). In the rat small intestine, they antagonize the spasmodic effect of acetylcholine, and in the uterus they antagonize the effect of $PGF_{2\alpha}$ [19]. In relatively high doses (60 mg/kg body weight), butylidenphthalide has shown an anti-anginous action in rats [15]. An anthelmintic effect has also been observed [17].

As with most essential oils, lovage oil has an antimicrobial effect. A fraction with a high boiling point was shown to be especially effective [3, 14].

Toxicology: Based on existing data, there is no acute or chronic toxicity with the regular use of lovage as a spice. The sensitization potential is small. Allergic reactions have only been observed very rarely [Ü39]. Phototoxic reactions have been documented [2].

Culinary use: Unlike celery, lovage can withstand long cooking times without a significant loss of aroma. Due to its intense taste, which can slightly overpower other spices, it should be measured carefully.

The leaves and the young stems, chopped, fresh or blanched, serve as a spice in salads (especially tomato- or paprika salad), herb sauces, marinades, meat stock, hearty soups (bean-, pea-, potato-, spring vegetable soup) and stews, especially rice- and noodle dishes, vegetable dishes (especially kohlrabi, cauliflower, and carrots), egg dishes (e.g. omelets), smoked or steamed fish and meat dishes (roast mutton, roast beef, ragouts, herb meatballs, as a component of meat fillings in beef rolls). The dried leaves, which taste a bit like yeast, serve the same purpose. The herb is also used in the production of lovage butter, which can be used for potato dishes, red beets and root vegetables. It is also suitable as a pickling spice for pickled vegetables and mushrooms. The finely chopped leaves taste good on quark- and cheese breads. The leaf stems can be candied for use as a decoration of baked goods [Ü2, Ü13, Ü47, Ü55, Ü65, Ü70, Ü74, Ü79].

The fruits are used as a spice in bread, cakes, crackers, pickles and sauces [Ü2, Ü74].

The ground roots are used as a spice in soups. The peeled roots are eaten as a vegetable, e.g. in Italy [Ü2].

The essential oil can be used as a component of spicy mustard, spice- and liqueur essences (especially herbal- and bitter liqueurs).

Combines well with: Basil, celery, chervil, garlic, lemon balm, marjoram, mints, onions, parsley, rosemary, tarragon, and thyme.

As a component of spice mixes and preparations: → Fish spice, → Gravy spice, → Herb vinegar, → Meat spice, → Sauce spice, → Soup spice, → Table mustard.

Similar culinary spices: → Celery.

Medicinal herb

Herbal drugs: Levistici radix, Lovage root (contains minimum 4.0 ml/kg of essential oil for the whole root and minimum 3.0 ml/kg for the cut root) [Ph Eur], Levistici fructus, Lovage fruit, Levistici herba, Lovage herb.

Indications: Inflammatory diseases of the lower urinary tract and for prevention of kidney gravel. Due to the diuretic effect, preparations of the root are used in these cases for irrigation therapy. The daily dose is 4 to 8 g of dried root, usually taken in the form of tea infusions (1.5 to 3.0 g per cup). Lovage root preparations should not be used in cases of acute inflammation of the renal parenchyma or with impaired kidney function, as well as in cases of edema due to impaired heart and kidney function. Due to potential phototoxic effects, exposure to ultraviolet light and intense sun bathing should be avoided after long-term application of lovage [16]. Other indications for use include digestive complaints such as eructation, heartburn and feeling of repletion [Ü12].

Noodles with lovage
400 g noodles, 1 teaspoon table salt, 2 teaspoons olive oil, 4 tablespoons plucked lovage leaves, 2 teaspoons butter.
Boil 4 l water with salt and oil and add the noodles. When the noodles are al dente, pour off almost all of the water with about 3 tablespoons remaining. Mix the lovage and the butter with the rest of the noodle-water, bring to a boil quickly, and pour the sauce over the noodles that have been placed in a heated tureen with lid. Let the dish stand for 3 minutes and serve it covered. Small sausages (bratwurst) or pan-fried meats and salad are excellent side dishes [Ü86].

In folk medicine, lovage root, fruit and herb are used for digestive pain and flatulence (for their secretion promoting and antispasmodic action) as well as for menstrual pains (possibly phytoestrogenic).

Literature

[1] Albulescu D. et al., Farmacia 23:159–165 (1975).

[2] Ashwood-Smith M.J. et al., Contact Dermatitis 26(5):356–357 (1992).

[3] Bauermann U. et al., Drogenreport 6(10): 24–30 (1993).

[4] Bjeldanes I.F., I.S. Kim, J. Food Sci. 43: 143–144 (1978).

[5] Blank I., P. Schieberle, Flavour Fragr. J. 8:191 (1993).

[6] Braun R., Dtsch. Heilpflanze 7:21 (1941).

[7] Cichy M. et al., Liebigs Ann. Chem. 397–400 (1984).

[8] Cu J.Q. et al., J. Ess. Oil Res. 2:53–59 (1990).

[9] Fehr D., Planta Med. (Suppl.) 34–40 (1980).

[10] Fischer F.C., A. Baerheim Svendsen, Phytochemistry 15:1079–1080 (1976).

[11] Genius O.B., Dtsch. Apoth. Ztg. 121:386–387 (1981).

[12] Gijbels M.J.M. et al., Rivista Italina EPPOS 61(7):335–341 (1979).

[13] Gijbels M.J.M. et al., Planta Med. 44: 207–211 (1981).

[14] Kemp M.S., Phytochemistry 17:10002 (1978).

[15] Ko W.Ch. et al., Planta Med. 64(3): 229–232 (1998).

[16] Kommission E beim BfArM, BAnz-Nr. 101 vom 01.06.1990.

[17] Lautenschläger L., Ber. Pharm. Ges. 31: 279 (1921).

[18] Mitsuhashi H. et al., Pharm. Bull. (Tokyo) 11:1317–1319 (1963).

[19] Mitsuhashi H. et al., Chem. Pharm. Bull. (Tokyo) 8:243–245 (1960).

[20] Naves Y.R., Helv. Chim. Acta 5: 1281–1295 (1943).

[21] Plouvier V., C. R. Acad. Sci., Paris, Ser. D 268(1):86–88 (1969).

[22] San Martin R., Farmacognosia 18: 179–186 (1958).

[23] Scheunert A., E. Theile, Pharmazie 7: 776–780 (1952).

[24] Scholz H., Natürlich 19(7):33–37 (1999).

[25] Stahl E. (Hrsg.): Chromatographische und mikroskopische Analyse von Drogen, Fischer Verlag Stuttgart, New York 1978.

[26] Toulemonde B., I. Noleau, in: Flavor Fragrances, A World Perspective (Eds. Lawrence et al.). Elsevier Science Publ. B.V., Amsterdam 1988, p. 641.

[27] Uhlig J.W. et al., J. Food Sciences 52:658–660 (1987).

[28] Vollmann C., Z. Phytother. 9(4):128 (1988).

[29] Vollmer H., K. Hübner, Arch. Exp. Path. 186:592–605 (1937).

[30] Weymar H., Buch der Doldengewächse, Neumann Verlag, Radebeul 1959.

Literature references identified by Ü can be found in the general listing of books and monographs at the back of this book.

Mints

Plant sources: The main mints that are used as culinary herbs include: *Mentha ×piperita* L. nm. *piperita*, peppermint, *M. spicata* L. emend. L. var. *crispa* BENTH., spearmint, *M. pulegium* L., European pennyroyal, *M. citrata* EHRH., lemon mint and *M. suaveolens* EHRH., apple mint. See below for information on other Mentha-species that are rarely used as culinary herbs.

Taxonomic classification: There are about 20 known Mentha-species. They hybridize easily (the botanical names of hybrids are denoted by the symbol × placed before the epithets, e.g. *Mentha ×piperita* L.), and are also distinguished by their chromosome number. Hybrids that share distinctive morphological properties are combined into subspecies, varieties or nothomorphs (abbreviated as nm., a nothomorph comprises hybrids from the same parents with different morphology). In total, approximately 600 species, subspecies, varieties and forms are known. For peppermint alone, there are over 100 known types.

Family: Mint family (Lamiaceae, synonym Labiatae).

Constituents: In mints used for seasoning, the following compounds are predominant in the essential oil:
- Monoterpenes of the *p*-menthane-type, particularly their
- 3-hydroxy derivatives, such as (–)-menthol, its stereoisomers and their esters, particularly acetates,
- 3-oxo derivatives, such as (–)-menthone and its stereoisomers, (+)-pulegone, piperitone and its derivatives,
- 2-oxo derivatives, such as (–)-carvone, dihydrocarvone,
- epoxides such as 1,8-cineole, menthofuran, piperitone oxide.

Minor constituents occurring rarely or in small amounts include:
- Other monoterpenes: e.g. linalool, linalyl acetate, limonene, β-ocimene, sabinene hydrate, terpinenol-4, terpinyl acetate, isopinocamphone (*cis*-pinocamphone),
- Sesquiterpenes, including, among others, elemol, viridiflorol, germacrene D, β-caryophyllene,
- Phenyl propane derivatives, with eugenol, among others.

The main composition of the essential oil, however, is not always a criterion for the aroma quality since odoriferous components occurring in only small amounts can influence the odor significantly. For the use in seasonings, different mint types are therefore interchangeable. Of particular importance for the aroma quality is the occurrence of menthol esters such as menthyl acetate and menthylisovalerate, as well as *cis*-jasmone and viridiflorol.

Cultivation: Mentha-species are without exception herbaceous perennial plants that form aboveground or subterranean runners (stolons). Hybrids are often sterile. Although they indeed flower, they do not produce viable seeds. Additionally, fertile hybrids may not be propagated by seed, because the descendents will not breed true to the properties of the hybrid. Therefore, propagation must be carried out with cuttings of the shoots or pieces of the stolons. The pure species (water mint, spearmint, and apple mint) can be propagated by seed.

History: Mint species have been used since antiquity. In 2000 BCE, cultivations of spearmint, among others, were already established in China and Egypt. Water mint (*M. aquatica* L) was probably cultivated by the Romans, 2000 years ago; they also used European pennyroyal to repel flies and fleas (*M. pulegium*, pulex = flea). In a government decree by Karl the Great, "Capitulare de villis" (authored in about 795 CE, see footnote under Anise) spearmint, watermint and horsemint were mentioned. In Central Europe, pennyroyal was mainly used in the 16th and 17th century. In 1696, peppermint was first described in England. In Germany and Holland, peppermint has been cultivated since 1770. Lemon mint was first documented about 200 years ago [U31, Ü92].

Culinary use: Mints are used as seasonings, for the most part spearmint and apple mint, and less often peppermint, predominantly in the UK, the USA, the Middle East, the Levant (Israel, Lebanon, Syria

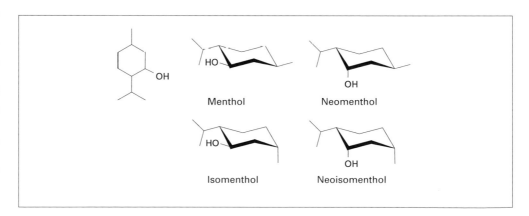

Menthol   Neomenthol

Isomenthol   Neoisomenthol

and Turkey), the Balkan countries, France, and India. Well known are the Anglo-Saxon mint sauces (green mint sauce, prepared with spearmint), which complement warm or cold roast -lamb or -mutton, chicken, duck, and ground meat dishes, but also peas, tomatoes, cucumbers, zucchini, and pumpkin, as well as Roquefort sauce and mint marmalade (mint jelly). In the USA and the UK, mint julep (see below) is a popular summer drink. In Turkey and Bulgaria, kabob, a dish made from roasted calf or lamb, among other dishes, is seasoned with mint leaves. In Germany, mint leaves play only a small role as a spice.

Spearmint or European pennyroyal appears to be especially suited as seasonings of salty dishes. Apple mint and peppermint are preferable for the seasoning of sweet dishes.

Due to their dominating aroma, one must carefully measure mints, especially peppermint. The finely chopped leaves should be sprinkled over the dish just shortly before serving. Fresh mint leaves are used as a spice of salty foods such as meat dishes with strong, characteristic taste (lamb, mutton, roast duck), vegetable-, mushroom-, pea-, tomato-, eggplant-, carrot-, cabbage- or rutabaga dishes, soups (especially fish soups), sauces (especially fish sauces), chutneys, relishes and marinades for grilled fish, of sweet dishes such as fruit salads, quark dishes, yogurt, ice cream as well as puddings and, especially in the UK and the USA, of beverages such as mint lemonade, mint ale, fruit juice-mint refreshing beverages, punch, and iced tea. Candied mint leaves serve as a garnish of pudding and pastry [Ü1, Ü13, Ü46, Ü71, Ü79, Ü91, Ü108].

Combines well with, carefully measured, sweet dishes with basil, salty dishes with chillies, coriander, garlic, or parsley, however mints are used preferably on their own rather than in combination.

As a component of spice mixes and preparations: (Peppermint or other mints) → Bouquet garni, → Chat masala, → Fish spice, → Harissa, → Herb vinegar.

Whiskey Julep
(2 portions)
6 peppermint leaves, crumbled between the fingers to release the aroma components, 2 peppermint twigs, 2 sugar cubes, 2 ice cubes (crushed), 2 miniature whiskey-bottles (bourbon).

Use ready-made crushed ice or place the ice cubes in a plastic bag on a solid surface and crush them with a rolling pin. Place one tablespoon of crushed ice into each whiskey-glass, add sugar, mint leaves and pour the whiskey on top. Stir the contents vigorously. Garnish the drink with the peppermint twigs and serve cold. This long drink is preferably drunk in an outdoors setting at sunset [Ü47].

Literature see → Apple mint.

Peppermint

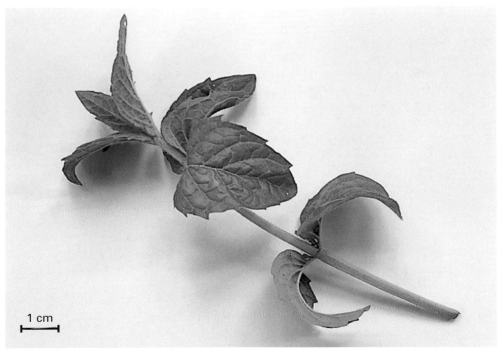

Fig. 1: Peppermint shoot tip

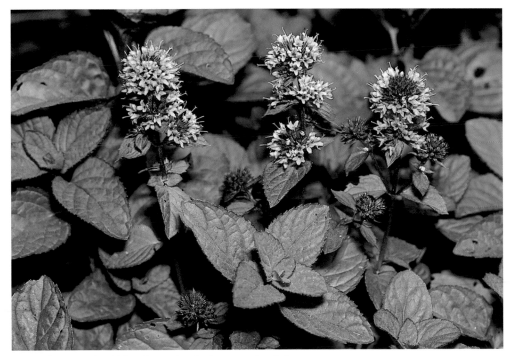

Fig. 2: Peppermint (*Mentha × piperita* L. nm. *piperita*)

Plant source: *Mentha × piperita* L. nm. *piperita.*

Synonym: *Mentha × piperita* L. var. *vulgaris* SOLE.

Taxonomic classification: *Mentha × piperita* L. is a sterile, hybrid derived from → *M. aquatica* L. and → *M. spicata* L.
The hybrids are differentiated by their habitus:
M. × piperita var. *piperita* f. *rubescens* (or *piperita*), dark green peppermint (black mint),
M. × piperita var. *piperita* f. *pallescens*, light green peppermint (white mint).

Common names: Engl.: peppermint; Fr.: menthe anglais, menthe poivrée; Ger.: Pfefferminze, Englische Minze, Edelminze, Teeminze.

Description: Perennial herb with stout rhizome forming long stolons, stem up to 90 cm in height, branched, quadrangular, often dark violet pruinose, with revolute trichomes in the upper part or glabrous, small shoots appear in the axils of the leaves. The leaves are decussate, all of them with petioles, oblong-ovate or lanceolate, 3 to 9 cm long, hairy or glabrous, with a serrate margin. The flowers are arranged in thick, elongate and cylindrical, spike-like, in the lower part mostly clustered inflorescences, or in axillary pseudowhorls; quinate calyx furrowed, corolla almost evenly quadrifid, pale-red or reddish-purple, 4 stamina of equal length, superior ovary, diphyllous, divided into 4 loculi. The fruit divides into 4, about 2 mm long, chestnut brown nutlets with one seed each. Many varieties are sterile. Flowering period is from July to September [100, Ü37].

Native origin: A cultivated hybrid plant, probably originating in England, and the Mediterranean countries.

Main cultivation areas: The USA, India, Europe (in Germany especially in Thuringia and Bavaria), Canada, Chile, Argentina, Brazil, Australia, Japan, as well as African countries such as Kenya, Tanzania, and Morocco.

Main suppliers: Bulgaria, Greece, Spain, and Hungary, and for peppermint essential oil, also the USA, and India.

Cultivation: Peppermint has no special soil type requirements. A high essential oil content and good aromatic quality are obtained from humus-rich, sandy, not too dry, loamy soil in warm, wind-protected sunny locations. The plant is self-incompatible, but it should also not be grown after other mint family plants on the same place (pause cultivation after 4- to 5 years). Propagation is carried out with runners or cuttings. Runners are obtained in the autumn after the last cutting either with a shaker sieve digger or shallow plough. The stolons are pulled apart by hand into 15 to 20 cm long pieces and then placed into 10 cm deep furrows, covered with soil and rolled over. Cuttings that have grown roots can be planted in the autumn or spring. In the garden, one should inhibit the rapid spreading of the stolons by cultivating inside of open-bottom containers that reach down at least 30 cm. The populations are productive for 1- to 3 years, followed by degeneration (self-incompatibility). Cultivated varieties of black mint include, among others, 'Mitcham' (decreasing importance), 'Multimentha' (= Polymentha, good rust resistance), 'Bulgarian 36 AQ', 'De Banat' and 'Mentola', and of white mint include, among others, 'Pfälzer Minze' and 'Grüne Minze' [Ü14, Ü21, Ü96]. For an evaluation of other varieties, see Lit. [88].

Culinary herb

Commercial forms: Peppermint leaf: dried leaves and the essential oil.

Production: Harvest takes place prior to the flowering period (June to July); hand cut on small farms, and on industrial farms it is mowed with a sidebar cutter or a combine harvester. A 2nd cutting, and possibly even a 3rd cutting, is possible in mid-September at the latest. The freshly harvested material is chopped and the leaf material is separated from the stems with an air separator or with sieves. In small-scale farming, removing the leaves and shoot tips with the uppermost 3 leaf pairs by hand is possible. Peppermint is dried on belt driers at temperatures up to a maximum of 42 °C. For personal household use, the fresh leaves should be harvested immediately before use [Ü21].

Forms used: For culinary use, the fresh leaves are used almost exclusively, as well as peppermint oil, and rarely the dried leaves.

Storage: The fresh leaves can be stored refrigerated in plastic bags or frozen with water in the ice tray. The dried leaves are kept in a cool place, in well-closed porcelain-, glass-, or suitable metal containers, protected from humidity and light.

Description. Whole leaf (Fig. 1)**:** Fresh leaves → plant description.

Cut dried leaf: Brittle, dark green to brownish leaf fragments with prominent nervature on the lower surface, glabrous or slightly pubescent [Ph Eur].

Powdered leaf: Characteristic are diacytic stomata, 6- to 8-celled, bent, articulate trichomes with granular or striated cuticula, less frequent short articulate trichomes and characteristic, typical labiate glandular scales with mostly 8 secretory cells, as well as short-stemmed, capitate glandular trichomes with enlarged oval head [Ph Eur].

Odor: Menthol-like, **Taste:** Aromatic-spicy, later cooling.

Constituents and Analysis

DIN- and ISO-Standards: ISO-Specification 2256 (Dried mint, Spearmint, *Mentha spicata* Linnaeus syn. *Mentha viridis* L.), ISO-Specification 5563 (Dried peppermint, *Mentha piperita* L.).

Constituents

- Essential oil: 0.5 to 6.0%, the main components are menthol ($(-)1R,3R,4S$-menthol, 15 to 68%), menthone ($(-)$-$1R,4S$-menthone, 15 to 76%), menthyl acetate (2 to 5%, in some provenances, up to 23%), 1,8-cineole (3 to 8%), menthofuran (0 to 7%), isomenthone (2 to 13%), neomenthol (2.5 to 5%), limonene (2 to 10%), pulegone (0.5 to 5%), β-caryophyllene (0.5 to 1.5%) and germacrene D (1 to 2%); also present are, among others, *trans*-sabinene hydrate, piperitenone, α- and β-pinene and viridiflorol; the distillation residue contains glycosidically bound terpene alcohols and aliphatic alcohols, e.g. glycosides of menthol, isomenthol, neomenthol, linalool, oct-1-ene-3-ols and octane-3-ols [2, 15, 25, 41, 55, 89, 91, 97].
- Hydroxycinnamic acid derivatives (labiate tannins): 3.5 to 6%, including, among others, rosmarinic acid (about 3%) [51].
- Flavonoids: Possibly up to 10%, glycosides of apigenin, diosmetin, luteolin and eriodictyol, particularly eriocitrin (eriodictyol-7-rutinoside) and luteolin-7-rutinoside, polymethoxylated flavones, including, among others, xanthomicrol, gardenin D, gardenin B and 5-O-demethylnobiletine [19, 35, 40, 43, 45, 98, 99].

- Triterpenes: Ursolic acid (0.1%), among others [11].

Tests for Identity: With sensoric, macroscopic and microscopic examination or TLC of the leaf extracts, that are extracted mainly with strongly lipophilic solvents [58, 87, Ü77, Ü102, Ü106, Ph Eur]. The identity and purity of the essential oil can be determined with TLC or GC [2, 28, Ph Eur].

Quantitative assay: The essential oil content is determined volumetrically with steam distillation and xylol in the graduated tube [Ph Eur]. Rosmarinic acid is quantitatively analyzed with HPLC [34], or after silylation with GC [77].

Adulterations, Misidentifications and Impurities are unlikely, since peppermint originates exclusively from cultivated sources and has a characteristic odor. Occasionally, peppermint oil is adulterated with mint oil obtained from Chinese mint (*M. arvensis* L. var. *piperascens* MALINV).

Actions and Uses

Actions: Due to its aromatic taste, peppermint causes a reflex action that stimulates the secretion of saliva, gastric juice and bile fluid, and therefore is has appetite stimulating and digestion promotion action. In animal experiments (rats), administration of freshly cut peppermint leaves caused elevated lipase- and amylase activity of the intestinal mucosa and of the lipase activity of the pancreas [82]. Peppermint has a choleretic effect [41, 101].

Aqueous-ethanolic extracts of peppermint leaf and peppermint oil have in vitro antagonistic activity on the isolated guinea pig ileum against the spasmodic effects of acetylcholine, histamine, serotonin and substance P, similar to the effect of atro-

pine. Aqueous solutions of isolated flavonoids from peppermint inhibited muscular contraction induced by $BaCl_2$. Intravenous injections of an aqueous solution of peppermint oil suppressed a morphine-induced spasm on Oddi's sphincter [18, 26–27, 66, 79]. The introduction of a diluted peppermint oil-suspension into the lumen of the colon with a colposcope led to the immediate relief of colonic spasms and made the insertion of the surgical instruments easier [57]. Following an urge to cough in guinea pigs induced by the spraying of citric acid from a nebulizer, cough frequency was reduced by the inhalation of menthol [53].

Intraperitoneal application of a vacuum concentrated aqueous-ethanolic extract of peppermint leaf showed anodyne action (Model: acetic acid-induced writhing and hot-plate test in mice). Oral application showed an antiinflammatory effect in the xylene-induced ear edema test model (mice) and cotton pellet granuloma test (rats).

Dry extracts of peppermint leaf, containing 3.3% flavonoids, 18.4% tannins and 1.2% essential oil, demonstrated a sedative effect in mice after initial stimulation, at a dose of 1 g/kg body weight [16].

Peppermint leaf and peppermint oil, on the basis of their menthol-content, stimulate cold receptors in the nasal mucosa, causing a cooling effect. This effect takes place through an influence on the calcium channels of the cold receptors [20, 21].

In a clinical study, the topical application of a 10% peppermint oil solution on patients with tension headaches caused a reduction in symptoms comparable to the oral administration of acetaminophen [30]. A meta-analysis of clinical studies carried out (up to 1998) concluded that peppermint oil has not yet been proven effective for the treatment of irritable bowel syndrome [76].

The antimicrobial effect of peppermint oil has been demonstrated repeatedly [3, 4,

13, 22, 59, 78, 81]. Among other effects, it was able, as a component of certain foods (used as models), to suppress the growth of *Salmonella enteritidis* and *Listeria monocytogenes*. Antiviral effects, observed in vitro for aqueous and ethanolic extracts of peppermint leaf [4, 40, 102], occur predominantly due the rosmarinic acid content and probably only with topical application.

Toxicology: Based on existing data, there is no acute or chronic toxicity with the normal use of the herb in beverage teas [18, 23]. Very high doses of peppermint oil can lead to headaches, heartburn, bradycardia, tremor and ataxia. The sensitization potential is low. Allergic reactions after the use of peppermint oil have been observed occasionally. Cross reactions with turpentine, Peru balsam and thymol have occurred [Ü39].

Culinary use: Peppermint can be used as a spice for fruit salads, groats, cold sweet soup, yogurt, and milk products [Ü90]. Peppermint oil is used in the liqueur- and confectionary industries (peppermint liqueur, peppermint bonbons, chewing gum, and other confectionary products).

Other uses: Peppermint oil is used extensively in cosmetics (toothpastes, mouthwashes, shaving- and body lotions) [Ü24].

Medicinal herb

Herbal drugs: Menthae piperitae folium, Peppermint leaf, contains not less than 12 ml/kg of essential oil in the whole leaf and not less than 9 ml/kg in the cut leaf [Ph Eur], Menthae piperitae aetheroleum, Peppermint oil, contains 30 to 55% menthol, 14 to 32% menthone, 2.8 to 10% menthyl acetate, 3.5 to 14% cineole, 1.0 to 9.0% menthofuran, 1.0 to 5.0% limonene, 1.5 to 10% isomenthone, maximum 4.0%

pulegone, and maximum 1.0% carvone [Ph Eur].

Indications: Peppermint is used in the form of tea infusions or extracts for treatment of gastrointestinal tract complaints as well as gallbladder and biliary duct problems. The dosage is 3 to 6 g of the dried leaf (1.5 g = 1 tbsp per cup) or 5 to 15 g of the tincture. In cases of convulsive gallstone pains, use only after consultation with a doctor [47]. Its use as a mild sedative appears to be conceivable [66]. In folk medicine, peppermint is also used for nausea, retching, vomiting, for common cold conditions, dysmenorrhea and as a sedative [66, Ü37, Ü106].

Peppermint oil is used internally for painful spasms in the upper gastrointestinal tract and of the biliary ducts, for irritable colon, catarrhs of the upper airway and inflammations of the oral mucosa. In cases of gallstone pains, use only after consultation with a doctor. Its use must be discontinued in cases of obstructed biliary ducts, inflammation of the gallbladder as well as in cases of liver damage. The average daily dose is 6 to 12 drops, for irritable colon 0.6 ml (single dose: 0.2 ml), in a gastric juice resistant (enteric-coated capsule) vehicle [66].

Peppermint oil is applied externally for the treatment of muscle pains, neuralgic type pains, headaches, catarrhs of the upper airway and head colds. It is applied by rubbing a few drops of the undiluted oil into the skin, in the form of 5- to 20% semi-solid or oily preparations, 1- to 5% nasal ointments, 5- to 10% aqueous-ethanolic solutions or inhalations (3 to 4 drops added to hot water). Menthol-containing preparations should not be applied on the faces of infants and toddlers (glottis cramps are possible) [31, 32, 49, 66].

Literature see → Apple mint.

Spearmint

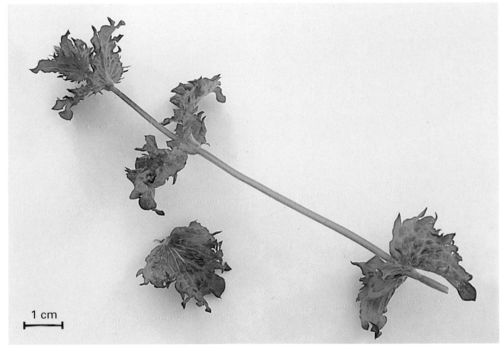

Fig. 1: Spearmint shoot tip

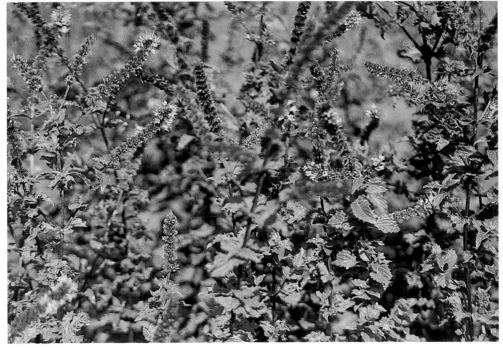

Fig. 2: Spearmint (*M. spicata* L. emend. L. var. *crispa* BENTH.)

Plant source: *M. spicata* L. emend. L. var. *crispa* BENTH.

Synonyms: *Mentha crispata* SCHRADER, *M. viridis* (L.) L., *M. spicata* var. *spicata* (SCHRAD.) BECK.

Taxonomic classification: Its origin is uncertain, but probably a hybrid of *M. longifolia* (L.) HUDS. and *M. suaveolens* EHRH.

Common names: Engl.: spearmint, curled mint, crisp mint, mackerel mint; Fr.: menthe verte, menthe douce, menthe crépue; Ger.: Krauseminze, Grüne Minze (some varieties of peppermint are also called green mint), Grüne Rossminze, Römische Minze.

Description: (Fig. 2). Stem up to 80 cm in height. Leaves decussate, sessile or almost sessile, oblong-ovate or lanceolate, 5 to 9 cm long, curled, glabrous to densely hairy, margin with pronounced and even double-serration, wavy. Flowers arranged in slender, loosely packed, spike-like inflorescences; calyx campanulate, glabrous or pubescent, furrowed, corolla pale-violet, pink or white, 4 stamina of equal length, superior ovary, diphyllous, divided into 4 locules. Fruit divided into 4 nutlets, containing one seed each. Flowering period is from July to September [100, Ü37].

Native origin: Unknown.

Main cultivation areas: The USA, China, India, England, and the Russian Federation.

Main suppliers: The main suppliers of the dried leaf are Egypt, Republics of the former Yugoslavia, and for the essential oil, the USA, China, and India.

Cultivation: Spearmint is grown in the same way as → Peppermint, also tolerating shady locations. Cultivated varieties include, among others, 'Erfurter', 'Mencris' (good rust resistance) and 'Misia' [Ü14]. Also belonging to the *M spicata* species are the varieties known as Moroccan spike mint, *M. spicata* L. 'Moroccan', and Tashkent-spike mint, *M. spicata* L. 'Tashkent'.

Production: Spearmint leaves are harvested during the flowering period.

Culinary herb

Commercial forms: Spearmint leaf: the dried leaves, spearmint essential oil (which is also obtained from other carvone-containing Mentha–species and –forms with curled leaves, in the USA including, among others, from *M. spicata* L. var. *tenuis* (MICHAUX) BRIQ., and in Russia obtained from *M. × verticillata* L.).

Forms used: The fresh or dried leaves and the essential oil.

Storage: → Peppermint.

Description. Whole herb (Fig. 1): Fresh leaves → plant description.

Cut dried leaf: Wrinkled, somewhat brittle leaf fragments, with blister-like expansions between the depressed veins; the leaf margin has long, acuminate teeth, which are bent and drawn out in a wavy fashion [EB 6].

Powdered leaf: Characteristic are the diacytic stomata, and the 1- to 6-celled, bent articulate trichomes, as well as the typical lamiaceous glandular scales with mostly 12 secretory cells [EB 6].

Odor: Intensely aromatic, caraway-like, **Taste:** Spicy (not cooling!).

Constituents and Analysis

Constituents

- Essential oil: 0.6 to 2.5%, the main components of the cultivated varieties are (–)-L-carvone (40 to 80%), dihydrocuminyl acetate (10 to 12%), both are mainly responsible for the odor, as well as (–)-limonene (5 to 15%), furthermore, among others, dihydrocarvone, dihydrocarveol, dihydrocarveol acetate, carvyl acetate and β-caryophyllene. Other races also contain carvone, in addition to 1,8-cineole (up to 20%), *trans*-sabinene hydrate (up to 22%), pulegone (up to 50%) or terpinenol-4 (up to 18%), among others. In the essential oil from the Russian Federation linalool (50 to 60%) dominates; also present are 1,8-cineole (about 20%). In other races, menthone/isomenthone + pulegone (together about 80%) are main components, or also menthone + isomenthone, piperitone + piperitenone, piperitenone oxide or piperitone oxide + piperitenone oxide [6, 9, 54, 62, 73, 85]. The plant also contains glycosidically bound volatile substances, e.g. glycosides of *cis*-carveol, eugenol and benzyl alcohol [7].
- Hydroxycinnamic acid derivatives (labiate tannins): About 6%, including, among others, rosmarinic acid (about 4%) [52]; another literature reference only claims about 0.001% [71].
- Flavonoids: Thymonin, among others [94].

Tests for Identity: Sensoric, macroscopic and microscopic analysis [Ü37], as well as TLC [Ü102, Ü106, DAC] or GC [according to PF X] of the essential oil.

Quantitative assay: The content of essential oil can be determined volumetrically with steam distillation [EB 6].

Adulterations, Misidentifications and Impurities have not been observed.

Actions and Uses

Actions: Due to its aromatic taste, spearmint has appetite stimulating and digestion promoting action. The essential oil has good antimicrobial activity [17, 42].

Toxicology: Based on existing data, there is no chronic or acute toxicity with the regular use of spearmint as a beverage tea or flavoring. The sensitization potential is only very small.

Culinary use: Fresh spearmint leaves are suitable for seasoning of meat dishes (especially of roast lamb) and fish dishes, salads, vegetables, sauces (e.g. of English mint sauce), soups (especially of cold peamint-soup) and stews (e.g. made from potatoes together with peas) [Ü17, Ü74]. In the Near East, predominantly the dried leaves are used, e.g. for quark fillings, yogurt dressings and sauces [Ü55].
Spearmint oil is used to a large extent as a flavor ingredient of mouthwashes, toothpastes and chewing gums.

Other uses: The essential oil is used extensively as a flavoring for mouthwashes, toothpastes and chewing gum.

Medicinal herb

Herbal drugs: Menthae viridis folium [PF X], feuille de menthe verte (Spearmint leaf), or Folia Menthae crispae [EB 6], Krausenminzblätter (Spearmint leaves), contains not less than 1% essential oil, Menthae crispae aetheroleum [DAC], Krauseminzöl (Spearmint oil), contains not less then 55% carvone.

Indications: In folk medicine, spearmint is used in the same way as → Peppermint for digestion problems. The single dose is 1.5 g per cup, several times daily, prepared as a tea infusion. The essential oil is recommended as an inhalant for common cold conditions [Ü106].

Literature see → Apple mint.

European pennyroyal

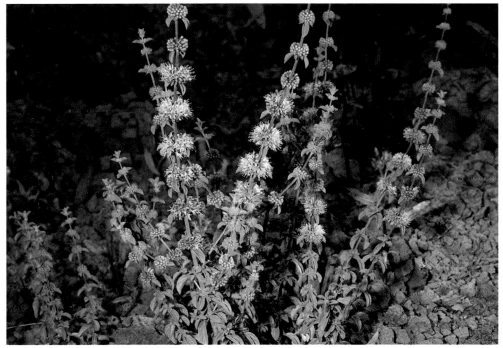

Fig. 1: European pennyroyal (*Mentha pulegium* L.)

Plant source: *Mentha pulegium* L.

Taxonomic classification: Varieties under cultivation include, among others: *Mentha pulegium* L. var. *erecta*, erect pennyroyal, and *Mentha pulegium* L. 'Cunningham Mint'.

Common names: Engl.: European pennyroyal, pennyroyal, pudding grass; Fr.: herbe aux puces, menthe pouliot; Ger.: Poleiminze, Flohkraut, Hirschminze, Polei.

Description (Fig. 1): Prostrate or ascending stem, up to 30 cm in height, sparsely pubescent or glabrous. Leaves decussate, short-petiolate, elliptic to narrowly ovate, up to 3 cm long, pubescent, entire-margined, or with up to 6 teeth along both sides. Flowers arranged in loose, globular, whorl-like inflorescences, calyx nearly bilabiate, bent, ciliated, with barbed throat, corolla violet, 4 equal stamina, superior ovary, diphyllous, divided into 4 loculi. The fruits separate into 4 one-seeded, about 0.5 mm long, shiny brown nutlets. The habitus of the plant is highly variable. Flowering period is from July to September [100, Ü37].

Native origin: Originally from the Mediterranean region, now also widely distributed in western-, southern- and central Europe, on the Canary Islands, and in western Asia.

Main cultivation areas: The USA, Morocco, and Spain.

Main suppliers: The herb is rarely traded. The essential oil is traded especially by the USA.

Cultivation: Propagation is carried out by sowing seed in spring or by root divisions in the autumn or spring. It prefers damp, sandy, acidic soil, and mild winters due to its high frost sensitivity. The (German) variety 'Erfurter Poleiminze' (Erfurter Pennyroyal) can be cultivated.

Culinary herb

Commercial forms: European pennyroyal: The dried herb and the essential oil.

Production: The plant is harvested prior to the flowering period.

Forms used: The fresh or dried herb.

Storage: → Peppermint.

Description. Whole herb: → Plant description.

Cut herb: Leaf fragments with soft pubescence on both sides, distinctly punctate, stem pieces and petioles also softly pubescent, flowers single or together in loose clusters, calices 2 to 6 mm long, tubular corolla with 4 lobes, bluish-pink, with hairs on the outside.

Powdered herb: Characteristic are the diacytic stomata, lamiaceous glandular scales with 8 to 10 secretory cells, capitate glandular hairs with single end cell, uni- and multicellular, articulate trichomes, fragments of the calyx and corolla, pollen grains with 6 pores, diameter 20 to 30 μm [Ü37].

Odor: Pungent and aromatic, **Taste:** Mint-like.

Constituents and Analysis

Constituents

- Essential oil: 1 to 5%, the main component of the commercial oil is mostly (R)-(+)-pulegone (14 to 90%); also present are, among others, menthone (10 to 31%), neoisomenthol (up to 21%), isomenthone (2 to 10%), piperitenone (0.5 to 2.5%), neoisomenthyl acetate (0.3 to 8%), 1,8-cineole and borneol. In plants from the wild, the ratios of the different ketones are highly variable; there are, among others, races in which the content of menthone or isomenthone is higher than the pulegone content, and there are others, which contain only little or no pulegone but are rich in piperitone + piperitenone (77 to 87%) instead [9, 14, 38, 69, 75].
- Hydroxycinnamic acid derivatives (labiate tannins): About 5%, particularly rosmarinic acid (about 3%) [52].
- Flavonoids: Diosmin, hesperidin, among others [Ü60].

Tests for Identity: Sensoric, macroscopic and microscopic analysis [Ü37], as well as TLC or GC of the essential oil [33].

Quantitative assay: Volumetric assay with steam distillation and xylol in the graduated tube [Ph Eur]. Determination of the volatile ketones using the sulfite method or oximation [Ü37].

Adulterations, Misidentifications and Impurities: It is possible that the essential oil from American pennyroyal is mistaken for the essential oil from European pennyroyal. The former originates from *Hedeoma pulegioides* (L.) PERS. (Lamiaceae) and is also rich in pulegone.

Actions and Uses

Actions: Due to its aromatic taste, European pennyroyal has appetite stimulating and digestion promoting action. The essential oil has insecticidal action [50].

Toxicology: Based on existing data, there is no acute or chronic toxicity with the normal use of European pennyroyal herb as a seasoning. The essential oil from European pennyroyal is hepatotoxic due to its pulegone content. Poisonings were observed after the intake of 5 g, lethal cases were documented with doses of 30 ml. The use of European pennyroyal as a beverage tea is not recommended [33, 60, 92, 93, Ü58].

Culinary use: European pennyroyal is used especially in Italy, similar to the way spearmint it used, e.g. as a seasoning component of fillings and piquant pies or pâtés. It is also recommended as a spice for blood sausages or hot herb sausages. Use sparingly! [Ü17, Ü74, Ü92].

Other uses: The essential oil is used as an insect repellent, and in the cosmetic industry, as a perfume ingredient in soap products.

Medicinal herb

Herbal drugs: Pulegii herba, European pennyroyal herb, Pulegii aetheroleum, European pennyroyal oil (obtained by steam distillation of the fresh herb).

Indications: In folk medicine, it is used the same as → Peppermint for digestive problems, but also for absence of menstrual period. The dosage is 1 to 4 g, t.i.d., prepared in the form of a tea infusion. The essential oil is misused as an abortifacient [Ü37].

Literature see → Apple mint.

Lemon mint

Plant source: *Mentha citrata* EHRH.

Synonym: *Mentha × piperita* L. nm. *citrata* (EHRH.) B. BOIVIN.

Taxonomic classification: Probably derived from *Mentha aquatica* L., also viewed as a nothomorph (nm.) of → *Mentha × piperita* L.

Common names: Engl.: lemon mint, bergamot mint, eau de Cologne mint; Fr.: eau de Cologne menthe; Ger.: Zitronenminze, Bergamotteminze, Orangenmize.

Description: Similar to water mint; the plant is sterile.

Native origin: A cultivated plant, becoming wild in Europe and North America.

Main cultivation areas: Italy, and the USA.

Main suppliers: Italy.

Cultivation: It is grown in the same way as → Peppermint. Cultivated varieties include 'Lemon' and 'Citrata'.

Culinary herb

Commercial forms: Lemon mint: dried leaves, lemon mint essential oil.

Production: The plant is harvested prior to the flowering period.

Forms used: The fresh leaves and the essential oil.

Storage: → Peppermint.

Description. Whole leaf: Leaves ovate to cordate, glabrous or sparsely pubescent, flowers in dense pseudo-whorls with inconspicuous bracts.

Odor: Lavender-like with slight lemon note, **Taste:** Somewhat soapy.

Constituents and Analysis

Constituents
- Essential oil: About 2.5%, with the main components linalool (30 to 55%) and linalyl acetate (15 to 40%); furthermore, among others, *cis*- and *trans*-linalool oxide, geraniol, geranyl acetate, citronellol, β-caryophyllene, elemol, viridiflorol [17, 65, 72, 83, 86] or limonene (up to 50%) and 1,8-cineole (up to 12%), as well as, among others, β-caryophyllene and germacrene D [64].

Actions and Uses

Actions: Due to its aromatic taste, lemon mint has appetite stimulating and digestion promoting action. The essential oil has antimicrobial activity [17]

Toxicology: Based on existing data, there is no acute or chronic toxicity with the normal use of lemon mint as a seasoning.

Culinary use: The fresh leaves of lemon mint are suitable for the seasoning of salads and mint butter (well fitting for grilled fish) [Ü74].

Other uses: In the perfume and cosmetic industries, similar to oil of lavender, as an aroma ingredient for soaps and cosmetic products.

Medicinal herb

Herbal drug: Mentha-citrata Oil, Lemon mint oil.

Indications: None known.

Literature see → Apple mint.

Apple mint

Plant source: *Mentha suaveolens* EHRH.

Synonym: *M. rotundifolia* auct. non (L.) HUDS.

Taxonomic classification: Cultivated varieties include:
Mentha suaveolens EHRH, var. *suaveolens*, apple mint,
Mentha suaveolens EHRH. "Variegata", pineapple mint.

Common names: Engl.: apple mint, round-leaved mint; Ger.: Apfelminze, Rundblättrige Minze.

Description: Stem up to 50 cm in height, pubescent-villous. Leaves decussate, sessile or short-petiolate, roundish-ovate, upper surface wrinkled, lower surface tomentose (var. *suaveolens*) or glabrescent (var. *glabrescens* (TIMB.) BÄSSLER), margin notched-serrate, in cv. "variegata" partially cream-colored. Flowers in thin, spike-like inflorescences, calyx almost regular 5-toothed, without fringe of hair, corolla pale lilac-colored, almost white, 4 equal stamina, superior ovary, diphyllous, divided into 4 loculi; the fruit separates into 4 one-seeded, about 2 mm long, chestnut brown-colored nutlets. Flowering period is from July to September [Ü85].

Native origin: Southern- and Western Europe.

Main cultivation areas: There is local cultivation in England.

Cultivation: → Peppermint.

Culinary herb

Commercial forms: Apple mint is not commercially traded.

Production: The leaves are harvested prior to the flowering period.

Forms used: The fresh leaves.

Storage: → Peppermint

Description. Whole leaf: See description of the plant.

Odor: Fruity, apple- or pineapple-like, **Taste:** Aromatic.

Constituents and Analysis

Constituents
- Essential oil: About 1%, in cultivated varieties, the main components are piperitenone oxide (about 13 to 87%) and *trans*-piperitone oxide (about 25 to 48%), in addition minor ones, such as *trans*-sabinene hydrate, germacrene D, terpinenol-4, (*Z*)-β-ocimene and β-pinene, among others. There are also essential oils from chemical races, in which carvone, dihydrocarvone or pulegone (up to 50%) + neoisopulegol dominate [6, 9].

Actions and Uses

Actions: Due to its aromatic taste, apple mint has appetite stimulating and digestion promoting action.

Toxicology: Based on existing data, there is no acute or chronic toxicity with the normal use of apple mint as a seasoning and beverage tea.

Culinary use: The fresh leaves of both types, due to their mild taste, are suitable especially as a spice ingredient of sweet dishes, compotes, jellies, jams, fruit salads, punches, bakery goods, but also of fresh cheese [Ü74 Ü81].

Other mint-species used as culinary herbs

Water mint (marsh mint, Ger.: Bachminze), *Mentha aquatica* L., native to Europe, western- and central Asia, northern-, eastern- and southern Africa, is not cultivated but is wild collected mainly in Macedonia and Romania. It contains 0.1 to 1% essential oil, of which the main components are menthofuran (20 to 90%), followed by, among others, 1,8-cineole (in some races up to 22%), menthone (about 18%), viridiflorol, β-caryophyllene, caryophyllene oxide, elemol, germacrene D and limonene [6, 37, 63, 90]. There are also chemical races in which the essential oil is dominated by elemol (about 25%), viridiflorol (about 27%) isopinocamphone (about 50%), linalool + linalyl acetate or menthol + menthyl acetate [6, 9, 36, 84]. The fresh or dried leaves are, albeit rarely, used as a seasoning similarly as peppermint.

Corn mint (Austrian mint, Carinthian mint, wild mint, Ger.: Ackerminze, Österreichische Minze, Kärntner Minze), *Mentha arvensis* L. (Synonym: *M. austriaca* JACQ.), is native to Europe and Asia and cultivated in northern Italy. The main components of its essential oil are menthol (up to 90%), menthone and isomenthone (up to 30%), menthofuran (up to 30%), pulegone (up to 50%), octan-3-one (up to 90%), β-caryophyllene (up to 32%), linalool, β-ocimene or isopulegol [2, 29, 67, Ü61]. It is used similarly as peppermint, e.g. as a seasoning of typical Austrian quark noodles [Ü46].

Chinese mint (Japanese peppermint, Ger.: Japanische Pfefferminze), *Mentha arvensis*

L. var. *piperascens* HOLMES ex CHRISTY, is native to and cultivated in eastern Asia. The essential oil contains 50 to 90% menthol. The commercial form of the essential oil (mint oil, partly dementholised) has its menthol content reduced by a crystallization process [74, Ü37]. Mint oil [Ph Eur] must contain 30 to 50% menthol, 17 to 35% menthone, 5 to 13% isomenthone, 1.5 to 7% menthyl acetate, 1.5 to 7% limonene, and not more than 1.5% 1,8-cineole, 2% carvone and 2% pulegone. It is used internally for treatment of meteorism, functional stomach-, intestinal- and biliary complaints, and externally for muscle pains, neuralgic problems, and catarrhs of the upper respiratory tract [49].

Mentha diemenica SPRENGEL, has essential oil that is dominated by menthone, neomenthyl acetate, pulegone, neomenthol, menthyl acetate, menthol and isomenthone [12].

Ginger mint (Australian mint, Ger.: Edelminze, Ingwerminze), *Mentha × gentilis* L. (Synonym: *M. × gracilis* SOLE, *M. cardiaca* GERARDE ex BAKER, a hybrid of *Mentha arvensis* L. and *M. spicata* L.), is cultivated in the USA in a large variety of forms. The main components of its essential oil are piperitenone oxide and pulegone [56] or eugenol, followed by, among others, methyl salicylate [95]. The essential oil is used mainly as a flavor enhancer for chewing gum [Ü61].

Scotch spearmint (Ger.: Schottische Krauseminze, Edelminze), *Mentha × gentilis* L. nm. *cardiaca* GERARDE ex BAKER, the source of Scotch spearmint oil (green mint oil), of which the main component is (–)-carvone, has a composition, which is very closely comparable to that of spearmint oil [Ü61].

Horse mint (long leaf mint, wild mint, biblical mint, Ger.: Rossminze, Langblättrige Minze, Wilde Minze), *Mentha longifolia* (L.) L. (Synonym: *M. asiatica* BORRISS., *M. spicata* L. var. *longifolia* L.). There are several subspecies of this species, including *M. longifolia* (L.) L. ssp. *longifolia*

which is distributed in Europe, native to western- and southern Europe as well as western Asia. It contains 0.1 to 3% essential oil of a composition that is quite variable, the main components are usually piperitone oxide (10 to 80%), followed by, among others, β-caryophyllene (2 to 15%), germacrene D (5 to 15%), 1,8-cineole (2 to 8%) and limonene (1 to 8%). In addition, there are chemical races with the main components (*R*)-(–)carvone (45 to 65%), linalool (50 to 60%), *trans*-sabinene hydrate (up to 90%), terpinenol-4 (about 40%) + *trans*-sabinene hydrate, α-terpinyl acetate (about 40%), piperitenene oxide (75 to 84%), piperitol, pulegone (about 70%), isomenthone, menthofuran, menthol, menthol + menthyl acetate, 1,8-cineole (26 to 35%) + menthone (10 to 16%) + pulegone (about 7%) + isomenthone (5 to 8%), 1,8-cineole (about 30%) + piperitone (about 15%) or piperitenone oxide (about 24%) + β-caryophyllene (about 23%) + piperitone oxide (about 18%) + germacrene D (about 17%) [1, 6, 8, 9, 24, 44, 46, 61, 70, 96]. The fresh leaves are used predominantly in Asian cooking, e.g. in Indian chutneys. Candied leaves are used as a garnish of sweet dishes. The essential oil serves as a flavoring ingredient of confectionery products [Ü61].

Corsican mint (Ger.: Korsische Minze), *Mentha requienii* BENTH., native to Corsica and Sardinia, the main components of its essential oil are pulegone (about 80%) and menthone (about 15%) [68, 80].

Bowles mint (foxtail mint, also known as apple mint, Ger.: Fuchsschwanzminze, Bowles-Minze, Ananasminze), *Mentha × villosa* var. *alopecuroides* (HULL.) BRIQ. (*M. alopecuroides* HULL., hybrid of *M. spicata* L. and *M. suaveolens* EHRH.), is cultivated in Great Britain where it is used as a spice in mint sauces [Ü61].

Korean mint (Chinese giant hyssop, Ger.: Koreanische Minze), *Agastache rugosa* (FISCH. et C.A. MEY.) KUNTZE, see → Anise, under other culinary herbs with an anise-like aroma.

Literature

[1] Abu-Al-Futuh I.M. et al., J. Ess. Oil Res. 12:530–532 (2000).

[2] Aflatuni A. et al., J. Ess. Oil Res. 12:462–466 (2000).

[3] Aktug S.E., M. Karapinar, Int. J. Food Microbiol. 3:349–354 (1986).

[4] Alwan A et al., Int. J. Crude Drug Res. 26:107–111 (1988).

[5] Atta A.H., A. Alkofahi, J. Ethnopharmacol. 60(2):117–124 (1998).

[6] Avato P. et al., Sci. Pharm. 63:223–230 (1995).

[7] Baerheim Svendsen A., I.J.M. Merkx, Planta Med. 55:38–40 (1989).

[8] Banthorpe D.V. et al., Egypt. J. Chem. 23:63–65 (1981).

[9] Baser K.H.C. et al., J. Ess. Oil Res. 11: 579 (1999).

[10] Boyd E.L., in: Adverse Effects of Herbal Drugs, Springer Verlag Berlin, Heidelberg, New York 1992, Bd. 1, p. 151–156.

[11] Brieskorn C.H. et al., Arch. Pharm. 285: 290–296 (1952).

[12] Brophy S. et al., J. Ess. Oil Res. 8(2):179–181 (1996).

[13] Büechi S., Dtsch. Apoth. Ztg. 138(14): 1265–1274 (1998).

[14] Chalchat J.C. et al., J. Ess. Oil Res. 12: 598–600 (2000).

[15] Croteau R., C. Martinkus, Plant Physiol. 64:169–175 (1979).

[16] Della Loggia R., A. Tubaro, Fitoterapia 61(3):215–221 (1990).

[17] Dikshit A., A. Husain, Fitoterapia 55:171–176 (1984).

[18] Dinckler K., Pharm. Zentralhalle 77:281 (1936).

[19] Duband F. et al., Ann. Pharm. Fr. 50:146 (1992).

[20] Eccles R., J. Pharm. Pharmacol. 46: 618–630 (1994).

[21] Eccles R., A.S. Jones, J. Laryngol. Otol. 97:705–709 (1983).

[22] El-Naghy M.A. et al., Zentralbl. Mikrobiol. 147(3/4):241–220 (1992).

[23] Erdmann W.D., Dtsch. Med. Wschr. 83: 2140 (1958).

[24] Fleisher Z., A. Fleisher, J. Ess. Oil Res. 10:647–648 (1998).

[25] Formacek V., K.H. Kubeczka, Essential Oils Analysis by Capillary Gas Chromatography and Carbon – 13 NMR Spectroscopy, John Wiley & Sons. Chicester etc., 1982.

[26] Forster H., Z. Allgemeinmed. 59: 1327–1331 (1983).

[27] Forster H.B. et al., Planta Med. 40(4): 309–319 (1980).

[28] Galle-Hoffmann U., W.A. König, Dtsch. Apoth. Ztg. 138(40):3793–3799 (1998).

[29] Gill L.S. et al., Bot. J. Linn. Soc. 67:213 (1973).

[30] Göbel H. et al., Nervenarzt 67(8): 672–681 (1996).

[31] Göbel H. et al., in: D. Loew, N. Reitbrock (Hrsg.): Phytopharmaka: Forschung und klinische Anwendung, Bd. 1, Steinkopf Verlag Stuttgart 1995, p. 177–184.

[32] Göbel H., G. Schmidt, Z. Phytother. 16(1):23–33 (1995).

[33] Gordon W.P. et al., Toxicol. Appl. Pharmacol. 65:413–424 (1982).

[34] Gracza L., P. Ruff, Arch. Pharmaz. 317: 339–345 (1984).

[35] Guedon D.J., B.P. Pasquier, J. Agric. Food Chem. 42:679 (1994).

[36] Guido S. et al., J. Ess. Oil Res. 9(4):455–457 (1997).

[37] Hefendehl F.W., Arch. Pharm. 300:438–448 (1967).

[38] Hefendehl F.W., Phytochemistry 9:1985–1995 (1970).

[39] Herrmann E.C. jr., L.S. Kucera, Proc. Soc. Exp. Biol. Med. 124:874–878 (1995).

[40] Hoffmann B.G., L.T. Lunder, Planta Med. 50:361 (1984).

[41] Hölzl J. et al., Dtsch. Apoth. Ztg. 114: 513–517 (1974).

[42] Janssen A.M. et al., Pharm. Weekbl. (Sci.) 10:277–280 (1988).

[43] Jullien F. et al., Phytochemistry 23:2972–2973 (1984).

[44] Karasawa D., S. Shimizu, Agric. Biol. Chem. 42:433 (1978).

[45] Karuza Ljiljana et al., Acta Pharm. (Zagreb) 46(4):315–320 (1996).

[46] Kokkini S. V.P. Papageorgiou, Planta Med. 54:59–69 (1988).

[47] Kommission E beim BfArM, BAnz-Nr. 223 vom 30.11.85 Berichtigung am 13.03.90 und 01.09.90.

[48] Kommission E beim BfArM, BAnz-Nr. 50 vom 13.03.1986.

[49] Kommission E beim BfArM, BAnz-Nr. 117a vom 24.09.1986.

[50] Konstantopoulou I. et al., Experientia 48: 616–619 (1992).

[51] Lamaison J.L. et al., Fitoterapia 62:166–171 (1991).

[52] Lamaison J.L. et al., Ann. Pharm. Franc. 46:103–108 (1990).

[53] Laude E.A. et al., Pulmon. Pharmacol. 7(3):179–184 (1994).

[54] Lawrence B.M., Perfum. Flavorist 5:6–16 (1980).

[55] Lawrence B.M., C.K. Shu, Perfum. Flavorist 14:21–30 (1989).

[56] Lawrence D. et al., Phytochemistry 11: 2638–2639 (1972).

[57] Leicester R.J., R.H. Hunt, Lancet 2(8305): 989 (1982).

[58] Lipták J. et al., Pharmazie 35(9):545–546 (1980).

[59] Lis-Balchin M. et al., Med. Sci. Res. 25: 151–152 (1997).

[60] Madyastha P. et al., Biochem. Biophys. Res. Comm. 128:921–927 (1985).

[61] Maffei M., Flavour Fragrance J. 3:23–26 (1988).

[62] Maffei M. et al., Flavour Fragrance J. 1:105–109 (1986).

[63] Malingre T.M., H. Maarse, Phytochemistry 13:1531–1535 (1974).

[64] Mikus B. et al., Drogenreport 10(18):68–73 (1997).

[65] Mikus B., J. Schaser, Drogenreport 8(13): 32–38 (1995).

[66] Mills S. et al. (Eds.): Principles and Practice of Phytotherapy, Churchill Livingstone, Edinburgh 2000.

[67] Mimica-Dukic N. et al., J. Ess. Oil Res. 10(5):502–506 (1998).

[68] Mucciarelli M., T. Sacco, J. Ess. Oil Res. 11:759–764 (1999).

[69] Müller-Ribau F.J. et al., J. Agric. Food Chem. 45(12):4821–4825 (1997).

[70] Nori-Sharg D. et al., J. Ess. Oil Res. 12:111–112 (2000).

[71] Omoto T. et al., Nippon Shokuhin Kagaku Gakkaishi 4(1):11–16 (1997).

[72] Pino J.A., J. Ess. Oil Res. 11:413–414 (1999).

[73] Pino J.A. et al., J. Ess. Oil Res. 10:657–659 (1998).

[74] Pino J.A. et al., J. Ess. Oil Res. 8(6):685–686 (1996).

[75] Pino J.A. et al., J. Ess. Oil Res. 8:295–296 (1996).

[76] Pittler M.H., E. Ernst, Am. J. Gastroenterol. 93(7):1131–1135 (1998).

[77] Reschke A., Z. Lebensm. Unters. Forsch. 176:116–119 (1983).

[78] Sarbhoy A.K. et al., Zentralbl. Bakteriol (Naturwiss.) 133(7):723–725 (1978).

[79] Schäfer D., W. Schäfer, Arzneim. Forsch. 31(1):82–86 (1981).

[80] Schnelle F.J., H. Hörster, Planta Med. 16:48–53 (1968).

[81] Shapiro S. et al., Oral Microbiol. Immunol. 9:202–208 (1994).

[82] Sharathchandra J.N.N. et al., Indian J. Pharmacol. 27(3):156–160 (1995).

[83] Sharma R.K. et al., Indian Perfum 32: 168–172 (1988).

[84] Shimizu S. et al., Agric. Biol. Chem. 30:200–201 (1966).

[85] Simandi B. et al., Planta Med. 59 (Suppl.): A 626 (1993).

[86] Singh S.B. et al., Phytochemistry 19:2466 (1980).

[87] Stahl E. (Hrsg.): Chromatographische und mikroskopische Analyse von Drogen, Fischer Verlag Stuttgart, New York 1978.

[88] Stahn T., U. Bomme, Herba Germanica 2(2):78–90 (1994).

[89] Stengele M., E. Stahl-Biskup, J. Ess. Oil Res. 5:13–19 (1993).

[90] Sticher O., H. Flück, Pharm. Acta Helv. 43:411–446 (1968).

[91] Stojanova A. et al., J. Ess. Oil Res. 12:438–440 (2000).

[92] Sullivan J.B. jr. et al., J. Am. Med. Assoc. 242:2873–2874 (1979).

[93] Thomassen D., et al., J. Pharmacol. Exp. Ther. 253:567–572 (1990).

[94] Tomás-Barberán F.A. et al., Biochem. Syst. Ecol. 16:43–46 (1988).

[95] Tsuneya T. et al., J. Ess. Oil Res. 10(5): 507–516 (1998).

[96] Venskutonis R., J. Ess. Oil Res. 8:91–94 (1996).

[97] Verzar-Petri G. et al., Sci. Pharm. 47(1):8–16 (1979).

[98] Voirin B., C. Bayer, Phytochemistry 31: 2299 (1992).

[99] Wagner H. et al., Chem. Ber. 102:2083–2088 (1969).

[100] Weymar H., Buch der Lippenblütler und Rauhblattgewächse, Neumann Verlag, Radebeul 1961.

[101] Yamahara J. et al., Jap. J. Pharmacol. 39:280 (1985).

[102] Yamasaki K. et al., Biol. Pharm. Bull. 21(8): 829–833 (1998).

Literature references identified by Ü can be found in the general listing of books and monographs at the back of this book.

Mugwort

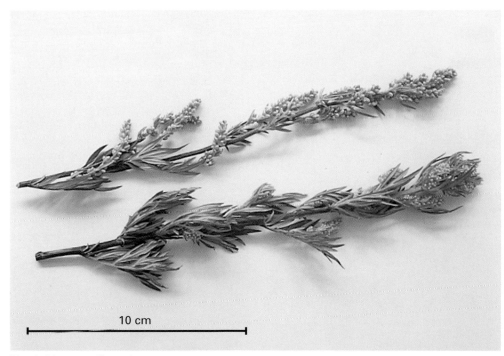

Fig. 1: Mugwort flowering tops

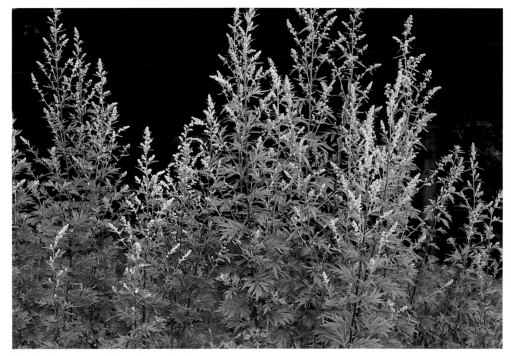

Fig. 2: Mugwort (*Artemisia vulgaris* L.)

Plant source: *Artemisia vulgaris* L.

Taxonomic classification: The species includes a wide variety of forms, and its subdivision into subspecies or varieties is practiced to some extent (e.g. *A. v.* ssp. *vulgaris* and *A. v.* ssp. *coarctata* (FORS.) LEMKE ex ROTHM., *A. v.* var. *vulgatissima*). Some authors consider species *A. indica* WILLD., occurring in Asia, as a variety of *A. v.*: *A. vulgaris* L. var. *indica* (WILLD.) MAXIM. (see below).

Family: Sunflower family (Asteraceae, synonym: Compositae).

Common names: Engl.: mugwort, bulwand wormwood, motherwort, sagebrush; Fr.: armoise, couronne de Saint-Jean; Ger.: Beifuß, Gemeiner Beifuß, Gewürz-Beifuß.

Description: A bushy perennial herb with erect and branched stems, up to 2 m high, reddish pruinose and sparsely pubescent; the above ground parts die at the end of growing season. The leaves are 10 cm long, mostly glabrous on the upper surface, whitish-tomentose on the lower surface, often somewhat revolute at the margins; the basal leaves are short petiolated, lyriform-pinnatilobate, with a large 3- to 5-lobed terminal segment; the upper leaves are sessile, singly pinnatisect with lanceolate segments and basal eared petioles. The 3 to 4 mm long and 2 mm wide anthodia are arranged in multi-branched panicles, the involucres have gray-felted outer surfaces; the receptaculum is leafless, the flowers are yellowish to reddish-brown; the marginal ones are female, the inner ones hermaphrodite. Flowering period is from July to September [35, Ü37].

Native origin: Probably native to Asia, today it is also widely distributed in Europe, northern Africa, in northern and central Asia, and in eastern North- and South America.

Main cultivation areas: Western and Central Europe, the Russian Federation, and Brazil.

Main exporting countries: The Balkan countries, Italy, France, and the Russian Federation.

Cultivation: Mugwort thrives in any soil type in sunny, dry locations. Propagation occurs mostly through preliminary cultivation in a greenhouse, but also through direct seeding in March or April (light requirements for germination!) or with root cuttings in the spring or autumn. There are no known cultivars. Plants are used for 4 to 5 years. For personal use, one plant is sufficient, purchased from a garden store in the springtime or collected from the wild. Because mugwort roots extend so deep, the plant is rarely removed from the garden once established, and therefore its location should be chosen carefully [7, Ü41, Ü91, Ü96].

Culinary herb

Commercial forms: Mugwort herb: dried, flowering tops, mostly separated from the leaves, harvested prior to the flowers opening.

Production: For use as a spice, the flowering tops are harvested, as long as the flowers are still closed. After the flowers open, the plant becomes strongly bitter in taste. Frequently, the flowering tops are freed from the leaves. For medicinal use, the tops, approximately 60 to 70 cm long aerial parts of the plant, are harvested during the flowering period. Due to its widespread occurrence in the wild, mugwort is collected on a large scale from wild populations.

Forms used: Fresh or dried flowering tops, harvested before bloom stage, or the inflorescence, separated from the leaves.

Storage: The fresh shoots can be stored in a plastic bag in the refrigerator for a few days. The dried herb is stored protected from moisture and light in suitable porcelain-, glass- or metal containers.

Description. Whole herb (Fig. 1): See description of the whole plant.

Cut herb, Powdered herb: Characteristic are the T-shaped trichomes with a 1 mm long, thin and often twisted transverse cell (Fig. 3). Glandular trichomes with a short biseriate, two-celled stalk and a two-celled head are rare [Ü94, Ü106].

Odor: Faintly aromatic, **Taste:** Spicy, harsh and somewhat bitter.

History: Mugwort was already used as a spice in China, 2000 BCE. In Europe, it was also used in ancient times as a spice, but also for rituals [Ü92].

Constituents and Analysis

Constituents

■ Essential oil: 0.03 to 0.3%, the main components depend on the chemotype; dominated mostly by 1,8-cineole, camphor, borneol, bornyl-acetate and/or linalool. Other constituents include among others, (–)-thujone, terpineol-4, α-cadinol, spathulenol, β-pinene, myr-

cene, vulgarol and γ-nonalactone [3, 10, 11, 18, 21, 22, 31]. In plants of Indian origin, (–)-thujone (about 56%) is the main component of the essential oil [19].

■ Sesquiterpene lactones: Vulgarin, psilostachyin, psilostachyin C, among others, which are responsible for the bitter taste [10].

■ Eudesmane-type sesquiterpene acids [10, 17].

■ Flavonoids: Quercetin-3-O-glucoside, rutin, isorhamnetin-3-O-glucoside, isorhamnetin-3-O-rhamnoglucoside, among others, including lipophilic methoxylated flavone derivatives, e.g. 5,3´-dihydroxy-3,7,4´-trimethoxyflavone [8, 30].

■ Hydroxycoumarins: About 1.9%, with aesculetin, umbelliferone, scopoletin, among others, including 6-methoxy-7,8-methylenedioxycoumarin [20].

■ Polyines: Centaur X_3 ((E,E)-heptadeca-1,7,9-triene-11,13,15-triyn), (E,E)-tetradeca-4,6-diene-8,10,12-triyn-1-ol, its acetate, (E)-tetradec-6-ene-8,10,12-triyn-3-one (also known as artemisia ketone), (E,E)-trideca-1,3,5-triene-7,9,11-triyn, its 3,4-epoxide (ponticaepoxide) and Z-dehydromatricaria ester ((Z)-dec-2-ene-4,6,8-triynic acid methyl ester) [5, 34, Ü31].

■ Triterpenes, sterols: β-Sitosterol, among others [15].

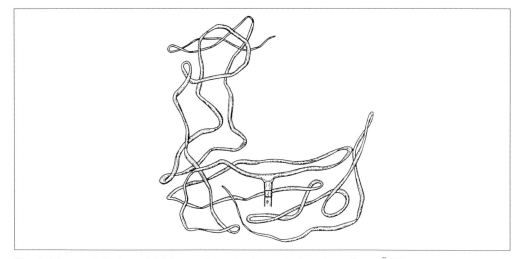

Fig. 3: Mugwort, T-shaped trichome from the lower leaf surface (from Ü29).

Vulgarin   Psilostachyin   Psilostachyin C

Absinthin

Tests for Identity: Macroscopic and microscopic examination or TLC analysis of the essential oil or flavonoids [12].

Quantitative assay: Following the Ph Eur procedure for the determination of the essential oil content, using steam distillation and xylol in the graduated tube.

Adulterations, Misidentifications and Impurities: Misidentification with wormwood, *Artemisia absinthium* L., is possible. This adulterant is significantly more bitter, and both leaf surfaces as well as the base of the inflorescences are pubescent. The transverse cells of the T-shaped trichomes from wormwood are significantly shorter than those of mugwort [Ü106].

Actions and Uses

Actions: On the basis of its aromatic-bitter taste, mugwort has appetizing and digestion promoting action. Its essential oil has a repellent effect on insects [10]. An ethanolic extract of mugwort has shown insecticide activity [26]. A bundle of mugwort, hung in a room, should repel flies and mosquitoes. Extracts of the plant and the essential oil have antimicrobial activity [4, 13].

Toxicology: Based on existing data, there is no acute or chronic toxicity with the regular use of this herb as a spice. The sensitization potential is very small. The literature describes only a few cases of contact allergies. Allergens such as the sesquiterpene lactones psilostachyin and psilostachyin C with exocyclic methylene groups, as well as macromolecular antigens, are considered to be responsible. Allergic reactions to mugwort pollen are relatively common. In most cases, cross reaction occurs with birch pollen, but also with certain umbelliferous food plants such as celery, carrots, anise, cumin, coriander and parsley as well as with sunflower oil and kiwi fruits [16, 29, 33, Ü39].

Culinary use: To maximize the full aromatic effect of mugwort, it should be added already at the start of cooking, preferably in the form of the flowering tops, and then removed from the pot before serving. Mugwort serves as a spice for fatty meats, especially roast goose, roast pork or roast venison, for goose- and duck-fat and for lard (mix dried herb into the fat while still hot), for sauces, fish dishes (e.g. eel soup, mackerel), legume-, mushroom- or cabbage dishes and salads [Ü45, Ü51, Ü74, Ü91, Ü92, Ü95].

Combines well with: Garlic, onions, and pepper.

As a component of spice mixes and preparations: → Picking spice, →Roast spice.

Medicinal herb

Herbal drug: Artemisiae herba, Mugwort herb [BHP 96, EB 6].

Indications: For loss of appetite, digestive complaints, anacid or subacid gastritis, for menstrual disturbances, colic, diarrhea, as a tonic and anthelmintic (0.5 to 2.0 g dried herb prepared as a tea infusion, t.i.d. before meals, as an appetite stimulant) [Ü106]. Because the efficacy of mugwort has not been substantiated, the German Commission E did not approve its therapeutic use [14]. [For the use of Artemisia-species in the traditional medicine systems of tropical countries, see Lit. 6].

Other Artemisia-species used as culinary herbs

Wormwood (absinthe), *Artemisia absinthium* L., native to the western Mediterranean region, eastward to southern Siberia and Kashmir, is cultivated, among other places, in the Mediterranean region, in the Balkan countries, the UK, France and in the USA. The main components of its essential oil, depending on the chemotype, are either (+)-thujone or (Z)-epoxyocimene (both types found in Italy), chrysanthenol acetate, *cis*-chrysanthenol or *trans*- and *cis*-sabinyl acetate (occurs in France), sabinene + myrcene + α-phellandrene (occurs in the USA, and is thujone-free) [1, 24, 25, 32]. Wormwood has a high content of sesquiterpene lactone bitter principles, especially absinthin (see formula) and artabsin [2, 28]. Also worth noting is the presence of homoditerpene peroxides, which, similar to artemisinin, are capable of killing malaria parasites, at very low concentrations (EC_{50} 1 µg/ml) in vitro [27]. Wormwood is used only rarely as a spice. Due to its strongly bitter taste, it must be used only very sparingly, e.g. in the preparation of sausage salads, goulash, pork knuckle and mutton dishes. Extracts are used in the production of wormwood wines and bitter liqueurs (Abtei, Alpenkräuterlikör, Boonekamp, Kartäuser, Stonsdorfer). The use of the essential oil in the alcoholic beverage industry, e.g. in the production of absinthe liqueur, is banned in many countries due to the high content of the neurotoxic component thujone (see page 7). High doses of wormwood extract can also lead to symptoms of poisoning [Ü30, Ü58, Ü92].

Indian wormwood, *Artemisia indica* WILLD. (Syn.: *A. vulgaris* L. var. *indica* (WILLD.) MAXIM.), is native to Southern- and Eastern Asia, where it is cultivated predominantly in gardens. The main components of its essential oil are chemotype-specific thujyl alcohol (about 75%), β-caryophyllene (about 24%) and β-cubebene (about 12%), (−)-thujone or 1,8-cineole + thujone [23, Ü31]. It is used similarly to mugwort (see above).

Roman wormwood, *Artemisia pontica* L., is native to Southern-, Central- and Eastern Europe, and eastward to western Siberia. It is cultivated, among other places, in France, Italy, Austria, Germany, Switzerland, the USA and southern Canada. The main components of its essential oil are *iso*-artemisia ketone (comprises about 47%) and (−)-thujone [9]. It is used similarly to wormwood (see above).

Lemon wormwood, *Artemisia balchanorum* H. KRASCH., is native to Turkmenistan, and is cultivated in the southern parts of the Russian Federation. The main components of its essential oil are citral (50 to 60%), linalool and geraniol. The essential oil is used primarily as an aromatic flavor component of baked goods [Ü92].

Alpine wormwood, *Artemisia mutellina* VILL. (Syn. *A. umbelliformis* LAM.), is native to the Alps, and mountains of southern Europe. The main components of its essential oil are (−)-thujone and (+)-thujone (up to 65%). It is used primarily as an aromatic flavor component of bitter liqueurs [Ü92].

Other Artemisia-species that are used as spices, mainly in the alcoholic beverage industry, include, among others, *Artemisia arborescens* L., *A. judaica* L., *A. maritima* L. (see Wormwood; contains santonin!) and *A. vallesciaca* ALL. (Valais wormwood; also contains santonin).

Other Artemisia-species with monographs in this book include → Southernwood, and → Tarragon.

Literature

[1] Arino A. et al., J. Essent. Oil Res. 11:182–184 (1999).

[2] Beauhaire J., J.L. Fourrey, Tetrahedron Lett:2751–2574 (1984).

[3] Carnat A.P. et al., Ann. Pharm. Fr. 43: 397–405 (1986).

[4] Chen P.C. et al., J. Ethnopharmacol. 27: 285–295 (1989).

[5] Drake D., J. Lam, Phytochemistry 13:455 ref. in Ü106 (1974).

[6] Dürbeck K., Drogenreport 9(14):47–51 (1996).

[7] Herold M., F. Pank, Drogenreport 4(6): 131 (1991).

[8] Hoffmann B., K. Herrmann, Z. Lebensm. Untersuch. Forsch. 174:211 (1982).

[9] Hurabielle M. et al., Planta Med. 31(2):97 (1977).

[10] Hwang Y.S. et al., J. Chem. Ecol. 11: 1297–1306 (1985).

[11] Jork H., S.M.K. Juell, Arch. Pharm. 312: 540–547 (1979).

[12] Kartnig T., A. Brantner, Sci. Pharm. 60: 129 (1992).

[13] Kaul V.K. et al., Indian J. Pharm. 38:21–22 (1976).

[14] Kommission E, BAnz-Nr. 122 vom 06.07. 1988.

[15] Kundu S.K, et al., J. Indian Chem. 46:584 (1969).

[16] Leitner A. et al., Allergy 53(1):36–41 (1998).

[17] Marco J.A. et al., Phytochemistry 30: 403–404 (1991).

[18] Michaelis K. et al., Z. Naturforsch. C: Biosc. 37c:152 (1982).

[19] Misra L.N., S.P. Singh, J. Nat. Prod. 49:941 (1986).

[20] Murray R.D.H., M. Stephanovic, J. Nat. Prod. 49:550 (1986).

[21] Naef-Mueller R. et al., Helv. Chim. Acta 64:1424 (1981).

[22] Nano G.M. et al., Planta Med. 30:211–215 (1976).

[23] Nguyen Xuan Dung et al., J. Essent. Oil Res. 4:433–434 (1992).

[24] Nin S. et al., J. Essent. Oil Res. 7(3): 271–277 (1995).

[25] Pino J.A. et al., J. Essent. Oil Res. 9(1): 87–89 (1997).

[26] Polos E. et al., Herba Hung 62:435 (1993), ref. in CA 119:1333473.

[27] Rücker G. et al., Phytochemistry: 31(1): 340–342 (1992).

[28] Schneider G., B. Mielke, Dtsch. Apoth. Ztg. 119:977–982 (1979).

[29] Stäger J. et al., Allergy 46:475–478 (1991).

[30] Stephanovic M. et al., Glas. Hem. Drus. (Beograd) 47:7 (1982), ref. in CA 96: 177968.

[31] Trumpowska M. et al., Acta pol. pharm. 25:313–318 (1968).

[32] Tucker A.O. et al., J. Essent. Oil Res. 5:239–242 (1993).

[33] Vallier, P. et al., Clin. Allergy 18(5):491–500 (1988).

[34] Wallnöfer B. et al., Phytochemistry 28(10):2687–2691 (1989).

[35] Weymar H., Buch der Korbblütler, Neumann Verlag, Radebeul 1957.

Literature references identified by Ü can be found in the general listing of books and monographs at the back of this book.

Nutmeg

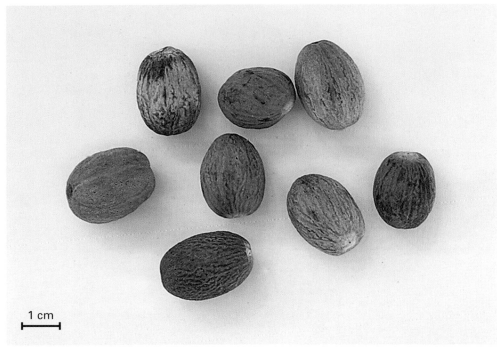

Fig. 1: Nutmeg

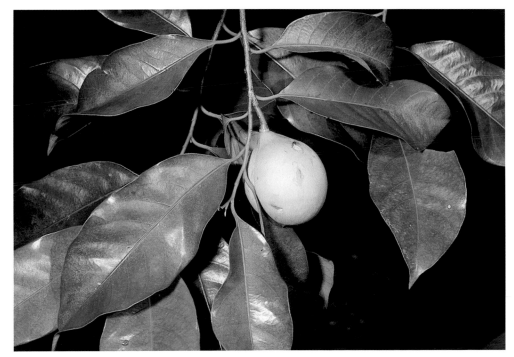

Fig. 2: Nutmeg (*Myristica fragrans* HOUTT.)

Plant source: *Myristica fragrans* HOUTT.

Family: Nutmeg family (Myristicaceae).

Common names: Engl.: nutmeg, nutmeg tree, Banda nutmeg; Fr.: muscade, muscadier, musque; Ger: Muskat, Muskatnussbaum, Bandanuss, Suppennuss.

Description: Dioecious, evergreen, up to 20 m tall tree. The leaves are leathery, ovate-elliptic, entire-margined, 4 to 8 cm long, 1.5 to 4 cm wide, with glandular punctations. The flowers are arranged in pauciflorous racemes or pseudoumbels. Female flowers mostly single, with 3-lobed perianth, yellowish-white, the superior ovary is monolocular; male flowers with 9 to 12 stamina, which are fused to form a tube. The fruit (Fig. 4) is an egg-shaped, light-yellow, fleshy and peach-like, 3 to 6 cm long, 2.5 to 5 cm broad, one-seeded berry, which, upon maturity, splits into two valves. The seeds have a hard, dark brown testa and are in a cup-like fashion enclosed by a bright red seed coat (arillus), which is finger-like slit at the top.

Native origin: Southern and Eastern Moluccas, the Banda Islands are the center of domestication.

Main cultivation areas: Indonesia (Aceh Province of Sumatra, Ambon, Banda Islands, Sula Islands, Sangihe Islands, Talaud Islands, Halmahera, Ternate), Grenada, as well as, among others, South India, Sri Lanka, Malaysia, Java, Thailand, New Guinea, Brazil, Republic of Guinea, Madagascar, Zanzibar, Mauritius, and Réunion.

Main exporting countries: Indonesia (the so-called East Indian provenances), and Grenada (the so-called West Indian provenances).

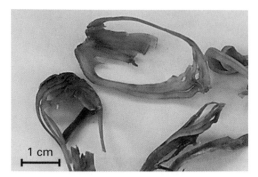

Fig. 3: Mace

Cultivation: Similar to the clove tree, the nutmeg tree prefers nutrient-rich, saturated yet well-drained soil at regular temperatures above 22 °C in humid lowland areas of the inner tropics in close proximity to water. With strong sunlight, it needs to be shaded by planting suitable shade trees, which also guarantee wind protection. Propagation is carried out by seed, which due to their short-lived germinating power over just a few days, are usually sown quickly in bamboo- or plastic baskets. After about one year, when they are about 30 cm in height, they are transplanted below shade trees that have been planted earlier. After about 6 to 8 years, at the time of the first bloom, for the most part the male trees are removed or are used as grafting stocks for female scions. In cultivation, in order to make harvesting easier, the height of the trees is limited to 6 m, maximum 9 m. The first harvest is possible after about 8 to 10 years. The peak harvests are reached between years 15 and 60. Healthy trees are still productive after 100 years. Nutmeg trees are very susceptible to insect pests and fungal diseases. Nutmeg seeds are also very easily infested by insects, especially the nutmeg-seed-burrowing-beetle (*Phlocosomos cribatus*) [69, Ü89].

Culinary herb

Commercial forms: Nutmeg: Dried, whole or ground seed kernels, sometimes coated with dried milk of lime. Best quality nutmeg comes from Grenada (about 11%

essential oil), and the islands of Banda (about 8% essential oil) and Siauw (6.5% essential oil). Nutmeg is classified in Grenada according to the number of nuts per English pound (lb = 453.6 g). So, for example, Grenada 65's means that 65 nuts weigh 1 lb. In Indonesia, it is customary to assign grades of nutmeg to Classes A through E. Sound, undamaged, large nuts (60's to 80's, which correspond roughly to Class A) have the highest value. Class E means 125 to 160 nuts/500 g. Class ABCD is an assortment of various sizes (unsorted). Substandard quality (broken, wormy and punky (BWP), grinders, defectives) is used for the production of oleoresin or essential oil [13, 47, Ü93].

Mace: Dried arillus, whole (whole pale, No. 1, No. 2), broken (No. 1 broken, No. 2 broken) or ground. Best qualities are Banda- and Java mace.

Nutmeg butter (balsam of nutmegs): A semi-solid mass obtained by exposing the nutmeg nuts to hydraulic pressure and heat, aside from fatty oil it contains 4% to 12% essential oil.

Nutmeg oil: Obtained by steam distillation of nutmeg or mace.

Mace oil: Obtained by steam distillation of the arillus.

Nutmeg oleoresin: Obtained by extraction of the seeds (about 30% essential oil) or of mace.

Production: When ripe, the fruits are plucked with a tool that is similar to an apple plucker (a long pole with a hook attached), more rarely they are knocked off the tree, or they are picked up from the ground after dropping from the tree. The fruit flesh is removed and then the aril and nut are separated.

To obtain mace, the arils are stripped from the nuts, without tearing them if possible, and then they are spread out in bamboo baskets or on mats to dry in the sun. Grenadian mace is cured by storage for about 8 months in crates that allow air to flow through. Sometimes mace is dried pressed between boards. During the drying process, mace loses its scarlet color and turns golden brown or yellowish. The seed kernels are dried in their shells in the

shade and/or in the morning sun in order to prevent the fats from melting (melting point 38 °C). After 6 to 8 weeks, when the seed kernels begin to rattle in their shells, the nuts are either cracked with mallets or they are mechanically cracked open to release the seed kernels. The nutmeg nut is not really a nut, but rather a part of the seed of a berry! Afterwards, the seed kernels are sometimes treated with lime whereby they are placed in a suspension of lime in seawater and then dried again. The lime treatment is supposed to prevent insect infestation, but originally it served the purpose of eliminating the possibility of germination and therefore protected the Dutch nutmeg cultivation monopoly. Lime treatment is practiced only rarely today [68, Ü89].

Forms used: Powdered nutmeg seeds, whole or powdered mace, nutmeg oil, and mace oil.

Storage: Nutmeg or mace is stored in airtight porcelain- or metal containers, protected from light and moisture. Nutmeg in powder form loses its aroma quickly during storage; comminuted mace is more suitable for storage.

Description

Nutmeg (Fig. 1): Dried, whole seed kernels, freed from the testa and arillus, sometimes covered with lime, brownish, obtuse-ovate to almost spherical, 2 to 2.5 cm long, 1.5 to 2 cm wide, having a weight of 5 to 10 g, occasionally the surface is light gray, whitish powdery due to the adhering

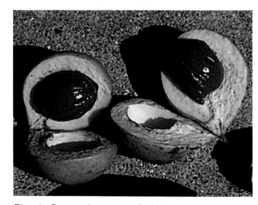

Fig. 4: Opened nutmeg fruits

Toxicology: Based on existing data, there is no acute or chronic toxicity with the normal use of nutmeg or mace as a spice [22].

Toxic effects: At high doses (5 g powdered nutmeg or higher, corresponding to one small nutmeg kernel), nutmeg is toxic [Ü58]. Symptoms arise a few hours after ingestion and include thirst, dryness of the mouth, nausea, dizziness, vomiting, reddening and swelling of the face, profuse perspiration, micturition, abdominal pain and headaches, weak pulse, hypothermia, tachycardia, insomnia, fear of dying, collapse and delirium. After about 12 h, deep sleep sets in. Fatal cases have been observed [9, 16, 20, 33, 40, 52, 74, 75, 79, 83, Ü58]. Poisonings usually take 2 to 4 days to clear up; what remains is an aversion to the taste of nutmeg [16, 20, 33]. Poisonings are usually due to the use of nutmeg as an intoxicant, abortive or aphrodisiac or as a result of folk medicinal applications in gastrointestinal illnesses [20, 83].
The essential oil from nutmeg reduces fertility in rats and has a mutagenic effect [54].
The sensitization potential is moderate [Ü39]. Inhalation of mace dust (paprika or coriander, respectively) led to asthma attacks in sensitized patients [66].

Psychotomimetic effects: Besides the symptoms described above, psychotomimetic effects occur due to the content of myristicine and elemicin, usually 2 to 5 h after the intake of 5 to 30 g of ground nutmeg or mace, respectively. Depressions of consciousness are associated with intense hallucinations, characterized by changes of spatial and time perceptions as well as sensations of weightlessness. Other symptoms include, among others, laughing-fits and incoherent speech [16, 33, Ü58, Ü100]. It is assumed that biotransformation in the human organism converts the phenyl propane derivatives to amphetamine- or mescaline-like substances [50, 74, Ü100]. However, the psychotomimetic effects of nutmeg have also been called in question [19].

Culinary use: For many years, Arabs have used ground nutmeg to season mutton and lamb. It is a standard seasoning in many Dutch recipes. In Holland, ground nutmeg is added especially to mashed potatoes, white cabbage, cauliflower, vegetable purees, macaroni and cooked meat. In Italy, nutmeg is a popular spice for veal, filled noodles (e.g. of fusilli with mushrooms and nutmeg, fillings for tortellini, ravioli and cannelloni), pasta sauces and vegetable plates. In France, nutmeg is used as a seasoning in béchamel- and bread sauces as well as in white puddings (small white sausages made from young chicken and cream), and in England in fish- and seafood stews, but also in cakes and sweet dishes. In Central European cooking, mace is only seldom used [Ü2, Ü73].
Prior to use, nutmegs are ground, finely grated, usually using a so-called nutmeg grater and less often with a nutmeg grinder. A coffee grinder is better for cutting mace. Nutmeg- and mace powder should be added to cooked dishes when finished cooking. One may also cook the dish with a matchstick-sized, uncut piece of mace, and then remove it before serving. Due to the pungent taste of nutmeg, it should be measured carefully.
Powdered nutmeg is used as a seasoning for meat dishes (e.g. lamb chops, veal ragout, poultry ragout, fillings), ground meat, fish dishes (e.g. trout, sole, rosefish), egg dishes (e.g. custard cubes), cheese dishes, baked puddings, sausage, soups (e.g. cream of asparagus soup, potato soup), stews, meat broths, vegetable juices, tomato juice, vegetable dishes as well as vegetable stews (especially cauliflower, Brussels sprouts, broccoli, savoy cabbage, kohlrabi, asparagus, carrot, leek), potato puree, spaghetti, spaetzle, semolina dumplings, rice dishes and sauces (e.g. béchamel-, onion-, tomato-, cheese-, bread sauces), chutneys and relishes [Ü2, Ü30, Ü51, Ü55, Ü61].
One can also use nutmeg to enhance the taste of sweet dishes and baked goods, such as fruit desserts (pear- and plum compotes), puddings, jams, fruitcakes, honey cakes and Swiss Leckerli. Grated nutmeg should lend an especially piquant note to

cherry- or apple cakes. Likewise, a tiny pinch of powdered nutmeg goes well in hot milk drinks or chocolate [Ü13, Ü68, Ü73, Ü90]. It is also used as a flavor component of alcoholic beverages such as mulled wine, fruit punch, rum punch, tea punch, eggnog, sangria (Spanish peach punch) and liqueurs [47].
Nutmeg is also used as a pickling spice [Ü1].
Mace is used similarly to nutmeg. Mace serves especially as a flavor enhancer of fine sausages (sausages for cooking in water, bratwurst, liver sausage), seasonal baked goods, especially ginger bread and "Printen" (specialty of Aachen), but also of fruit salads, fruit jellies, compotes, creams, some puddings and punch drinks [47, Ü13, Ü30].
Nutmeg oil, mace oil and the oleoresin are used mainly as flavor components of herbal- and fruit liqueurs, for the production of spice essences and for flavoring tobacco [47, Ü30, Ü92].

Combines well with: Bay leaf, cardamom, cinnamon, clove, ginger, and pepper.

As a component of spice mixes and preparations.

Nutmeg → Almond biscuit spice, → Apple cake spice, → Baharat, → Bologna spice mix, → Curry powder, → English pudding spice, → Garam masala, → Gingerbread spice, → Grill spice, → La kama, → Masala, → Meat spice, → Mélange classique, → Mulled wine spice, → Parisian pepper, → Pickling spice, → Poultry spice, → Quatre épices, → Ras el hanout, → Sambal manis, → Sauce spice, → Sausage spice, → Scappis spice mix, → Soup spice, → Stollen spice, → Table mustard, → Tomato ketchup, → Vegetable spice.

Mace → Curry powder, → Grill spice, → Masala, → Plum jam spice, → Ras el hanout, → Sausage spice, → Stollen spice, → Vegetable spice.

Other uses: In Malaysia, Grenada and Indonesia, the fruit pulp (pericarp) is candied, pickled or used for the manufacture of jam and nutmeg jelly. On the Moluccas, the fermented pulp serves as a raw material for the manufacture of a popular nutmeg liquor. Nutmeg essential oil is used in the perfume and cosmetic industries, for example as an aroma ingredient of toothpastes and soaps [68, Ü89]. In addition it is used as tobacco flavoring in the tobacco industry [47]. Due to the good antimicrobial effects of nutmeg extracts, it is also applied as a preservative in fruit juices [12].

Medicinal herb

Herbal drugs: Myristicae semen, Nutmeg, contains minimum 5% essential oil [EB 6], Mace, contains minimum 4.5% essential oil [EB 6], Myristicae oleum expressum (Oleum Nusticae, Oleum Myristicae), Nutmeg balsam (nutmeg butter) [DAB 6], Myristicae fragrantis aetheroleum, Nutmeg oil [Ph Eur].

Indications: For illnesses and complaints in the area of the gastrointestinal tract, such as diarrhea, stomach cramps, intestinal catarrh and flatulence. Because efficacy has not been sufficiently substantiated and due to the possible risks, the German Commission E of the BfArM did not approve its therapeutic use [35]. In Ayurvedic medicine, mace is also used for treating mild fever and asthma. In Indonesia, nutmeg is used for stomach pains, stomach cramps, diarrhea, rheumatism, nervousness, vomiting, sleep disturbances in children and pertussis. In Malaysian medicine, nutmeg serves as an aphrodisiac (also in India, in Arab countries as well as in Europe during the 18th and 19th centuries). Applied to the temples or taken internally (1 drop per cup of tea), nutmeg oil is supposed to alleviate headaches [19, 83].

Spice herbs with uses similar to nutmeg

Long nutmeg, Macassar mace (Papua nutmeg, Macassar nut, male nutmeg), obtained from *Myristica argentea* WARB., native to the Bombarai peninsula (in southwestern New Guinea), and cultivated in western New Guinea and in Papua New Guinea. The seed kernel contains 2 to 6% essential oil and the arillus contains about 7%, with a relatively high safrole content, little elemicin and no myristicin. Furthermore, β-phellandrene and *p*-cymene, among others, are present. It is mainly the arillus that is used as a spice [47, Ü61, Ü92].

Bombay nutmeg, Bombay mace, obtained from *Myristica malabarica* LAM., native to the west coast of India (Malabar Coast), and cultivated in gardens in the Antilles. It is mainly the arillus (0.7% essential oil) that is used as a spice; the seed kernel contains almost no essential oil [Ü92].

Otoba nutmeg, the seeds of *Myristica otoba* H. et B. (*Dialyanthera otoba* H. et B.) WARB.), native to Columbia. The seed kernels contain about 7% essential oil [Ü31].

Batjang nutmeg (Pala Maba), the seed kernels of *Myristica speciosa* WARB., native to the Moluccas.

Halmahera nutmeg (sometimes also described as Batjang nutmeg), the seeds of *Myristica succedeana* BLUME, native to the northern Moluccas (Ternate, Tidore, Batjan), cultivated on a small scale in Ternate (Moluccas), the arillus contains about 7% essential oil and the seed kernels about 5% [Ü31, Ü37, Ü61].

Calabash nutmeg (Calabash nutmeg seed, nutmeg beans), the seed kernels of *Monodora myristica* (GAERTN.) DUNAL (Annonaceae), native to West- and Central Africa, contain about 2 to 7% essential oil, of which the main components include limonene, β-phellandrene and 1,8-cineole [38, Ü43].

Chilean nutmeg (Chilean laurel), the seeds of *Laurelia sempervirens* (RUIZ et PAV.) TULASNE (Monimiaceae).

Brazilian nutmeg, the seeds of *Cryptocarya moschata* NEES et MART. (Lauraceae), native to Brazil [Ü92].
California nutmeg, the seeds of *Torreya californica* TORR. (*Torreya myristica* HOOKER, Taxaceae), native to the California coastal region.

Madagascar nutmeg (Madagascan nutmeg, Ravensara nut), the seeds of *Ravensara aromatica* SONN. (*Agathophyllum aromaticum* WILLD., Lauraceae), native to Madagascar, and cultivated in Mauritius and Sri Lanka [Ü92].

Plum nutmeg, the seeds of *Atherosperma moschatum* LABILL. (Monimiaceae), native to Australia.

Large mace bean (Pichurim bean), seeds of the pichurim tree, *Ocotea puchurymajor* MART. (*Acrodiclidium puchurymajor* (MART.) MEZ., *Licaria puchurymajor* (MART.) KOSTERM., Lauraceae), native to Brazil, contain about 5% essential oil, of which the main components include eugenol, methyleugenol, safrole, anethole, 1,8-cineole, α-terpineol, terpinen-4-ol, geraniol, limonene, γ-terpinene and linalool [26].

Spice-Cheese-Pudding

4 tablespoons of sugar, 1 tablespoon of grated Swiss cheese, 3 tablespoons of flour, 100 ml milk, 1/2 teaspoon of freshly ground nutmeg, ground caraway, white pepper, 4 egg yolks, 6 egg whites, salt, 125 g grated cheese (Parmesan or Emmentaler).

Grease the casserole with butter and sprinkle with grated Swiss cheese. Heat the remaining butter, add the flour to form a thick sauce and fill up with milk while mixing the ingredients; add the spices, heat again to a boil and mix in the egg yolks. Beat the egg whites until stiff, add a bit of salt, and combine 1/4 of the egg white with the previous mixture. Stir in the grated cheese and the remaining egg white and pour the mixture into the casserole. Bake at 180 °C for about 30 minutes until the surface is nicely brown. Serve immediately [Ü9].

Literature

[1] Al-Khatib I.M.H. et al., J. Food Compos. Analysis 1:59–64 (1987).

[2] Archer A.W., J. Chromatogr. 438: 117–121 (1988).

[3] Banerjee S. et al., Nutrition and Cancer 21(3):263–269 (1994).

[4] Barrowman J.A. et al., Brit. Med. J. 3:11–12 (1975).

[5] Bejnarowicz E.A., E.R. Kirch, J. Pharm. Sci. 52:988–993 (1963).

[6] Bennett A. et al., N. Engl. J. Med. 290: 110–111 (1974).

[7] Braun U., D.A. Kalbhen, Pharmacol. 9: 312–316 (1973).

[8] Chandrashekar K. et al., J. Food Sci. Technol. 32(5):403–405 (1995).

[9] Cushny A.R., Proc. Royal Soc. Med. 1908 – I C:39 (1908).

[10] Davis D.V., R.G. Cooks, J. Agric. Food Chem. 30:495–504 (1982).

[11] Dorman H.J., S.G. Deans, J. Appl. Microbiol. 88(2):308–316 (2000).

[12] Ejechi B.O. et al., J. Food Prot. 61(6): 725–727 (1998).

[13] Flach M., Meded Landbouwhogeschool Wageningen 66(1):1–84 (1966).

[14] Forrest J.E. et al., J. Chromatogr. 69:115–121 (1972).

[15] Forrest J.E. et al., J. Chem. Soc. Perkin. Trans. I:205–209 (1974).

[16] Forrest J.E., R.A. Heacock, Lloydia 35: 440–449 (1972).

[17] Forrest J.E., R.A. Heacock, J. Chromatogr. 89:113–117 (1974).

[18] Forrest T.P. et al., Naturwissenschaften 60(5):257 (1973).

[19] Gils van C., P.A. Cox, J. Ethnopharmacol. 42(2):117–124 (1994).

[20] Green R.C., J. Am. Med. Assoc. 171: 1342–1344 (1959).

[21] Hada S. et al., Phytochemistry 27:563 (1988).

[22] Hallström H., A. Thuvander, Nat. Toxins 5(5):186–192 (1997).

[23] Harvey D.J., J. Chromatogr. 110:91–102 (1975).

[24] Hattori M. et al., Chem. Pharm. Bull. 35: 668–674, 3315–3322 und 36:648 (1987).

[25] Hattori M. et al., Chem. Pharm. Bull. 34:3885–3893 (1986).

[26] Himejima M., I. Kubo, J. Nat. Prod. 55:620–625 (1992).

[27] Huhtanen C.N., J. Food Protection 43:195–196 (1980).

[28] Hussain S.P., A.R. Rao, Cancer Lett. 56(3):231–234 (1991).

[29] Isogai A. et al., Agr. Biol. Chem. 37:193–194, 889–895, 1479–1486 (1973).

[30] Jannsen J. et al., J. Ethnopharmacol. 29: 179–188 (1990).

[31] Jannu L.N. et al., Cancer Lett. 56(1):59–63 (1991).

[32] Joseph J., J. Plantation Crops. 8(2):61–72 (1980).

[33] Kalbhen D.A., Angew. Chem. 83(11): 392–396, Angew. Chem. Int. Ed. 10(6): 370–374 (1971).

[34] Kim Y.B. et al., Arch. Pharmacol. Res. 14:1–6 (1991).

[35] Kommission E beim BfArM, BAnz-Nr. 173 vom 18.09.1986.

[36] Kumari M.V.R., A.R. Rao, Anticancer Res. 8:1056 (1988).

[37] Kumari M.V.R., A.R. Rao, Cancer Lett. 46(2):87–91 (1989).

[38] Lamaty G. et al., Flavour Fragrance J. 2:91–94 (1987).

[39] Lawrence B.M., Perfumer Flavorist 15:62–64 (1990).

[40] McCord J.A., L.P. Jervey, J.S.C. Med. Ass. 58:436 (1962).

[41] Misra V. et al., Indian J. Med. Res. 67:482–484 (1978).

[42] Mitra C.R., Riechstoffe, Aromen, Körperpflegemittel 26:252 (1976).

[43] Miyazawa M. et al., Nat. Prod. Lett. 8(1):25–26 (1996).

[44] Mobarak Z. et al., Forens. Sci. 4:161–169 (1974).

[45] Nakamura N. et al., Chem. Pharm. Bull. 36:2685–2688 (1988).

[46] Nakatani et al., Phytochemistry 27:3127–3129 (1988).

[47] Oberdieck R., Fleischwirtschaft 69:1648–1664 (1989).

[48] Olajide O.A. et al., Phytother. Res. 13(4):344–345 (1999).

[49] Orabi K.Y. et al., J. Nat. Prod. 54(3): 856–859 (1991).

[50] Oswald E.O. et al., Biochem. Biophys. Acta 244:322 (1971).

[51] Ozaki Y. et al., Jap. J. Pharmacol. 49(2): 155–16 (1989).

[52] Painter J.C. et al., Clin. Toxicol. 4:1–4 (1971).

[53] Pathak R.K. et al., Indian Drugs Pharm. Ind. 14:7 (1979).

[54] Pecevski J. et al., Toxicol. Lett. 7:239 (1981).

[55] Perez C., C. Anesini, Am. J. Clin. Med. 22(2):169–174 (1994).

[56] Power F.B., H.H. Salway, J. Chem. Soc. 93:1653 (1908).

[57] Purushotaman K.K. et al., J. Chem. Soc. Perkin Trans I:587–588 (1977).

[58] Purushothaman K.K., A. Sarada, Indian J. Chem. 19B:236–237 (1980).

[59] Ram A. et al., J. Ethnopharmacol. 55(1): 49–53 (1996).

[60] Rasheed A., J. Pharm. (Lahore):6:41–50 (1985).

[61] Rasheed A. et al., Planta Med. 50:222–226 (1984).

[62] Reynolds J.E.F. (Ed.) Martindale: The Extra Pharmacopoeia, The Royal Pharmaceutical Society of Great Britain, 32. Edition, The Pharmaceutical Press, London 1999.

[63] Salzer U.J., Fleischwirtschaft 62:885–887 (1982).

[64] Sammy G.M., W.W. Nawar, Chem. Ind. 1279–1280 (1968).

[65] Sarath-Kumara S.J. et al., J. Sci. Food Agr. 36:93–100 (1985).

[66] Sastre J. et al., Allergy 51(2):117–120 (1996).

[67] Schenk H.P., D. Lamparsky, J. Chromatogr. 204:391–395 (1981).

[68] Scholz H., Natürlich 19(1):31–37 (1999).

[69] Seidemann J., Drogenreport 11(20):68–75 (1998).

[70] Shafran I. et al., N. Engl. J. Med. 296:694 (1977).

[71] Sharma A. et al., Indian J. Physiol. Pharmacol. 39(4):407–410 (1995).

[72] Shidore P.P. et al., Indian J. Pharm. Sci. 47:188–190 (1985).

[73] Shin K.H. et al., Arch. Pharm. Res. 11: 240–243 (1988).

[74] Shulgin A.T., Nature 210:380–383 (1966).

[75] Shulgin A.T. et al., Nature 189:1011 (1961).

[76] Shulgin A.T., H.O. Kerlinger, Naturwissenschaften 51:360 (1964).

[77] Stahl E. (Hrsg.): Chromatographische und mikroskopische Analyse von Drogen, Fischer Verlag Stuttgart, New York 1978.

[78] Truitt E.B. et al., Proc. Exp. Biol. Med. 112:647–650 (1963).

[79] Truitt E.B. et al., J. Neuropsychiat. 2:205–210 (1961).

[80] Variyar P.S., C. Bandyopadhyay, PAFAI J. 17(1):19–25 (1995).

[81] Varshney I.P., S.C. Sharma, Indian J. Chem. 6:474 (1968).

[82] Warburg O., Die Muskatnuß. Ihre Geschichte, Botanik, Kultur, Handel und Verwertung sowie ihre Surrogate. Zugleich ein Beitrag zur Kulturgeschichte der Banda-Inseln, Leipzig 1897.

[83] Weil A.T., Econ. Bot. 19:194–217 (1965).

Literature references identified by Ü can be found in the general listing of books and monographs at the back of this book.

Olive

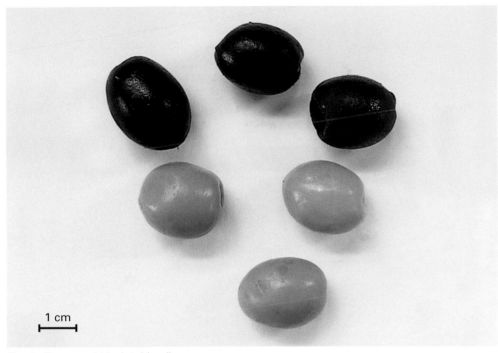

Fig. 1: Green and black table olives

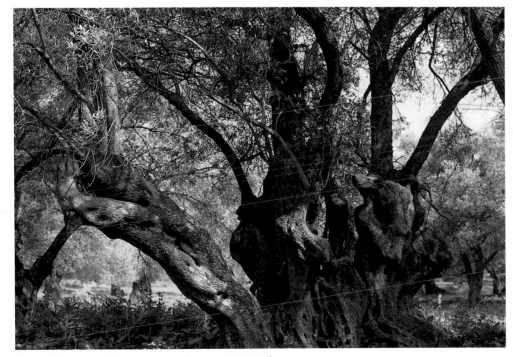

Fig. 2: Olive tree (*Olea europaea* L. var. *europaea*)

Plant source: *Olea europaea* L. var. *europaea*.

Synonyms: *Olea officinarum* CRANTZ, *O. sativa* HOFFMGG. et LINK.

Taxonomic classification: The species *O. europaea* can be subdivided into three varieties or subspecies: *O. europaea* L. var. *europaea*, *O. europaea* L. var. *silvestris* BROT. (Synonym: *O. europaea* ssp. *oleaster* (HOFFMGG. et LINK) NEGODI, also regarded as a separate species: *Olea oleaster* HOFFMGG. et LINK) and *O. europaea* L. var. *africana* (MILL.) P.S. GREEN (also regarded as a separate species: *O. africana* MILL.).
The cultivated form is *O. europaea* L. var. *europaea*. From this form there are over 300 races, of which about 30 are cultivated on a large scale. The fruits of the cultivated varieties that are used as table olives are more pulpy and lower in oil than the smaller, firm oil olives. The other two varieties are wild- or escaped forms, which sometimes are used as grafting stock for the cultivated form.

Family: Olive family (Oleaceae).

Common names: Engl.: olive, olive tree; Fr.: olivier; Ger: Olive, Ölbaum, Olivenbaum.

Description: Evergreen tree, up to 20 m tall, with gnarled trunk and light colored bark; in cultivation, the trees are cut back to a height of 5 to 8 m to facilitate harvest. The base of the trunk forms subterranean outgrowths with emerging stolons and adventitious roots, just below the soil's surface; the trunk above the surface also produces roundish outgrowths, which can be separated for suitable, vegetative propagation. The twigs are rod-shaped, first with a felt-like surface, with or without thorns.

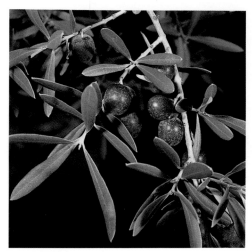
Fig. 3: Olive twig with fruits

The leaves are opposite, 3 to 8 cm long, narrow-elliptic to lanceolate or cordate, mucronate, entire-margined, leathery, with dark green upper surface, glabrous or with scattered peltate hairs, the lower surface is silvery, shiny due to aforementioned peltate hairs. Flowers are arranged in small, axillary composite racemes; calyx with 4 teeth, 4-lobed corolla, white, 2 stamina, superior ovary, 2-chambered. The stone fruit bears one seed, more rarely two, resembling a prune, up to 3.5 cm long, first green, and when mature, depending on the cultivar greenish, reddish, brown, violet, dark brown or black [Ü26, Ü42].

Native origin: Only known in cultivation.

Main cultivation areas: Cultivated throughout the entire Mediterranean region and Portugal, especially Spain and Italy, furthermore Greece, Algeria, and Turkey, to a lesser extent in the Russian Federation, in the USA (California, Florida), Mexico, Ethiopia, South Africa, Angola, Pakistan, India, Japan, Australia, Peru, Chile, Argentina, in the Bermudas, and Jamaica

Main producing countries: Spain (Andalusia, Seville, Córdoba, Málaga, Jaén, Extramadura), and to a lesser extent in France, Italy, Greece, and California.

Cultivation: The olive tree prefers neutral to slightly calcareous, not too humus soil in sunny, dry, protected slopes at altitudes up to 600 m above sea level. It also succeeds in very poor, stony soil. Growing regions with balanced climates with an average annual temperature between 15 and 22 °C are favorable. This corresponds to Mediterranean regions between the 46th and 24th degrees of latitude. At 0 °C the olive tree suffers somewhat, at –8 °C it suffers severe frost damage, and temperatures below –10 °C will kill the tree. Due to the risk of genetic dispersion, propagation is carried out by grafting or with cuttings, and rarely also with detached shoots. The grafting stocks are grown from the seeds [Ü89].

Culinary herb

Commercial forms. Table olives (marinated olives): Table olives are unripe fermented, ripe fermented or ripe unfermented fruits, cured in a salt solution, each described according to their origin and method of preparation including, among others, Aragón-olives (Northern Spain, black), Arbequina-olives (Northern Spain, dark brownish-green, often flavored with rosemary or thyme), Cailletti-er-olives (France, Nice, reddish, very small), Conservolea-olives (Greece, black, slightly bitter), Gordal-olives (Königin-olives, Southern Spain, Seville, green or black, thick, pulpy), Hojiblanca-olives (Southern Spain, Jaén, Cordoba, fibrous, not very palatable), Kalamata-olives (Greece, Peloponnesian, black, large, juicy), Lucque-olives (France, Languedoc, green, very tasty), Manzillos (Southern Spain, Andalusia, green, very delicious), Megaritki-olives (Greece, preserved in dry salt, quite shriveled, raisin-like appearance, salty), Mission-olives (USA, California, medium-sized), Picholine-olives (France, Languedoc, Provence, green, long, thin, stabilized with oak wood ash, very delicious), Salonenque-olives (France, Hérault, Aude, green), Taggiasca-olives (Italy, Ligurian, small, black) and Tanche-olives (France, Nyon, black, slightly wrinkled) [35].

Olive oil: Extra virgin (extra native olive oil, first cold pressing, light yellow or greenish, less than 1% free fatty acids), virgin (native olive oil, fine quality, not more than 2% acid content), refined (usually warm pressed, then refined), pure (olive oil, mixture of refined and cold pressed oil). Sweet oil is obtained from the pressed cake, however it may not be designated as olive oil (maximum 1.5% acids) [35, Ü2]. Similar to wine, olive oils have special trademarks from different cultivation operations and oil mills [for an overview of marks and qualities, see Lit. 35].

Production: Under favorable conditions, the first harvest can already take place during the third to fifth years, but often not until after the 20th year. In the Mediterranean region, the main harvest season is from November to January. The harvest of unripe fruits is done by hand, harvest of the ripe fruits is usually carried out with a mechanical olive picker (by collecting the individual olives or by a suction device), stripped off with rakes, shaken off (mechanical tree shaker) or by picking up the fallen fruits from the ground or from spread out cloth or nets [15, 35, Ü26].

Green, lactic acid-cured olives: The fruits are harvested when they are yellowish-green to yellow and for 6 to 10 hours are placed in a solution of 1.3 to 2.6% caustic soda. This strongly increases the permeability of the exocarp and hydrolyzes most of the bitter oleuropein. After that the olives are washed and then left to ferment in a 10 to 12% salt solution. The main fermentation stimulating germs are *Pediococcus*-, *Leuconostoc*- and *Lactobacillus*-species as well as yeasts. After fermentation is completed, the olives are usually pitted and filled with paprika, anchovies, almonds, capers or onions, pasteurized and packed into glass- or plastic containers. The pH-value of the finished product amounts to 3.8 to 4.2, the lactic acid content 0.8 to 1.2%, and the sodium chloride content 7 to 8% [Ü8].

Black, lactic acidic olives: The ripe fruits are harvested and after washing in an 8 to

10% salt solution they are left for 1 to 3 months duration of spontaneous fermentation. The main fermentation stimulators are *Lactobacillus*-species and yeast. Following fermentation they are pasteurized and filled into glass- or plastic containers. The pH-value of the finished product amounts to 4.5 to 4.8, the lactic acid content 0.1 to 0.6%, and the sodium chloride content 6 to 9% [Ü8].

Black, non-fermented olives: The ripe fruits are incubated 3 to 5 times in well-ventilated (phenol oxidation!) 1 to 2% solution of caustic soda. To stabilize the color iron gluconate is added to the final wash water. After that they are placed in a 3% salt solution, sterilized and packed. The pH-value of the finished product amounts to 5.8 to 7.9, the sodium chloride content 1 to 3% [Ü8, for an overview of fermentation, see Lit. 19].

Forms used: Marinated table olives, whole, crushed or pureed.

Storage: Loose bought olives should be consumed within 3 days. Preserved olives can be kept in closed containers for a few years. After the container has been opened, they need to be stored in the refrigerator.

Description. Whole fruit (Fig. 1): Drupes 2 to 3.5 cm long, smooth, green when unripe, purple to black when ripe, stone very hard, oblique-elongated or club-shaped, somewhat compressed, wrinkled or furrowed, light brown, seeds oblong, compressed, 9 to 11 mm long, with much nutritive tissue and straight embryo [Ü29, Ü42].

Cross section of the fruit: The exocarp consists of thick-walled, polyhedral cells with granular content, which is dark in the ripe fruits. The mesocarp contains thin-walled parenchyma cells with dark granular content and large amounts of fatty oil. Between the parenchyma cells are numerous barrel-shaped, dotted stone cells with antler-like projections. The endocarp consists mostly of elongated, spindle-shaped or isodiametric, stone cells, which are dot-ted as well; the seeds mostly contain small, thin-walled parenchyma cells with aleuron grains and are rich in fatty oil and oxalate raphides [Ü29].

Odor: Preserved table olives have a faintly sour odor, **Taste:** The untreated fruit is very bitter and therefore unpalatable. The treated fruits are aromatic and depending on the type of curing faintly to somewhat bitter, salty or sourish.

History: Olive trees have probably been cultivated since the early Bronze Age. By the middle of the 3rd century BCE, their cultivation in Greece and Palestine has been documented. Greek mythology and Bible texts also mention olive trees repeatedly. From Greece, the cultivation of olive trees spread to Italy, and from Central Persia to Phoenicia, Egypt, Tunisia, Algeria, Morocco, Spain and Portugal. Spanish Franciscan monks introduced olive trees to California in the mid 18th century. Canned olives were introduced at the beginning of the 19th century [Ü61, for a historical overview, see Lit. 35].

Constituents and Analysis

Constituents

- Fatty oil: In the whole fruit 15 to 40%, in the fruit pulp (65 to 85% of the total fruit weight) 12 to 60 (and up to 75)%, in the seed (15 to 35% of the total fruit weight) 20 to 33% [Ü8]. The main fatty acids of olive oil vary, depending on the origin: 55 to 83% oleic acid, 7.5 to 20% palmitic acid, 3.5 to 21% linolic acid and 0.5 to 3.5% stearic acid [12, Ü26].

- Secoiridoid glucosides (bitter): In unripe fruits particularly oleuropein (oleuropeoside, up to 2%), olacein (artifact: from the cleavage of oleuropein or demethyloleuropein, respectively), elenolic acid glucoside (oleoside-11-methyl ester), ligstroside (ligustroside, only in very young fruits), cornoside (from which the artifact halleridone develops) and in a few races demethyloleuropein. The content of elenolic acid- and demethyloleuropein glucoside increases during ripening while the content of oleuropein diminishes; in the ripe fruits oleuropein is practically absent [2, 7, 18, 25, 27, 31, 37].

Decomposition products of oleuropein, which arise during the processing of table olives, are elenolic acid glucoside and hydroxytyrosol as well as cleavage products of the oleuropein aglycone, such as dialdehydes, including olacein, among others [21].

- Monoterpene acid esters: 6-*O*-oleuropeylsaccharose [31, 37].

- Phenols: In the ripe fruits tyrosol (4-hydroxyphenylethanol, cleavage product of ligstroside), hydroxytyrosol (3,4-dihydroxyphenylethanol, dopanol, cleavage product of oleuropein), 3,4-dihydroxyphenylglycol, hydroxytyrosol glucoside), furthermore pyrocatechol [6, 33, 40], in the seeds salidroside, nuezhenide and nuezhenide oleoside [30].

- Phenolcarboxylic acids: Protocatechuic acid, vanillic acid [10].

- Phenylacrylic acids and their glucosides: *p*-Coumaric acid, caffeic acid, 1-*O*-caffeoyl glucose, verbascoside (orobanchin, in traces in the fruits), ferulic acid [3, 7, 10, 31].

- Flavonoids: Particularly quercetin and quercetin glycosides [3, 40, 42].

- Anthocyans: As pigments in the ripe fruit, mainly cyanidin-3-*O*-glycosides besides paeonidin-3-*O*-glycosides and their acyl derivatives, in addition to delphinidin-3-*O*-rhamnosylglucoside-7-*O*-xyloside [11, 40, Ü43].

- Mono- and oligosaccharides, alditols: In the fruit pulp, especially D-glucose, as well as D-fructose, saccharose and mannitol [Ü37].

- Fruit acids: Malic acid, citric acid and oxalic acid [Ü37].

- Estrogens: 0.35 mg/100 g estrone were detected in the seeds [1].

- Triterpenes: Mainly oleanolic acid (especially in the wax of the fruit wall), as well as squalene, in the green olives uvaol and erythrodiol (oleandiols), whose content diminishes during ripening. In the stored fruits also maslinic acid (crataegolic acid, 2α-hydroxy-oleanolic acid, possibly an artifact) [5].

- Wax components: In the wax of the fruit wall, triacylglycerols, as well as free fatty acids, triterpenes (see above) and long chained alkans, alkanols, alkyl esters and alkanals, among others [5].

Tests for Identity: Detection of oleuropein with TLC [Ü101] and of the flavonoids and other polyphenols with HPLC, HPLC/MS and HPLC/DAD [4, 36].

Quantitative assay: The fatty acids of the oil are determined with GC or HPLC [9, 38, 39]; the content of oleuropein and the flavonoids are analyzed with HPLC [20].

Adulterations, Misidentifications and Impurities: Not known.

Actions and Uses

Actions: Due to their aromatic, sour and slightly bitter taste, table olives are taken for appetite stimulant and digestive promoting effects.

In animal tests, oleuropein has shown antihypertonic action [32], probably on the basis of negatively inotropic and negatively chronotropic effects on the heart [17], antiarrhythmic [32], antidiabetic [23] and antihypercholesterolemic effects [13]. Olacein is a strongly active inhibitor of ACE (angiotensin converting enzyme) and therefore it also has antihypertonic activity [24]. Hydroxytyrosol has shown calcium antagonist activity [34]. Oleuropein and hydroxytyrosol inhibit blood platelet aggregation and improve flexibility of erythrocytes [16]. The combined effects of these substances with different mechanisms of action are probably jointly responsible for the antihypertonic and antiarteriosclerotic effect of the green organs of the olive [Ü38]. Furthermore, oleuropein and hydroxytyrosol have good antioxidative [41, 28], antimicrobial [8] and insecticidal action [26].

Toxicology: Based on existing data, there is no acute or chronic toxicity with the normal use of olives as a flavoring, snack or condiment. Sensitization to olives and

Oleuropein R$_1$= CH$_3$, R$_2$= OH
Demethyloleuropein R$_1$=H, R$_2$= OH
Ligstroside R$_1$=CH$_3$, R$_2$= H

Hydroxytyrosol

Elenolic acid glucoside

Olacein

Cornoside

Halleridone

olive oil only occurs rarely. The pollen of olive trees (wind pollination!) frequently leads to serious allergies (runny nose, conjunctivitis, bronchial asthma) [29]. Their allergens (proteins) have similar epitopes as birch-, mugwort-, pine- and cypress pollen [22].

Use as a spice, side dish or snack: Olives are used predominantly in the Mediterranean region as hors d'oeuvres, in salads, noodle sauces, pizzas, in strong meat-, poultry- and fish dishes, used as a side dish with eggplant fruits, tomatoes and paprika fruits or baked with Italian and Greek-Cypriot style breads.

Black or dark violet olives have a more intense taste than green olives and are better suited for seasoning cooked dishes. To improve the aroma of marinated olives it is recommended to drain them, rinse them off, add crushed garlic, dried oregano and crushed pepper corns, pour over a mixture of vinegar and olive oil, and allow to penetrate for a week before use. Olive oil, which is commercially available in numer-

ous different tasting varieties, is also used as a seasoning due to its characteristic taste [Ü2, Ü55].

Olives serve as decorative and spicy additions to pizzas, paellas, canapés (small pieces of roasted, piquant covered white bread), cold plates and salads (e.g. French Nicoise salads, Greek salads, Spanish style orange salads) [35, Ü55].

Pureed olives, mixed with olive oil, serve as a seasoning of meat stews, vegetable casseroles and tomato sauces. Olive puree, cold or warm, serves as a delicious pasta sauce [Ü55].

Tapénade, a Provencal dip sauce, is prepared from black, pitted olives, anchovy fillets, capers, garlic, and ground black pepper (→ Capers). Tapénade is suitable as an ingredient for toasts, cooked eggs, raw vegetables or pastas [Ü55].

Marinated olives can be pitted using an olive stoner and filled with anchovy butter [Ü55].

Olives are consumed as snacks with aperitif, e.g. speared on a cocktail stick, with croutons, ham- or cheese cubes [35].

Olive oil is used to enhance, among others, salad dressings, mayonnaises and baked potatoes [Ü2].

Combines well with: Capers, coriander, garlic, and thyme.

As a component of spice mixes and preparations: → Tartar sauce.

Other uses: The pulp or the comminuted whole olives are used for the manufacture of olive oil. For pharmaceutical use, only the oil that is cold-pressed or obtained by other mechanical means (for example by centrifuging a homogeneous mixture of the whole processed fruits [14, 15]) is official [Ph Eur].

Medicinal herb

Herbal drugs: Oleae fructus, Olive fruits, Oleae folium, Olive leaves [Ph Eur], Olivae oleum raffinatum, Refined olive oil [Ph Eur], Olivae oleum virginale, Native olive oil [Ph Eur].

Indications: In the folk medicine of the table olive-producing countries, olives are used for loss of appetite and digestive problems.
Extracts of the leaves are used for hypertension (dose: 20 to 30 g/d), among other conditions [Ü37]. Due to the insufficiently substantiated efficacy of this medication and the extremely low level of pharmacologically active constituents in table olives (decreasing with ripeness, decomposition with long treatment and fermentation) and due to the low quantity of fruits that are ingested, a pharmacological effect from the use of table olives can hardly be expected.

Similar fruits

Chinese olives, a collective term for fatty fruits of the *Canarium* genus, e.g. *Canarium pimela* K.D. KOENIG (Burseraceae), native to and grown in China and Vietnam. They are consumed fresh, cooked or salted, and the seeds are roasted [Ü61, Ü98].

Wild olive (Ceylon olive, elephant apple), a very vitamin C-rich, oil-containing fruit of the tree *Elaeocarpus floribundus* BLUME (Elaeocarpaceae), native in India (East Bengal) to Java, and grown in India (Bengal, Assam). The fruits, raw or cooked, are preserved in vinegar and taste similar to marinated olives [Ü61, Ü98].

Herb butter Provencal with olives
120 g soft butter, 1 to 2 tablespoons finely minced black olives, 1/2 to 1 teaspoon crushed herbes de Provence, lemon juice.

Stir the butter until foamy, mix with olives and herbs and season to taste with lemon juice.

Literature

[1] Amin E.S., A.R. Bassiouny, Phytochemistry 18:344 (1979).
[2] Amiot M.J. et al., Phytochemistry 28(1): 67–69 (1989).
[3] Amiot M.J. et al., J. Agric. Food Chem. 34:823–826 (1986).
[4] Baldi A. et al., Colloq. – Inst. Natl. Rech. Agron 69 (Polyphenol 94):269–270 (1995), ref. in CA 124:028268w.
[5] Bianchi G. et al., Phytochemistry 31: 3503–3506 (1992).
[6] Bianchi G., N. Pozzi, Phytochemistry 35(5):1335–1337 (1994).
[7] Bianco A. et al., Phytochemistry 32: 455–457 (1993).
[8] Bisignano G. et al., J. Pharm. Pharmacol. 51(8):971–974 (1999).
[9] Bizzozero N. et al., Ind. Aliment. (Pinerolo, Italy) 37(367):187–190 (1998), ref. CA 128:229594f.
[10] Brenes-Balbuena M. et al., J. Agric. Food Chem. 40:1192–1196 (1992).
[11] Camurati F. et al., Riv. Ital. Sost. Grasse 58:541–547 (1981).
[12] Conte L., O. Koprivnjak, Food Technol. Biotechnol. 35(1):75–81 (1997).
[13] DePasquale R. et al., Plant Méd. Phytothér. 25:134–140 (1991), ref. Ü37-
[14] Demicheli M.C. et al., Fresenius Environ. Bull. 6(5/6):240–247 (1997).
[15] Di Giovacchino L., Ol. Crops. Gras., Lipides 4(5):359–362 (1997), ref. CA 128: 114107g.
[16] Driss F. et al., Ol. Crops. Gras., Lipides 3(6):448–451 (1996), ref. CA 126: 211458n.
[17] Duarte J. et al., Planta Med. 59(4):318–322 (1993).
[18] Esti M., L. Cinquanta, E.L. Notte, J. Agric. Food Chem. 46(1):32–35 (1998).
[19] Fernandez A. et al., Biotechnology (2nd Ed.) 9:593–627 (1995).

[20] Ficarra P. et al., Farmaco 46(6):803–815 (1991).

[21] Gil M. et al., Phytochemistry 49(5): 1311–1315 (1998).

[22] Gonzales E.M. et al., Allergy 55(7): 658–663 (2000).

[23] Gonzales M. et al., Planta Med. 58: 513–515 (1992).

[24] Hansen K. et al., Phytomedicine 2: 319–325 (1996).

[25] Inouye H. et al., Tetrahedron 30:201–209 (1974).

[26] Kubo A. et al., J. Chem. Ecol. 11:251 (1985).

[27] Kubo J. et al., J. Agric. Food Chem. 32:687–688 (1984).

[28] Le Tutour B., D. Guedon, Phytochemistry 31:1173–1178 (1992).

[29] Liccardi G. et al., Int. Arch. Allergy Immunol. 111(3):210–217 (1996).

[30] Maestro-Duran R. et al., Grasas Aceite (Seville) 45(5):332–335 (1994), ref. CA 123:165064v.

[31] Panizzi L. et al., Gazz. Chim. Ital. 95: 1279–1292 (1965).

[32] Petkov V. et al., Arzneim. Forsch. 22:1476 (1972).

[33] Ragazzi E., G. Veronese, Ann. Chim. 57:1386–1397 (1967).

[34] Rauwald H.W. et al., Phytother. Res. 8:135–140 (1994).

[35] Ridgway J., Olivenöl, ein Handbuch für Genießer, Benedikt Taschen Verlag GmbH, Köln 1998.

[36] Romani A. et al., J. Agric. Food Chem. 47(3):964–967 (1999).

[37] Scarpati M.L., C. Trogolo, Tetrahedron Lett. 5673–5674 (1966).

[38] Stefanoudaki E. et al., Food Chem. 60(3): 425–432 (1997).

[39] Tava A., Ind. Aliment (Pinerolo, Italy) 37(366):28–32 (1998), ref. CA 128: 229610h.

[40] Vazquez Roncero A. et al., Grasas Aceites 25:269–279 (1974), zit. Ü37.

[41] Visioli F., C. Galli, Life Sci. 55:1965–1971 (1994).

[42] Vlahov G., J. Sci. Food Agric. 58:157–159 (1992).

Literature references identified by Ü can be found in the general listing of books and monographs at the back of this book.

Onion

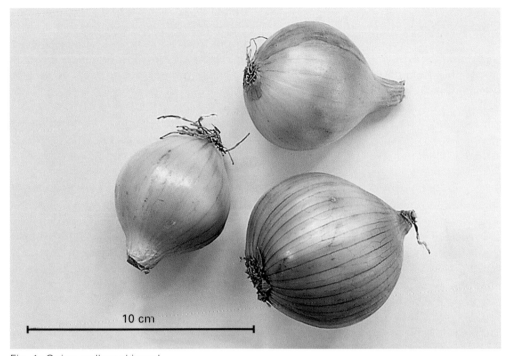

Fig. 1: Onion, yellow-skinned

Plant source: *Allium cepa* L. var. *cepa*.

Synonym: *Allium cepa* L.

Taxonomic classification: The species is subdivided into numerous varieties, of which a few are also considered to be separate species or hybrids. Of particular importance are:
Allium cepa L. var. *cepa,* onion, summer onion,
Allium cepa L. var. *ascalonicum* BACKER, → Shallot,
Allium cepa L. var. *cepiforme* REGEL (*A. fistulosum* L.) → Scallion,
Allium cepa L. var. *viviparum* (METZG.) ALEF. (Synonym: *A. cepa* L. var. *proliferum* (MOENCH) ALEF. ex WILLD., *A.* × *proliferum* (MOENCH) SCHRAD. ex WILLD.) → Triploid viviparous onion (see: → Scallion).

Family: Allium plants (Alliaceae; in older literature the genus Allium was placed in the lily family, Liliaceae).

Common names: Engl.: onion; Fr.: oignon, ciboule; Ger.: Speisezwiebel, Zwiebel, Sommer-Zwiebel, Küchen-Zwiebel, Bolle, Rams, Zipolle, Zipelln.

Description: Perennial plant, flowering after a cold spell only, 0.6 to 1.2 m tall. Shape and color of the bulb depend on cultivar and environmental conditions and are very variable. Offset bulbs are mostly absent. The basal unifacial leaves are tubiform or inflated, glabrous, shorter than the inflorescence axis, which is inflated below the middle. The inflorescence is a globose pseudoumbel; its coat is 2- to 4-valvate. The 6 perigone leaves are white or bright violet, the 6 stamina are taller than the

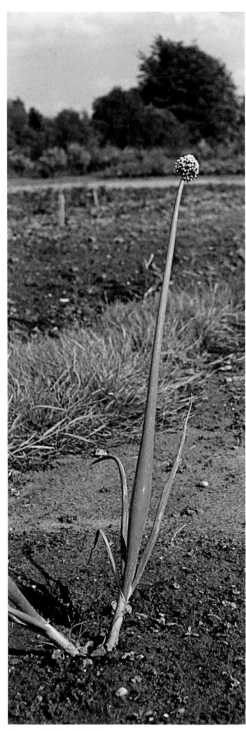

Fig. 2: Onion (*Allium cepa* L. var. *cepa*)

perigone. The ovary is three chambered. The fruit is a globose capsule with trigonous seeds. Flowering period is from June to August [Ü42, Ü85].

Native origin: Only known in cultivation, its domestication center of origin is probably Central Asia (Northwestern India, Afghanistan).

Main cultivation areas: Cultivated worldwide.

Main exporting countries: European producers include Spain, Italy, Cyprus, Austria, Poland, Hungary, the Netherlands, Germany (particularly in Rhineland-Palatinate, Hesse, Bavaria and Lower Saxony), and Bulgaria, furthermore Egypt, Asian countries, Mexico, Peru, Argentina, and the USA.

Cultivation: Onions prefer deep, loosened-up, humus soil in sunny locations. They must be irrigated well, however stagnant moisture is not tolerated. Propagation is carried out in March either by sowing, about 1 cm deep, with row spacing of 20 to 30 cm, later the seedlings are pricked off and spaced at 5 cm, or by planting seed bulbs, with row spacing of about 25 cm, about 10 cm distance from one another, nearly pressed against each other! To cover requirements in the spring and early summer, one sows or plants in August and then allows the plants to overwinter mounded up and covered. Salad onions must be planted in advance. They are planted already in February under glass (at about 15 °C), pricked out after about 8 to 9 weeks and planted in the outdoors in May.

There are over 300 known cultivars. Cultivated varieties include **yellow- to brown-skinned onions**, e.g. 'Ajax', 'Alamo', 'Clipper', 'Copra', 'Django', 'Elsa', 'Lagergold', 'Maraton', 'Stuttgarter Riesen' and 'Zittauer Gelbe', **red-skinned onions**, e.g. 'Braunschweiger dunkelrote', 'Piroska', 'Proska', 'Red Baron', 'Rijnsburger', 'Tango' and 'Zerti', **white-skinned onions**, e.g. 'Albion', **green-skinned onions**, e.g. 'Greenella', **overwintering onions**, e.g.

'Alix', 'Express Yellow' and 'Martina', **salad onions**, e.g. 'Ailsa Craig', 'The Kelsea' and 'Exhibition', **green onions**, e.g. 'Elody', 'Sperlings Toga (red)' as well as **white-skinned early onions**, 'Southport', 'White Globe' and 'Zur' [Ü15].

Culinary Herb

Commercial forms: Onions (pickling onions, transverse diameter 2 to 3 cm, household onions, transverse diameter 3 to 6 cm, and meat- or industrial onions, transverse diameter over 6 cm, yellow-, brown-, white-, red-violet or green-skinned), **salad onions** (very large, mildly-sweetish), **green onions** (bundled whole fresh plant with young, small, still green bulbs), **dried onions** (in pieces = kibbled onion, in rings, granules, flakes and powder), **roasted onions** (in pieces or in rings), **onion juice concentrate** (fresh onion and broiler onion flavor concentrate, liquid or dried onto a carrier, e.g. sodium chloride or glucose) and **onion oleoresin**.

Production: Fresh onion greens can be taken throughout the entire year. Onions sown in the spring can be harvested in August, and if seed bulbs are planted the harvest can take place already in July. With overwintering, the onion harvest is possible already by May. For the production of dry products, the roots and the outer onion skins are removed after a first drying phase, and then they are washed and cut into slices. Then they are dried in the tunnel dryer until they attain a residual

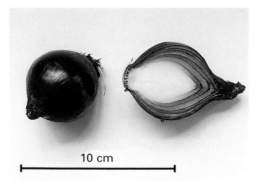

10 cm

Fig. 3: Onion, red-violet skinned

water content of 4% or they are freeze-dried. Processing causes considerable loss of aroma, which is minimized with freeze-drying. The aroma loss can be partially compensated for by the admixing of cysteine. Admixing of calcium- or magnesium stearate is supposed to prevent agglutination of powdered onion [Ü30, Ü93].

Forms used: Fresh onions, dried or roasted onions in slices, rings, granules, flakes or powder, onion greens (leaves of the onion).

Storage: Green onions are intended for immediate use. Onions suitable for storage should be stored in a cool and dry place, hung up on the dried leaves, or stored in nets or wide-meshed bags. They can be stored for about 6 months at a storage temperature of 1 to 2 °C and 2 to 3 months at room temperature. At temperatures above 4 °C, they germinate prematurely. Good varieties for storage include, among others, 'Copra', 'Piroska', 'Lagergold', 'Red Baron', 'Rijnsburger', 'Stuttgarter Riesen' and 'Zerti'. Dried products obtained from onions are hygroscopic and must be stored protected from moisture, in airtight glass or porcelain containers.

Description. Whole bulb (Figs. 1 and 3): Onions consist of 10 to 12 thick and fleshy, helically arranged, fused scale leaves, which are situated on top of a disciform axis (basal plate of bulb, remains of the reduced rhizome). The outer paper-thin scale leaves (tunic) are yellow, brown, white, red-violet or green. The shape is discoid-obloid and subglobular, flattened, globose, pyriform or bottle-shaped [Ü37].

Odor: Odorless if unbruised, after bruising pungent, causing tearing of the eyes, **Taste:** Sweet, aromatic, depending on the cultivar, from mild (salad onion) to pungent.

History: The onion was already taken into cultivation in Egypt and Asia Minor, more than 5000 years ago. The Romans introduced it to Central Europe. From there, it was brought to North America and Australia [30, Ü92].

Constituents and Analysis

DIN- and ISO-Standards: ISO-Standard 5559 (Dried onions, specification).

Constituents

- Alliins (*S*-alk(en)ylcysteine sulfoxides) in the unbruised plant, particularly *trans*-(+)-*S*-(prop-1-enyl)-L-cysteine sulfoxide, isoalliin, about 0.2%, furthermore (+)-*S*-methyl-L-cysteine sulfoxide and (+)-*S*-propyl-L-cysteine sulfoxide [Ü83].

- Alliaceous oils: Upon tissue injury, the non-volatile alliins come into contact with the enzyme alliinase and are transformed to the volatile alk(en)ylsulfenic acids, which spontaneously convert to the alliaceous smelling, odor determining reaction products, the alk(en)yl-alkane/alkenethiosulfinates (Fig. 10, → General section). (*Z*)-thiopropanal-*S*-oxide (volatile, lachrymatory principle of the onion) is however also formed from prop-1-enyl-sulfenic acid through rearrangement [14].
  The thiosulfinates transform, especially upon heating, into the dialk(ene)yl-di- and trisulfides, the cepaenes 1 and 2 and to cycloalliin. Relevant aroma- and flavor components of cooked or sautéed onions are the monoalk(en)ylhydrosulfides (e.g. prop-1-enylthiol, sweet tasting), dialk(en)ylsulfides, dialk(en)yldisulfides and dialk(en)yltrisulfides, particularly diprop-1-enyl-di- and trisulfides, dipropyldi- and trisulfide, propyl-prop-1-enyl-sulfide, in addition to 3,5-diethyl-1,2,4-trithional, 5,6-dihydro-2,4,6-triethyl-4*H*-1,3,5-dithiazine, methyl-prop-1-enyl-trisulfide, in sautéed onions, as sugar breakdown products, there are furan derivatives present (with sweet taste) [7–9, 22–25, 48, 62, 65, 66, 68, Ü83].
  Also detected, besides thiopropanal-*S*-oxide were, among others, (*E,Z*)-prop-1-enyl-propane-thiosulfinate (10 to 33%), (*E*)-methyl-prop-1-enethiosulfinate (14 to 26%), propyl-propanethiosulfinate (5 to 14%), (*E*)-propyl-prop-1-enethiosulfinate (10 to 12%) and *cis*- or *trans*-zwiebelane (14 to 20% or 6 to 8%, respectively) [10].

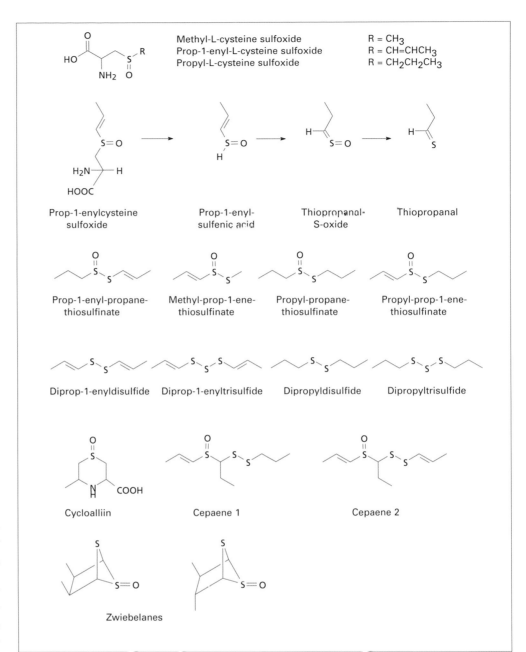

Methyl-L-cysteine sulfoxide R = CH₃
Prop-1-enyl-L-cysteine sulfoxide R = CH=CHCH₃
Propyl-L-cysteine sulfoxide R = CH₂CH₂CH₃

Prop-1-enylcysteine sulfoxide → Prop-1-enyl-sulfenic acid → Thiopropanal-S-oxide → Thiopropanal

Prop-1-enyl-propane-thiosulfinate   Methyl-prop-1-ene-thiosulfinate   Propyl-propane-thiosulfinate   Propyl-prop-1-ene-thiosulfinate

Diprop-1-enyldisulfide   Diprop-1-enyltrisulfide   Dipropyldisulfide   Dipropyltrisulfide

Cycloalliin   Cepaene 1   Cepaene 2

Zwiebelanes

- γ-Glutamyl peptides of the alliins, particularly, γ-glutamyl-*trans*-S-(prop-1-enyl)-L-(+)-cysteine sulfoxide (about 0.2%), which, upon tissue injury, catalyzed by peptidase, can be cleaved into the alliins and glutamic acid. The alliins are further converted to the alliaceous oils (see above). Also present are γ-glutamyl peptides of sulfur-free and sulfur-containing amino acids. In the latter, sulfur is partially replaced by selenium [59, 68].

- Flavonoids: Quercetin glycosides, particularly quercetin-3,4′-diglucoside (about 50 to 1300 mg/kg) and quercetin-4′-β-D-glucoside (spiraeoside, 36 to 394 mg/kg), furthermore, among others, quercetin-7,4′-diglucoside, isorhamnetin-4′-glucoside and rutin, in the outer dry skins 2.5 to 6.5% quercetin-glycosides, in the red-skinned varieties also, quercetin-3,7,4′-triglucoside and cyanidin glycosides, e.g., cyanidin-3-(6″-malonyl-3″glucosylglucoside), among others [26, 27, 32, 53–56].

- Phenolcarboxylic acids: Particularly protocatechuic acid (1 to 2% in the outer skins of the yellow variety) [56].
- Steroid saponins: About 0.04%, alliospirosides A to D, ceposides A to F [overview in Lit. 41].
- Sterols: Cholesterol, cycloartenol, lophenol, β-sitosterol, among others [33].
- Cyclopentane derivatives: 5-Octyl-cyclo-penta-1,3-dione and 5-hexyl-cyclo-penta-1,3-dione, also known as tsibulins, they are phytoalexins, only formed in onions which have been infected with fungi [63].
- Polysaccharides: Fructosanes (about 10 to 40%), monosaccharides (10 to 15%), saccharose (5 to 8%) and other oligosaccharides; total carbohydrate content about 9% (fresh weight) [58, 60].

The occurrence of diphenylamine is questionable (insecticide residue).

Depending on the cultivar, the total dry weight of the onion is 8 to 21% [60, Ü82].

Tests for Identity: With TLC [Ü102], analysis of the thiosulfinates with GC-MS [10] or HPLC [45], and of the alliaceous oils with TLC [6], of the flavonoids with HPLC or TLC [17, 26, 52].

Quantitative assay: Analysis of the thiosulfinates with HPLC [45], GC/MS [10] or by immobilized alliinase [43], of the flavonoids with HPLC [17, 36].

Adulterations, Misidentifications and Impurities: Since the onion is cultivated, misidentification can be usually avoided. The literature describes poisonings with narcissus bulbs and bulbs of other amaryllis plants [Ü100]. These bulbs are easily distinguished from onions due to absence of the alliaceous aroma.

Actions and Uses

Actions: Due to the pungent taste of raw onions as well as the irritant effect of the alliaceous oils on the gastric mucosa and the aromatic odor and taste of cooked or fried onions, they are appetizing and digestion promoting.

Other actions of onions are similar to those of → Garlic. The strength of action may be somewhat less than that of garlic. The effects can be explained in part by the antioxidative actions of the alliaceous oils.

Antiatherosclerotic action: Raw onions have antiatherosclerotic action through thrombocyte aggregation inhibition, fibrinolytic, antioxidative as well as blood lipid level and blood pressure lowering activity and prevent infarction. The degree of inhibition of thrombocyte aggregation increased with the content of sulfurous constituents. An inhibition of the formation of thromboxanes, which promote thrombocyte aggregation, could be demonstrated in rats with onion extract or thiosulfinates. Heating the extract diminished the effect [4, 11, 21, 29]. Administration of onion alliaceous oils increased fibrinolytic activity (measured by euglobulin lysis time) in humans. The same effect was attainable with cycloalliin (250 mg/d) [2, 49]. In animal experiments (rabbits), onions lowered the blood lipid level despite the animals being fed a lipid diet and averted the occurrence of arterial lesions [64]. After meals with fried onions, onion flavonoids were detected in the blood plasma of healthy subjects. The occurrence of these flavonoids in the blood were combined with a decrease in the occurrence of indicators for oxidative stress including, among others, reduced urinary excretion of 2-hydroxy-2´-desoxyguanosine (indicator fur oxidative attacks on the DNA) and an increased resistance of lymphocyte DNA strand breakage [12].

Antiasthmatic action: A strong diminution of allergen-induced broncho-constriction in humans with the administration of an ethanolic onion extract (corresponding to 2 × 200 g fresh onions) could be demonstrated and therefore an antasthmatic action [20, Ü103]. This effect probably takes place by inhibition of cyclooxygenase and 5-lipoxygenase, which has been shown in vitro with thiosulfinates and cepaenes [67].

Antihyperglycemic action: Onions have a blood sugar lowering effect in healthy and diabetic individuals. In diabetic rats, hypoglycemic activity and an increase of serum-insulin-level were also attained with high doses of S-methyl-L-cysteine sulfoxide (or S-allyl-L-cysteine sulfoxide, 200 or 250 mg/kg body weight) [13, 34, 35, 39, 44, 57].

Antitumor action: Epidemiological studies have shown that the risk of getting gastric- or esophageal- cancer is reduced by eating onions (same as for garlic, scallion, and Chinese chives) [18, 28]. As numerous studies prove, the ingestion of onions, similar to that of garlic, also acts against numerous other forms of tumors (see: → Garlic). In in-vitro studies it could be shown that extracts of onions (as well as extracts of a few other vegetables) were able to detoxify cancerogenic nitrosamines and counteract their cytotoxic activity [46]. In the AMES-test, extracts of onions antagonized the mutagenic effect of 4-nitroquinoline-N-oxide and 2-aminofluorene [50].

Antimicrobial action: Pressed juice and extracts of fresh onions have antimicrobial action. Heating these preparations destroys the antibiotic activity. Onion oil obtained by steam distillation also has antimicrobial action. It is active against pathogenic oral bacteria including, among others, *Streptococcus mutans* and *S. sobrinus* [1, 15, 18, 38, 51, 69, 71].

Other activities: In mice, aqueous extracts of onion are androgenic (increase of sperm count, weight gain in the testicles and epididymis) [3]. In the Carrageenan rat paw edema test, onion extracts have shown an antiphlogistic effect [47]. Peroral administration of onion extracts in rabbits has immunosuppressive action [16].

Toxicology: Based on existing data, there is no chronic or acute toxicity in healthy individuals with the normal use of onions. In animal tests, p.o.- or i.p. application of onion extracts (50 mg/kg body weight) did not lead to liver and lung damage [61].

Especially in sensitive individuals, large doses of raw onions can cause stomach complaints, heartburn, colic and diarrhea due to the irritant effects of the alliaceous oils on the gastric mucosa [39]. Patients suffering from gastric and duodenal ulcers should therefore not eat raw onions [40]. Cooked or sautéed onions often cause flatulence and meteorism. The lachrymatory action of thiopropanal-S-oxides is possibly caused by its breakdown to propion aldehyde and sulfuric acid, in presence of water [Ü30].

The sensitization potential for onions is low. However, with frequent contact, hand eczema occurs, as well as allergic asthma with contact with onion dust [5, 15, 37 Ü39].

Culinary use: Large amounts of onions are used particularly in English, German, French, Italian, Arabian, Hungarian and Spanish cooking. Important onion dishes include, among others, the French onion soup, Indian 'doh peaazah' and numerous Venetian dishes.

In order to avoid irritation of the eyes, the onions should be peeled under cold, running water and also sliced under water. Very small onions, e.g. pearl onions, are immersed in boiling water for 10 to 15 seconds in order to make peeling easier. After removing the parchment-like skins, the onions can be cut into slices, which can be pulled apart into rings, chopped or grated. Cut onions are often briefly roasted before use. Chopped onion can only be stored for a short time in the refrigerator wrapped in aluminum foil. They turn stale rapidly. For soup pots, whole small onions with their brown skins can be used in order to give the dish a brown appearance. Smoked onions with clove are used as a seasoning of stews and broths. Onions are added already at the start of cooking time.

Cooked or fried with the dishes, onions are suitable as an integral seasoning for almost all salty foods including, among others, as a seasoning for broths, sauces, marinades,

soups, rich stews, pizzas, fried hamburger meat, liver, meat-, fish- and vegetable dishes, mushrooms, fried potatoes and egg dishes. Onions are also used to season or supplement bakery goods, e.g. onion bread or onion cake (see below) [Ü2, Ü55, Ü95].

Sliced onions, with finely chopped mushrooms or herbs quickly fried, are a good side dish for grilled or fried steaks. Steamed with herbs in wine, they do justice to braised meat [Ü55].

Mild varieties of onions (e.g. salad onions) and green onions are used raw, cut into slices or cubed, and used for flavoring of salads, e.g. of tomato salad or green salad, of hamburger meat and quark. Due to their sumptuous color, red onions are preferred in those dishes. The color dissipates during cooking [Ü2].

Pickling onions, used in whole form, can be preserved frozen or in vinegar. They also serve as an accompaniment of sour preserves, e.g. mixed pickles and cucumbers. They can also, however, be added to stews and braised meat dishes.

Meat- or industrial-onions are used as a sausage seasoning, among other uses, e.g. for seasoning of onion liverwurst and lard. Onions are also consumed as a vegetable, cooked or baked as a single dish and with white sauces or cheese sauces [Ü2].

Onion greens are used in the same way as → Chives.

Combines well with all other spices.

As a component of spice mixes and preparations: → A.1 sauce, → Bologna spice mix, → Bomboe, → Bread spice, → Café de Paris spice mixture, → Cajun spice, → Chili powder, → Chilli sauce, → Fish spice, → Hamburger meat spice, → Herb salt, → Ketchup, → Masala, → Meat spice, → Pickling spice, → Poultry spice, → Quark spice, → Salsa, → Sambal, → Sauce spice, → Tai-ping China, → Tartar sauce, → Tomato ketchup, → Vegetable spice.

Other uses: The outer skins of the onion were formerly used as a colorant for wool or silk, and today they are sometimes still used for the coloring Easter eggs yellow.

Medicinal herb

Herbal drug: Allii cepae bulbus

Indications: For loss of appetite and for prevention of age-related vascular changes (average daily dose 50 g fresh, 20 g dried onions, in the form of cut onions, pressed juice or other preparations) [42].

In folk medicine, onions are used in the form of sweetened decoctions or in the form of syrups for coughs and bronchitis, fresh onions or fresh pressed juice of onions for asthma, to simulate biliary function, to bring on menstruation, as a vermifuge in cases of roundworm and for diarrhea. Fresh onions are used externally for treatment of insect bites, mild burns, wound and effusion of blood, among other uses [Ü37].

Similar bulbous species

Pearl onion: A collective term used for small, round, skinned offset bulbs (up to 15 mm diameter) of various Allium-species: → Shallot, → Serpent garlic (see: → Garlic), → Mild chives (see: → Chives). They are used mainly as an addition to pickled aseptic preserves, e.g. mixed pickles, or in marinated form as a garnish of meat- and fish dishes as well as of delicatessen salads and glazed as a vegetable side dish. It is also well suited as a flavoring of soups and stews. In French cooking it is a component of Boeuf à la bourguinonne and Coq au vin [Ü2, Ü98].

Silver skin onion: (Also described as → Pearl onion): small, round offset bulbs of → *Allium porrum* var. *sectivum* F.H.H. LUEDER, among others. The term is not unequivocally defined. Other small varieties of onions which are planted densely together, e.g. → Onions, forming small bulbs, are often described as silver skin onion.

Ansur-onion: *Allium stipitatum* REGEL (native to Afghanistan, Pakistan, and Central Asian Republics of the Russian Federation, where it is also cultivated), usually a collective term for these species, *Allium giganteum* REGEL (Himalayas, Central Asia) and *A. suvorovii* REGEL (Russian Federation), wild collected, used in the same way as onion, usually marinated [Ü98].

Allium cernuum Roth., native to North America, used in the same way as onions [Ü61].

Allium grayi REGEL, native to Japan, occurs escaped from cultivation in China, the main components are probably *S*-propyl-L-cysteine disulfide and *S*-methyl-L-cysteine sulfoxide, as breakdown products in the liquid fraction, dipropyldisulfide has been found [31]; these types of onions are used in the same way as regular onions, especially for salads [Ü61].

Onion cake

Dough: 200 g flour, 10 g yeast, 4 tablespoons of oil, 1 egg yolk, salt. Topping: 750 g onions, 40 g butter, 4 eggs, 1 tablespoon quark, 1 teaspoon salt, 1 teaspoon caraway.

Prepare soft dough from flour, yeast, oil, egg yolk, salt and warm water (about 3 tablespoons) and let the dough rest in the oven at 50 °C for 30 minutes. Spread the dough on a round, greased baking tin (diameter about 26 cm, with rim). Peel the onions and finely dice, then sauté in butter for 10 minutes while stirring until light brown. Egg, quark, caraway and salt are mixed, added to the onions and placed evenly on the dough. The onion cake is placed in the oven at 200 °C and baked for 40 minutes. Serve hot [Ü56].

Literature

[1] Abdou L. et al., Qual. Plant. Mater. Veg. 22:29–35 (1972).

[2] Agarwal R.H., Atherosclerosis 27: 347–351 (1977).

[3] Al-Bekairi A.M. et al., Fitoterapia 62: 117–125 (1991).

[4] Ali M. et al., Prostaglandins Leukot. Ess. Fatty Acids 60(1):43–4 (1999).

[5] Anibarro B. et al., J. Allergy Clin. Immunol. 100(6 Pt):734–738 (1997).

[6] Bandyopadhyay C. et al., J. Chromatogr. 47:400 (1970).

[7] Bayer T. et al., J. Am. Chem. Soc. 111: 3085 (1989), zit. bei S. Ferary, J. Auger (s.u.).

[8] Bayer Th et al., Phytochemistry 28: 2373–2377 (1989).

[9] Block E. et al., J. Am. Chem. Soc. 101:2200 (1979), zit. bei S. Ferary, J. Auger (s.u.).

[10] Block E. et al., J. Agric. Food Chem. 40:2431–2438 (1992).

[11] Bordia T. et al., Prostglandins Leukotrienes Fatty Acids 54(3):183–186 (1996).

[12] Boyle S.P. et al., Eur. J. Nutr. 39(5):213–223 (2000).

[13] Brahmachari H.D., K.T. Augusti, J. Pharm. Pharmacol. 13:128 (1962).

[14] Brodnitz M.H., J.V. Pascale, J. Agr. Food Chem. 19:269 (1971).

[15] Bruynzeel D.P., Contact Dermatitis 37(2): 70–77 (1997).

[16] Chisty M.M. et al., Bangladesh Med. Res. Counc Bull. 22(2):81–85 (1996).

[17] Crozier A. et al., J. Chromatogr, A. 761(1+2):315–321 (1997).

[18] Dankert J. et al., Zentralbl. Bakteriol. (Orig. A) 245(1/2):229–239 (1979).

[19] Dorant E. et al., Gastroenterology 110(1): 12–20 (1996).

[20] Dorsch W. et al., Allergologie 8:316–323 (1987).

[21] Dorsch W. et al., Allergologie 9:388–396 (1989).

[22] Ettala T., A.I. Virtanen, Acta Chem. Scand. 16:2061 (1962).

[23] Farkas P. et al., Z. Lebensm. Unters. Forsch. 195:459–462 (1992).

[24] Fenwick G.R. et al., CRC Crit. Rev. Food Sci. Nutr. 22:199–377 (1985).

[25] Ferary S., J. Auger, J. Chromatogr. A. 750(1/2), 4th Intern. Symp. on Hyphenated Techniques in Chromatography and Hyphenated Chromtographic Analyzers, 1996): 63–74 (1996), ref. CA: 126: 059106n.

[26] Fossen T. et al., Phytochemistry 47(2): 281–285 (1998).

[27] Fossen T. et al., J. Food Sci. 61(4):703–706 (1996).

[28] Gao C.M. et al., Jpn. J. Cancer Res. 90(6): 614–621 (1999).

[29] Goldman I.L. et al., Thromb. Haemostasis 76(3):450–452 (1996).

[30] Hanelt P., Drogenreport 7(11):17–25 (1994).

[31] Hashimoto S. et al., J. Sci. Food Agric. 35:353 (1984), ref. in Ü43.

[32] Herrmann K., Qual. Plant.-Plant Foods Hum. Nutr. 25:231 (1976), zit. Ü37.

[33] Itoh T. et al., Phytochemistry 16:140 (1977), ref. in Ü43.

[34] Jain R.C., K.N. Sachdev, Curr. Med. Pract. 15:901–902 (1971).

[35] Janot M.M., J. Laurin, Compt. Rend. Hebd. Acad. Sci. 191:1098–1100 (1930).

[36] Justesen U. et al., J. Chromatogr. A., 799(1/2):101–110 (1998).

[37] Kawane H., J. Allergy Clin. Immunol. 96(4):568 (1995).

[38] Kim J.H., J. Nihon Univ. Sch. Dent. 39(3): 136–141 (1997).

[39] Koch H.P., Z. Phytother. 13(6):177–188 (1992).

[40] Koch H.P., Dtsch. Apoth. Ztg. 132(27): 1419–1428 (1992).

[41] Koch H.P., Dtsch. Apoth. Ztg. 133(41): 3733–3743 (1993).

[42] Kommission E beim BGA., BAnz-Nr. 50 vom 13.03.86 (1986).

[43] Krest I. et al., Pharm. Pharmocol Lett. 7(4):145–147 (1997).

[44] Kumari K., K.T. Augusti, Planta Med. 61(1):72–74 (1995).

[45] Mandon N. et al., Biomed. Chromatogr. 14(1):53–55 (2000).

[46] Martinez A. et al., J. Agric. Food Chem. 46(2):585–589 (1998).

[47] Mascolo N. et al., Phytother. Res. 1:28–31 (1987).

[48] Matikakla E.J., A. Virtanen, Acta Chem. Scand. 21:2891 (1967).

[49] Menon I.S. et al., Brit. Med. J. 3:351 (1968).

[50] Noriega-Ponce, P. et al., Cienc. Cult. (Sao Paulo) 48(5/6):364–366 (1996), ref. CA 126:130744b.

[51] Ohta T., K. Takatori, Bokin Bobai 24(9): 587–591 (1996), ref. CA 125:216778g.

[52] Park Y.K., C.Y. Lee, Colloq. Inst. Natl. Rech. Agron. 69(Polyphenols 94): 265–266 (1995), ref. CA 123:283885m.

[53] Park Y.K., Ch.Y. Lee, J. Agric. Food Chem. 44(1):34–36 (1996).

[54] Perkin A.G., J.J. Hummel, J. Chem. Soc. 69:1295 (1986), zit. Ü37.

[55] Price K.R., M.J.C. Rhodes, J. Sci. Food Agric. 74(3):331–339 (1997).

[56] Schmidtlein H., K. Herrmann, Z. Lebensm. Unters. Forsch. 159:257 (1975).

[57] Sheela C.G. et al., Planta Med. 61(4): 356–357 (1995).

[58] Shiomi N. et al., New Phytol. 136(1): 105–113 (1997).

[59] Shrift A., Ann. Rev. Plant Physiol. 20:475 (1969).

[60] Stahl B. et al., Anal. Biochem. 246(2): 195–204 (1997).

[61] Thomson M. et al., J. Ethnopharmacol. 61(2):91–99 (1998).

[62] Tokitomo Y, Nippon Shokuhin Kagaku Kogaku Kaishi 42(4):279–287 (1995), ref. CA 123:008281w.

[63] Tverskoy L. et al., Phytochemistry 30: 799–800 (1991).

[64] Vatsala T.M., M. Singh, Artery 7(6):519 (1980).

[65] Velisek J. et al., Spec. Publ. R. Soc. Chem. 197(Flavour Science):258–261 (1996), ref. CA: 126:237607m.

[66] Virtanen A.I., Angew. Chem. Int. Ed. Eng. 1:299, zit. bei S. Ferary, J. Auger (s.o.) (1962).

[67] Wagner H. et al., Prostaglandins, Leukotrienes and Essential Fatty Acids 39:59–62 (1990).

[68] Whitaker J., Adv. Food Res. 22:73–133 (1976).

[69] Yin M.C., W.S. Cheng, J. Food Prot. 61(1):123–125 (1998).

[70] Yin M.C., S.M. Tsao, Int. J. Food Microbiol. 49(1/2):49–56 (1999).

[71] Zohri AN et al., Microbiol. Res. 150(2): 167–172 (1995).

Literature references identified by Ü can be found in the general listing of books and monographs at the back of this book.

Oregano

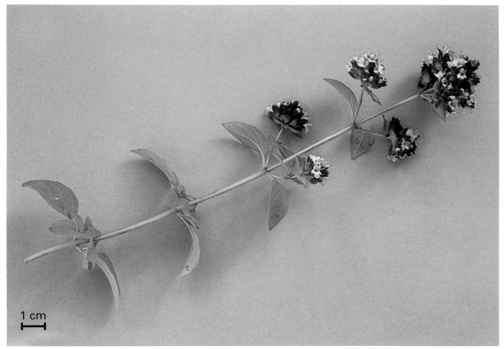

Fig. 1: Oregano, shoot tip

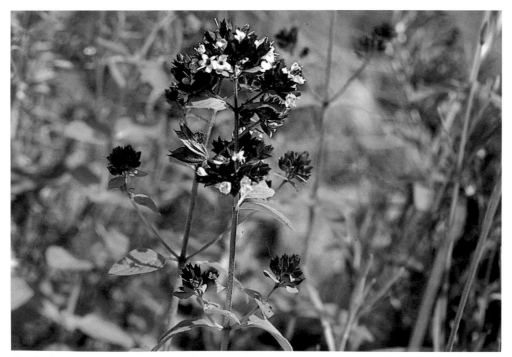

Fig. 2: Oregano (*Origanum vulgare* L. ssp. *vulgare*)

Plant sources: Oregano originates mostly from *Origanum vulgare* L. ssp. *vulgare*, but under the common name "Oregano", in a broad sense, a range of other culinary herbs with an oregano-like aroma from plant sources of several families and genera are also referred (see below).

Taxonomic classification: *O. vulgare* L. is usually subdivided into 6 subspecies, among others, *O. v.* L. ssp. *hirtum* (LINK) IETSWAART, *O. v.* L. ssp. *gracile* (KOCH) IETSWAART, *O. v.* L. ssp. *virens* (HOFF-MANGG. et LINK) IETSWAART and *O. v.* L. ssp. *viridulum* (MARTIN-DONOS) NYMAN. In literature references that do not provide the subspecies name, usually it is understood to be *O. v.* L. ssp. *vulgare*.

Family: Plants of the mint family (Lamiaceae, synonym Labiatae).

Common names: Engl.: oregano, wild marjoram, organy; Fr.: marjolaine sauvage, origan vulgaire; Ger.: Echter Dost, Gemeiner Dost, Dorant, Wilder Majoran, Griechischer Majoran, Badkraut, Berghopfen, Spanischer Hopfen, Orangenkraut, Oregano, Origano.

Description: Perennial stoloniferous herb, up to 50 cm (sometimes 1.2 m) tall, erect, quadrangular stem, branched, often reddish pruinose, with soft, velvety or bristly hairs, rarely glabrous. Leaves ovate, short petioled, up to 5 cm long and 2.5 cm wide, entire margined or indistinctly serrate, glabrous or pubescent, with glandular punctuations on the lower surface. The flowers are arranged in false whorls with 4 to 5 mm long bracts, elliptic, often with dark red coloration; the corolla is red-violet, pale-pink, rarely white, 4 to 7 mm long and the 4 stamina are white, calyx with 5 teeth, superior ovary, diphyllous, divided into 4 chambers, which, in the ripe fruit, separate into 4 brown, 1 mm long locules, containing one seed each. Flowering period is from July to September [30, Ü37].

Native origin: Europe, temperate Asia, and introduced into North America.

Main cultivation areas: Especially France, Greece, Spain, Italy, Mexico, and the USA. It is also wild collected.

Main exporting countries: Countries of Central- and Southern Europe, especially Turkey, Scandinavia, Asia, North America, Russian Federation, Scotland, Mexico, and Chile.

Cultivation: Oregano prefers dry, humus, permeable soil in warm, sunny locations protected from wind. Propagation takes place through direct seeding from the end of April, plants spaced 50 × 50 cm. It is possible to start advance planting indoors in February or plant root divisions in the spring. Commercially available seeds are usually a mixture of forms of different aromatic qualities. For personal use, it is recommended to plant 2 to 3 plants in a rock garden or in a spice bed. The wild plants found in Central Europe have little aromatic quality [Ü21].

Culinary herb

Commercial forms: Oregano: dried herb freed from the thicker parts of the stems, rubbed herb, essential oil of oregano, oregano oleoresin.

Production: In the 1st year the crop can be cut at the start of the flowering period in July. In the 2nd year, two cuts are possible, July and September, and the crop is productive for 3 to 5 years. For personal use, the leaves and the young shoot tips can be plucked from spring to autumn [Ü21].

Forms used: The fresh leaves, the dried and rubbed herb, and milled herb.

Storage: The fresh leaves or the fresh herb can be stored in plastic bags in the refrigerator for a few days, or frozen with little water in the deep freezer. The best way to extend shelf life, however, is by drying the herb and storing it in airtight glass-, porcelain- or suitable metal containers, protected from light, heat and moisture. In this way, oregano can be stored for several years without significant loss of aroma.

Description. Whole herb (Fig. 1): Consisting of leaves and fragments of the inflorescences with flowers and often stem pieces, see description of the whole plant.

Powdered herb: The powdered herb has characteristic 3- to 8-celled, straight and acuminate, thick-walled, articulate trichomes with distinctly granular cuticula as well as bicellular trichomes particularly at the margins of the fragments of bracts and calyx, with the top cell broken off. Also typical are the 8-celled lamiaceous, scale-like trichomes and the spherical pollen grains, about 30 μm in diameter, with an exine with 6 slit-like pores [EB 6].

Odor: Pleasantly aromatic, **Taste:** Spicy and aromatic, slightly bitter and peppery, weakly astringent.

History: Oregano is an ancient spice plant. It was already used during antiquity and was frequently described in medieval herbal literature [Ü92].

Constituents and Analysis

DIN- and ISO-Standards: ISO-Standard 7925 (Oregano).

Constituents

- Essential oil: 0.3 to 1.5% (up to 4%); the main components depend on the chemotype and time of harvest. Most often, carvacrol is the principle constituent (40 to 70%), besides γ-terpinene (8 to 10%), p-cymene (5 to 10%) as well as α-pinene, myrcene and thymol, among others. There are other chemotypes with mostly thymol (60 to 80%), thymol (about 32%) + carvacrol (about 17%) + p-cymene (about 12%) + γ-terpinene (about 10%), thymol (about 32%) + trans-β-ocimene (about 23%) + p-cymene (about 10%) + carvacrol (about 9%), β-phellandrene (about 22%) + β-caryophyllene (about 10%) + elemene (about 6%) + trans-β-ocimene (about 5%), linalool (about 24%) + myrcene (about 18%) + β-caryophyllene (about 9%) + germacrene D (about 7%) + terpinenol-4 (about 4%), linalool (about 37%) + β-caryophyllene (about 9%) + carvacrol (about 7%), germacrene D (about 34%) or linalool + terpinenol-4 [1, 4, 5, 7, 15, 19, 20, 29]. In a chemical race from the Himalayans, the main components detected were γ-muurolene, in addition to elemol (about 6%) and δ-cadinene (about 5%) [22]. Headspace analysis led to the identification of the heat sensitive cis-sabinene hydrate (2 to 44%, within the headspace), which, during steam distillation, converts to terpinenol-4, α-terpinene, γ-terpinene and limonene, among others; this component contributes significantly to the aroma [31].
  The main components in samples from the subspecies O. v. L. ssp. *hirtum* were found to be carvacrol (up to 70%), thymol or p-cymene; the main components in the subspecies O. v. L. ssp. *gracile* are β-caryophyllene (about 18%) + germacrene D (about 13%); the main components in the subspecies O. v. L. ssp. *viride* are terpinenol-4 (about 17%) + germacrene D (about 16%); and in the subspecies O. v. L. ssp. *viridulum* thymol (about 69%) + carvacrol (about 10%) [5, 15, 25].
- Flavonoids: Particularly glycosides of luteolin, apigenin and naringenin [2, 32].
- Hydroxycinnamic acid derivatives (labiate tannins): About 7%, with 5% rosmarinic acid, among others [12, 17, 18].

Tests for Identity: According to organoleptic, macroscopic and microscopic analyses as well as TLC and GC assays of the extract or essential oil [4, 9, 14, 20, 21].

Quantitative assay: The content of rosmarinic acid can be determined with HPLC [11] or after silylation with GC [23].

Adulterations, Misidentifications and Impurities: Admixtures and substitutions with other Mediterranean oregano species are possible.

Actions and Uses

Actions: On the basis of its aromatic and bitter taste, it has an appetite stimulating and digestion promoting activity. Oregano and its essential oil have shown a good antimicrobial effect [3, 4, 8, 10, 13, 24].

Toxicology: Based on existing data, there is no acute or chronic toxicity with the regular use of oregano as a spice. Sensitization to this herb is rare, but possible [6].

Culinary use: Oregano is not only a favorite spice in Italian cooking, but also in Greek, Spanish, French, South American and more recently in North American cooking. Before the 1950's, oregano was almost completely unknown in Germany. It arrived in Central Europe with the Italian restaurants and pizza. Due to its strong aroma, oregano should be used sparingly and due to the volatility of its aromatic components it should be added at just about 10 minutes before the meal is finished cooking. Before using dried oregano, it should be soaked in a little oil or alcohol in order to improve its aromatic quality.
Fresh oregano leaves are used especially in mixed salads, marinades, dressings and dips (e.g. avocado dip).
Fresh or dried oregano, similar to the herb of *O. heracleoticum* and *O. onites* (see: Marjoram) is used mainly as a pizza spice. It is exquisitely suited as an aromatic component for dishes made with tomatoes (e.g. sugo), paprika spice, eggplant (e.g. moussaka) or zucchini, cheese, beans, mushrooms (e.g. agarics), pilaf, risotto, noodle dishes, fried potatoes, sauces (e.g. Bologna sauce), grill marinades, soups, stew pots, meat dishes (roasted, especially roast lamb, grill meat, rissole), ground meat, fish dishes (grilled or roasted scampi, mussels, cuttlefish soup) and egg dishes (e.g. omelets) [Ü13, Ü17, Ü30, Ü56, Ü93, Ü108]. In Sweden, oregano is strewn over the traditional Thursday pea soup [Ü97]. In Italy, it is also used as a baking spice for small cookies [Ü81]. In Russia, oregano is used for making kvass or homemade beer [Ü81].

Combines well with: Basil, garlic, olives, rosemary, and thyme (but not with marjoram).

As a component of spice mixes and preparations: → Chili con carne spice, → Chili powder, → Herbes de Provence, → Pizza spice, → Tofu spice.

Other uses: The use of oregano extract as a brown colorant for textiles is being considered [28]. The essential oil of oregano is used in the perfume industry.

Medicinal herb

Herbal drug: Origani herba, Oregano, dried leaves and flowers separated from the stems of *Origanum vulgare* L. ssp. *hirtum* (LINK) IETSWAART, or *Origanum onites* L., or a mixture of both species. The essential oil content is minimum 0.25% with minimum 1.5% of carvacrol and thymol combined [Ph Eur].

Indications: In folk medicine, oregano is used as an appetite stimulant, for gastrointestinal pains, e.g. for flatulence and insufficient bile production, as an expectorant, for diseases of the urinary tract, dysmenorrhea and rheumatic diseases. It is used in the form of a tea infusion (1 heaping tablespoonful per 250 ml water). For digestive problems the tea should be taken unsweetened. As an expectorant, the tea is prepared with sugar or honey and drunk as hot as possible in small portions. The infusion can also be used as a gargle for inflammations of the oral mucosa and throat. The essential oil (5 to 6 drops on a sugar cube, 2 to 3 times daily) is taken for indigestion [Ü37]. Because its efficacy has not been proven, Germany's Commission E does not recommend its therapeutic use [16].

Similar culinary herbs

Indian mint, *Plectranthus amboinicus* (LOUR.) SPRENG. (Syn.: *Coleus amboinicus* LOUR.) and *P. glandulosus* J.D. HOOK. (Lamiaceae), native to tropical Africa, and cultivated in India, Indonesia, Malaysia, Sri Lanka, and the Philippines, among other countries. The main components of the essential oil are carvacrol (16 to 18%), Δ^3-carene (15 to 20%), camphor (15 to 19%), *p*-cymene (5 to 10%), and γ-terpinene (5 to 10%) [26, 27]. It is used, mostly fresh, as a spice for fish- and mutton dishes as well as for salads. In India, it is also used as an ingredient in beer [Ü92].

Other herbs, referred as "Oregano": There are about 60 other plant sources from 17 genera and 6 families, having a strong, characteristic aroma predominantly due to their carvacrol content. These herbs and mixtures of them are likewise described with the common name "Oregano". Within this group of plant sources are, among others, 38 species of *Origanum*, e.g. → *O. dictamnus* L. (Cretan dittany, see → Marjoram), → *O. heracleoticum* L. (Greek oregano, see → Marjoram), → *O. onites* BENTH. (Pot marjoram, Cretan oregano, see → Marjoram) and → *O. syriacum* L. (Syrian oregano, see → Marjoram). Furthermore there are other Lamiaceae such as *Thymus capitatus* (L.) HOFFM. (Spanish oregano), → *Monarda fistulosa* L. (wild bergamot beebalm) and → Plectranthus species (e.g. *Plectranthus amboinicus* (LOUR.) SPRENG., Indian borage, see above) as well plants from the Verbenaceae family such as → *Lippia graveolens* H.B.K. (Mexican oregano, see → Lemon verbena), *L. parmeri* WATS., *L. micromera* SCHAU. (Spanish thyme) and *Aloysia triphylla* (L'HÉRIT.) BRITTON (Lemon verbena, see → Lemon verbena) [Ü37].
These plants have a strong taste and an intensively pepper-like aroma. They serve, especially, as spices for pizzas, tomato dishes, meat- and fish recipes as well as for anchovies and noodle and rice dishes. In Italy it is often combined with basil and capers.

Neapolitan Tomato Pizza

Pizza dough: 350 g flour, 20 g yeast, 1 teaspoon sugar, 3 to 4 tablespoons milk, 2 eggs, table salt, 40 g butter or margarine. Toppings: 2 to 3 tablespoons olive oil, 125 g mozzarella, 300 g tomatoes, table salt, black pepper, 1 tablespoon ground oregano, 50 g anchovies.

Place 2/3 of the flour in a deep bowl, add the crumbs of yeast, sugar, some milk, eggs, a pinch of salt and warm butter or margarine; mix thoroughly while adding the remaining milk and flour until the dough separates from the bowl. Shape the dough into a ball and let it sit in a warm oven for 30 minutes. Spread the dough on a greased cookie sheet or baking tin (diameter 30 to 35 cm) and let it stand for another 25 minutes. Brush the dough with olive oil and place the cheese on top. Shortly boil the tomatoes and peel them; place the slices on top of the cheese and sprinkle the pizza with black pepper and oregano. Evenly distribute the anchovies on the surface of the pizza. Bake for 25 to 35 minutes at 190 to 200 °C or until brown. Serve hot with red wine [Ü23].

Literature

[1] Afshaypuor S., Planta Med. 62, Abstracts of the 44th Ann. Congress of GA, 133 (1996).

[2] Antonescu V. et al., Farmacia (Bukarest) 30:201–208 (1982).

[3] Aureli P. et al., J. Food Prot. 55:344–348 (1992).

[4] Baratta Z.M. et al., J. Ess. Oil Res. 10:618–627 (1998).

[5] Baser K.H.C. et al., J. Ess. Oil Res. 5:619–623 (1993).

[6] Benito M. et al., Ann. Allergy Asthma Immunol. 76(5):416–418 (1996).

[7] Carmo M.M, et al., J. Ess. Oil Res. 2:69–71 (1989).

[8] Conner D.E., L.R. Beuchat, J. Food Sci. 49:429–443 (1984).

[9] Daferra D.J. et al., J. Agric. Food Chem. 48(6):2576–2581 (2000).

[10] Dorman H.J., S.G. Deans, J. Appl. Microbiol. 88(2):308–316 (2000).

[11] Gracza L., P. Ruff, Arch. Pharmaz. 317: 339–345 (1984).

[12] Herrmann K., Pharmazie 11:433–448 (1956).

[13] Ismaiel A.A., M.D. Pierson, J. Food Prot. 53:755–758 (1990).

[14] Kaul V.K. et al., J. Ess. Oil Res. 8:101–103 (1996).

[15] Kokkini S. et al., Phytochemistry 44(5): 883–886 (1997).

[16] Kommission E beim BfArM, BAnz-Nr. 122 vom 06.07.88.

[17] Lamaison J.L. et al., Pharm. Acta Helv. 66(7):185–188 (1991).

[18] Lamaison J.L. et al., Ann. Pharm. Franc. 48:103–108 (1990).

[19] Maarse H., F.H.L. Van Os, Flavour Ind. 4:477–481, 481–484 (1973).

[20] Nykänen I., Z. Lebensm. Unters. Forsch. 183:267–272 (1986).

[21] Oberdieck R., Fleischwirtschaft 70:391–398 (1990).

[22] Pande C.H. et al., J. Ess. Oil Res. 12: 441–442 (2000).

[23] Reschke A., Z. Lebensm. Unters. Forsch. 176:116–119 (1983).

[24] Salmeron J. et al., J. Food Prot. 53: 697–700 (1990).

[25] Sezik E. et al., J. Ess. Oil Res. 5:425–431 (1993).

[26] Vahirua-Lechat I. et al., Rlv. Ital. EPPOS 1997 (Spec. Num., 15th Journees Internat. Huiles Essentielles, 1996): p.704–711 (1997).

[27] Vera R. et al., Planta Med. 59(2):182–183 (1993).

[28] Vetter A. et al., Drogenreport 13(23): 12–15 (2000).

[29] Werker E. et al., Ann. Bot. 55:793–801 (1985).

[30] Weymar H., Buch der Lippenblütler und Raublattgewächse, Neumann Verlag, Radebeul 1961.

[31] Wilkins C., J. Madsen, Z. Lebensm. Unters. Forsch. 192:214–219 (1991).

[32] Zheng Sh. et al., Indian J. Chem., Sect. B: Org. Chem. Incl. Med. Chem. 36B(1): 104–106 (1997), ref. CA 127:092675r.

Literature references identified by Ü can be found in the general listing of books and monographs at the back of this book.

Oswego tea

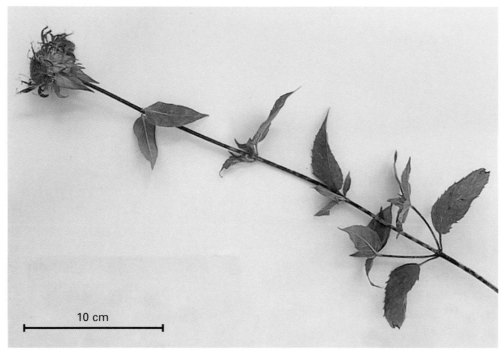

Fig. 1: Oswego tea flowering top

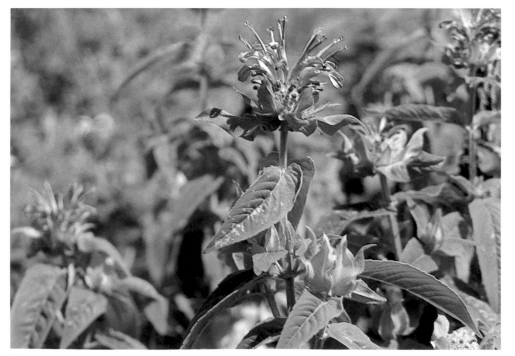

Fig. 2: Oswego tea (*Monarda didyma* L.)

Plant source: *Monarda didyma* L.

Synonym: *Monarda fistulosa* SIMS non L.

Family: Mint family (Lamiaceae, synonym Labiatae).

Common names: Engl.: Oswego tea, bee balm, bergamot; Fr.: monarde; Ger.: Monarde, Indianernessel, Scharlachrote Monarde, Sharlach-Monarde, Gold-melisse, Rote Melisse, Oswego-Tee, Etagenblume, Bienenbalsam, Bergamotte, Pferdeminze.

Description: Perennial herb, up to 90 cm tall, quadrangular stem, pubescent and often reddish pruinose. The leaves are petioled, ovate-lanceolate, longish acuminate, 4 to 7 cm in length, often reddish pruinose, pubescent especially along the veins, leaf margin mucronate-serrate. The numerous flowers are arranged in 1 to 3 false whorls often with colored bracts and subtending leaves, corolla 3.5 to 6 mm in length, with long, slightly bent upper lip and shorter lower lip, light- to purple-red, often supported by bracteoles of the same color, 2 stamina, long calyx, with 10 nerves and 5 short teeth. Flowering period is from July to September [7, Ü60, Ü92].

Native origin: USA (New York to Michigan, south to Georgia, and Tennessee), widely distributed as an ornamental plant.

Main cultivation areas: Southwestern USA, and South America.

Main suppliers: USA.

Cultivation: The plant prefers damp, loosely packed, deep, nutrient-rich, humus soil in sunny to half-shaded locations. During dry spells, it must be irrigated intensively. The plant is hardy in Central Europe.

Propagation is carried out using cuttings or runners in the spring or autumn, spaced at intervals of 50 × 40 cm, but direct seeding is also possible. Plants grown from seed however do not remain true to color. Oswego tea is also grown as an ornamental plant (scarlet red-flowering 'Cambridge Scarlet', 'Prairie Fire', 'Squaw', purple-flowering 'Blue Stockings', and pink-flowering 'Croftway Pink'). For production of the dried herb the scarlet red varieties should be selected. After 3 to 4 years, transplanting to a new location is beneficial [Ü21, Ü96].

Culinary herb

Commercial forms: Oswego tea: dried leaves.

Production: The young, fresh leaves (Fig. 1) can be picked at any stage. The shoot tips are harvested and dried during the flowering period. The flowers are plucked from the whorl-like inflorescences [Ü21].

Forms used: The fresh or dried leaves, collected during the flowering period, and the fresh or candied flowers.

Storage: The fresh flowers and leaves can be stored refrigerated in plastic bags for a few days. Candied flowers are kept wrapped in foil in the refrigerator. The dried leaves are stored in a cool place, protected from moisture and light, in airtight porcelain-, glass- or suitable metal containers.

Description. Whole leaf: Dried leaves, see description of the whole plant.

Odor: Aromatic, lemon-like, **Taste:** Somewhat spicy, bitter.

History: The plant was already used by Native Americans, particularly the Oswego Indians, among other tribes, as a medicinal plant and spice as well as for the preparation of beverage teas. The white settlers of North America adopted the use of Oswego tea from the native population after the so-called "Boston tea party" of 1773, wherein tea bales were thrown overboard to protest against the tariffs on tea shipments which had been imposed by the British parliament [Ü17].

Constituents and Analysis

Constituents

- Essential oil: In the herb 0.1 to 0.3%, in the leaves up to 1.3%; the main components are linalool and linalyl acetate, in addition to limonene, β-ocimene, α-pinene, camphene, Δ^3-carene, carvacrol and thymol [1, 4].
- Bitter substances: Possibly diterpenes.
- Flavonoids: Didymin (isosakunaretin-7-rhamnoglucoside), naringenin-7-rhamnoglucoside, linarin, glucogenkwanin, isosakuranetin, among others [1, 6].
- Hydroxycinnamic acid derivatives (labiate tannins): About 5%, particularly rosmarinic acid (2%) [2].
- Triterpenes, sterols: β-Sitosterin, ursolic acid [1].

Tests for Identity: Can be carried out using sensoric, macroscopic and microscopic analysis.

Quantitative assay: The essential oil content can be determined volumetrically with steam distillation and xylol in the graduated tube [according to Ph Eur].

Adulterations, Misidentifications and Impurities: Accidental substitutions with the herb from *Monarda fistulosa* L, wild bergamot beebalm, are possible; the adulterant has a densely pubescent, white, violet-dotted or violet-red corolla.

Actions and Uses

Actions: On the basis of its aromatic and slightly bitter taste, it is appetizing and digestion promoting.
Inhalation of Oswego tea essential oil (0.1 to 0.5 mg/m³) improved the therapeutic outcome in the treatment of chronic bronchitis [5]. Inhalation of the essential oil in rabbits (01. to 0.2 mg/ m³ air) inhibited the development of arteriosclerotic plaque in the aorta [3]. The author is not aware of any clinical studies investigating its febrifuge action.

Toxicology: Based on existing data, there is no acute or chronic toxicity with the normal use of the herb as a spice or in form of beverage teas at typical dosages. The sensitization potential is not known.

Culinary use: The young, fresh leaves serve as a seasoning of salads, salsas, stuffings, stews and meat dishes, especially roast pork, and also used sparingly to season cream cheese. The leaves and flowers are also used to garnish fruit drinks, summer punches and salads.

One fresh leaf added to a cup of freshly brewed Chinese tea suggests the aroma of an Earl Grey mixture.

The dried herb is used to prepare the beverage tea known as Oswego Tea [Ü2, Ü17, Ü55, Ü92].

Other uses: The essential oil is used as a perfume in sun tan oils and lotions [Ü2].

Medicinal herb

Herbal drug: Monardae herba, Monarda herb, may also be obtained from *Monarda fistulosa* L.

Indications: In folk medicine, especially in the USA, it is used for digestive problems and fever (formerly as a quinine substitute).

Other Monarda-species used as culinary herbs

Wild bergamot beebalm, *Monarda fistulosa* L., in Mexico also known as oregano, native to southern Canada south to Mexico, and cultivated in the USA. Carvacrol is the main component of its essential oil [Ü43, Ü61].

Lemon monarda (prairie bergamot, lemonmint), *Monarda citriodora* CERV., is native to the USA and Mexico and cultivated in the USA. The main components of its essential oil are thymol and carvacrol [Ü43, Ü61].

Literature

[1] Brieskorn C.H., G. Meisters, Arch. Pharmaz. 298:435–440 (1965).
[2] Lamaison J.L. et al., Ann. Pharm. Franc 48:103–108 (1990).
[3] Nikolaevskii V.V. et al., Patol. Fiziol. Exsp. Ter. (5):52–53 (1990).
[4] Scora R.W., Am. J. Bot. 54:446–452 (1967).
[5] Shubina L.P. et al., Vrach. Delo. (5):66–67 (1990).
[6] Wagner H. et al., Chem. Ber. 101(2): 445–449 (1968).
[7] Weymar H., Buch der Lippenblütler und Rauhblattgewächse, Neumann Verlag, Radebeul 1961.

Literature references identified by Ü can be found in the general listing of books and monographs at the back of this book.

Paprika

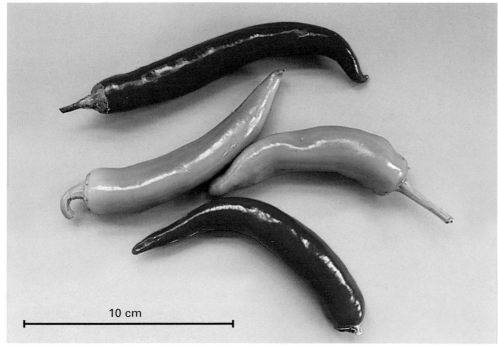

Fig. 1: Paprika, green and red fruits

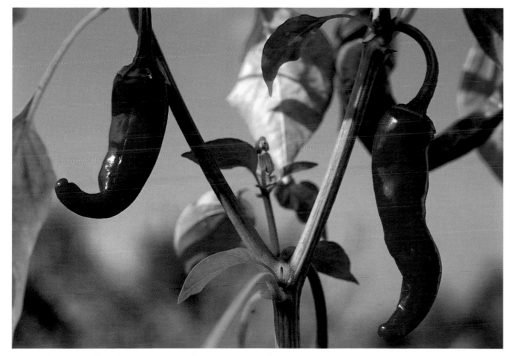

Fig. 2: Paprika (*Capsicum annuum* L. var. *annuum*)

Plant source: *Capsicum annuum* L. var. *annuum*.

Synonyms: *Capsicum annuum* L. var. *longum* (DC.) SENDTN., *C. annuum* var. *minimum* (MILLER) HEISER.

Taxonomic classification: There are over 200 cultivated varieties of the genus Capsicum in existence, which are differentiated mainly on the basis of the shape, color, size and pungency of their fruits. The great variety of cultivars makes precise species classification complicated or often impossible without knowledge of the plant's past history. Due to varieties, which overlap species boundaries, it is also very difficult to determine from studies published in the scientific literature just which Capsicum species the referenced fruits originate from [2].

Zander´s Dictionary of Plant Names [Ü22, 17th ed., 2002) proposed to group the cultivars as follows:
– Cerasiforme-group: Cherry pepper (small fruited),
– Conoioides-group: Cone pepper,
– Fasciculatum group: Red cone pepper,
– Grossum-group: Bell pepper, pim(i)ento, sweet pepper (vegetable varieties),
– Longum-group: Cayenne pepper, chilli pepper.

Family: Nightshade family (Solanaceae).

Common names: Engl.: paprika, red pepper, green pepper; Fr. poivre d'Espagne, poivre d'Inde, poivre de cayenne, piment annuel, paprika; Ger.: Gewürzpaprika, Gemeiner Paprika, Mexikanischer Paprika, Brasilianischer Pfeffer, Indianischer Pfeffer, Indischer Pfeffer, Spanischer Pfeffer, Türkischer Pfeffer, Roter Pfeffer, Piemento, Beißbeere, Schotenpfeffer.

Very pungent varieties of *C. annuum* and *C. frutescens* (hot pepper, Tabasco pepper) are referred to as chili peppers (some authors also include the fruits of *C. baccatum* L., aji pepper, *C. chinense* JACQ., habañero pepper, and *C. pubescens* RUIZ. ET PAV. (apple chile, tree pepper). The terms paprika, Spanish pepper and chili are very often used interchangeably in the literature.

Description: Annual cultivated, up to 80 cm high (sometimes 1.8 m), bushy, perennial in the tropics and when grown in green houses. The stems are angular, glabrous, somewhat woody at the base. The leaves are mostly single, about 4 cm long and 2 cm wide, petiolated, longish-ovate, partially ending in a blunt tip, having a conical base, with an entire or slightly wavy margin. The flowers appear most often singly in the axils of the leaves (in C. *frutescens* in groups of 2 to 5 per axil); the calyx is hemispherical and 5 to 7 dentate, corolla well-shaped, short-tubular, diameter about 2.5 cm, 5 to 9 white lobes, rarely with violet tips, or yellowish-white, 5 to 6 stamina with dark-gray to black anthers additionally 5 small, papillose staminodes, superior ovary, undivided in the upper part, the lower part is divided into 2 or 3 compartments, filiform style with multiple lobed, yellowish stigma. The inflated fruits are berries (sometimes erroneously called "pods") with a rather leathery and not very fleshy skin and numerous seeds. The pungent paprika varieties used as spices have elongated, conical, rarely round, 6 to 12 cm (rarely 20 cm) long and up to 4 cm thick, bright red, reddish-brown, orange, yellow or green, hanging fruits. The non-pungent, mild varieties used for vegetable dishes and salads have thick-fleshed, longish-round, globular or conical fruits, yellow, green, red or orange or more rarely black, white or purple. The seeds of all cultivars are yellowish-white, disk-shaped with a diameter of 3 to 5 mm and a thickness of 0.5 to 1 mm, having a pitted surface (Ü37, Ü41, Ü42].

Native origin: Paprika is a cultivated plant. The wild form is probably *C. annuum* L. var. *glabriusculum* (DUNAL) HEISER et PICKERSVILLE (Synonym: *C. annuum* var.

aviculare (DIERBACH) D'ARCY et ESCHBAUGH), native to southern USA, and Mexico to northwestern South America.

Main cultivation areas: Southwestern States of the USA, especially California and New Mexico, southern Europe, especially Hungary, Spain, Italy, Republics of the former Yugoslavia, Bulgaria and Romania, as well as the Russian Federation, Morocco, Central American countries, and Brazil.

Main exporting countries: Hungary, Spain, Brazil, Republics of the former Yugoslavia, Bulgaria, and Romania.

Cultivation: Paprika requires nutrient- and humus rich, medium-heavy soil in full sun locations. It does not tolerate stagnant moisture. It is possible to grow it in gardens in Central Europe, but with only moderate yields. For optimal utilization of the short summer vegetation period in Central Europe, seeds can be started in a plastic covered planter box in mid February to early March, for the first time at temperatures between 22 and 24 °C. The seeds should only be lightly covered with soil (their germination requires light). After about 14 days the seedlings should be pricked and further grown at 16 to 18 °C. At the end of May to early June, they can be transplanted outdoors in a protected location at 50 cm lines × 50 cm apart. For industrial cultivation in Europe, northern to eastern Austria, suitable vegetable varieties come from, among other locations, from the Hungarian plant breeding station Szegedi and Kaloscsai, they are characterized using numbers, e.g. 'Szegedi 47-25', 'Szegedi F03' and 'Kaloscai Cs 631' (medium hot), or 'Kalocsai 621' (hot). Other varieties, among others, are named 'De Cayenne', 'Escort', 'Torito', 'Westlandia', 'Wulkan' and 'Negral' [Ü16, Ü21, Ü96].

Culinary herb

Commercial forms: Paprika: dried fruit, almost always ground, varieties: **Heat-free Paprika** (placenta and seeds removed,

fiery red, fine aroma, without pungency, capsaicin content below 5 mg/100 g), **Top Quality Paprika** (first quality, fully ripe, select fruits, with placenta, seeds, calyx, stems and tips removed, fire red, mildly fruity, very finely ground, capsaicin content 6 to 8 mg/100 g), **Edelsüß-Paprika** (contains up to 30 to 40% seeds, dark red, mild, with milder pungency, capsaicin content 12 to 14 mg/100 g), **Semisweet-** or **Goulash-Paprika** (ground with placenta, less intense color than the above named varieties, pungent and spicy, capsaicin content 12 to 25 mg/100 g), **Rose Quality Paprika** (ground whole fruits, reddish brown, pungent, capsaicin content 80 to 150 mg/100 g), **Pungent-**, **Mercantile-** or **Königs-Paprika** (powdered whole fruits admixed with up to 10% chili powder or seeds and placenta of other fruits, brownish-red, biting pungency, capsaicin content about 250 mg/100 g), **Paprika Oleoresin** (deep red, viscous, solvent-free extract, obtained through extraction with organic solvents or supercritical CO_2, yields 8 to 16%, varieties "heat-free" and "pungent", pigment units 40,000, 80,000 and 100,000) [67, Ü89, Ü92, Ü98]. Occasionally, paprika fruits, especially chili peppers, are classified according to pungency grades 1 to 10 or according to the Scoville-Index, 0 to 300,000 Scoville heat units = SU (ISO-Standard 3513). Uncut fresh fruits, or fruits packed in vinegar, are also commercially available [83, Ü68].

Production: Paprika is harvested by hand or with a mechanical harvester (similar to a mechanical bean harvester), when the fruits are red (in Southern Europe from August to September). Because the fruits do not ripen simultaneously, they must be plucked repeatedly. The fruits are occasionally stored for a few days to mature. Smallholdings hang them up on strings to dry, and larger companies dry them in ventilated drying chambers at temperatures below 35 °C. By complete or partial removal of the placenta, which is the plant part with the highest concentration of pungent compounds, the flavor strength can be regulated. The removed plant parts are added to other commercial varieties, those which a higher pungency is desired. Added crushed seeds (containing 30% fatty oil) function as solubilizers for the carotenoids [67, Ü89]. For personal use, one can also harvest the green fruits in July or August [Ü96].

Forms used: Fresh or dried fruits, ground, rarely whole, shredded or in flakes.

Storage: Fresh paprika fruits are stored in plastic bags in the refrigerator. Dried fruits can be kept in whole or cut form in airtight porcelain- or glass containers protected from light and moisture. Ground paprika loses its color (oxidation of the carotenoids by peroxidases), aroma and pungency rather quickly. Bleaching can be inhibited by addition of suitable antioxidants.

Description. Whole fruits (Fig. 1): Conical, green, orange, brown- to dark red, about 6 to 12 cm long fruits with a 4 cm wide base having a flattened, gray-green, pentadentate calyx, and often bearing the remains of the bent and hollow pedicle. The fruit wall is brittle, shiny on the outside, smooth indistinctly cross-striped and with punctiform protrusions; the fruit in the upper part is undivided, in the lower part di- or trilocular. Seeds are pale yellow, discoid, almost circular, diameter 3 to 5 mm, 0.5 to 1 mm thick, with a granular surface, in the upper part of the fruit, they are falsely parietal situated, in the lower part, they are attached to the longitudinal ridges representing the parietal placenta.

Powdered fruits: Yellowish-red to dark-red powder; characteristic are the fragments of the endocarp with clusters of cells with beaded, lignified walls (so called "rosary" cells), the thick-walled epidermal cells of the testa with robust, yellowish green thickenings and distinct striations (so-called "mesentery cells", see Fig. 3) including thick, collenchymatic or thin-walled cells of the mesocarp with yellowish-red oil drops and red granules. Also present are fragments of the endosperm and embryo, gray-green remains of the calyx with stomata and glandular trichomes as well as fiber-like parts of the pedicle [Ü49].

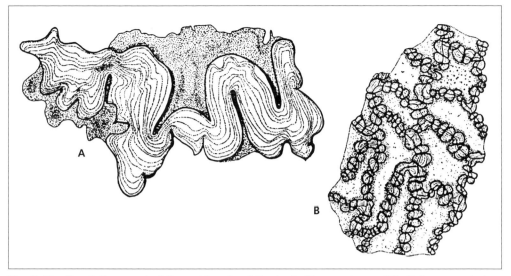

Fig. 3: Paprika. **A** Fragment of the epidermis of the testa ("mesentery cell"), **B** A group of elongated sclereids of the endocarp ("rosary cells"). From Ü49.

Odor: Uncomminuted fruit practically odorless, powder with typical odor, **Taste:** Depending on the variety mild, fruity or intensely pungent and burning.

History: The use of paprika can be traced back to Peru, around 2000 BCE, and in 700 BCE, it was also documented in Central America. Columbus brought first samples of paprika back to Spain in 1514. The first cultivation in Germany was reported as early as 1542. In 1569, the author Monardes extensively described this plant and its cultivation in Spain. In Greece, it was also grown in the 16th century. From there, it reached Turkey, and with the expansion of the Ottoman Empire, Bulgaria and Hungary where large-scale cultivations were established by the 19th century. Europeans introduced it to India and China [78, Ü42, Ü89, Ü97].

Constituents and Analysis

DIN- and ISO-Standards: DIN Standard 10234 (Determination of capsaicinoid content in paprika), ISO-Standard 972 (Chillies and capsicums, whole or ground (powdered): Specification), ISO-Standard 7540 (Ground (powdered) paprika, 3 grades of powdered paprika are specified based on their capsaicin content, among other standards: I: 0 to 10 mg/100 g, II: maximum 20 mg/100 g, III: maximum 30 mg/ 100 g, furthermore the specifications include the grade of comminution, total ash content and acid insoluble ash content as well as natural pigment content (2.5, 2.0 or 1.5 g/kg)), ISO-Standard 7541 (Ground (powdered) paprika–Determination of total natural colouring matter content), ISO-Standard 7542 (Ground (powdered) paprika: Microscopical examination), ISO-Standard 7543-1 (Chillies and chilli oleoresins: Determination of total capsaicinoid content, Part 1: Spectrometric method), ISO-Standard 7543-2 (Chillies and chilli oleoresins: Determination of total capsaicinoid content, Part 2: HPLC method), ISO-Standard 3513 (Chillies: Determination of Scoville index).

Constituents

■ Acid amides: Capsaicin and capsaicinoids (amides of vanillylamine = 4-hydroxy-3-methoxy-benzylamine with saturated or mono-unsaturated C_8- to C_{10}-fatty acids or methyl fatty acids): 0.03 to 0.35% (up to 0.7%), dissolved in the oily secretions in the subcuticular spaces of the seed-bearing placenta. The main components are capsaicin (32 to 49%, (*E*)-capsaicin, *trans*-form), dihydrocapsaicin (18 to 52%) and nordihydrocapsaicin (7 to 17%); furthermore, homocapsaicins I and II, homodihydrocapsaicins I and II, nonivamide, caprylic acid vanillyl amide, decylic acid vanillyl amide, among others [7, 16, 40–42, 44, 45, 59, Ü30].

▪ Carotenoids: 0.1 to 0.8%, mostly capsanthin (35 to 50%), β-carotene (10 to 18%), violaxanthin (7 to 10%), β-cryptoxanthin (4 to 12%), capsorubin (6 to 10%); also present, among others, are lutein, zeaxanthin, cucurbitaxanthins A and B, carpoxanthin, cycloviolaxanthin, antheraxanthin, capsanthone and nigroxanthin as well as epoxides and fatty acid mono and diesters (particularly 3,3′-lauroylmyristoylcapsanthin) [20, 30, 31, 69, 95, Ü30].

▪ Volatile compounds: 0.05 to 1.1%, the major odoriferous components in the green fruits are 2-methoxy-3-isobutylpyrazine and capsiamide (N-(13-methyltetradecyl)acetamide; they cannot be detected in the dried fruits. A variety of volatile constituents have been found in the material of commerce which mostly arise from breakdown processes and from the smoke used during drying; they include acetic acid, 2-methylbutanal and 3-methylbutanal, ethyl acetate, 1,3-butandiol, 2,3-butandiol, acetoin (3-hydroxy-2-butanone), phenol, p-cresol and dimethoxyphenol [11, 47, 61].

▪ Steroid saponins: In the seeds, they include capsicoside A to D (capsicoside A = 22-hydroxyfurostanol bisdesmoside), proto-degalactotigonine, among others [92, 98].

▪ Flavonoids: Including apiin, luteolin-7-O-glucoside, eriocitrin, hesperidine [75].

▪ Mono- and oligosaccharides: such as fructose (5 to 9%), glucose (1 to 3%), saccharose (0.4 to 2%) [67, 73].

▪ Fatty oil: About 30% in the seeds [67].

▪ Proteins: About 4% [Ü98].

▪ Vitamins, particularly vitamin C: In paprika used for seasoning up to 100 mg/100 g (fresh weight), vegetable paprika 60 to 300 mg/100 g (fresh weight) [55, Ü82].

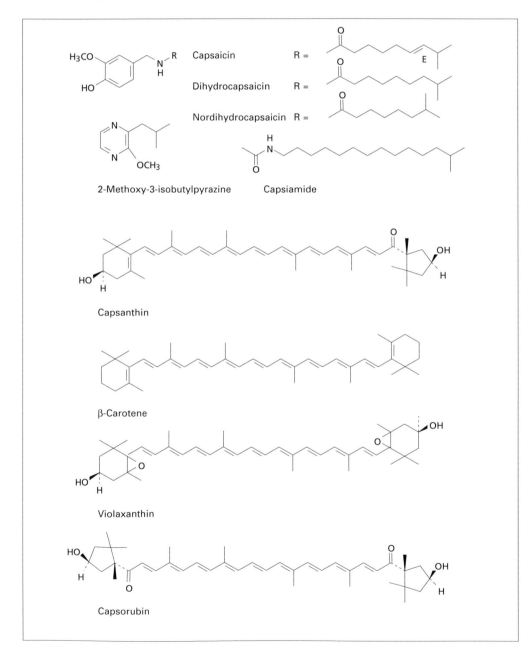

Capsaicin   R =

Dihydrocapsaicin   R =

Nordihydrocapsaicin   R =

2-Methoxy-3-isobutylpyrazine   Capsiamide

Capsanthin

β-Carotene

Violaxanthin

Capsorubin

Tests for Identity: According to organoleptic, macroscopic and microscopic assays, as well as TLC [29, 81, 82, 89, Ü102, Ph Eur].

Quantitative assay: Determination of the capsaicinoids in the fruits or oleoresin with spectrophotometry or colorimetry after separation with liquid chromatography (DAB, Cayenne pepper), TLC or column chromatography, respectively [36, 39, 74, 80, Ph Eur, Ph Helv, ÖAB], or with GC [22, 32, 45, 76, 90] and HPLC [15–17, 33, 35, 43, 58, 59, 71, 84]. Analysis of the carotenoids with TLC or HPLC according to [6, 10, 12, 18, 19, 26, 27, 95, 96].

Adulterations, Misidentifications and Impurities. Accidental adulterations with fruits from other Capsicum species can occur. The fruits from. C. frutescens are usually smaller (1 to 7 cm long). The microscopic examination does not allow for a distinction between different species in powder form. Some information on the botanical origin can be obtained based on the capsaicin/nordihydrocapsaicin ratio [41, 42]. Also described is the adulteration with azo-dyes as a colorant, the admixture of synthetic n-vanillylnonamide to augment the spicy aroma, and the addition of antioxidants to increase color stability; such impurities can be detected with TLC or HPLC [Ü93].

Actions and Uses

Actions: Paprika has digestive promoting activity and accelerates metabolism. With oral ingestion, the pungent, burning taste of the capsaicinoids, leads to a reflective increase in the secretion of saliva and gastric juice and to stimulation of digestive organs motility, but this is also triggered by direct contact of the capsaicinoids with the gastric mucosa [21, 53, 93, Ü38, Ü99]. In animal experiments (rats), capsaicin elevated the intestinal lipase-, saccharase- and maltase activity [70]. Feeding of capsaicin (15 mg/100 g in feed of rats) for 8 weeks led to increased activity of pancreas lipase, pancreas amylase, trypsin and chymotrypsin. Single doses had no effect [72]. Carbohydrate metabolism (measured as the respiratory quotient and blood lactate levels) was significantly elevated in the human body [52]. Nevertheless the addition of paprika or chilies to test meals decreased desire of human subjects to eat [100].

Epidemiological evidence shows that the regular consumption of paprika as a spice in typical amounts seems to protect against stomach ulcers: the frequency of occurrence of stomach ulcers was lower in the group that often uses chilies as a spice compared to the group that avoids or rarely uses this spice (elimination of *Helicobacter pylori*?) [46]. Chili powder has also been shown to protect against aspirin-induced (600 mg) gastroduodenal mucosal injury [99].

Capsaicinoids cause an activation of peripheral nociceptive neurons (polymodal nociceptors, C-fibers and Aδ-fibers) via reaction with specific receptors ("vanilloid receptor 1 = VR1", which is also activated by strong heat) [13, 88]. These neurons are responsible for the per-

ception of damaging warm- and pain stimuli. Their activation is transmitted to the central nervous system and induces in addition the release of an undeca-peptide substance P, of calcitonin gene-related peptide (CGRP), somatostatin and vasoactive polypeptides. At the same time, the biosynthesis and reuptake of substance P is inhibited. This is followed by a local neurogenic inflammation that is triggered by the mediators of substance P (histamine, bradykinin, prostaglandins) [23, 54, 65, Ü38]. Application of capsaicinoids to the skin leads to painful burning and hyperemia (erythema) caused by vasodilatation. Subsequent depletion of substance P induces insensitivity (analgesia!). Chronic use of capsaicin leads to damage of the affected neurons. They become insensitive to physiological activation. This results in an analgesic and antiphlogistic effect that lasts for hours to weeks. Repeated use can lead to complete desensitization [4, 8, 37, 66, Ü99].

Capsicum-carotenoids suppress in vitro the mutagenic effect of nitroarens (1-nitropyrene, 1,6-dinitropyrene and 1,8-dinitropyrene) in the AMES-Test. Capsicum extracts inhibited their mutagenicity by about 90%. The extract was more active than β–carotene [34]. Capsaicin protects against experimentally-induced mutagenesis and tumorigenesis [85].

Aqueous extracts of various Capsicum-species or capsaicin have a variable, and some only moderate, antibacterial effect [14, 63].

Toxicology: Paprika and its preparations strongly irritate the skin and mucous membranes and cause a painful, burning sensation. Avoid skin and particularly eye contact [49]. The internal use of high doses can lead to gastritis, gall bladder spasms and kidney damage. After the intake of 0.1 to 1.5 g paprika by humans in test meals, elevated pepsin production, microhemorrhages as well as cell loss of the mucous membrane of stomach were reported, which were comparable to the damaging effects of aspirin on the gastric mucosa [64]. The gastric introduction of 1 mg capsaicin in physiological solution increased

the development of stomach ulcers in rats [60]. The administration of paprika extracts, or ethanolic capsaicin solution (1 mg/kg body weight, p. o.), respectively, to rats over 3 to 9 months, led to degeneration of mucous producing cells and therefore to loss of the mucus layer of the stomach, to edema of the mucosa and submucosa as well as to stomach hemorrhages [25] (which contradicts the gastroprotective effect, see above; these different results could possibly be due to a dose-dependent activity).

The reports of co-carcinogenic and carcinogenic effects are also contradictory. In some animal test models, capsaicin was a co-carcinogenic and a weak carcinogenic [1, 48]. In mice, which were fed a diet containing 1% (!) capsaicin for 35 days, the incidence of duodenal adeno-carcinoma was increased [5, 91]. In an epidemiological study from India, the consumption of chilies (including high rice intake and hot meals) has been described as a risk factor for stomach cancer [62]. Other authors could not observe any co-carcinogenic and carcinogenic effects in mice [68]. Anti-carcinogenic activities have also been postulated.

In vitro assays to measure the mutagenic effects of paprika extracts and capsaicin, respectively, showed contradictory results [overview in Lit. 86, 87].

Some authors recommend moderate use of paprika seasoning and chilies until the risk has been clarified [24].

External application of high concentration or to broken skin can cause blisters and damage of the sensitive nerve endings. In animal tests (rats, ferrets, rabbits, guinea pigs) a single, topical application of 1% capsaicin in olive oil in the area of the Nervus saphenus led to a decreased sensitivity even after 3 months. The authors therefore postulate that the C-fibers, which were destroyed by capsaicin, are only partially regenerated [57].

Allergic sensitization to paprika and chilies is relatively rare. Observed symptoms, particularly in people with occupational exposure, include urticaria, rhinoconjunctivitis and asthma. It is assumed the antigens are proteins, among other allergens, with cross-reaction to antibodies against proteins in celery and birch pollen [7, 28, 38, 49, 51, 94]. Capsaicin is also postulated to have allergenic activity [97].

Culinary use of fruits of Capsicum-species: In tropical countries, paprika and chilies are frequently used as spices, e.g. in India and Southeastern Asia as a spice for rice, in Mexico and in the Southern USA as a spice in beans, corn, Mexican mole (traditional sauce) or chili con carne, in South America to spice cassava (pudding from detoxified roots of *Manihot esculenta* CRANTZ, manioc) and in China, among others, as a spice in Hoisin sauces. In Spain, paprika is used to improve the taste of salted cod à la vicaina, romesco sauce and chorizo sausage, and in Italy for piquant noodle dishes. Generally well known are Hungarian dishes spiced with paprika such as Szegediner goulash, Szegediner kraut or roast shepherd's spits. Throughout the entire Mediterranean region green olives are packed with pieces of paprika [83, Ü56, Ü68, Ü73]. The great era of paprika in Central Europe began after the Second World War, and the use of chilies has begun only in recent years.

Use caution when handling paprika or chilies. Do not get them near the lips or eyes. With sensitive skin, wear rubber gloves. When finished, hands and equipment should be washed thoroughly. As an antidote for intense burning in the throat, cream, milk or yogurt is recommended (water is not helpful). Paprika should be added only near the end of cooking time. It should never be added to hot fat, because through caramelization the sugars form bitter breakdown products [Ü92].

Paprika powder serves as a spice of soups (e.g. goulash-, tomato-, vegetable- and fish soups), sauces (roasted meat- and salad sauces), meat dishes (especially goulash, veal and lamb), poultry dishes (e.g. chicken and turkey), fish dishes (red sea bass), game, ground meat, seafood, baked potatoes, quark, cheese (e.g. Liptauer cheese), mayonnaise, as well as rice dishes, egg dishes and cream sauces, cooked or steamed vegetables (e.g. tomatoes, eggplants, mushrooms, cucumbers, white beans, leeks, sauerkraut, red cabbage), salads (with the exception of sweet salads) and marinades [Ü30, Ü59, Ü89, Ü90, Ü95].

In the food industry paprika powder is added to sausages, ketchup, dressings, cheese biscuits, potato chips, mixed pickles and gherkins, besides others. Paprika oleoresin serves for flavoring of sausages, canned fish and cheeses, heat-free oleoresins for coloring of farinaceous products or butter [Ü89, Ü92, Ü98].

Whole paprika fruits or chilies (fruits dried after soaking) have the stem attachment, the seeds and the placenta removed, and are cut into strips. Fresh chilies with a thick skin are skinned after being fried (5 seconds in hot vegetable oil) or roasted (after being rubbed with oil, in the oven for 1 to 2 minutes at 200 ºC) and afterwards steamed (5 to 10 minutes wrapped in a damp cloth). The cut fruits are used as a spice for pizzas, pot roast dishes, soups (e.g. fish soups), hot sauces, moles, salsas, stews, sea foods, salads, mixed pickles, vinegar (chili vinegar), oil (chili oil), pickled gherkins and other foods. Connoisseurs use a special variety for each dish [83, Ü55, Ü93].

The preparation of appetizing snacks by pickling fresh chilies or cayenne fruits in vinegar is practiced especially in Mexico, the USA, and Italy [Ü55, Ü68].

To prepare chili vinegar, one puts the fruits in a bottle and fills it with vinegar. After 2 weeks the vinegar can be used as a seasoning.

Combines well with: Basil, black pepper, caraway, cardamom, cinnamon, clove, coriander, cumin, fennel, fenugreek, garlic, ginger, marjoram, onions, oregano, parsley, and thyme.

As a component of spice mixes and preparations: → Barbecue spice, → Bologna spice mix, → Bomboe, → Cajun spice, → Chili con carne spice, → Curry powder, → Egg spice, → Fish spice, → Grill spice, → Hamburger meat spice, → Masala, → Meat spice, → Pepper bouquet, → Pepper sauce, → Pickling spice, → Pizza spice, → Poultry spice, → Quark spice, → Roast spice, → Salami spice, → Seven-seas-spice, → Soup spice, → Tika-paste, → Tschubritza, → Tai-ping China, → Vegetable spice, → Venison spice, → Zhug.

Other uses: Capsaicin is also employed as an ingredient in hair waters (0.001 to 0.003%) or in ointments against frostbites [Ü24]. Capsanthin and capsorubin (as E160c) are approved colorants for food and cosmetics [Ü24]. Paprika has been used as an additive to chicken feed in order to obtain reddish yellow yolks. The oleoresin is a component of pepper sprays (OC-sprays, OC = **O**leoresin **C**apsicum) used in self-defense [for a toxicology of pepper spray products, see Lit. 11].

Medicinal herb

Herbal drugs: Capsici fructus, Cayenne pepper, contains minimum 0.4% of total capsaicinoids, expressed as capsaicin, dried ripe fruits of *Capsicum annuum* L. var. *minimum* (MILLER) HEISER and small-fruited varieties of *Capsicum frutescens* L. [Ph Eur] and Capsici frutescentis fructus, Cayennepfeffer (cayenne pepper), minimum 0.4% capsaicinoids [Ph Helv], fruit of *C. frutescens* s.l. (see below).

Indications: Germany's Commission E did not approve the oral administration of cayenne for medicinal purposes [49]. Cayenne extracts or capsaicin are approved as topical analgesics for painful muscle spasms in the cervicobrachial (shoulder and arm) region as well as in the region of the spinal column, for rheumatic complaints, neuralgia (e.g. post-herpetic neuralgia, diabetic neuropathy) and for local frost damage. The most commonly used dosage forms are tinctures, fluid preparations corresponding to 0.005–0.01% capsaicinoids and semi-solid preparations corresponding to 0.02–0.05% capsaicinoids, as well as plasters corresponding to 10 to 40 µg capsaicinoids per cm^2. External use should be limited to no longer than 2 days, and 14 days must pass before a new application can be applied to the same skin area [3, 49]. Capsaicin solution may be helpful in cases of neurogenic bladder evacuation problems [79].

In folk medicine, paprika with low capsaicin content is taken internally as a supportive remedy for digestive problems, stomach and intestinal complaints, as well as a dehydrating agent and to improve cardiac and circulatory functions. Because efficacy has not been substantiated, its use for these conditions has not been approved [50].

Additional Capsicum-species in use

Chili (plural: chilis, chilies, also chilli, chili, chile, aji, Tabasco pepper, peperoni, in ground form as cayenne pepper or Guinea pepper; Fr.: piments, poivron; Ger.: Chilly, Chili, Tabasco), fruits of *Capsicum frutescens* L. (Synonym: *C. fastigiatum* BL., *C. annuum* L. var. *frutescens* sensu O. KUNTZE non L.). The wild form is a perennial, 0.5 to 1.5 m high subshrub with greenish or dull whitish petals and erect standing fruits that are about 1 to 3 cm long and 0.3 to 1.0 cm wide. Numerous cultivated forms of the plant are grown, some of which have considerably larger fruits. The wild form is native to the Amazon region, especially Guyana. Cultivation takes place from the USA to northern South America, in Africa (Nigeria, Kenya, Uganda) and Southeastern Asia (India, Pakistan, China, Thailand). To some extent, there are also plants in the wild that have escaped cultivation. The main exporting countries are China, Pakistan and India.

Constituents include 0.3 to 1.5% capsaicinoids, especially capsaicin (63 to 77%), dihydrocapsaicin (20 to 32%) and nordihydrocapsaicin (1 to 8%) [7, 41, 56, 59, Ü61, Ü93, Ü106]. For its uses, see above.

The following are the main commercially traded varieties, ripe or unripe, fresh and freshly pureed as well as dried whole, ground or crushed (range of heat levels in parenthesis): Aji pepper (7 to 8), Amatisa (7, also sold fresh), Anaheim (2 to 3, also sold fresh), Ancho (3 to 5, dried Poblano), Banana chili (2 to 3, also sold fresh), Casabel (4), Cayenne (8, variable pungency), Chawa (3 to 4, also sold fresh), Chilaca (3 to 4, Chile negro, also sold fresh), Chipotle (6, dried and smoked Jalapeno), Choricero (0 to 1), Fiesta (6 to 8), Fresno (6 to 7, also sold fresh), Guajillo (2 to 4), Güero (4 to 6, term used collectively for yellow chillies, also sold fresh or marinated), Guindilla (3), Guntur (5, also sold fresh), Habañero (10, also sold fresh), Huachinango (5 to 6, also sold fresh), Jalapeno (5 to 6, also sold fresh or marinated), Manzana (6 to 8, also sold fresh), Mulato (3), New Mexico (2 to 4, also sold fresh, trade names NuMex Big Jim, New Mexico No. 6 to 4, Espanola improved), Nyora (1 to 2), Poblano (3, labeled as Ancho when dried), Pasado (3, roasted, peeled), Pasilla (4, usually traded in powdered form), Rocotillo (7, also sold fresh), Red chillies (2 to 4), Serrano (7, also traded as Balin, Tipico, Largo, and Hidalgo), Tabasco (9, also sold fresh), Tepin (8, also sold fresh), Hungarian kirsch paprika (1 to 3) and Birdseye chillies (7 to 8, Thailand chili, Thai chili, also sold fresh) [Ü55, Ü73, Ü80]. For more varieties and details, see Lit. [83].

Whole fruits in vinegar are also commercially available: e.g. Jalapenò, Cherry paprika, Güero, Chili puree and Cayenne pepper (powder of dried, ground pungent fruits, e.g. of Birdseye chillies), as well as oleoresins of various varieties (Chipotle and Jalapeno, among others, water- or oil-soluble) [Ü55, Ü73].

Chillies are components of the following spice mixtures and preparations, among others: → Baharat, → Barbecue spice, → Cajun spice, → Chat masala, → Chili powder, → Chili sauce, → Cocktail sauce, → Curry powder, → Green masala, → Grill spice, → Harissa, → Ketchup, → Mélanche classique, → Mixed pickles spice, → Nam prik, → Pickling spice, → Sambal, → Sambhar powder, → Shichimi tograrashi, → Soup spice, → Tabasco sauce, → Tabil, → Zhug.

Habañero pepper, fruits of *Capsicum chinense* JACQ. (Closely related to *C. frutescens*, possibly a cultivated form of this species), also known as bonnet pepper, includes a great variety of forms of cultivated plants whose fruits have high capsaicin content. Cultivation takes place in the Americas from Mexico and Florida in the North to Bolivia, Chile and Brazil in the South. The fruits are used as chillies [Ü73].

Aji pepper (Peruvian pepper, Brown's pepper), fruits of *Capsicum baccatum* L. var. *pendulum* (WILLD.) ESHBAUGH (petals are white, each with 2 basal yellowish-green spots), is a cultivated plant, fruits 1.5 to 2.0 cm long, 4 mm wide, almost spherical yellow or red, grown in Argentina, Bolivia, Brazil, Chile, Japan, Columbia, Ecuador, Peru, Central Africa, USA, Hawaii, India, Japan and Europe. The very pungent fruits contain 0.1 to 0.25% capsaicinoids, of which the main constituents are capsaicin (32 to 66%) and dihydrocapsaicin (26 to 51%) [59], and is used the same as paprika, especially as a spice in hot Latin American dishes such as tamales, picadillo and chili con carne. Due to their thick flesh layer the fruits are very rarely dried, but frequently used in the preparation of paprika purée, spice pastes and spice sauces (e.g. Tabasco sauce) [Ü45, Ü61].

Tree pepper (Rocoto), fruits of *Capsicum pubescens* RUIZ ET PAV. (Petals are violet with a white center), only known in cultivation; grown in the mountains and highlands from Mexico to Southern Bolivia. It is used the same as paprika [41, Ü61] and contains 0.12 to 0.36% capsaicinoids, of which the main constituents are dihydrocapsaicin (49 to 54%), capsaicin (26 to 36%) and nordihydrocapsaicin (5 to 15%) [7, 59].

Obatzda

1 small onion, 200 g Camembert, 100 g cottage cheese, salt, black pepper, cayenne pepper, cumin, 1 teaspoon of sweet paprika, 1 tablespoon of freshly cut chives.

Dice the peeled onion into cubes. Squash the Camembert with a fork and incorporate it into the cottage cheese. Add the onion cubes and season with salt, black pepper and a pinch of cayenne, cumin as well as paprika. Place the obatzda in a small bowl and sprinkle with chives (or garnish with chopped walnuts and radish). Serve with freshly baked farmer's bread [Ü90].

Literature

[1] Agrawal R.C. et al., Int. J. Cancer 38: 689–695 (1986).

[2] Andrews J., Peppers, the Domesticated Capsicums, Univ. Texas Press, Austin 1984.

[3] Anonym, Dtsch. Apoth. Ztg. 137(13): 1027–1028 (1997).

[4] Anonym, Dtsch. Apoth. Ztg. 139(40): 3859 (1999).

[5] Balachandra B., V.M. Sivaramkrishnan, Indian J. Cancer 32(3):104–109 (1995).

[6] Baranyai M. et al., Acta Alimentaria 11:309–323 (1982).

[7] Becker H., Pharmazie i. u. Zeit 10:75–80 (1981).

[8] Bevan S., J. Szolcsanyi, TIPS 11/8: 330–333 (1990).

[9] Biacs P.A. et al., J. Agric. Food Chem. 37:350–353 (1989).

[10] Busker R.W., H.P. van Helden, Am. J. Forensic Med. Pathol. 19(4):309–316 (1998).

[11] Buttery R.G. et al., J. Agric. Food Chem. 17:1322–1327 (1968).

[12] Camara B., R. Monéger, Phytochemistry 17:91–93 (1978).

[13] Caterina M.J. et al., Nature 389(6653): 816–824 (1997).

[14] Cichewicz R.H., P.A. Thorpe, J. Ethnopharmacol. 52(2):61–70 (1996).

[15] Constant H.L., G.A. Cordell, J. Nat. Prod. 58(12):1925–1928 (1995).

[16] Constant H.L., G.A. Cordell, J. Nat. Prod. 59(4):425–426 (1996).

[17] Cooper T.H. et al., J. Agric. Food Chem. 39:225 (1991).

[18] Cserhati T. et al., J. Chromatogr. A896 (1/2):69–73 (2000).

[19] Czinkotai B. et al., J. Liquid Chromatogr. 12:2707–2717 (1989).

[20] Deli J., G. Toth, Z. Lebensm. Untersuch. Forsch. A205(5):388–391 (1997).

[21] Desai H.G. et al., Indian J. Med. Res. 66:440–448 (1977).

[22] DiCecco J.J., J. Assoc. Off. Anal. Chem. 59(1):1–4 (1976).

[23] DiSclafani A., J.K. Wilkin, Cutis 31:523–530 (1983).

[24] Diaz Barriga Arceo S. et al., Mutat. Res. 345(3/4):105–109 (1995).

[25] Ekandem G.J., Diss. Abstr. in B39:491, p. 116 (1978) ref. Ü37.

[26] Fekete M. et al., Z. Lebensm. Unters. Forsch. 161(1):31–33 (1976).

[27] Fisher C. et al., J. Agric. Food Chem. 35:55–57 (1987).

[28] Foti C. et al., Contact Dermatitis 37(3): 135 (1997).

[29] Glasl H., M. Ihrig, Pharm. Ztg. 129(11): 609–612 (1984).

[30] Goda Y. et al., Tennen Yuki Kagobutsu Toronkai Koen Yoshishu 38th:343–348 (1996), ref. CA 126:018000e.

[31] Govindarajan V.S., CRC Crit. Rev. Food Sci. Nutr. 24:245–355 (1986).

[32] Grushka E., P. Kapral, Separation Science 12(4):415 (1977).

[33] Heresch F., J. Jurenitsch, Chromatographia 12:647 (1979).

[34] Hernadez Qu. et al., Tecnol. Aliment 31(6):15–21 (1997), ref. CA 127:064838c

[35] Hoffmann P.G. et al., J. Agric. Food Chem. 31(6):1326–1330 (1983).

[36] Holló J. et al., Fette, Seifen, Anstrichmittel 59:1048–1049 (1957).

[37] Jancsó G., Nature 270:741–743 (1977).

[38] Jensen-Jarolim E. et al., Int. Arch. Allergy Immunol. 116(2):103–109 (1998).

[39] Jentzsch K. et al., Scientia pharmacol. (Wien) 38:50–58 (1969).

[40] Jurenitsch J., Sci. pharmaceut. 50:64–70 (1982).

[41] Jurenitsch J. et al., Planta Med. 35: 174–183 (1979).

[42] Jurenitsch J. et al., Planta Med. 36(1):61–67 (1979).

[43] Jurenitsch J, I. Kampelmühler, J. Chromatogr. 193:101–110 (1980).

[44] Jurentisch J. et al., Planta Med. 36(1):54–60 (1979).

[45] Jurentisch J. et al., Sci. pharmaceut. 46(4):307–318 (1978).

[46] Kang J.Y. et al., Dig. Dis. Sci. 40(3): 576–579 (1995).

[47] Keller U. et al., ACS Symp. Ser. No. 31, p. 137–146 (1982).

[48] Kim J.P. et al., Japan. J. Surg. 15:427–437 (1985).

[49] Kommision E beim BfArM, BAnz Nr. 22A vom 01.02.90.

[50] Kommission E beim BfArM, BAnz 80 vom 27.04.89.

[51] Leitner A. et al., Allergy 53(1):36–41 (1998).

[52] Lim K. et al., Med. Sci. Sports Exercise 29(3):355–361 (1997).

[53] Limlomwongse L. et al., J. Nutr. 109(5): 773–777 (1979).

[54] Loew D., Z. Phytother. 18(6):332–340 (1998).

[55] Lopez-Hernandez J. et al., Food Chem. 57(4):557–559 (1996).

[56] Lopez-Hernandez J. et al., Dtsch. Lebensm.-Rundsch. 92(12):393–395 (1996).

[57] Lynn B., Acta Physiol. Hung 69:287–294 (1987).

[58] Maillard M.N. et al., Riv. Ital. EPPOS (Spec. Num., 15th Journees Internat Huiles Essentielles): 577–582 (2997), ref. CA 128:012654r.

[59] Maillard M.N. et al., Flavour Fragrance J. 12(6):409–413 (1997).

[60] Makara G.B. et al., Acta Medica Hung XXI:213–216 (1965).

[61] Mateo J. et al., J. Food Compos. Anal. 10(3):225–232 (1997).

[62] Mathew A. et al., Eur. J. Cancer Prev. 9(2):89–97 (2000).

[63] Molina-Torres J. et al., J. Ethnopharmacol. 64(3):241–248 (1999).

[64] Myers B.M. et al., Am. J. Gastroenterol. 82(3):211–214 (1987).

[65] Nakamura A., H. Shiomi, Jpn. J. Pharmacol. 79(4):427–431 (1999).

[66] Neeck G. et al., Z. Phys. Med. Baln. Med. Klim. 16:383–388 (1987).

[67] Oberdieck R., Fleischwirtschaft 68:1086–1096 (1988).

[68] Park K.K. et al., Anticancer Res. 18(6A): 4201–4205 (1998).

[69] Parkes K.E.B. et al., Tetrahedron Lett.: 2535–2538 (1968).

[70] Platel K., K. Srinivasan, Int. J. Food Sci. Nutr. 47(1):55–59 (1996).

[71] Peusch M. et al., Lebensmittelchemie 50(5):112–115 (1996).

[72] Platel K., K. Srinivasan, Nahrung 44(1): 42–46 (2000).

[73] Polacsek-Racz M. et al., Z. Lebensm. Unters. Forsch. 172:115–117 (1981).

[74] Rangoonwala R., Dtsch. Apoth. Ztg. 109:273–274 (1969).

[75] Rangoonwala R., H. Friedrich, Naturwissenschaften 54:368 (1967).

[76] Sagara K. et al., Chem. Pharm. Bull. 28(9): 2796–2799 (1980).

[77] Sastre J. et al., Allergy 51(2):117–120 (1996).

[78] Scholz H., Natürlich 18(2):32–39 (1998).

[79] Siebert-Wellnhofer A., Dtsch. Apoth. Ztg. 138(48):4622–4624 (1998).

[80] Spanyar P., M. Blazovich, Analyst 94 (125): 1084–1089 (1969).

[81] Stahl E. (Hrsg.), Chromatographische und mikroskopische Analyse von Drogen, Fischer Verlag Stuttgart, New York 1978.

[82] Stahl E., L.J. Kraus, Arzneim. Forsch. 19:684 (1969).

[83] Steer, G., Chiliküche, 100 feurige Rezepte, Könemann Verlagsgesellschaft mbH, Köln 1996.

[84] Sticher O. et al., J. Chromatogr. 166: 221–231 (1978).

[85] Surh Y., Mutat. Res. 428(1/2):305–327 (1999).

[86] Surh Y.J. et al., Food Chem. Toxicol. 34(3):313–316 (1996).

[87] Surh Y.J. et al., Mutat. Res. 402(1/2): 259–267 (1996).

[88] Szallasi A., P.M. Blumberg, Pain 68(2,3): 195–208 (1996).

[89] Todd P. Jr. et al., J. Chromatogr. 13(12): 577–579 (1975).

[90] Todd P. Jr. et al., J. Food Sci. 42:660 (1977).

[91] Toth N.N., Anticancer Res. 4:117 (1984).

[92] Tschesche R., H. Gutwinski, Chem. Ber. 108(1):265–272 (1975).

[93] Vasudevan K. et al., Indian J. Gastroenterol. 19(2):53–56 (2000).

[94] Vega de la Osada F. et al., Med. Clin. (Barc) 111(7):263–266 (1998).

[95] Versper H., S. Nitz, Advance Food Science 19(3/4):124–130 (1997).

[96] Weissenberg M. et al., J. Chromatogr. A757(1/2):89–95 (1997).

[97] Williams S.R. et al., Ann. Emerg. Med. 25(5):713–715 (1995).

[98] Yahara S. et al., Phytochemistry 37(3): 831–835 (1994).

[99] Yeoh K.G. et al., Dig. Dis. Sci. 40(3): 580–583 (1995).

[100] Yoshioka M. et al., Br. J. Nutr. 82(2): 115–123 (1999).

Literature references identified by Ü can be found in the general listing of books and monographs at the back of this book.

Parsley

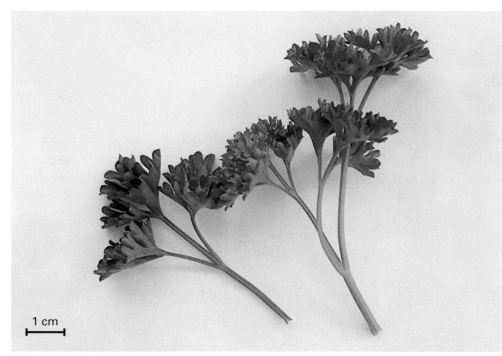

Fig. 1: Parsley leaf, curled-leaf form

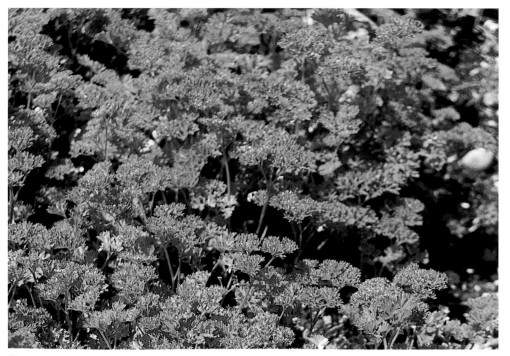

Fig. 2: Parsley (*Petroselinum crispum* (MILL.) NYM. ex A.W. HILL.), curled-leaf form

Plant source: *Petroselinum crispum* (MILL.) NYM. ex A.W. HILL.

Synonyms: *Petroselinum sativum* HOFFM., *Petroselinum hortense* auct. non HOFFM.

Taxonomic classification: The species can be subdivided as follows: *Petroselinum crispum* convar. *crispum* (Synonym: *P. c.* ssp. *foliosum* (ALEF.) THELL.), leaf- or cut parsley, with flat- or curled-leaf forms, *Petroselinum crispum* convar. *radicosum* (ALEF.) DANERT (Synonym: *P. c.* ssp. *tuberosum* BERNH. ex RCHB.), turnip-rooted parsley, Hamburg parsley.

Family: Umbelliferous plants (Apiaceae, synonym Umbelliferae).

Common names: Engl.: parsley; Fr.: persil, jaubert; Ger.: Petersilie, Garten-Petersilie, Garteneppich, Petersil, Peterle, Peterlein, Peterling, Peterli, Bittersilche, for turnip-rooted parsley Fr.: persil à grosse racine; Ger.: Wurzelpetersilie, Petersilienwurzel, Suppenwurzel.

Description: Biennial plant, about 60 to 120 cm in height, flowering not before the second year. *P. c.* convar. *radicosum* has a turnip-shaped root. The petiolate basal leaves are dark-green, in their contours triangular, 2- to 3-times pinnately divided, cartilaginous dentate, dependent on the cultivated form smooth or more or less crispate. Flowers are arranged in 10- to 20-rayed compound umbels with no or 1 to 3 involucres and only a few involucels. The small greenish yellow or reddish pruinose flowers are radiate, partly gynandrous, partly male, with 5 petals, 5 stamina, 2 styles and a two-chambered inferior ovary. The bipartite schizocarp fruit (diachene) disintegrates in 2 mericarps. Flowering period is from June to July.

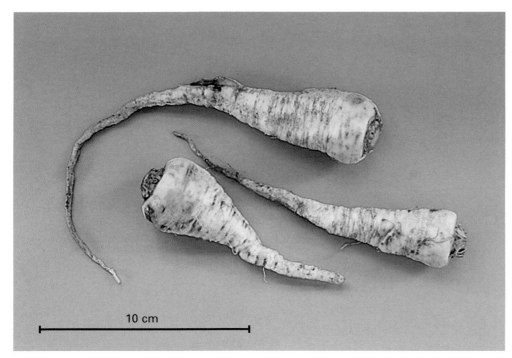

Fig. 3: Parsley root

Native origin: Southwestern Europe to Western Asia.

Main cultivation areas: All European countries, especially Germany, France, Russian Federation, and the Balkan States, as well as Northern- and Eastern Africa, Asia (India, Malaysia, Indonesia, China, Philippines), and America (Chile, Argentina, Brazil, USA).

Main exporting countries: The fresh leaf material that is used in Germany originates almost exclusively from domestic cultivation. Parsley root also comes from the Czech Republic, Slovakia, and Hungary, and the dried leaf predominantly from France.

Cultivation: Parsley prefers deep, humus rich, damp soil in sunny or half shaded locations. Seeds can be sown in March, spaced at 25 to 30 cm apart. The soil cover should not be more than 1 cm. Later, leaf parsley must be thinned to 10 to 15 cm apart in the row, and root parsley to 25 cm apart. Due to self-incompatibility parsley should not be sown for more than one season in the same location. Because the sprouts do not emerge until about 4 to 8 weeks, in order to carry out weeding a companion marker crop is useful, e.g. radishes or spinach. Soaking the fruits for 24 hours in warm water before sowing should accelerate germination. For domestic use, sowing in the autumn is also possible in our latitude. During drought parsley must be irrigated. The first cut is possible in June, and additional cuts can follow in August and October. For one's personal demand, parsley can be continuously harvested, even in the winter, with careful protection of the basal leaves, if one covers the plants with foil or conifer prunings. Cultivation in a flowerpot is sensible, especially for winter use. Parsley root is harvested in October or November. Varieties of the flat-leaf cut parsley that are permitted for cultivation in Germany include 'Hamburger Schnitt', 'Festival 68' and 'Gigante d Italia', of the curled-leaf varieties are, among others, 'Mooskrause 2', 'Bravour', 'Clivi', 'Curlina', 'Darki', 'Decora', 'Gekrulde/Triplex', 'Frisé vert foncé', 'Grüne Perle' and 'Kruse', of the turnip-rooted parsley varieties are 'Halblange/-Perfecta' and 'Halblange/Berliner' [Ü14, Ü17, Ü21, Ü41, Ü46, Ü86].

Culinary herb

Commercial forms: Parsley leaf: dried, sometimes freeze-dried, whole or rubbed leaves, deep-frozen, chopped leaves; Parsley root: cut or ground, dried roots, in the fresh produce trade the fresh leaves, rarely also the whole fresh roots, alone or as a component of so-called soup greens; Parsley seed oleoresin.

Production: The harvest of the leaves is carried with a loader-combine with conveyer or with a spinach combine-harvester, for the fresh market the leaves are hand harvested. The roots are dug with an elevator digger or with a trough-uprooter. For medicinal purposes, the roots may also be harvested in the spring after overwintering [Ü21, Ü41].

Forms used: The fresh, frozen or rarely also dried leaves of *P. c.* convar. *crispum*, whole or chopped or cut (the leaves of convar. *radicosum* can be used as well, but have a less characteristic aroma), the fresh or dried root of *P. c.* convar. *radicosum*.

Storage: The fresh leaves with the attached, cut stems can be kept immersed in water or wrapped in wet paper-towels for a few days or plastic bags, at –1 to +2 °C up to 8 weeks in the refrigerator. The leaves, after the stalks have been removed, can also be finely cut, frozen with water in the ice-tray stored for 9 to 12 months. Frozen parsley, however, is less flavorful than the fresh herb. Also, frozen parsley turns flaccid after it has been thawed and is therefore no longer suitable for garnishing. Drying of the leaves leads to a considerable aroma loss and is not recommended. The fresh roots can be stored in a sufficiently ventilated area with a relative humidity of 60 to 95%, at 2 to 7 °C for 6 months. The dried roots are stored in well-closed metal- or glass containers, protected from light and moisture.

Description.

Leaf (Fig. 1 and 4): For the fresh leaves, see description of the whole plant. The

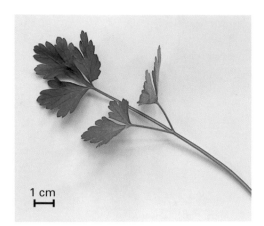

Fig. 4: Parsley leaf, flat-leaf form

dried leaves mostly consist of leaf fragments from which the coarse stem pieces have been removed. The epidermis on both leaf surfaces is undulate-sinuate, only straight-walled above the nerves, axially stretched with distinctly striated cuticula; anomocytic stomata can be found in lower epidermis. Trichomes are absent. **Odor** and **Taste:** Characteristically spicy.

Root (Fig. 3): Fresh roots yellowish, carrot-shaped, with yellowish-white to reddish-yellow cross section, up to 20 cm long, up to 5 cm wide at the top; the cut, dried root consists of yellowish-white to reddish-yellow pieces or strips with roughly wrin-

kled surface and sometimes fine, brown-striated transverse girdling; in the bark, dark-brown and shiny oil cells are present, the xylem is lemon-yellow on the outside and white on the inside. The bark and the xylem show radial striations due to the brown medullary rays. **Odor:** Characteristically aromatic, **Taste:** Sweetish, somewhat pungent.

History: Parsley has been known in Mediterranean region for about 2000 years, where it was cultivated first and foremost as a medicinal plant; the Greeks also used it for ritual purposes. Hippocrates (466 to 375 BCE) and his students recommended it as a diuretic. The Romans introduced parsley to Central Europe. In a government decree by Karl the Great, "Capitulare de villis" (authored in about 795 CE, see footnote → Anise), its cultivation was made mandatory. In England, it has only been cultivated since the 16th century [Ü92, for history and mythology Ü86, Ü97].

Constituents and Analysis

Constituents of the leaf

- Essential oil: 0.02 to 0.9%, the main components are the phenyl propane derivatives myristicine and apiol (to-

gether up to 80%, myristicine mostly dominating) and monoterpenes, particularly β-phellandrene (2 to 12%), p-mentha-1,3,8-triene (up to 50% in the flat-leaf form, and less in the curled-leaf varieties) and 4-isopropenyl-1-methyl-benzene (about 7%), which all contribute to the odor. Also present are, among others, α- and β-pinene, myrcene, α-phellandrene, p-cymenene and terpinolene, as well as small amounts of sesquiterpenes (up to 4%), including (E)-β-farnesene, germacrene D and angelic acid esters (crispan, crsipanone). Although only occurring in very low concentrations, the following substances also contribute to the typical parsley odor: e.g. methyl-2-methyl-butanoate, oct-1-en-3-one, (Z)-octa-1,5-diene-3-one, 2-(p-tolyl)propane-2-ol, 2-isopropenyl-3-methoxypyrazine, 2-sec-butyl-3-methoxypyrazine, p-mentha-1,3,8-triene, (Z)-dec-6-enal, deca-2(E),4(E)-dienal, myrcene, linalool, citronellol and β-ionone [2, 9, 12, 16, 17, 25, 26, 28, 31]. The cabbage-like note is due to dimethyldisulfide, methyl-propanal, 2- and 3-methylbutanal, respectively. The hay-like scent upon drying of the leaves is caused by the formation of 3-methylnona-2,4-dione [20].

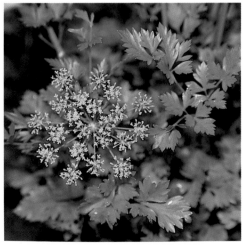

Fig. 5: Parsley (*P. crispum* (MILL.) NYM. ex A.W. HILL.), flat-leaf form with inflorescence

Myristicine

Apiol

β-Phellandrene

p-Mentha-1,3,8-triene

4-Isopropenyl-1-methylbenzene

- Flavonoids: 1.9 to 6.6%, with the main component apiin (apigenin-7-O-(6-O-apiosyl)glucoside), furthermore luteolin-7-apiosylglucoside, apigenin-7-glucoside, 6''-acetylapiin, isorhamnetin-3,7-diglucoside, chrysoeriol-7-apiosylglucoside, among others [11, 24, 35].
- Furanocoumarins: Up to 0.2%, the main components are oxypeucedanin and bergaptene (5-methoxypsoralene), as well as xanthotoxin (8-methoxypsoralene), psoralene, imperatorin and isopimpinellin [1, 3, 5, Ü100].
- Vitamins: Vitamin C (0.12 to 0.4%, calculated with reference to the fresh leaves), among others [8, 18, 27].

Constituents of the root

- Essential oil: In *P. c.* convar. *radicosum* 0.1 to 0.3%, the main components of the steam-distilled essential oil are β-pinene (21 to 40%), β-phellandrene (7 to 14%), apiol (15 to 42%) and myristicine (5 to 15%); in the essential oil obtained by extraction polyines (see below) dominate. *P. c.* convar. *crispum* contains 0.2 to 0.75% essential oil with the main components terpinolene (7 to 43%), β-pinene (4 to 30%), apiol (20 to 57%) and myristicine (4 to 21%); also present are small amounts of elemicin and other mono- as well as sesquiterpenes [9, 10, 31].
- Flavonoids: 0.2 to 1.6% with the main component apiin [32].
- Coumarin derivatives: Up to 0.1%, the main components are oxypeucedanin and, among others, bergaptene, imperatorin, isopimpinellin and xanthotoxin [3, 5].
- Phthalides: Ligustilide, senkyunolide, butylphthalide (very low concentrations but also contributing to the odor) [10].
- Polyines: Falcarinol and falcarindiol, in the essential oil obtained by extraction with diethylether 30 and 9%, respectively [4, 23].

The fruits contain 1 to 6% essential oil; the main components, depending on the race, are apiol, myristicine or 1-allyl-2,3,4,5-tetramethoxybenzene. The essential oil is only used rarely, e.g. for the manufacturing of spice essences in the food industry.

Tests for Identity: With organoleptic, macroscopic and microscopic examination as well as with the following analytical methods:

Herb: TLC [BHP 90, described in lit. Ü37], HPLC [32, described in lit. Ü37] and TLC [Ü101], GC [Ü37] or, after obtaining the essential oil, with GC/MS and FID-GC, respectively [17].

Root: TLC [32, AB-DDR, described in lit. Ü37] and, after obtaining the essential oil, with TLC [Ü101] or GC [Ü37].

Quantitative assay: As described in the European Pharmacopoeia the content of essential oil can be determined volumetrically with steam distillation and xylol in the graduated tube [Ph Eur]. The flavonoid content is analyzed with HPLC [described in Lit. Ü37].

Adulterations, Misidentifications and Impurities: Adulteration of the leaves from the flat-leaf parsley variety with fool's parsley, *Aethusa cynapium* L. (considered poisonous), or with the leaves of the poison hemlock (*Conium maculatum* L.) have been documented. The foliage leaves from dog parsley have a lighter colored lower surface and smell disagreeable upon rubbing; the flowers have white petals and 3 noticeable, secund, outward weeping, relatively long involucels. The stalk of poison hemlock has mostly brownred spots, the leaves have a disagreeable smell upon rubbing, the petals are white and the involucre is polyphyllous. Parsley roots are sometimes confused with those of parsnip. In contrast to parsnip, the cortex of parsley root takes on a red color upon contact with $FeSO_4$ solution [Ü106].

Actions and Uses

Actions: On the basis of its essential oil content, parsley is supposed to promote the secretion of bile and gastric juices and thereby good digestion.

According to older studies in mice and rats the essential oil of parsley has diuretic action [19]. A diuretic and spasmolytic

effect of the flavonoids has been postulated and is quite probable [13, Ü37].

In rat brain homogenates, extracts of parsley leaves were able to inhibit lipid peroxidation [7]. With the addition of parsley to food over a 2-week period in humans, the activity of oxygen free radical inactivating enzymes (glutathione reductase, superoxide dismutase) was increased [22].

In estrogen-dependent tumor cells, methanolic extracts of parsley demonstrated estrogenic effects. Additionally, oral application of the extracts could restore the uterus weight reduced after ovariectomy. It has been postulated that apigenin (EC_{50}, i.e. growth increase of estrogen-dependent cells by 50% = 1.0 μM) is an active principle. With regard to estrogenic effects, in this model apigenin and also diosmetin (2.9 μM) as well as kaempferol (0.56 μM) were comparable to the isoflavone glycosides of soybeans (genistein 0.60 μM, daidzein 0.61 μM) [35].

In animal experiments with mice, myristicine strongly inhibited benz[a]pyrene-induced tumor genesis. The inhibition probably takes place through stimulating the production of detoxification enzymes (glutathione-S-transferase) in the liver and in the small intestine mucosa [36].

Freeze-dried parsley leaves have shown an antibacterial effect in quantities of 0.12 to 8% in agar, e.g. inhibiting the growth of *E. coli*, *Listeria monocytogenes*, *Listeria innocua* and *Erwinia carotovora*, but not of *Pseudomonas fragi* [18].

Toxicology: Based on existing data, there is no acute or chronic toxicity with normal dosages of parsley leaves and root as a spice. Parsley fruits should not be used as a spice due to the high levels of phenyl propane derivatives, which are toxic in high doses.

Based on older research, myristicine (0.01 to 0.05 ml/l), apiol (50 to 100 mg/l) and the essential oil from parsley fruits increased the tonus and triggered contractions in isolated guinea-pig uterus [6]. These effects explain the use of parsley fruits and parsley oil as an abortifacient [21, Ü100]. At high doses (such as in abortion attempts), the essential oil of parsley is acutely toxic, leading to gastroenteritis, headache, kidney and liver damage, shock and coma [Ü100]. Due to the low levels of essential oil in the leaves and roots, such effects can be excluded if parsley is used as a spice [14].

The plant has a low sensitization potential. Allergic reactions are possible though, particularly in individuals who show allergic reactions upon contact with other umbelliferous plants (e.g. celery, carrots and caraway) or with the composite mugwort (celery-mugwort-spice-syndrome) [29, 34]. In housewives and garden workers, photodermatosis due to furanocoumarins was observed after intense contact with the fresh plant [30, Ü39].

Culinary use: Parsley is used in all temperate zones of the world. In German cooking, it is undoubtedly the most commonly used kitchen herb. In Turkey, parsley omelets are very popular, in the Near East tabbouleh, a salad made from shredded wheat and parsley. In Italy, parsley is an indispensable component of Ossobuco alla Milanese (Milan veal shank) and in France of Omelette Fines Herbes.

Because the flat-leaf parsley has an essentially stronger aroma than the curled-leaf forms, its culinary use is preferred. The chopped, fresh leaves of the curled-leaf varieties should be added to cooked dishes just prior to serving because they will lose their aroma during cooking. The leaves of the flat-leaf varieties are often cooked with the meal. Parsley leaf stalks can also be used as to spice. They are bundled and added at the start of cooking and removed before serving. Parsley root can also be cooked with the food. The leaves of the curled-leaf varieties are used especially as a garnish (e.g. for cold meat plates, sausage plates or light à la carte dishes). Parsley leaves can be used to season almost all strong, salty cooked dishes: In white sauces (e.g. for steamed fish), broths, soups, stews, meat-, fish-, poultry-, vegetable-, potato-, rice and noodle dishes, crustaceans, mushrooms and dumplings (e.g. parsley dumplings, bread dumplings, semolina dumplings). Likewise, parsley can be added to braised meat in the frying

pan or, it can be rapidly fried in hot butter until crispy and added to grilled or pan-fried meat. It is also suitable as an accompaniment to salads (e.g. tomato salad), cheeses (soft cheese, cottage cheese), herb butter, ground meat, fillings (for chicken, duck, goose), soufflés, egg dishes (e.g. omelets), quark and, alone or mixed with chopped chives, as a topping of buttered breads [Ü13, Ü33, Ü51, Ü79, Ü91, Ü95].

It is recommended to deep-fry parsley leaf stalks in oil and serve with seafood [Ü51] or to eat them baked in wine batter [Ü90]. Fresh parsley roots are used raw in salads grated or, added before cooking as a seasoning of soups and stews. In cooked, pureed form, they are well suited as a flavoring of potato puree. Parsley root is also eaten on its own as a vegetable cut into slices (especially in Great Britain) or cooked together with other vegetables. Leeks, celery tubers and carrots make up so-called soup greens. Herb soup mixes contain the dried root [Ü55, Ü70, Ü74].

Combines well with: Borage, chervil, chives, cress, dill, garlic, lemon balm, onions, and pepper.

As a component of spice mixes and preparations: → Baking spice, → Bouquet garni, → Café de Paris spice mix, → Cocktail sauce, → Fines herbes, → Fish spice, → Frankfurter green sauce, → Gremolata, → Herb butter, → Herb salt, → Meat spice, → Parsley butter, → Persillade, → Quark spice, → Ravigotte, → Salad spice, → Sauce spice, → Soup greens, → Tartar sauce, → Vegetable spice.

Other uses: The essential oil is used in the perfume industry.

Medicinal herb

Herbal drugs: Petroselini radix, Parsley root [EB 6], Petroselini herba, Parsley herb.

Indications: For diseases of the lower urinary tract and for prevention of renal gravel, it is used in the context of irrigation

therapy [14]. It is prepared in the form of aqueous infusions of the dried herb or of the dried cut root (2 g / cup of tea, the daily dose is 6 g of the dried herb or root) as well as in the form of liquid extracts (also dry extracts: flavonoids as the primary active principles) as a component of prepared medicines. An ample intake of fluids must be observed with its use. It is contraindicated in pregnancy, inflammatory kidney diseases and edema caused by impaired cardiac or renal function [14].

In folk medicine, parsley herb and root are used as a remedy for the treatment of flatulence and of menstrual difficulties. (The therapeutic use of parsley fruit was not approved by the Commission E of Germany's BfArM because of insufficient evidence of efficacy and possible risks [15]).

Similar culinary herbs

Honewort (Japanese parsley), *Cryptotaenia canadensis* (L.) DC. ssp. *japonica* (HASSK.) HAND.-MAZZ. (Apiaceae), is native to Japan, Korea and China, where it is cultivated as well as in Indonesia.

Italian Parsley Spaghetti
500 g spaghetti, 1 onion, 2 garlic cloves, 7 tablespoons olive oil, 2 bundles of parsley (flat variety), 300 ml white wine, salt, pepper, 50 g butter, Parmesan cheese to sprinkle on top.

Boil the spaghetti in a sufficient amount of water for about 8 minutes or until al-dente. Meanwhile finely chop the onion and garlic cloves and sauté in olive oil. Wash the parsley, spot dry with a towel and slightly shake. Place 2/3 of the parsley into the pan with the oil, add the white wine and let the sauce thicken to half of its volume; season to taste. Mix the well-drained spaghetti with butter, sauce and the remaining parsley. Before serving, sprinkle with Parmesan cheese [Ü91].

Its essential oil contains, among other components, pinene, limonene, dimethyl sulfide, methylethyl sulfide, α- and β-selinene, cuparene and eremophilene [Ü43]. The leaves and stems are used in Japan similarly as parsley; the bleached stems are also used as a vegetable [Ü61].

Literature

[1] Ashraf M. et al., Pakistan J. Sci. Ind. Res. 23:&hsp’;128–129 (1980).

[2] Bauermann U. et al., Drogenreport 6(10): 24–30 (1993).

[3] Baumann U. et al., Mit. Geb. Lebensm. Hyg. 79:112–129 (1988).

[4] Bohlmann F., Chem. Ber. 100:3454–3456 (1967).

[5] Chaudhary S.K. et al., Planta Med. 52: 462–464 (1986).

[6] Christomanos A.A., Arch. Exp. Pathol. Pharmakol. 123:252–258 (1927).

[7] Fejes S. et al., Phytother. Res. 14(5): 362–365 (2000).

[8] Feldheim W., Dtsch. Apoth. Ztg. 139(15): 1552–1557 (1999).

[9] Franz C., H. Glasl, Qualitas Plantarum – Plant Foods Hum. Nutr. 24:175–182 (1974).

[10] Gijbels M.J.M. et al., Fitoterapia 56:17 (1985).

[11] Grisebach H., W. Bilhuber, Z. Naturforsch. 22b:746–751 (1967).

[12] Jung H.P. et al., Lebensm. Wiss. Technol. 25:55–60 (1992).

[13] Kaczmarek F. et al., Roslin Leczinczych 8:111–117 (1968), ref. CA 68:14589g.

[14] Kommission E beim BfArM., BAnz-Nr. 43 vom 02.03.89.

[15] Kommission E beim BfArM., BAnz-Nr. 43 vom 02.03.89.

[16] Lawrence B.M., Perfum. Flavorist 6:43–48 (1982), 11:78–80 (1986) und 16:81–83 (1990).

[17] MacLeod A.J. et al., Phytochemistry 24(11):2623–2627 (1985).

[18] Manderfeld M.M. et al., J. Food Prot. 60(1):72–77 (1997).

[19] Marri R., Chem. Zbl. 1:562 (1944).

[20] Masanetz C., Grosch W., Z. Lebensm. Unters. Forsch. A. 206(2):114–120 (1998).

[21] Mele V., Folia Med. 51:601–613 (1968).

[22] Nielsen S.E. et al., Br. J. Nutr. 81(6):447–455 (1999).

[23] Nitz S. et al., J. Agric. Food Chem. 38: 1445–1447 (1990).

[24] Nordström K. et al., Chemistry Industry 85 (1953).

[25] Pino J.A. et al., J. Ess. Oil Res. 9(2):241–242 (1997).

[26] Porter N.G., Flavour Fragrance 4:207–219 (1989).

[27] Scheunert A., E. Theile, Pharmazie 7:776–780 (1952).

[28] Spraul M.H. et al., Chem. Mikrobiol. Technol. Lebensm. 13:178 (1991).

[29] Stäger J. et al., Allergy 46:475–478 (1991).

[30] Stransky L. et al., Contact Dermatitis 6(3):233–234 (1980).

[31] Warncke D., Z. Phytother. 15(1):50–58 (1994).

[32] Warncke D., K.H. Kubeczka: Posterpräsentation, 35. Jahrestagung der Ges. für Arzneiplanzenforsch., Leiden Niederlande 1987, ref. Ü37.

[33] Weymar H., Buch der Doldengewächse, Neumann Verlag, Radebeul 1959.

[34] Wüthrich B., T. Hofer, Dtsch. Med. Wschr. 109:981–986 (1984).

[35] Yoshikawa M. et al., Chem. Pharm. Bull. 48(7):1039–1044 (2000).

[36] Zheng G.Q. et al., J. Agric. Food Chem. 40(1):107 (1992).

Literature references identified by Ü can be found in the general listing of books and monographs at the back of this book.

Pepper

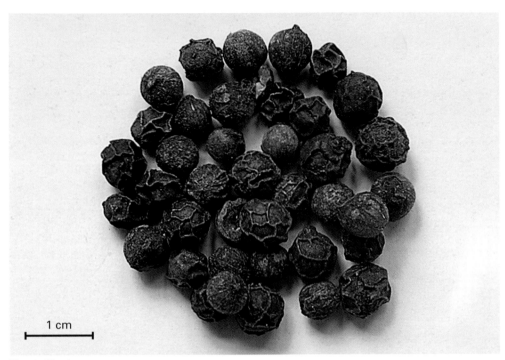

Fig. 1: Black pepper

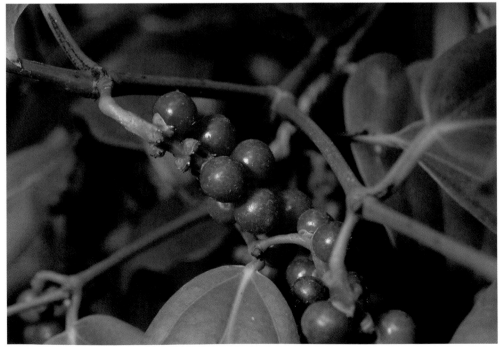

Fig. 2: Pepper (*Piper nigrum* L.)

Plant source: *Piper nigrum* L.

Synonym: *Piper aromaticum* LAM.

Taxonomic classification: Numerous cultivated taxa are in existence, which are differentiated, among other considerations, by their number of chromosomes, habitus, size and shape of the leaves, infructescences and fruits as well as by their aroma and pungency. A new US-American variety, Charleston Hot, is 25-times as pungent as typical pepper [Ü61, Ü92].

Family: Pepper family (Piperaceae).

Common names: Engl.: black pepper, white pepper, green pepper; Fr.: poivre noir, poivre blanc, poivre vert; Ger: Pfeffer, schwarzer Pfeffer, weißer Pfeffer, grüner Pfeffer, Pfefferkorn.

Description: Climber, diameter of the lignified stalks in the lower part about 2 cm, nodes with adventitious roots, climbing up to 10 m. Foliage leaves alternate, entire-margined, the lower ones roundish-ovate, the upper ones oblong-ovate, acuminate, 7 to 18 cm in length, 5 to 10 cm in breadth. Up to 50 flowers are arranged in 5 to 16 cm long hanging spikes. Cultivated forms have inconspicuous unisexual flowers without perianth, with 2 stamina, a unilocular ovary with 5 stigmata but no stylus. The pollination is carried out by the wind or by self-fertilization. The one-seeded ripe fruits are red [Ü76, Ü89].

Native origin: Probably in the spur of the Himalayas (Assam, Myanmar) and/or Southwestern India (Malabar Coast), widely distributed throughout tropical Asia.

Main cultivation areas: India (Malabar Coast, especially in the State of Kerala),

Indonesia (especially in Kalimantan, Sumatra, and Bangka), Malaysia (Sarawak = Administrative Province of Northwest Kalimantan), Brazil (especially in Pará Province), China (Taiwan, Southern Provinces), Thailand (Districts of Thon and Buri), and Sri Lanka (Dunbara-Valley, Matale District), furthermore cultivated in Myanmar, Cambodia, Laos, Vietnam, New Guinea, on many of the Pacific Islands, the Antilles, Madagascar, Zanzibar, and in West Africa (Ghana to Angola) [51].

Main exporting countries: Indonesia, Malaysia, Brazil, Madagascar, China, Sri Lanka, Thailand, Vietnam, and India.

Cultivation: Pepper is a tropical plant. It thrives in aqueous, but well-drained, humus-rich soil near the coast with high atmospheric humidity, constant temperatures and about 2500 mm of rainfall spread out as evenly as possible throughout the year. Propagation through seeds is complex and does not result in uniform plant material, therefore it is carried out almost exclusively by stem cuttings. With propagation by stem cutting the first harvest is possible after 3 to 4 years, with propagation by seeds the first harvest is considerably later. After 7 to 8 years the peak harvest is attained. After 15 to 20 years, the yield decreases. The plants are usually replaced after the 10th year. To facilitate climbing the cuttings are set out near wooden posts, wire netting or trees. The plants are kept at 3 to 5 m tall by pruning. Because it is a costly and labor-intensive crop to maintain and harvest (pruning, soil husbandry, hand harvest), it is mostly grown on small plantations, so-called pepper gardens [64, Ü89].

Culinary herb

Commercial forms. Black pepper: harvested unripe, dried fruits, usually named according to their origin or to the port from which they are shipped as, among other designations, Tellicherry-, Goa-, Aleppi- or Malabar-pepper (India), Lampong-pepper (Indonesia), Cambodia-pepper, Sarawak-pepper (Malaysia) and Brazilian-pepper, **White pepper:** harvested ripe, fruits with the outer part of the pericarp removed, Muntok- as well as Batavia-pepper (Indonesia), Brazilian-pepper (Belem pepper) and Sarawak-pepper, among others, **Green pepper:** harvested unripe, air-dried, freeze-dried, quick-frozen or fruits preserved in brine, **Decorticated black pepper:** peeled black pepper, **Red pepper:** fruits harvested when mature (rarely exported, not to be confused with Pink pepper, **Pepper-oleoresin:** pepper extracts, from white or black pepper, using ethanol and/or acetone as solvents, and **Pepper essential oil.**

Production: During harvesting the spikes are cut off or pinched off by hand. Ripe fruits that have dropped to the ground are gathered up. At what stage of ripeness the fruits are harvested and into which commercial form they will be processed is often dependent on the tradition in the region where they were grown

Black pepper: Produced by harvesting the whole spikes when the lowest fruits begin to turn red. After harvesting the berries are often dipped in boiling water for a few minutes. Then they are dried during the day on mats or drying surfaces, and in the evenings they are raked together and covered with canvas. Afterwards the fruits are separated from the rachis by rubbing over sieves, hitting with sticks or stepping on them with bare feet, screened and packed into sacks. In the production of black pepper, cell mortification occurs through the treatment with hot water, which, subsequently leads to enzyme-catalyzed reactions, especially to oxidation and spontaneous polymerization of the orthodiphenolic constituents, e.g. of the 3,4-dihydroxyphenylethanolglycosides, their aglycone and 3,4-dihydroxy-6-(N-ethyl amino)-benzamide by o-diphenoloxidase to black polymers [7, 77].

Decorticated black pepper: Produced by removing the skin of black pepper in a machine [51, Ü89].

Green pepper: Obtained from fruits that are harvested almost mature, but still green, and after separation from the rachis they are preserved immediately in brine (sodium chloride, 7 to 9%, acidified with vinegar or citric acid) or in vinegar. Lyophilized or dried green fruits (obtained partially from preserved peppers, partially by classical drying) are also commercially available, whole or ground.

Red pepper: Obtained from the mature fruits in the same manner as green pepper.

White pepper: Obtained from the mature fruits. The fruits are separated from the rachis, filled into sacks and placed into cold, preferably flowing water until about 7 to 10 days after which the outer skin (exocarp and mesocarp) dissolves from the endocarp. By rubbing, threshing or processing with a decorticator the pulp is loosened and under running water it is washed off. Afterwards they are dried on mats or on a cement floor.

Forms used: Dried pepper corns, whole, cracked or ground, whole fresh or preserved fruits.

Storage: Dried peppercorns can be stored for a long time in airtight, opaque porcelain- or glass containers, protected from light and moisture. Ground pepper loses its aroma very quickly during storage. Pickled green or red pepper should be stored in the refrigerator after opening of the containers.

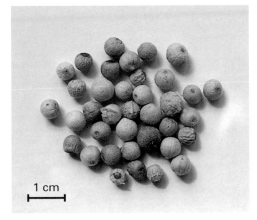

Fig. 3: White pepper

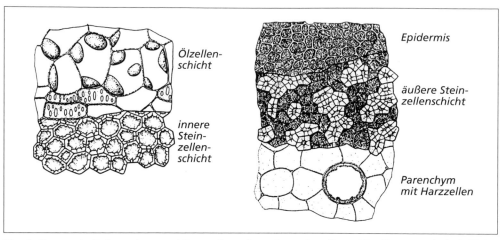

Fig. 4: Pepper. Left: inner layers of the pericarp in surface view (found in all pepper fruits). Right: outer layers of the pericarp in surface view (only in black, red and green pepper). From Ü29.

Description. Whole fruit:

Black pepper (Fig. 1): Dark-brown to black, globose, coarsely rugose, diameter 3 to 6 mm, sometimes crowned with remains of the stigmas at the apex. The thin pericarp consists of the epidermis with thick cuticula, which covers the small polygonal cells with dark brown content, the hypoderm (outer layer with square shaped to radially elongated stone cells, interrupted by parenchymatic cells), a layer of large-celled, parenchymatic tissue with scattered resin cells and few stone cells, a layer of small parenchymatic cells with vascular bundles, the layer of oil cells and the endocarp (inner, continuous layer of stone cells). The pericarp encloses and is fused to the seed (see below, white pepper) [Ü29].

Green pepper: Fruits globose, diameter 3 to 7 mm, light green when fresh, dark green if pickled in salt brine, smooth, rugose when dried.

Red pepper: Fruits red, globose, diameter 3 to 7 mm.

White pepper (Fig. 3): Gray-white to pale gray-yellow, globose, smooth, diameter 2 to 5 mm. The seed is covered with the remains of the pericarp that consists of an inner stone cell ring and the zone with vascular bundles (see above); the rest of this zone shows the vascular bundles extending from top to bottom. The seed contains a large starch-filled mealy perisperm, hollow on the inside, with a horn-like outer surface; situated at the pointed end is the starch-free endosperm with embryo [EB 6].

Powdered fruit:

White pepper: Pale gray-yellow powder. The chloral hydrate preparation is characterized by interconnected polygonal stone cells of the endocarp, thickened all around, and shreds of the parenchymatic tissue with pieces of the oil cell layer (Fig. 4, left). The hydrated mount shows the prominent shreds of perisperm with tightly filled starch cells and free or aggregated, small starch grains [Ü29, EB 6].

Black pepper: Dirty gray powder, with the same tissue parts as white pepper, but also containing fragments of the exocarp, particularly dark brown fragments from the outer layer of stone cells, which never form a continuous layer but are scattered in clustered groups (Fig. 4, right and left) [Ü29].

Odor: Spicy, **Taste:** Spicy, in black pepper strongly spicy and in green or white pepper, less pungent.

History: Pepper was already mentioned 3000 years ago in old Indian texts. It was also used in the Mediterranean regions during antiquity and was especially valued by the Romans and Greeks. It first reached Europe through Arab and Phoenician merchants. The occupation of Egypt by the Romans (30 BCE) opened the trade routes for Roman traders to India and Malaysia. An important trading center for the Romans was what is now Aden in Yemen and later also Adulis (now Zula) in Ethiopia. In contrast to the (West) Roman Empire, the Byzantine Empire traded pepper via overland route (e.g. silk route). It is likely that long pepper (see below) was first preferred for import but later black pepper was also traded, which was less expensive at that time. After the fall of the Byzantine Empire, the coastal cities of Italy, in particular Venice, were taking over the pepper trade with the Orient. The search for a sea-route to the pepper-producing countries was a main motive for the European powers to explore the oceans to the east and west. At the end of the 14th century, the Portuguese started to dominate the pepper trade, followed by Holland in the 16th century. It was not until the 18th century, when the Dutch spice trade monopoly was broken up by the British and French [8, 51, 63, Ü89, Ü97].

Constituents and Analysis

DIN- and ISO-Standards: DIN-Standard 10200-1 (Black and white pepper, technical specifications), DIN-Standard 10200-2 (Black and white pepper, determination of the number of light berries), DIN-Standard 10200-3 (Black and white pepper, determinations of nitrogen content in methylene chloride extract, Kjeldahl-method), ISO 959-1 (Black pepper, whole or ground), ISO 959-2 (White pepper, whole or ground), ISO 5564 (Black and white pepper, determination of piperine content), ISO 10621 (Dehydrated green pepper), and DIN/ISO 11027 (Black and white pepper, determination of piperine content using HPLC).

Constituents

- Essential oil: In black pepper 1.2 to 3.9%, in white pepper 1.0 to 3.8%. The ratios of the different components significantly depend on the type of cultivar, the climate conditions and harvest methods [50, 61]. The main components can be β-caryophyllene (12 to 47%), α-pinene (2 to 25%), sabinene (0 to 25%), (+)-limonene (9 to 23%), Δ³-carene (0.1 to 20%), β-pinene (2 to 15%), α-phellandrene (0.1 to 10%) and myrcene (0 to 8%). Also present may be α- and γ-terpinene, terpinolene, p-cymene, β-bisabolene, α-caryophyllene, caryophyllene epoxide, δ-elemene, α-copaene, α-caryophyllene (humulene), δ-cadinene, terpinenol-4, pinocarveol, myrtanol and safrole, among others [12, 18, 19, 23, 24, 38, 39, 47, 54, 75, 80].

- Acid amides: 5 to 10%, especially piperine (4.5 to 7.5%, *all-trans*, pungent tasting, light exposure causes isomerization into the tasteless *cis-trans*-diene isochavicin; also present are, among others, piperyline (trichostachine), piperatinine (4,5-dihydropiperine), piperolein A and B, piperide, piperettine and guineensine, as well as analogs with methoxy-groups at the aromatic ring, such as piperlongumine, with only one hydroxy-group, in cumaperine, or with one hydroxy- and one methoxy-group, in feruperine and dihydroferuperine [25, 27, Ü43]. Aliphatic acid amides (alkamides) also occur in pepper fruits, e.g. *N*-isobutyl-octadeca-*trans*-2-*cis*-4-dienamide (pipericine) and *N*-isobutyl-eicosa-*trans*-2-*trans*-4-dienamide [19, 57, 69].

- Flavonoids: Kaempferol-, rhamnetin- and quercetin glycosides [79].

- Fatty oil: 6 to 10%, which include, besides the usual fatty acids, vernolic, malvinic and sterculic acid [11].

- Starch: 40 to 55% [Ü60].

Tests for Identity: Based on morphological and anatomical characteristics, as well as with TLC [51, Ü102] or GC [51].

Quantitative assay: The essential oil content is determined volumetrically with

Piperine

Piperyline

Piperolein A   n = 3
Piperolein B   n = 5

Pipercide   n = 4
Guineensine   n = 6

Piperlongumine

steam distillation [DAB 6], its components are assayed with GC or GC/MS [50, 54]; the acid amides are detected with UV-spectroscopy by measuring the absorption of piperine, in a dichlormethane extract, at 343 nm [42]; directly by TLC [22], HPLC [4, 51, 58, DIN/ISO 11027], capillary-GC or GC/MS [23]; also possible is the colorimetric determination of the formaldehyde, which develops from acidic cleavage of the methylenedioxy-group, after reaction with chromotropic acid or p-dimethyl-aminobenzaldehyde [Ü38].

Adulterations, Misidentifications and Impurities: The whole peppercorns are sometimes confused or adulterated with fruits from other Piper-species or with other pungent tasting fruits of similar size, e.g. from Xylopia- or Schinus-species. Declaration of decorticated black pepper as white pepper is considered an adulteration. Adulteration of powdered pepper with pepper husks (from the processing of black decorticated pepper, see above), with so called "pin-heads" (hollow corns without seeds), or with a high content of fruit stalks, occur rarely. The dilution of pepper powder with flour from different grains and ground nutshells etc., is a rarity these days [51, Ü37].

Actions and Uses

Actions: Due to its pungent, aromatic taste, pepper stimulates the secretion of saliva, gastric juices, intestinal enzymes and the excretion of biliary fluid. Therefore it has appetite stimulant and digestive promoting action. Feeding of black pepper to rats (0.2 or 0.4% in feed) or piperine (0.01 or 0.02% in feed) over the course of 4 weeks increased the excreted quantity of biliary fluid but not the excreted quantity of cholesterol and bile acid [20]. Feeding of piperine (20 mg % in feed) for 8 weeks led to stimulation of pancreatic lipase activity, pancreatic amylase, trypsin and chymotrypsin. A single dose, however, had no effect [55].

Black pepper and piperine influence the detoxification capacity of the liver. Feeding of black pepper to mice (0.5 or 2% in feed, 20 days) dose-dependently increased glutathione-*S*-transferase activity and the content of acid-soluble sulfhydryl compounds as well as cytochrome b_5 and cytochrome P-450 in the liver thereby increasing its detoxification capacity [70]. Piperine did not evoke this effect in rats [2]. Conversely, piperine (25 mg/kg body weight, orally) inhibited the activity of some cytochrome P-450 dependent enzymes in the lungs [59]. Clearly the hepatic detoxification capacity is induced by the essential oil. In animal tests (mice), however, piperine protected against tert-butyl hydroperoxide and carbon tetrachloride hepatotoxicity by reducing lipid peroxidation, releasing of liver enzymes, and by preventing the depletion of GSH and total thiols. By comparison, piperine showed less activity than that of silymarin [33].

Ethanolic extracts of pepper or pepper essential oil have antibacterial action (e.g. MHK-value for *Clostridium botulinum* 0.125 mg drug / 100 ml) [13, 26, 28, 53]. Also the propagation of protozoon such as amoeba [21] and *Leishmania* [31] were inhibited. Administration of pepper extract (obtained from long pepper fruits) or piperine also cured 90% or 40% of rats with experimentally induced intestinal amoebiasis [21]. The growth of mycotoxigenic molds was not, however, significantly influenced, because pepper can hold high concentrations of aflatoxins (e.g. 1.2 μg/g) [15, 60]. However, a substance of unknown structure (Cp2), isolated from black pepper extracts, inhibited the activation of a gene (beta-glucuronidase reporter gene) of *Aspergillus parasiticus* at the transcriptional level, whose product is a key enzyme involved in aflatoxin biosynthesis. Cp2 did not inhibit mycelial growth [3].

In preparations that are rich in fat made from pork or beef, black pepper acts as an antioxidant whereby it inhibits lipid peroxidation [44].

Numerous studies on the activity of piperine are available, from which here below only a brief summary can be provided. As studies in rats have shown, piperine can stop inflammatory processes that are experimentally induced by Croton oil, among others [48]. Piperine increases the absorption of various medicinal- and natural substances. This action probably takes place because the lipophilic constituent piperine, which itself is easily absorbed, forms apolar complexes with other substances thereby improving their absorption [32, 43, 67]. Piperine has shown antimutagenic action in vitro [62], and in the AMES-Test pepper increased the number of revertants [72]. Furthermore it has been postulated that piperine has central sedative, analgesic, antipyretic and spasmolytic activity [40, 66]. Piperine, pipercide, dihydropipercide, guineensine and a few other acid amides of pepper have insecticide action, and in some cases, have shown activity surpassing that of pyrethrine [46, 73].

Toxicology: Based on existing data, there is no acute or chronic toxicity with the use of black pepper as a spice in typical doses. Intake of very high doses (50 to 60 g) lead to thirst, burning in the mouth, throat and pharynx, as well as stomach pains, palescence, fever, laryngitis, loss of consciousness, convulsions, vomiting and urticaria. Fatal outcomes of inexpert "pepper-cures" have been described in older literature [Ü58].

There are contradictory results with regard to the cancerogenic effects of large doses. Application of a black pepper extract in mice (2 mg for 3 d/week, p.o., corresponding to a human dose of 5 g) for 3 months, led to an increase of tumor-bearing animals. Doses of vitamin A-palmitate (5 or 10 mg, respectively, twice a week) cancelled this effect. Pepper extracts (2 mg, thrice/week for 5 months, applied sub- or percutaneously) or ground, black pepper (applied p.o.) had cancerogenic effects in toads. Particularly liver tumors with metastasis in the intestine, kidneys and spleen (due to aflatoxin content?) were observed [16, 17]. In other tests, 50 g pepper powder/3 kg feed, given to mice over a 3-month period, had no effect on the frequency of tumors [68]. Similar results were obtained from another test (total amount of 28 mg extract/animal, distributed over 3 months) [9].

The intensity of the sensitizing effect is not known. Immunological investigations, however, led to the detection of antibodies against pepper antigens in the blood from patients with celery-birch-mugwort-spice allergy [41].

Culinary use: Pepper is a universal spice. It is a component of nearly every spice mixture (see below) that is used for the seasoning of salty foods. However, pepper can also be used to season sweet dishes.

Black and white pepper are added to cooked- or baked meals when finished cooking, preferably freshly ground (in a pepper mill) or powdered (crushed in a plastic bag with a rolling pin or mashed in a mortar and pestle). The adding of whole peppercorns in a steel tea ball or small cloth bag during cooking is practiced. The whole peppercorns are used not only in marinades, broths, sauces and vinegar conserves, but also in a few types of sausage. Green- and red pepper are almost always used in preparations in an unground form. Meals that contain a lot of pepper should be prepared with care. The rising vapors can irritate the nose, eyes and respiratory tract.

Whole pepper in a pepper mill or ground pepper can also be kept at the table for re-seasoning the meal.

Black and white pepper primarily serve as seasonings for all meat dishes and fish dishes, meat fillings, egg dishes, cheese dishes, mussels, mushrooms, one-dish meals (e.g. of legumes), soufflés, potato purees, vegetables, sausages, ham, sauces, relishes, chutneys, marinades, soups, salads and vinegar conserves (e.g. seasoned pickles). White pepper is preferred as a seasoning for white meat, fish, light dishes and white sauces, probably only on a basis of visual appearance [Ü1, Ü30, Ü68, Ü91, Ü98].

The flavor of sweet dishes and fruits can also be enhanced with white or black pepper, e.g. fruit bread, gingerbread cookies, strawberries, banana slices baked in butter, marmalades, jams and fruit jellies [Ü1, Ü68].

Green pepper is especially suitable for creamy sauces (e.g. whipped cream sauce, butter sauce, pepper sauce), soups (e.g. pea soup, pepper soup), rice, steaks, tartar, poultry (e.g. duck), cheese, salads and tomato soups. It is rarely used as a seasoning for sweet dishes. Preserved green pepper is rinsed off with water prior to use, for butter- and cream sauces it is crushed [Ü13, Ü30, Ü45, Ü55, Ü74].

Combines well with: All spices suitable for seasoning of salty meals, but it should not be combined with paprika or chillies.

As a component of spice mixes and preparations: → Arabian spice mix, → Baharat, → Barbecue spice, → Bologna spice mix, → Bomboe sajoer lodeh, → Café de Paris spice mix, → Cajun spice, → Chat masala, → Chemen, → Cocktail sauce, → Curry powder, → Dukkah, → Egg spice, → Fish spice, → Garam masala, → Grill spice, → Hamburger spice, → La kama, → Lemon pepper, → Meat spice, → Mélange classique, → Mignonette pepper, → Multi-colored pepper, → Parisian pepper, → Parsley butter, → Pepper bouquet, → Pickling spice, → Pizza spice, → Poultry spice, → Quark spice, → Ras el hanout, → Roast spice, → Salsa comum, → Sambal badjak, → Sambhar powder, → Sauce spice, → Sausage spice, → Soup spice, → Table mustard, → Tika paste, → Tomato ketchup, → Tridschataka, → Vegetable spice, → Venison spice.

Medicinal herb

Herbal drugs: Piperis nigri fructus, Black pepper [ÖAB, DAB 6], Piperis albi fructus, White pepper [EB 6].

Indications: As a digestive-promoting remedy (single-dose 0.3 to 0.6 g, daily dose 1.5 g). However, pepper is rarely used today for this indication, but rather it is used more widely as a spice. In folk medicine, pepper was formerly used for cholera and skin diseases as well as externally in the form of pepper ointments for treating scabies [5, Ü60].

Similar culinary herbs

Ashanti pepper (Guinea pepper, West African black pepper, Ethiopian pepper, false cubeb, Congo cubeb, kissi pepper), dried, globose, 3.5 to 4 mm long, with up to 5 mm long stalks bearing fruits of *Piper guineense* SCHUM. et THONN. (Synonym: *Piper clusii* (MIQ.) C. DC.), native to tropical West- and Central Africa, where it is also cultivated in some areas. The main aroma- and taste components are about 10% essential oil, with, among others, myristicine, elemicin, safrole and dillapiol as well as acid amides, among others piperine (5 to 8 %), piperyline (trichostachine), piperanine, guineensine, piperolein B, wisanine, okolasine (wisanidine) and dihydrowisanidine [10, 14, 19, Ü43]. In its countries of origin, it is used

in the same way as black pepper. The leaves are also used as a spice [Ü61, Ü81, Ü92].

Cubeb pepper (tailed pepper, Java pepper), harvested immature, blackish-brown after drying, globose, 4 to 5 mm long fruits with 5 to 10 mm long stalk-like apophysis of *Piper cubeba* L. f. (Synonym: *P. officinalis* RAFF.), native to Indonesia (Greater Sunda Islands), where it is cultivated as well as in India, Sri Lanka, and Malaysia, aroma components 5 to 18% essential oil of which the main components are β-cubebene, copaene, cubebol, δ-cadinene, α-cubebene and α-caryophyllene (humulene) [37]. Furthermore the fruits contain, among others, lignan derivatives, especially (−)-cubebine (responsible for the red color of powder of fruits after treatment with 80% sulfuric acid) [28]. Acid amides are probably absent. In its countries of origin, especially in Malaysia, cubeb pepper is used as a seasoning of rice, vegetables and sea foods. In Europe, it is sometimes used, as well as its essential oil, as a flavoring of spice sauces, liqueurs (Aromatique, Stonsdorfer, Goldwasser), tobaccos and soap perfumes. It is a component of a few gingerbread spices (e.g. Ulmer gingerbread spice). In folk medicine it is used internally as a urinary disinfectant, expectorant, and for headaches [51, Ü37, Ü81].

Java pepper (Javanese long pepper), immature, dried infructescence and dried, ripe fruits of *Piper retrofactum* VAHL (Synonym: *P. officinarum* VAHL), native to Indonesia, the Philippines, Vietnam, and Malaysia, cultivated in Java, among other locations. The main aroma- and taste components are the essential oil (0.6 to 0.7%) and acid amides, among others, piperine, piperlongumine and retrofactamide B [49, Ü43, Ü61].

Bengal pepper (long pepper, pole pepper, Indian long pepper, pippali pepper, fly pepper), immature, upon drying turns very dark brown, spadiceous infructescences of *Piper longum* L., native to the Himalaya region, cultivated in India, Bangladesh and

Sri Lanka. Aroma component about 1% essential oil, among others, with β-caryophyllene (10 to 17%), germacrene D (up to 17%), pentadecan (about 18%), heptadec-8-ene (up to 19%), heptadecan (up to 10%), β-bisabolene (about 11%) and αr-curcumene (about 5%) [1, 65, 75]. As pungent compounds it contains, among others, piperine (4 to 6%), piperlongumine (piplartine), piperlonguminine, pipercide, dihydropipernonaline, piperundecaline, guineensine, brachyamide A, brachyamide B, brachystine, longamide and pipernonaline as well as alkamides, e.g. *N*-isobutyl-eicosa-*trans*-2-*trans*-4-dien-amide [34, 74]. Bengal pepper is not as pungent as black pepper. In Southeast Asian countries, but also in Great Britain, Canada, Australia and in the USA, it is used just like black pepper, e.g. to season meals, pickles and preserves. In India, it is also a component of curry powder. In Central Europe, it is rarely used [51, Ü61, Ü74, Ü81, Ü98].

Other Piper-species, of which the fruits or leaves are used as spices include, among others, *P. aduncum* L. (big pepper, spiked pepper, cultivated in Southern Mexico and South America), *P. betle* L. (betel pepper, native to Malaysia, cultivated in tropical Asia, Coastal Africa, West Indies, its leaves serve as a component of betel chew [Ü99, Ü100]. *P. elongatum* VAHL (Synonym: *P. angustifolium* RUIZ et PAV.), matiko, native to the Northern Andes region, cultivated in Argentina, Columbia, Tanzania, the leaves are used as a cocoa spice), *P. peepuloides* (A. DIETR.) ROXB. (Cultivated in India), *P. saigonense* C. DC. (lolo, cultivated in Vietnam), *P. schmidtii* J.D. HOOK. (Nilgiri pepper, cultivated in India), and *P. trichostachyon* (MIQ.) C. DC. (Bag pepper, cultivated in India) [Ü61].

Kumba pepper (kani, African pepper, Guinea pepper, Ethiopian pepper, burro pepper, Egyptian pepper, grains of selim, Xylopia pepper, African cubeb, also described as Melegueta pepper and grains-of-paradise), bean-shaped, 2.5 to 5 cm long, 4 to 8 mm wide, dried seeds of various Xylopia-species (Annonaceae): *Xylopia aethiopica* (DUNAL) RICH. (Synonym: *Annona aethiopica* DUNAL), Ethiopian pepper (kani, Melegueta pepper, spice tree), aroma component is the essential oil, of which the main components are α-pinene (4 to 18%), sabinene (3 to 36%), β-pinene (11 to 42%), 1,8-cineole (traces up to 15%), (Z)-β-ocimene (traces up to 18%), terpinenol-4 (7 to 15%), α-phellandrene (traces up to 8%), germacrene D (3 to 7%) and linalool (up to 4%) [6, 30, 52, 56, 76], furthermore the fruits contain, among others, acid amides, lignan amides and ent-kaurene-type diterpenes [36], *X. quintasii* ENGL. ET DIELS (Synonym: *Xylopia striata* ENGL.), striped pepper (grains of selim), native to and cultivated as well in tropical West Africa, and *X. aromatica* (LAM.) MART., burro pepper, native to the West Indies, Costa Rica, Venezuela and Southern Brazil, in its countries of origin it is used in the same manner as black pepper, its essential oil is dominated by spathulenol (about 65%) [Ü61, Ü98].

Monk's pepper, globose to oblong, 3 to 5 mm in size, very dark brown fruits of *Vitex agnus-castus* L., chaste tree berry (Ger: Mönchspfeffer, Keuschlamm or Abrahamsstrauch) (Verbenaceae), native to the Mediterranean region and Central Asia, aroma- and taste components about 0.8 to 1.2% essential oil, of which the main components are 1,8-cineole, sabinene, limonene, α- and β-pinene, β-phellandrene, cadinene, (E)-β-farnesene, β-caryophyllene, β-caryophyllene epoxide, α-terpinyl acetate and germacrene B [35, 45, 71, 81], cultivated in Georgia, monk's pepper is used as a pepper substitute. In the Middle Ages, it was used as an anaphrodisiac (hence its name), in modern medicine, it is used for premenstrual complaints, menstrual cycle irregularities and mastodynia [78, Ü37, Ü92, Ü98].

See also → Allspice, → Grains-of-paradise, Peruvian pepper, Spanish pepper and Cayenne pepper (→ Paprika), → Pink pepper, and → Sichuan pepper.

Pepper Steak

Ingredients per person: 1 teaspoon white peppercorns, 1 round flank steak or sirloin tip, a pad of butter, salt, one small glass of brandy, 1 teaspoon of heavy cream.

Crush the whole peppercorns and sprinkle the coarse powder on a plate. Place the meat on top and press it against the crushed peppercorns; turn the steak around and cover the other side with pepper in the same way. Heat the butter in the pan, add salt and start to sauté the meat on both sides. Pour the brandy into the pan and flambé; let the steak simmer for 10 minutes. At the end, mix in the heavy cream [8].

Literature

[1] Achenbach H., W. Karl, Chem. Ber. 104:1468–1477 (1986).

[2] Allameh A. et al., Cancer Lett. 61(3):195–199 (1992).

[3] Annis S.L. et al., J. Agric. Food Chem. 48(10):4656–466 (2000).

[4] Archer A.W., J. Chromatogr. 351:595–598 (1986).

[5] Arseculeratne S.N. et al., J. Ethnopharmacol. 13:323–335 (1985).

[6] Ayedoun A.M. et al., Flavour Fragrance J. 11(4):245–250 (1996).

[7] Bandyopadhyay C. et al., J. Agric. Food Chem. 38:1696–1699 (1990).

[8] Bosi R., Pfeffer und Peperoni, Droemersche Verlagsanstalt Th. Knaur Nachf., München 1997.

[9] Concon J.M. et al., Nutr. Cancer 1:22–26 (1979).

[10] Das B. et al., Planta Med. 62(6):582 (1996).

[11] Daulatabad C.D. et al., Fett Wiss. Technol. 97(12):453–454 (1995).

[12] Debrauwere J., M. Verzele, J. Sci. Food Agric. 26:1887–1892 (1976).

[13] Dorman H.J., S.G. Deans, J. Appl. Microbiol. 88(2):308–316 (2000).

[14] Dwuma-Badu D. et al., Lloydia 39(1):60–64 (1976).

[15] El-Kady I.A. et al., Folia Microbiol. (Prague):40(3):297–398 (1995).

[16] El-Mofty M.M. et al., Oncology 45(3):247–252 (1988).

[17] El-Mofty M.M. et al., Oncology 48(4):347–350 (1991).

[18] Farag S.E.A., Abo-Zeid M., Nahrung 41(6):359–361 (1997).

[19] Freist W., Chemie i.u. Zeit 23(3):135–142 (1991).

[20] Ganesh B.B., N. Chandrasekhara, Nahrung 31:913–916 (1987).

[21] Ghosal S. et al., J. Ethnopharmacol. 50(3):167–170 (1996).

[22] Glasl H., M. Ihrig, Dtsch. Lebensm. Rundschau 80:111–113 (1984).

[23] Gopalakrishnan M. et al., J. Ess. Oil Res. 5:247–253 (1993).

[24] Govindarajan V.S., Critical Reviews Food Sci. Nutr. 9(2):115–225 (1977).

[25] Grewe R. et al., Chem. Ber. 103:3752–3770 (1970).

[26] Huhtanen C.N., J. Food Prot. 43:195–196 (1980).

[27] Inatani R. et al., Agric. Biol. Chem. 45(3): 667 (1981).

[28] Ismaiel A.A., M.D. Pierson, J. Food Prot. 53:755–758 (1990).

[29] Jensen S., J. Hansen, P.M. Boll, Phytochemistry 33:523–530 (1993).

[30] Jirovetz L. et al., Ernährung (Wien):21(7/8):324–325 (1997).

[31] Kapil A., Planta Med. 59(5):474 (1993).

[32] Khajuria A. et al., Indian J. Exp. Biol. 36(1):46–50 (1998).

[33] Koul I.B., A. Kapil, Planta Med. 59(5): 413–417 (1993).

[34] Koul S.K. et al., Phytochemistry 27:3523 (1988).

[35] Kustrac D. et al., Planta Med. 58(7):A681 (1992).

[36] Lajide L. et al., Phytochemistry 40(4):1105–1112 (1995).

[37] Lawrence B.M., Perfum. Flavorist 5:28 (1980).

[38] Lawrence B.M., Perfum. and Flavorist 17:67 (1992).

[39] Lawrence B.M., R.J. Reynolds, Perfum. Flavorist 20(2):49–59 (1995).

[40] Lee E. et al., Arch. Pharmacol. Res. 7:127 (1984).

[41] Leitner A. et al., Allergy 53(1):36–41 (1998).

[42] Lupina T., H. Cripps, J. Assoc. Off. Anal. Chem. 70:112–112 (1987).

[43] Majeed M. et al., U.S. US 5, 744, 161 (Cl. 424–464;A6F2/02), 28 Apr. 1998, US Appl. 393,738, 24 Febr. 1995, 13 pp, ref. CA 128:326500c.

[44] Milivojevic J., Tehnol. Mesa. 37(1):32–34 (1996), ref. CA 128:139911c.

[45] Mischurova S.S. et al., Rastitelnye Resurcy 22:526–530 (1986), ref. CA 106:1164956.

[46] Miyakado M. et al., Agric. Biol. Chem. 43:1609, zit. Ü43 (1979).

[47] Möllenbeck S. et al., Flavour Fragrance J:12(2):63–69 (1997).

[48] Mujumdar A.M. et al., Jpn. J. Med. Sci. Biol. 43(3):95–100 (1990).

[49] Nakatami N. et al., Environ. Health Perspect. 67:135–142 (1986).

[50] Nirmala Menon A. et al., J. Ess. Oil Res. 12:431–434 (2000).

[51] Oberdieck R., Fleischwirtschaft 72:1–7 (1992).

[52] Onayade-Sontan O.A., Analysis of the essential oils of some plants used in traditional medicine in Nigeria, Dissertationsschrift, Universität Leiden 1991.

[53] Perez C., Anesini C., Am. J. Clin. Med. 22(2):169–174 (1994).

[54] Pino J. et al., Nahrung 34:555–560 (1990).

[55] Platel K., K. Srinivasan, Nahrung 44(1): 42–46 (2000).

[56] Poitou F., J. Ess. Oil Res. 8(3):329–330 (1996).

[57] Raina M.L. et al., Planta Med. 30(2):198–200 (1976).

[58] Rathnawathie M., K.A. Buckle, J. Chromatogr. 264(2):316–320 (1983).

[59] Reen R.K., J. Singh, Indian J. Exp. Biol. 29(6):568–573 (1991).

[60] Roy A.K. et al., Appl. Environ. Microbiol. 54(3):842–843 (1988).

[61] Sankar K.U., J. Sci. Food Agric. 48:483, (1989).

[62] Schimmer O., Dtsch. Apoth. Ztg. 139(19): 1947–1956 (1999).

[63] Scholz H., Natürlich 17(4):40–45 (1997).

[64] Seidemann J., Drogenreport 13(23):65–68 (2000).

[65] Shankaracharya N.B. et al., J. Food Sci. Technol. 34(1):73–75 (1997).

[66] Shin K.H., S. Woo, Recent Adv. Nat. Prod. Res., Proc. Int. Symp, Eds: Woo W.S., Hoon B., Seoul Natl. Univ. Press, Seoul, Korea 1980.

[67] Shoba G. et al., Planta Med. 64(4): 353–356 (1998).

[68] Shwaireb M.H. et al., Exp. Pathol. 40(4):233–238 (1990).

[69] Siddiqui B.S. et al., Phytochemistry 45(8):1617–1619 (1997).

[70] Singh A., A.R. Rao, Cancer Lett. 72:5–9 (1993).

[71] Sorensen J.M., S.Th. Katsiotis, J. Ess. Oil Res. 11:599–605 (1999).

[72] Soudamini K.K. et al., Indian Physiol. Pharmacol. 39(4):347–353 (1995).

[73] Su H,C,F., R. Horvat , J. Agric. Food Chem. 29:115–118 (1981).

[74] Tabuneng W. et al., Chem. Pharm. Bull. 31:3562–3565 (1983).

[75] Tewtrakul S. et al., J. Ess. Oil Res. 12:603–608 (2000).

[76] Tomi F. et al., J. Ess. Oil Res. 8(4):429–431 (1996).

[77] Variyar P.S. et al., Phytochemistry 27(3): 715–717 (1988).

[78] Vonarburg B., Natürlich 20(2):60–63 (2000).

[79] Vösgen B., K. Herrmann, Z. Lebensm. Unters. Forsch. 170:204–207 (1980).

[80] Wrolstad R.E., W.G. Jennings, J. Food Sci. 30:274–279 (1965).

[81] Zwaving J.H., R. Bos, Planta Med. 62(1):83–84 (1997).

Literature references identified by Ü can be found in the general listing of books and monographs at the back of this book.

Pink pepper

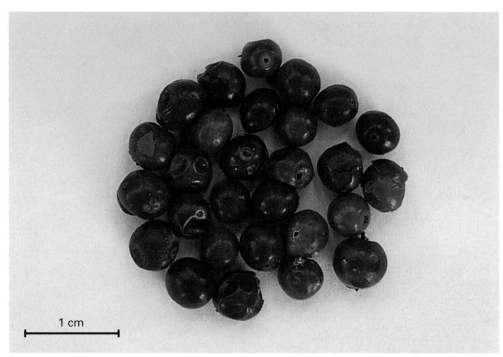

1 cm

Fig. 1: Pink pepper

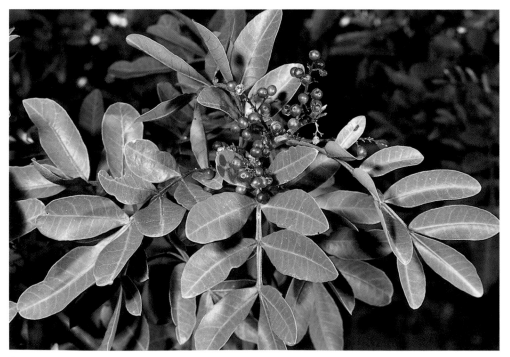

Fig. 2: Brazilian pink pepper (*Schinus terebinthifolius* RADDI)

Plant sources: *Schinus terebinthifolius* RADDI and *Schinus molle* L.

Family: Sumac family (Anacardiaceae).

Brazilian pink pepper

Plant source: *Schinus terebinthifolius* RADDI.

Taxonomic classification: The species can be subdivided into 4 varieties, which are differentiated mainly based on the shape and size of the leaves. The material that is used in Europe originates predominantly from the variety *S. terebinthifolius* RADDI var. *radianus* ENGL. [20].

Common names: Engl.: Brazilian pepper tree, Christmas berry tree, pink berry tree, pink peppercorn tree; Fr.: encens, baies roses de Bourbon, poivrier rose, faux poivrier, poivrier de Brézil, sorbier; Ger: Brasilianischer Rosa Pfeffer, Brasilianischer Pfefferbaum, Turbitobaum.

Description: Shrub or tree, height up to 12 m, evergreen or semi-evergreen, dioecious, the branches do not hang over. Leaves up to 40 cm long, imparipinnate, with 7 to 13, usually 9, up to 8 cm long, 1 to 2 cm wide pinnules. The small flowers are arranged in up to 15 cm long multiflorous panicles. They have 5 ivory-colored or greenish-white petals, 10 stamina and a 5-lobed calyx. The one-seeded drupes are globose, bright-pink to red and shiny, diameter up to 5 mm [Ü37].

Native origin: Central- and South America, mainly Brazil and Paraguay, rapidly spread after cultivation in the 1st half of the 20th century in the Southern USA [17].

Main cultivation areas: Réunion, Mediterranean region (especially Spain), USA (Florida and California), Africa, and Southern Asia.

Main exporting countries: France, originated from Réunion Island.

Cultivation: Propagation is carried out by seed or with cuttings. In Central Europe the plant is not winter-hardy.

Culinary herb

Commercial forms: Rose pepper (Brazilian pink pepper): dried fruits, whole or cut, and the fresh fruits preserved in salt water.

Production: The fruits are harvested when ripe and air-dried, freeze-dried or preserved in a saline solution [Ü68].

Forms used: Dried, whole, crushed or ground fruits, preserved fruits.

Storage: The ripe dried fruits should be stored in well-closed metal- or glass containers, protected from light and moisture. The aroma of the comminuted fruits is rapidly lost.

Description. Whole fruit (Fig. 1): Bright pink to red, shiny, single-seeded drupes, diameter 3 to 5 mm. The pericarp easily separates or loosely encloses the stone. Typical is the structure of the exocarp, which consists of the very regular arranged small, roundish cells with strongly thickened and not dotted cell walls; the primary wall is not clearly outlined (in contrast to the fruits of *Schinus molle*, see below, Fig. 3). The cells of the mesocarp are thin-walled and only moderately punctate; in the mesocarp, there are numerous secretory canals. The endocarp consists of several layers of palisade-like stone cells [20].

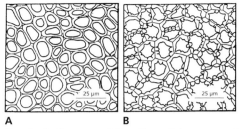

Fig. 3: **A** Exocarp of Brazilian pink pepper, **B** Exocarp of Peruvian pink pepper.

Powdered fruit: The powder is characterized by the fragments of the endocarp and exocarp (see above) [20].

Odor: Flowery and turpentine-like after crushing, **Taste:** Sweet, turpentine-like, with peppery aftertaste, seeds bitter.

History: → Peruvian pink pepper.

Constituents and Analysis

Constituents

- Essential oil: 1.5 to 6%, the main components are α-phellandrene (16 to 22%), limonene (11 to 16%), β-phellandrene (8 to 15%), α-pinene (about 25%), β-pinene (1 to 7%), *p*-cymene (about 7%) and Δ³-carene (traces to 50%, high amounts were detected in fruits from Florida), furthermore sabinene, α-terpinene, γ-terpinene, terpinolene and β-caryophyllene, among others [12, 13, 20]. Essential oil from fruits of Indian origin contained the following components: 43% α-pinene, 19% α-phellandrene, 2% β-pinene, 2% sabinene and 1% terpinolene [15, 27].
- *n*-Alkenylphenols: About 0.08%, including cardanol 15:1 (n-7), content 0.025 to 0.05%, cardanol 15:3 (n-1), cardanol 15:2 (n-4), cardanol 15:1 (n-7), cardanol 15:0, cardol 15:3 (n-1), cardol 15:2 (n-4), cardol 15:1 (n-7), cardol 15:0 and 2-methylcardolene [2, 21, 23, 27].
- Flavonoids: Including, among others, the biflavonoids amentoflavone, II-2,3-dihydromentoflavone and tetrahydro-amentoflavone [21, 24].
- Triterpenes: Masticadienonic acid, among others, possibly as the main components of the balsamic secretion [13].
- Fatty oil: 23 to 60% in the seeds [Ü43].

Tests for Identity: With TLC [26] or TLC-fingerprint, which is also suitable for the distinction of the fruits from *Sch. molle* [20].

Quantitative assay: Based on the determination of the essential oil content using the method of the European Pharmacopoeia; the composition of the essential oil and the content of Δ³-carene can be analyzed with GC [1, 14, 20, Ph Eur].

Adulterations, Misidentifications and Impurities are possible with the fruits of other *Schinus* species, which, however, are below 4 mm in size, brown, bluish or black [Ü98].

Cardanols   Cardols

R = -(CH₂)₁₄-CH₃   15 : 0
R = -(CH₂)₇-CH=CH-(CH₂)5-CH3   15 : 1 (n-7)
R = -(CH₂)₇-CH=CH-CH₂-CH=CH-(CH₂)₂-CH₃   15 : 2 (n-4)
R = -(CH₂)₇-CH=CH-CH₂-CH=CH-CH₂-CH=CH₂   15 : 3 (n-1)

Actions and Uses

Actions: Due to its pungent taste, pink pepper has appetizing and digestion promoting action. The essential oil and extracts of the dried fruit have good antimicrobial activity [8, 16, 22].

Toxicology: Based on existing data, there is no acute or chronic toxicity with the use of Brazilian pink pepper as a spice at normal doses [5, 20, 23].

n-Alkylphenols are skin-irritants after a longer latent period (ID$_{50}$, mouse ear, cardanol 15:1 (n-7) 4 µg/ear) [23]. Together with the essential oil (particularly if the content of Δ^3-carene is high), they are responsible for the irritating effects on the buccal mucous membranes after prolonged chewing of the fruits, or for the symptoms of intoxication such as nausea, vertigo, vomiting and skin rashes after intake of high doses of Brazilian pink pepper. It is claimed that these symptoms can occur in children who have only ingested a few fresh fruits [17, 26, 27, 29].

Based on the content of n-alkenylphenols, which are responsible for the sensitizing properties of Toxicodendron species, e.g. poison sumach [Ü39, Ü100], such effects can also be expected from the fruits of pink pepper. Cases of allergic reactions (skin rashes and swellings) after contact with the fresh fruits have only been observed in the USA, possibly because the population there is frequently sensitized against n-alkenylphenols due to contact with Toxicodendron species [17, 26, 27].

Culinary use: Pink pepper plays a role especially in Mediterranean region cooking. But in the last few years it has entered Central European cooking, particularly due to its decorative effect. Because of the possible sensitization properties, pink pepper originating from *Schinus terebinthifolius* should be used sparingly, not more than 12 to 15 fruits per meal [Ü68]. A few authors also advise that this spice should not be used at all and that it should be substituted with juniper berries [26].

The pulverized or whole fruits are suitable for the seasoning or decoration of steaks, roast, poultry, game dishes, sauces, dressings, and fish dishes [11, 26, Ü68].

Combines well with: Pepper.

As a component of spice mixes and preparations: → Multi-colored pepper.

Other uses: The fruits are used as a pepper adulterant in some countries, or pickled in vinegar as a substitute for pepper. The gum resin isolated from the trunk bark (aroeira resin) is used medicinally in Mexico, Central America and South America, particularly as a strong-acting laxative. The branches with decorative berries are used in the Southern USA as Christmas decorations (Christmas berry, Florida holly) [Ü37, Ü100].

Medicinal herb

Herbal drug: Schini terebinthifolii fructus, Schinus-terebinthifolius-fruit.

Indications: In the folk medicine of Central- and South America, it is taken internally in the form of tea infusions as a diuretic remedy and for the treatment of tumors as well as externally in the form of decoctions for the treatment of wounds and ulcers [Ü37].

Peruvian pink pepper

Plant source: *Schinus molle* L.

Synonym: *Schinus areira* L.

Taxonomic classification: The species can be subdivided into 2 varieties. The material that is used as a spice originates almost exclusively from the variety *Schinus molle* L. var. *areira* DC.

Common names: Engl.: Peruvian pepper tree, Australian pepper tree, California pepper tree, false pepper; Fr.: faux poivrier, poivrier d'Amérique, poivre du Pérou; Ger: Peruanischer Pfefferbaum, Amerikanischer Pfefferbaum, Mollebaum.

Description: Tree, height up to 15 m, evergreen, dioecious, with overhanging branches. Leaves are up to 25 cm long, imparipinnate, with 17 to 35, up to 6 cm long, 2 to 8 mm wide pinnules, dotted with oil glands. The small flowers are arranged in up to 30 cm long multiflorous panicles. They have 5 yellowish-white petals, 10 stamina and a 5-lobed calyx. The one-seeded drupes are globose, bright pink to red and shiny, diameter up to 7 mm [Ü37].

Native origin: Temperate America, originally Peru, now occurring from Bolivia to Northern Argentina, naturalized in southern North America, from Mexico to California, also in the Mediterranean region, mainly along the coast of Italy, widely distributed as an ornamental tree.

Main cultivation areas: Southern Australia, South Africa, Southern Europe, Costa Rica and California, cultivated mostly as an ornamental shrub.

Main exporting countries: South America, mainly Peru, also Southern India.

Cultivation: Propagation is carried out by seed or with cuttings. In Central Europe the plant is not winter-hardy, but it is sometimes kept indoors as a tub plant.

Culinary herb

Commercial forms: Pink pepper (Peruvian pink pepper): dried fruits, whole or cut.

Production: The fruits are harvested when ripe and air-dried or freeze-dried.

Forms used: Whole or crushed fruits.

Storage: The ripe dried fruits should be stored in well-closed metal- or glass containers, protected from light and moisture. The aroma of the comminuted fruits is quickly lost.

Description. Whole fruit: Bright pink to red, more rarely pale yellow, shiny, one-seeded drupes, diameter 4.5 to 6 mm. The pericarp easily separates or loosely encloses the stone. The exocarp shows, in contrast to the fruits of *Sch. terebinthifolius*, strongly punctate cell walls with clearly recognizable primary walls (Fig. 3). The mesocarp cells below are thin-walled and only moderately punctate; there are numerous secretory canals in the mesocarp. The endocarp consists of 3 layers of palisade-like stone cells [20].

Powdered fruit: The powder is characterized by the fragments of the endocarp and exocarp (see above) [20].

Odor: After crushing flowery and turpentine-like, **Taste:** Sweetish, turpentine-like, with peppery aftertaste, seeds bitter.

History: Plantlets and seeds reached Europe already in the 16th century. In the early 1950's, the brown, wrinkled fruits, freed from the exocarp, appeared as a substitute and adulterant of pepper in the spice trade. Since the 1970's, pink pepper is offered individually, or mixed with different forms of pepper as a decorative spice mixture for pepper mills. Its use in Central European kitchens has also increased significantly [5, 18, 20, 25, 26, Ü93].

Constituents and Analysis

Constituents

- Essential oil: 2.0 to 5.2%, the main components are α- and β-phellandrene, limonene, α- and β-pinene; furthermore camphene, carvacrol, *p*-cymene, 2-ethylphenol, myrcene, β-spathulene, viridiflorene, viridiflorol [4, 12, 14, 20, 28]. In fruits of Turkish origin, the main components of the essential oil were: 22 to 38% α-phellandrene, 10 to 12% β-phellandrene, 10 to 12% limonene, 6 to 7% cadinol, 3 to 5% methyl octanoate [3].
- Flavonoids: Biflavonoids, among others.
- Triterpenes: Masticadienonic acid, isomasticadienonic acid, isomasticadienonalic acid, 3-epiisomasticadienonalic acid, 3-epiisomasticadienonolic acid, probably mostly as components of the balsam-like secretion [13, 19].
- Fatty oil: 6 to 14% in the seeds [Ü43].
- *n*-Alkenylphenols have not yet been detected in the fruits [26, Ü43].

Tests for Identity: With TLC-fingerprint, which is also suitable for the distinction of the fruits from *Sch. terebinthifolius* [20, 26].

Quantitative assay: The content of Δ^3-carene in the essential oil is determined by capillary-GC [1, 20]. Essential oil levels are determined, according to the Swiss and Austrian food codex, with the diffusion-oxidation method (similar to the Widmark-method for the analysis of blood alcohol levels), by releasing the fruit's components with water at 103 to 105 °C, followed by iodometric absorption measurements in potassium dichromate solution [9].

Adulterations, Misidentifications and Impurities are possible, with the fruits from other Schinus species, which, however, are smaller than 4 mm and brown, bluish or black [Ü98].

Actions and Uses

Actions: On the basis of its pungent taste, pink pepper has appetizing and digestion promoting action. The balsam of the fruit is supposed to have a laxative effect [Ü37]. Aqueous extracts of the dried fruit inhibit in vitro the activity of angiotensin-converting-enzyme (ACE). This effect is attributed to the triterpenes contained in the extract [19]. Healing of inflammations of the vaginal mucosa and of the opening of the uterus can be brought about with aqueous-alcoholic extracts of the dried fruit due to their antibiotic and antiphlogistic activity [6]. The fungicidal action of the essential oil is also considerable. In concentrations of 200 to 900 ppm, it kills pathogenic and storage-spoiling fungi [7, 10]. The antibacterial action is also significant [10].

Toxicology: Based on existing data, there is no acute or chronic toxicity with the normal use as a spice at normal doses. Older reports indicate that higher amounts could lead to nausea, vomiting, diarrhea, gastroenteritis, exhaustion and headache, particularly in children. Poisonings have not been reported [29]. The sensitization potential is not known.

Culinary use: Peruvian pink pepper is used in the same way as Brazilian pink pepper (see above).

Other uses: The fermented fruits are used for the manufacture of alcoholic beverages, e.g. in Peru, Chile, Mexico, Greece and other countries, for the Peruvian "Chica de molle" and the Mexican "Capalote", among others. In Mexico, the fruits are also a component of "Pulque". Fermentation to obtain vinegar is also practiced [Ü37, Ü61]. The gum resin isolated from the trunk bark (aroeira resin) is used medicinally in Mexico, Central America and South America, particularly as a strong-acting laxative. The bark itself is also used as a traditional medicine in Central- and South America [Ü37].

Medicinal herb

Herbal drug: Schini mollis fructus, Schinus-molle-fruit.

Indications: In Mexico, it is taken internally for loss of appetite and indigestion. In the folk medicine of Central- and South America, it is used internally in the form of tea infusions as a diuretic remedy, among other uses, externally in the form of cataplasms for nausea and vomiting and in the form of tinctures as a rub for rheumatic pains [Ü37].

Literature

[1] Anonym, Ernährung 14:158–167 (1990), 15:451–452 (1991).

[2] Anonym, Dtsch. Apoth. Ztg. 127: 1345–1346 (1987).

[3] Baser K.H.C et al., J. Ess. Oil Res. 9:693–696 (1997).

[4] Bernhard R.A. et al., J. Agric. Food Chem. 31:463–466 (1983).

[5] Campello J.P. et al., Phytochemistry 13: 659–660 (1974).

[6] Carneiro Wanik M., W., Ejacyrema Alves, Rev. Inst. Antibiot. (Recife) 14(1/2):105–106 (1974).

[7] Dikshit A. et al., Appl. Environ. Microbiol. 51(5):1085–1088 (1986).

[8] Fariq S.R. et al., Pak. J. Sci. Ind. Res. 38(9–10):358–361 (1995), ref. CA 126: 303577e.

[9] Frühwirth H., F. Krempler, Ernährung 3:26–35 (1979).

[10] Gunddidza M., Centr. Afr. J. Med. 39(11):231–234 (1993).

[11] Jaspersen-Schib R., Dtsch. Apoth. Ztg. 132(13):621–625 (1992).

[12] Lawrence B.M., Perfum. Flavorist 65–69 (1984).

[13] Lloyd H.A. et al., Phytochemistry 16: 1301–1302 (1977).

[14] Maffei M., F. Chialva, Flav. Fragrance J. 5:49–52 (1990).

[15] Malik M.S.H. et al., Sci. Int. (Lahore) 6(4):351–352 (1994), ref. CA 123: 251323k.

[16] Martinez M.J. et al., J. Ethnopharmacol. 52(3):171–174 (1996).

[17] Morton J.F., Econ. Botany 32:353–359 (1978).

[18] Oberdieck R., Fleischwirtschaft 72:1–7 (1992).

[19] Olafsson K. et al., Planta Med. 63(4): 352–355 (1997).

[20] Schrutka-Rechtenstamm R. et al., Ernährung 12:541–547 (1988).

[21] Schwenker G., G. Skopp, Dtsch. Apoth. Ztg. 127:1345–1346 (1987).

[22] Siddiqui R.F. et al., Pak. J. Sci. Ind. Res. 38(9–10):358–361 (1995), ref. CA 126: 303577e.

[23] Skopp G. et al., Z. Naturforsch. 42c:7–16 (1987).

[24] Skopp G. et al., Z. Naturforsch. 41b: 1479–1482 (1986).

[25] Soos E., M. Hausknost, Sci. Pharm. 19: 213–219 (1951).

[26] Stahl E., Dtsch. Apoth. Ztg. 122(7): 337–340 (1982).

[27] Stahl E. et al., Planta Med. 48:5–9 (1983).

[28] Terhune S.J. et al., Phytochemistry 13: 865–866 (1974).

[29] Watt J.M., Meyer-Brandwijk M.G., The Medicinal and Poisonous Plant of Southern and Eastern Africa, E. & S. Livingstone Ltd., Edinburgh, London 1962.

Literature references identified by Ü can be found in the general listing of books and monographs at the back of this book.

Ramsons

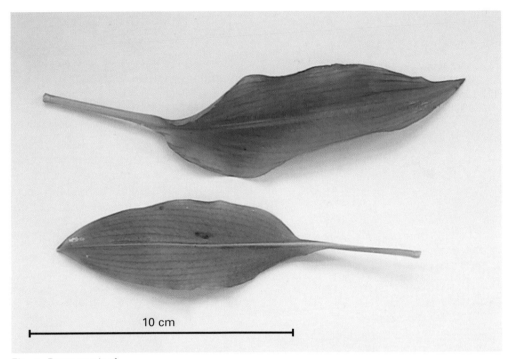

Fig. 1: Ramsons leaf

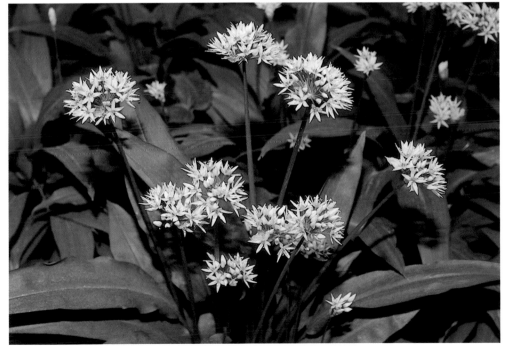

Fig. 2: Ramsons (*Allium ursinum* L.)

Plant source: *Allium ursinum* L.

Family: Allium plants (Alliaceae; in older literature this species was placed in the lily family, Liliaceae).

Common names: Engl.: ramsons, wild garlic, bear's garlic, hog's garlic, broad-leaved garlic, wood garlic, gipsy onion; Fr.: ail des ours, ail des bois; Ger.: Bärlauch, Bärenlauch, Hexenzwiebel, Judenzwiebel, Rams, Ramsell, Ramseren, Ränsel, Waldlauch, Waldknoblauch, Waldknofel, Wilder Knoblauch, Wilder Knofel, Zigeunerzwiebel.

Description: Perennial herb, 20 to 50 cm high, with an elongated bulb, almost cylindrical, 2 to 4 cm long, about 1 cm wide, in the young plant surrounded by a paper-like membrane, which later on disappears with a few bristles remaining, without or with only a few offset bulbs. The plant has 2, rarely 3, basal leaves, flat, elliptic-lanceolate, 6 to 20 cm long, up to 8 cm wide, narrowing into a 5 to 20 mm long petiole. The peduncle of the inflorescence is mostly triangular or almost roundish and compact. The coat of the inflorescence is 1- to 2-lobed, with 2 to 3 clefts, deciduous. The inflorescence is a loose pseudoumbel, always without bulblets; the flower stalk is as long or double the size of the star-shaped flowers, 6 perigone leaves, pure white, 6 stamina, about half as long as the perigone leaves, toothless, ovary 3-parted with 3 deep furrows. The fruit is a spherical capsule with black, roundish seeds. Flowering period is from April to June [Ü42].

Native origin: Probably Asia. Today it is widely distributed throughout nearly all of Europe, up to 64 degrees in latitude (with the exception of the Hungarian Plains and evergreen regions of the Mediterranean region), Asia Minor, Caucasia, Siberia, and North America.

Methyl-L-cysteine sulfoxide   R = CH₃

Alliin (allyl-L-cysteine sulfoxide)   R = CH₂CH=CH₂

Allyl-prop-2-ene-thiosulfinate (Allicin)

Allyl-methane-thiosulfinate

Methyl-methane-thiosulfinate

$R^1 = R^2 = CH_2–CH=CH_2$ Ajoene

$R^1 = CH_3$ $R^2 = CH_2–CH=CH_2$ Methylajoene

$R^1 = R^2 = CH_3$ Dimethylajoene

Methylallyl-trisulfide

Main cultivation areas: Grown only in small tracts or in gardens.

Main exporting countries: The supply is mostly wild collected in Eastern European countries.

Cultivation: Ramsons prefers damp, humus rich, preferably calcareous soil in shade or half-shaded locations, thrives in the garden, but also in sandy soil. It is a cold germinator, requiring the influence of frosty weather for vernalization. Therefore, sowing must take place from August to March. If sowing must occur later than March, it is then necessary to mix the seeds with damp sand and store in plastic bags for at least three weeks at 15 to 20 °C, and then another 4 to 6 weeks in the refrigerator at maximum +4 °C. After that, the seeds can be cultivated at 10 to 12 °C. Propagation with the bulbs is also possible. They can be planted out with 8 to 10 clusters/m². Although ramsons is an impressive plant, it is only rarely tolerated in the garden due to its intensive garlic-like odor and its tendency to rapidly spread out [Ü96].

Culinary Herb

Commercial forms: Ramsons: dried lower part of the plant (lower sections of the leaves and the bulb).

Production: The fresh leaves are harvested from April to May, and the bulbs are harvested after the flowering period up until the autumn [Ü96].

Forms used: Fresh leaves, fresh bulbs, rarely also the flowers, dried lower plant parts.

Storage: The leaves should be used fresh; they can be stored in the refrigerator in a plastic bag for 1 to 2 weeks. Deep freeze storage of the plant material is recommended. Drying leads to an almost complete loss of aroma.

Description. Whole leaf (Fig. 1): Leaves and bulbs, see description of plant.

Odor: Garlic-like, **Taste:** Faintly pungent and reminiscent of garlic.

History: Ramsons seeds were found in human dwellings of the Neolithic period along the lakes of the subalpine zone. The ancient Germans as well as the Romans and Gauls used ramsons. In the Middle Ages, it was preferably cultivated in cloister gardens and near fortresses. The occurrence of ramsons today can be traced back to these cultivation areas [8].

Constituents and Analysis

Constituents

- Alliins: (*S*-Alk(ene)ylcysteine sulfoxides): In the bulb and leaves (+)-*S*-methyl-L-cysteine sulfoxide and alliin (*S*-(+)-allyl-L-cysteine sulfoxide), as well their γ-glutamyl-derivatives [12].
- Alliaceous oils: The non-volatile alliins come into contact with the enzyme alliinase when the plant tissue is damaged, and thus convert to volatile alk(ene) sulfenic acids, which spontaneously transform into the alliaceous aroma components, the alk(ene)yl-alkane/-alkene thiosulfinates (see Fig. 10 in the General Section).
  After extraction, 0.18 to 0.43% allicin (allyl-prop-2-enthiosulfinate) was detected in the bulb and 0.07% in the leaves, as well as allyl-methane-thiosulfinate, methyl-prop-2-ene-thiosulfinate and methyl-methane-thiosulfinate; also present are the breakdown products ajoene and ajoene homologs, such as methyl-ajoene, dimethyl-ajoene, 2-vinyl-(4H)-1,3-dithiin and 3-vinyl-(4H)-1,2-dithiin. After steam distillation, mostly methyl-allyl-trisulfide as well as diallyl-disulfide and diallyl-trisulfide were found [10, 12].
- Flavonoids: Kaempferol glycosides, partially esterified with phenylacrylic acids, e.g. kaempferol-3-*O*-β-neohesperidoside-7-*O*-[2-*O*-(*trans-p*-coumaroyl)]-β-D-glucoside [1, 2].
- Saponins: One component has been structurally identified as a pregnadiene-olon-tetraoside [3].
- Polysaccharides: Fructans, about 30 to 90% [6].

Tests for Identity: → Onion, see also Lit. [12].

Quantitative assay: → Onion, see also Lit. [12].

Adulterations, Misidentifications and Impurities: The leaves of autumn crocus (*Colchicum autumnale* L.), have been mistaken for ramsons, resulting in poisonings, some of which were fatal [4, Ü27]. Misidentification of the leaves from lily-of-the-valley (*Convallaria majalis* L.) is also possible. By their alliaceous odor and taste, the leaves of ramsons, however, are easily recognized.

Actions and Uses

Actions: Due to its pungent taste as well as the stimulating effect of its oil on the gastric mucosa, ramsons has an appetite stimulating and digestion promoting action.
2% pulverized ramsons leaves in the standard chow of rats had a cardioprotective effect. The incidence of ventricular fibrillation after occlusion of the descending branch of the left coronary artery was lower than in the hearts of the control group (20% vs. 88%) [5]. Extracts of ramsons inhibited in vitro 5-lipoxygenase, cyclooxygenase, angiotensin-I-converting enzyme (ACE) and thrombocyte aggregation. The results suggest that ramsons exhibit the same effects as → Garlic [9, 11, 12].

Toxicology: Based on existing data on healthy individuals, there is no acute or chronic toxicity with the regular use of ramsons as a culinary herb. It can be assumed that high doses lead to gastric irritation in susceptible people.

Culinary use: The fresh, finely chopped leaves or the chopped bulbs are used, similar to chives, as a spice for salads, cottage cheese, soft cheese (especially sheep's milk cheese and goat's milk cheese), herb but-

ter, ground meats, sauces, herb-, vegetable- and fish soups, herb omelets, vegetable dishes, meat courses, e.g. roast veal and roast lamb, or spaetzle (pasta) dough. The whole or cut leaves are also quite delicious on buttered bread or with cottage cheese on an open face sandwich. Occasionally, the flowers are used as a spicy and decorative salad topping [7, 8, Ü46, Ü66, Ü90].
The leaves can be steamed and eaten as a vegetable or they can be used as an ingredient in risotto or pasta [7, Ü51, Ü71].

As a component of spice mixes and preparations: → Pesto.

Similar tasting spices: → Chives, → Garlic.

Ramsons-Pizza
Dough: 200 g flour, 10 g yeast, 3 tablespoons of vegetable oil, some lukewarm milk, salt.

Prepare smooth and elastic dough from the above ingredients, and let it set for 30 minutes in an oven at 50 °C. Spread the dough in a layer of 0.5 cm on a lightly oiled sheet.

Topping: 100 g fresh ramsons leaves, 75 g smoked bacon, 30 g butter, 4 eggs, 1 cup of sour cream, 50 g graded cheese, salt, pepper, a pinch of caraway.

The bacon is diced into small cubes and pan-fried. The washed leaves are cut into 1 cm wide strips, and steamed together with butter and bacon for 5 minutes. The eggs are shortly beaten in a large bowl and then mixed well with the steamed ramsons, fried bacon pieces, sour cream, cheese and spices.
Distribute the topping mixture evenly on the pizza dough, and bake at 200 °C for 45 minutes [Ü56].

Medicinal herb

Herbal drug: Allii ursini herba, Ramsons herb, Allii ursini bulbus, Ramsons bulb.

Indications: In folk medicine, it is used for gastrointestinal complaints, such as fermentative dyspepsia and flatulence, but also for high blood pressure and for prevention of arteriosclerosis [Ü106]. Ramsons milk (pour milk over finely chopped leaves and bulbs and steep for three hours) is recommended for gastrointestinal disturbances [7].

Literature

[1] Carotenuto A. et al., Gazz. Chim. Ital. 127(9):523–536 (1998).
[2] Carotenuto A. et al., Phytochemistry 41:531–536 (1996).
[3] Janeczko Z. et al., Acta Pol. Pharm. 57(2):131–133 (2000).
[4] Klintschar M. et al., Forensic Sci. Int. 106(3):191–200 (1999).
[5] Rietz B. et al., Mol. Cell Biochem. 119 (1/2):143–150 (1993).
[6] Rubat de Mérac ML, Recherches sur le métabolisme glucidique du genre Allium et en particulier d'Allium ursinum L, Theses (Sci. nat.) Univ. Paris 1949, ref. in Ü43.
[7] Scholz H., Natürlich 18(3):46–51 (1998).
[8] Scholz H., Natürlich 20(4):30–34 (2000).
[9] Sendl A. et al., Planta Med. 58(1):1–7 (1992).
[10] Sendl A., H. Wagner, Planta Med. 57:361–362 (1991).
[11] Wagner H. et al., Pharm. Pharmacol. Letters 1(1):15–18 (1991).
[12] Wagner H., A. Sendl, Dtsch. Apoth. Ztg. 130(33):1809–1815 (1990).

Literature references identified by Ü can be found in the general listing of books and monographs at the back of this book.

Rosemary

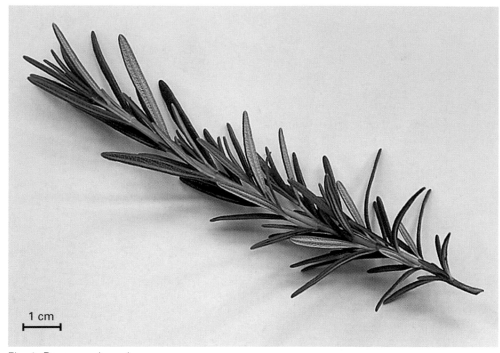

Fig. 1: Rosemary branch

1 cm

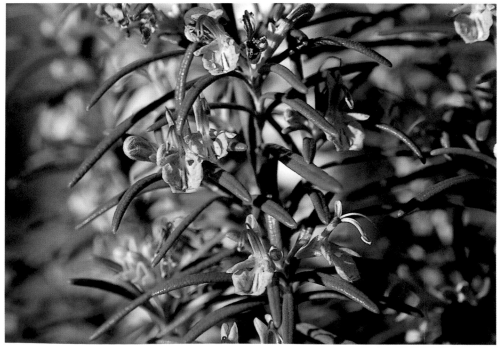

Fig. 2: Rosemary (*Rosmarinus officinalis* L.)

Plant source: *Rosmarinus officinalis* L.

Taxonomic classification: The species is morphologically very diverse. Some authors have divided it into several varieties and forms.

Family: Mint family (Lamiaceae, synonym Labiatae).

Common names: Engl.: rosemary; Fr.: rosmarin, romarin; Ger.: Rosmarin, Kranzenkraut.

Description: Evergreen shrub, about 2 m in height, bearing sessile, narrowly linear, almost acicular, coriaceous, up to 4 cm long leaves with a revolute margin and covered with a white tomentum on the inferior side. The axillary, labiaceous flowers are pale bluish, light bluish violet or white, with the 2 stamina extending well beyond the corolla [Ü106].

Native origin: Southern Europe, particularly the coastal regions of the Mediterranean Sea: Spain, Southern France, Italy, Greece, Turkey, Morocco to Tunisia, and in the Caucasus region.

Main cultivation areas: Mediterranean region (Spain, Portugal, Southern France, Northern Africa), Russian Federation (on the Crimea), India, the Philippines, Antilles, South Africa, Australia, the USA, and Mexico.

Main exporting countries: Spain, Turkey, France, Italy, Morocco, and Tunisia. A significant amount of the supply originates from wild collections, particularly in Spain.

Cultivation: Soil requirements for rosemary are very low. It will also grow in soils that are not suitable for agricultural use. Sandy loam soil in sunny, warm, dry, wind-protected locations has proven to be favorable. Because of its low cold-resistance, it is only possible to grow rosemary as a perennial crop in warm southern locations in Central Europe (a Hungarian strain of rosemary that can endure freezing temperatures down to –25 °C has been described [24]). Propagation can be carried out by seeds or with tip cuttings. Seeding is done in a cold frame. At the end of May, the plantlets can be transplanted into the open field. For personal use it is recommended to grow rosemary in pots, which from May until October can be left outside and during the winter kept in light rooms at about 10 °C. The plant needs only a little watering in the winter, but the root balls should never become completely dry. Older plants should only be repotted in intervals of a few years. Upright growing varieties include, among others, 'Suffolk Blue' (blue flowering), 'Majorca Pink' (pink flowering), 'Albus' (white flowering), 'Miss Jessup's Upright' (pale blue flowering), procumbent or semi-prostrate varieties include 'Prostratus' and 'Severn Sea' [Ü41, Ü47, Ü96].

Culinary herb

Commercial forms: Rosemary: dried leaves, rosemary extract (largely free of essential oil), rosemary essential oil and rosemary oleoresin.

Production: Harvested during or after the blooming period. Generally the branches are collected and then the leaves are separated by hand or after drying by threshing [Ü41]. For individual need, the leaves and shoot tips can be harvested throughout the year.

Forms used: The fresh or, if not available, the dried leaves or branches, rarely the flowers.

Storage: The fresh leaves or herb can be stored for a few days in plastic bags in the refrigerator, or minced and deep-frozen in water. The dried herb should be stored in a cool place, protected from light and moisture, in air-tight porcelain-, glass- or suitable metal containers; in this way, rosemary can be kept for several years without significant aroma loss. Ground rosemary quickly loses its aroma.

Description. Whole leaf (Fig. 1): 2 to 4 cm long, 0.2 to 0.4 cm wide, acicular, sessile, entire-margined, gray-green and brittle leaves, having a hairy lower surface with very prominent midrib, which is most always unrecognizable due to the revolute leaf margin; flowers and fragments thereof can also be present [Ü37].

Powdered leaf: Characteristic of the microscopic mount are the particularly numerous multiple-branched trichomes, small glandular trichomes, lamiaceous glandular scales (Fig. 3) and leaf fragments with epidermal cells having a thick-walled cuticula [Ü49].

Odor: Spicy, somewhat camphorous, **Taste:** Aromatic, bitter, astringent.

History: Rosemary was already used in Egypt during antiquity. The Benedictine monks brought this plant to Central Europe in the 9th century. In the government decree by Karl the Great "Capitulare de villis" regulating agricultural practices (authored about 795 CE, see footnote → Anise), its cultivation was made mandatory [20, 70, Ü92, Ü97].

Constituents and Analysis

DIN- and ISO-Standards. ISO Specification 11164 (Dried rosemary).

Constituents
- Essential oil: 0.1 to 3.0%, the ratio of the individual components is race-specific and strongly depends on the developmental stage of the plant. The main components can be 1,8-cineole (3 to 60%), α-pinene (1 to 57%), camphene (1 to 57%), camphor (10 to 35%), borneol (1 to 18%), bornyl acetate (1 to 21%), verbenone (0 to 28%), p-cymene (0.5 to 10%) or myrcene (0.5 to 12%);

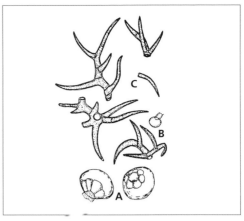

Fig. 3: Rosemary. **A** Lamiaceous glandular scales **B** Multiple-branched trichomes and fragments thereof, **C** Small glandular trichome. From Ü49.

also present are, among others, β-caryophyllene, limonene, linalool, β-pinene, sabinene, γ-terpinene, α-terpineol and terpinenol-4. The occurrence of octane-3-one (up to 10%) is disputed [8, 10, 12–14, 22, 24, 29, 50, 53, 57–59, 63–66, 74, 77–79].
The European Pharmacopoeia allows an essential oil composition of provenances from Spain of 16 to 25% 1,8-cineole, 18 to 26% α-pinene, 13 to 21% camphor and of 8 to 12% camphene, among others, of provenances from Morocco or Tunisia 38 to 55% 1,8-cineole, 9 to 14% α-pinene, 5 to 15% camphor and 2.5 to 6% camphene, among others [Ph Eur].
- Diterpene phenols: Mainly carnosolic acid (about 0.35%, readily transformed to carnosol = picrosalvin and rosmanol), as well as isorosmanol, rosmadial, rosmaridiphenol, rosmariquinone (miltirone) and 7-methoxyrosmanol [7, 42, 60, 80].
- Hydroxycinnamic acid derivatives (known as "labiate tannins"): About 3.5%, mainly rosmarinic acid (about 1.1 to 2.5%) [37, 41, 51, 52, 67].
- Flavonoids: Including, among others, the glycosides cirsimarin, diosmin, hesperidin, homoplantiginin, eupafolin-3′-glucoside, luteolin-3′-glucuronide as well as its 4″- and 3″-acetate and the aglycones of these compounds [1, 15, 17, 61].

Carnosolic acid   Carnosol   Rosmanol

Rosmadial   Rosmariquinone   Rosmadiphenol

Rosmarinic acid

■ Triterpenes, sterols: Oleanolic and ursolic acid, their 3-acetates, as well as α- and β-amyrin, rofficerone [16, 32, 45].

Tests for Identity: With sensoric, macroscopic and microscopic examination as well as TLC of the extract [DAC 86, PF X, see Lit. Ü37, Ü102] or essential oil [Ph Eur see Lit. Ü37, Ü77], and GC of the essential oil [27, 29, 38].

Quantitative assay: The content of essential oil can be determined, according to the European Pharmacopoeia, with the steam distillation assay using a prefilled graduated tube with xylol [Ph Eur]. The quantitative composition of the essential oil is determined with GC [DAB]. Other assays include HPLC methods for the antioxidative diterpene phenols [71] and rosmarinic acid [33], which also can be determined with GC after silylation [67].

Adulterations, Misidentifications and Impurities have been observed, with the leaves from *Ledum palustre* L. (wild rose-

mary, Labrador tea). The essential oil of commerce is sometimes adulterated with oil of turpentine, eucalyptus oil or camphor oil fractions and, in some cases, adjusted to certain specification requirements by the addition of 1,8-cineole, borneol or bornyl acetate [Ü37].

Actions and Uses

Actions: Due to their aromatic and bitter taste, rosemary leaves are appetizing and digestion promoting.

Ethanolic and aqueous extracts of the rosemary plant, especially of the young branches have shown dose-dependent choleretic action. The extracts also have hepatoprotective action. Pretreatment of experimental animals with extracts before application of carbon tetrachloride (hepatotoxic agent) lessened liver damage (measured as plasma glutamic-pyruvic transaminase levels, among other parameters). Administration after the application of carbon tetrachloride had no effect. The

mutagenic effect of cyclophosphamide in mice could also be suppressed [26, 40].

Aqueous-alcoholic extracts of rosemary are also able to inhibit the induction of ethanol-, indomethacin- or reserpine-induced gastric ulcers in rats [23].

Ethanolic extracts of the herb exhibit antispasmodic action in vitro in isolated guinea pig intestine with acetylcholine or histamine used as the spasmogens [30]. Rosemary oil has also demonstrated spasmolytic activity in vitro in electro-stimulated guinea pig longitudinal smooth muscle of the ileum, although only at relatively high concentrations (ED_{50} 130 mg/l). The borneol component was shown to be more effective than the essential oil itself (ED_{50} 8 mg/l) [76]. Similar results were shown in preparations of guinea pig trachea [5, 6].

Supplementation of rosemary powder to rats (1% mixed in the feed) for 2 weeks reduced by 76% the binding of carcinogenic 7,12-dimethylbenz[a]anthracene in the cells. The formation of carcinogen-induced mammary tumors was strongly reduced [4, 73]. Cocarcinogen (TPA)- and carcinogen (7,12-dimethylbenz[a]anthracene and benzo[a]pyrene)induced formation of skin tumors in mice could be strongly limited by the application of rosemary extracts on the skin [43].

The observed in vitro antiviral action of rosemary extracts [69], which depends mainly on the rosmarinic acid content but possibly also on the diterpene phenols content, is probably only relevant in topical application.

Inhalation of rosemary oil of the cineole-type increases locomotor activity in mice [49].

Rosemary oil has antibacterial [11, 24, 44, 56, 62, 75] and fungistatic [21] activity. Rosemary extracts have a strong antioxidative effect due to the diterpene phenols and flavonoids that function as hydrogen donators and free radical scavengers [2, 9, 19, 31, 34, 36, 68].

Toxicology: Based on existing data, there is no acute or chronic toxicity with the use of rosemary leaves as a spice or essential oil at normal doses (up to 20 drops/d).

In mice, an accelerated metabolism of estrogens (estradiol, estrone) by hydroxylation and glucuronidation has been observed if the feed contained 2% of a methanolic rosemary extract [82]. Whether these effects are related to the misuse of rosemary preparations as an abortifacient remains unclear. Even though animal experiments with rats showed that rosemary extracts cannot induce abortion [54], high doses of rosemary preparations should be avoided during pregnancy until the potential risks have been clarified.

Allergic reactions have been observed occasionally with the use of rosemary leaves [28, 39] and rarely with the use of the essential oil [Ü39].

Culinary use: Rosemary is a typical spice of Italian, Spanish and Provençal cooking, but is also used in English cooking, as well as cooking of the Balkan- and Caucasus countries, the USA and Mexico. Rosemary is an integral component of the Mexican national dish "Rosmeritas" (corn meal with crabs).

For culinary use the young leaves are finely chopped or ground in a mortar. They are then filled into a small cloth sack or steel tea ball and cooked with the meal or added 10 minutes before the end of cooking (keeping rosemary for too long in the meal may lead to the occurrence of a bitter off-taste). Less often the adding of fresh or dried rosemary branches when cooking or roasting is recommended. The leaves usually fall off and then must be individually removed before serving. For grilling, a branch can be laid on the fire and/or the grilled pieces of meat can be rubbed with it. Woody branches, defoliated in the lower part, can be used as grill spears. For dishes from which the leaves cannot be removed before serving, e.g. salads, freshly prepared rosemary powder (spice mill) is used. Because of its intense taste, rosemary should be dosed reservedly. A small branch is enough for one dish.

The fresh or dried leaves are used as a seasoning of meat dishes, (especially of lamb, but also of pork, game and poultry), of fatty fish dishes (e.g. of mackerel or sardines), liver (of liver pastes and chicken liver), of sausage products, pizzas and, carefully measured, also of soups (e.g. of potato soup), sauces (especially of tomato-based sauces for fish), salads (e.g. cheese salad), vegetables (of peas, green beans, asparagus, broccoli, cauliflower, zucchini, spinach and rutabaga), tomato- and eggplant dishes, baked potatoes, mushrooms, omelets, farinaceous pastes, marinades (especially for grilled dishes, fish dishes or brats) and sheep cheese [Ü2, Ü13, Ü45, Ü65, Ü79, Ü93].

Rosemary is also used as a spice of sweet dishes, e.g. of marmalades and jellies (of sour cherry-, apricot- and strawberry marmalade as well as apple jelly), and baked goods [Ü71, Ü79].

Likewise rosemary is suitable as a flavoring of herb vinegar and is it quite suitable as a salad seasoning [Ü51].

The flowers are used as a salad garnish [Ü30, Ü55, Ü74, Ü92].

The essential oil is used in the liqueur industry (Benedictine, Danziger Goldwasser) and in the perfume industry, e.g. for perfuming of soaps, but also in the production of air fresheners.

Rosemary extracts, especially the essential oil-free rosemary extract, are used as antioxidants for increasing the shelf life of fat-containing foods (also declared on the label as a spice extract) [55, 72, Ü98].

Combines well with: Bay, caraway, garlic, marjoram, onions, parsley, sage, tarragon, and thyme.

As a component of spice mixes and preparations: → Bouquet garni, → Café de Paris spice mix, → Fines herbes, → Fish spice, → Grill spice, → Herb butter, → Herb salt, → Herb vinegar, → Herbes de Provence, → Meat spice, → Mélange classique, → Parisian pepper, → Pizza spice, → Venison spice.

Other uses: Rosemary extracts are used in cosmetics and as components of hair lotions and bath additives; rosemary oil is used as a perfume in soaps, eau de Cologne and skin oils [Ü24].

Medicinal herb

Herbal drugs: Rosmarini folium, Rosemary leaves, minimum 1.2% essential oil and minimum 3% hydroxycinnamic acid derivatives [Ph Eur], Rosmarini aetheroleum, Rosemary oil, specifications see above [Ph Eur].

Indications: Rosemary leaves and rosemary oil are taken internally for problems with digestion, externally as supportive therapy in the treatment of rheumatic diseases and circulatory disorders [47], as well as in baths for supportive treatment of conditions of exhaustion [46]. The internal use of rosemary leaves is in the form of tea infusions (single dose 2 g/150 ml, daily dose 4 to 6 g) and tinctures as per the EB 6 monograph (daily dose 2.5 to 7.5 g) or externally in the form of baths (50 g per full bath). Rosemary oil is orally ingested in pure form (3 to 4 drops, 3 to 4 times daily with sugar), externally in the form of 5 to 10 per cent ointments, skin oils and spirits or of baths (minimum 0.01 g/l). Internal rosemary oil should not be given during pregnancy. For baths the common restrictions must be observed [46].

Furthermore rosemary leaf can be taken internally for improvement of hepatic- and biliary function and externally for promotion of wound healing [25].

In folk medicine, rosemary serves, among other uses, to promote digestion, as a treatment for headaches, migraines, bronchitis, colic, respiratory tract infections, urinary tract disorders and dysmenorrhea, and is used externally for the treatment of alopecia. Rosemary wine is popularly used for menstrual complaints, heart problems and nervousness. Rosemary oil is used in the form of ointments, embrocations or baths for rheumatic pains, circulatory problems, conditions of exhaustion, bruises, strains and sprains [8, 35, 70, 83, Ü37].

Similar culinary herbs

Lavender, *Lavandula angustifolia* MILL., native to the coastal regions of the Mediterranean Sea, cultivation takes place particularly in Southern France, Spain, Albania, Hungary, Bulgaria and the former Yugoslavia. The main components of its essential oil are $(R)(-)$-linalool (20 to 50%) and $(R)(-)$-linalyl acetate (30 to 55%), followed by, among others, 1,8-cineole, camphor and β-caryophyllene epoxide. The inflorescences, flowers and leaves are used as a flavoring of sweet and salty dishes, especially in France, Spain and Italy, but also in England. For example, they are added as a seasoning of marmalades, ice creams, pudding and sorbets, as well as roast mutton, pheasant, fish (especially trout), fish soups and salad marinades. Lavender is also used for the production of lavender oil or vinegar (for seasoning of salads), of lavender flower syrup (for flavoring of fruit salads), cream for desserts and of herb butter. When grilling meat, a few branches can also be placed on the charcoal. Lavender should be measured very carefully. Too much lavender will bestow a perfume-like off-taste to the meal. Because of their lower essential oil content, the leaves can be dosed more liberally than the flowers. Lavender is a component of spice mixes including → Fines herbs, → Herbes de Provence, and → Ras el hanout. Small cloth sacks filled with lavender flowers can be hung in the closet for a pleasant odor and to protect against moths [3, 18, Ü1, Ü2, Ü17, Ü46, Ü93]. For therapeutic use, lavender is taken internally in the form of tea infusions (1 to 2 teaspoons/cup) for mood disorders such as conditions of restlessness, insomnia and functional upper abdominal complaints (nervous stomach irritations, Roehmheld syndrome, meteorism, nervous intestinal discomfort) as well as in balneotherapy for functional circulatory disorders [48].

Literature

[1] Aeschbach R. et al., Bull. Liaison – Groupe Polyphénols 13:56–58 (1986), ref. Ü37.

[2] Aeschbach R., E. Prior, J. Agric. Food Chem. 44(1):131–135 (1996).

[3] Agnel H., P. Teisseire, Perfum. Flavorist 9:53–56 (1984).

Rosemary marmalade with cranberries

250 g rosemary leaves, 1/2 l orange juice, 2 lemons, 2 small packs of vanilla sugar, 1 kg sugar (premixed with pectin), 250 g cooked cranberries.

Combine the rosemary leaves with the orange juice in a large pot, bring to a boil and allow the mixture to rest on medium heat for 10 to 15 minutes; then, remove the pot from the flame and pass the content through a strainer or sieve. Mix the obtained filtrate with lemon juice and vanilla sugar, and then stir in the premixed sugar with pectin. Bring the whole mixture to a boil and let it bubble for 5 to 6 minutes under constant stirring. Mix in the cooked cranberries and again bring to a boil. Fill the hot mixture into canning jars, apply the seal and allow to cool to room temperature [Ü1].

[4] Amagase H. et al., J. Nutr. 126(5): 1475–1480 (1996).

[5] Ammon H.P.T., Z. Phytother. 10(6): 167–174 (1989).

[6] Aqel M., J. Ethnopharmacol. 33:57–62 (1991).

[7] Arisawa M. et al., J. Nat. Prod. 50:1165–1166 (1987).

[8] Arnold N. et al., J. Ess. Oil Res. 9:167–175 (1997).

[9] Aruoma O.I. et al., Food Chem. Toxicol. 34(5):449–456 (1996).

[10] Baratta Z.M. et al., J. Ess. Oil Res. 10:618–627 (1998).

[11] Benjilali B. et al., J. Food Prot. 47:748–752 (1984).

[12] Boelens M.H., Perfum. Flavorist 10:21–24, 26 et 28–37 (1985).

[13] Boutekedjiret C. et al., J. Ess. Oil Res. 10:680–682 (1998).

[14] Boutekedjiret C. et al., J. Ess. Oil Res. 11:238–240 (1999).

[15] Brieskorn C.H. et al., Dtsch. Lebensm. Rdsch 69:245–246 (1973).

[16] Brieskorn C.H. et al., Arch. Pharm. 286: 501–506 (1953).

[17] Brieskorn C.H., H.J. Dömling, Arch. Pharm. 300:1042–1044 (1967).

[18] Canaud F., M.O. Martineu, Bull. Union Physiciens 90(789, Cahier 1):1941–1950 (1996).

[19] Cuvelier M.E. et al., J. Ess. Oil Chem. 73(5):645–652 (1996).

[20] Czygan I., F.C. Czygan, Z. Phytother. 18(3):182–186 (1997).

[21] Daferera D.J. et al., J. Agric. Food Chem. 48(6):2576–2581 (2000).

[22] Dellacassa E. et al., J. Ess. Oil Res. 11:27–30 (1999).

[23] Dias P.C. et al., J. Ethnopharmacol. 69(1):57–62 (2000).

[24] Domokos J. et al., J. Ess. Oil Res. 9(1):41–45 (1997).

[25] ESCOP, ESCOP Monographs, Rosmarini folium cum flores, Rosemary (1997).

[26] Fahim F.A. et al., Int. J. Food Sci. Nutr. 50(6):413–427 (1999).

[27] Fehr D., G. Stenzhorn, Pharm. Ztg. 124: 2342–2349 (1979).

[28] Fernandez L. et al., Contact Dermatitis 37(5):248–249 (1997).

[29] Formacék, V., K.H. Kubeczka, Essential Oils Analysis by Capillary Gas Chromatography and Carbon–13-NMR Spectroscopy, John Wiley & Sons, Chicester, New York, Brisbane, Toronto, Singapore 1982.

[30] Forster H.B. et al., Planta Med. 40(4): 309–319 (1980).

[31] Fränkel E.N. et al., J. Agric. Food Chem. 44:131–316 (1996).

[32] Ganeva Y. et al., Planta Med. 59(3):276 –277 (1993).

[33] Gracza L., Ruff P., Arch. Pharmaz. 317: 339–345 (1984).

[34] Hall III C.A. et al., J. Am. Oil Chem. Soc. 75(9):1147–1154 (1998).

[35] Haloui M. et al., J. Ethnopharmacol. 71(3):465–472 (2000).

[36] Haraguchi H. et al., Planta Med. 61(4): 333–33 (1995).

[37] Herrmann K., Z. Lebensm. Unters. Forsch. 116:224–228 (1961).

[38] Hethelyi E. et al., Acta Pharm. Hung. 57:159–169 (1987).

[39] Hjorther A.B. et al., Contact Dermatitis 37(3):99–10 (1997).

[40] Hoefler C. et al., J. Ethnopharmacol. 19: 133–143 (1987).

[41] Hohmann J. et al., Planta Med. 65(6): 576–578 (1999).

[42] Houlihan C.M. et al., J. Am. Oil Chem. Soc. 62:96–99 (1985).

[43] Huang M.T. et al., Cancer Res. 54(3): 701–708 (1994).

[44] Janssen A.M. et al., Pharm. Weekbl. 10: 277–280 (1988).

[45] Kojima H., H. Ogura, Phytochemistry 28: 1703–1710 (1989).

[46] Kommission B8 beim BfArM., BAnz Nr. 48 vom 10.03.1992 (1992).

[47] Kommission E beim BfArM., BAnz 223 vom 30.11.85, Berichtigung vom 13.03. 1990.

[48] Kommission E beim BfArM., BAnz-Nr. 228 vom 05.12.1984, Berichtigung vom 13.03.1990.

[49] Kovar K.A. et al., Planta Med. 53: 315–318 (1987).

[50] Kreis P. et al., Dtsch. Apoth. Ztg. 131(39):1984–1987 (1991).

[51] Lamaison J.L. et al., Pharm. Acta Helv 66(7):185–188 (1991).

[52] Lamaison J.L. et al., Ann. Pharm. Franc 48:103–108 (1990).

[53] Lamparsky D., H.P. Schenk, in: K.H. Kubeczka (Hrsg.): Ätherische Öle, Thieme Verlag, Stuttgart 1982, p, 136–148 (1982).

[54] Lemonica I.P. et al., Braz. J. Med. Biol. Res. 29(2):223–227 (1996).

[55] Lindberg Madsen H. et al., Z. Lebensm. Unters. Forsch. 203(4):333–338 (1996).

[56] Mangena T., N.Y. Muyima, Lett. Appl. Microbiol. 28(4):291–296 (1999).

[57] Mastelic J. et al., Acta Pharm. (Zagreb) 47(2):139–142 (1997).

[58] Moretti M.D.L. et al., J. Ess. Oil Res. 10(1):111–112 (1998).

[59] Moretti M.D.L. et al., J. Ess. Oil Res. 10(3):261–267 (1997).

[60] Nakatani N., R. Inatani, Agric. Biol. Chem. 48:2081–2085 (1984).

[61] Okamura N. et al., Phytochemistry 37(5): 1463–1466 (1994).

[62] Pellecuer J. et al., Plant Méd. Phytothér. 9:99–106 (1975).

[63] Pérez-Alonso M.J. et al., J. Ess. Oil Res. 7(1):73–75 (1995).

[64] Pino J.A. et al., J. Ess. Oil Res. 10(1):111–112 (1997).

[65] Porte A. et al., J. Ess. Oil Res. 12:577–580 (2000).

[66] Ravid U. et al., Flavour Fragrance J. 12(2): 109–112 (1997).

[67] Reschke A., Z. Lebensm. Unters. Forsch. 176:116–119 (1983).

[68] Richheimer S.L. et al., J. Am. Oil Chem. Soc. 73(4):507 514 (1996).

[69] Romero E. et al., Mitt. Gebiete Lebensm. Hyg. 80:113–119 (1989).

[70] Scholz H., Natürlich 19(10):54–59 (1999).

[71] Schwarz K., W. Ternes, Z. Lebensm. Unters. Forsch. 195:95–98, 99–103, 104–107 (1992).

[72] Shahidi F. et al., J. Food Lipids 2(3): 145–153 (1995).

[73] Singletary K. et al., Cancer Lett. (Shanon, Israel) 104(1):43–48 (1996), ref. CA 125: 048538h.

[74] Soriano Cano M.C. et al., J. Ess. Oil Res. 5:243–246 (1993).

[75] Steinmetz M.D. et al., Mycoses 31:40–51 (1988).

[76] Taddei I. et al., Fitoterapia 59:463–468 (1988).

[77] Tomei P.E. et al., J. Ess. Oil Res. 7(3): 279–282 (1995).

[78] Tuberoso C.I.G. et al., J. Ess. Oil Res. 10:660–664 (1998).

[79] Tucker A.O., M.J. Maciarello, Flav. Fragr. J. 1:137–142 (1986).

[80] Wenkert E. et al., J. Org. Chem. 30:2931–2934 (1965).

[81] Weymar H., Buch der Lippenblütler und Rauhblattgewächse, Neumann Verlag, Radebeul 1961.

[82] Zhu B.T. et al., Carcinogenesis 19(10): 1821–1827 (1998).

[83] al-Sereiti M.R. et al., Indian J. Exp. Biol. 37(2):124–130 (1999).

Literature references identified by Ü can be found in the general listing of books and monographs at the back of this book.

Rue

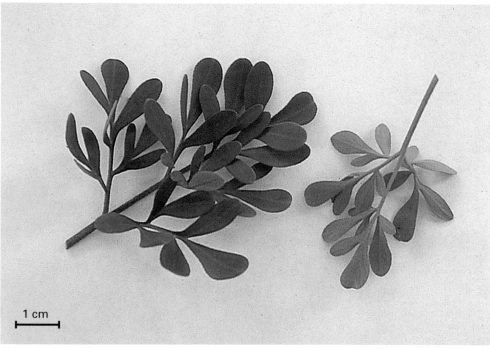

1 cm

Fig. 1: Rue leaves

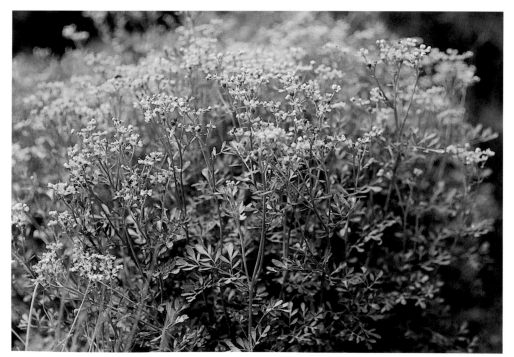

Fig. 2: Rue (*Ruta graveolens* L.)

Plant source: *Ruta graveolens* L.

Taxonomic classification: The species can be divided into 2 subspecies:
R. g. ssp. *hortensis* (MILLER) GAMS (*R. g.* var. *vulgaris* WILLK., *R. hortensis* MILL.), the cultivated subspecies,
R. g. ssp. *divaricata* (TENORE) GAMS (*R. divaricata* TENORE), apparently the wild form of *R. g.* ssp. *hortensis*.

Family: Rue family (Rutaceae).

Common names: Engl.: rue, common rue, vine-rue, garden rue; Fr.: rue, rue de jardins, rue puante; Ger.: Weinraute, Raute, Garten-Raute, Wiesen-Raute, Edel-Raute, Kreuz-Raute, Gnadenkraut.

Description: Perennial plant or subshrub, 20 to 90 cm tall, stem cylindrical, in the lower part woody, with dot-shaped, protruding wart-like oil glands. The bluish-green (ssp. *hortensis*) or faint-yellow (ssp. *divaricata*), glabrous leaves are alternate arranged, up to 10 cm long, up to 6 cm wide, imparipinnate, pinnate leaves are pinnately cleft, the terminal lobes are spatulate, their contours are nearly three-cornered, the leaves bear many dot-shaped translucent wart-like oil glands. The flowers, arranged in cymes, are radial, the terminal ones are quinate, the other ones quadrate; the green calyx is connate in the lower part; the petals are greenish-yellow, bearing a hood-shaped top, 8 or 10 stamina are present; the 5 carpels of the lobed superior ovary show many oil glands. The capsular fruit contains many black-gray angular seeds. Flowering period is from June to August [Ü42].

Native origin: Mediterranean region, in Southern Europe, and naturalized in both American continents.

Main cultivation areas: Worldwide, albeit always cultivated on a small scale

Main exporting countries: France, Spain, Italy, and the former Yugoslavia.

Cultivation: Attention! Due to phototoxicity, avoid skin contact with the plant in all stages of development. It should not be planted alongside of ways!
Rue prefers loose to semi-heavy soil in protected, warm, sunny to half-shaded locations. Rue is cultivated as a perennial plant (3 to 4 years). Propagation is carried out either by direct drilling in April to May, or better yet by advance planting after sowing in March in cold frames in the greenhouse or in hotbeds and planting outdoors in May in a row width of 30×25 cm. The plants are cut several times annually in order to avoid the formation of seeds on the costa of the herbage. For personal use, one plant is sufficient, for which also the non-lignified shoot cuttings can be grown. In rough climates it should be mounded up somewhat in the winter. Rue is also grown as an ornamental plant. Varieties include, among others, 'Großblättrige Späte', 'Kleinblättrige Mittelfrühe', 'Jackman's Blue' (leaves bluish, propagated only by cuttings) and 'Variegata' (leaves in spring with white spots) [55, Ü41, Ü66, Ü96].

Culinary herb

Commercial forms: Rue: dried leaves, whole or ground, rue essential oil.

Production: For culinary use the herb is harvested before the flowering period, wide as a hand above the ground. It is shade dried or dried at about 35 °C [Ü41]. The German Drug Codex [DAC 86] requires however that the aerial part of the plant should be collected and dried during the flowering period.

Forms used: Fresh leaves and shoot tips, ground, dried leaves.

Storage: The fresh leaves or shoot tips stay fresh in a plastic bag for a few days in the refrigerator. They can also be frozen in freezer-bags or frozen in water in the ice-tray. The dried leaves are stored in a cool place, protected from light and moisture, in airtight porcelain-, glass- or suitable metal containers.

Description. Whole leaf (Fig. 1): See description of the whole plant.

Cut leaf: Green, brittle, revolute and lobed leaflets, rolled down, wrinkled on the upper side, glandular punctate pinnate on the lower surface; the official leaf material also contains cylindrical, pithy, dotted fragments of the stem [DAC 86].

Powdered leaf: Microscopic examination of the light green powder reveals the leaf fragments with epidermis, having undate-flexuous side walls, anomocytic stomata and many large, round, schizolysigenous secretory ducts with 4 small covering cells in the upper epidermis. Calcium oxalate druses occur scattered to frequent. The official material also contains stem fragments, remains of the petals and pollen grains with 3 pores, visible as pronounced depressions [DAC 86].

Odor: Characteristic, harshly aromatic, rose-like after drying, **Taste:** Spicy-pungent, bitter.

History: Rue was already known in ancient Rome and Greece as a spice and medicinal plant (particularly in ocular diseases to "strengthen eyesight"). The bible also mentions this plant. Dioscorides (2nd half of the 1st century) described the plant and its use extensively. The Romans brought it to Central Europe and England. In the agricultural decree "Capitulare de villis" by Karl the Great (authored in about 795, see footnote → Anise), its cultivation was made mandatory [for an overview of its history, see Lit. 3, 4].

Constituents and Analysis

Constituents

- Essential oil: 0.4 to 1.2% (high yield with steam distillation of the fresh plant), the main components are nonan-2-one (methylheptyl ketone, 3 to 60%) or undecan-2-one (methylnonyl ketone, 5 to 85%, the ratios of both of the components varies considerably, chemical races?), 2-nonyl-acetate and 2-undecyl acetate; also present are, among others, decan-2-one, ?-undecylpropionate, 2-nonylisobutyrate, 2-nonyl-2-methylbutyrate, pregeierene, hexadecanoic acid and curcuphenol [9, 29, 30, 31, 43, 57, 59, 60, 68, Ü31, Ü38].
- Coumarin, hydroxycoumarin derivatives: Coumarin, umbelliferone, herniarin, gravelliferone, rutacultin, 8-methoxygravelliferone and 3-(1,1'-dimethylallyl)-herniarin, among others, [17, 45], in addition to dimeric hydroxycoumarins, e.g. daphnoretin and its glucoside daphnorin [46].
- Furanocoumarins: The main components are bergaptene (0.01 to 0.12%), psoralene (0.01 to 0.07%), xanthotoxin (0.005 to 0.05%), as well as prenylated constituents, among others, such as chalepensin and 5-geranyloxypsoralene [34, 44, 51].
- Dihydrofuranocoumarins: Mainly rutarin (about 0.9%, rutaretinglucoside), rutaretin (about 0.2%) and rutamarin (chalepinacetate, up to 0.1%) [47, 56].
- Pyranocoumarins: Xanthyletin, among others [48].
- Quinoline alkaloids (0.2 to 1.4%), including the following types, among others:
- Quinoline-type: Graveolinin, graveolin, among others,
- Furo- and dihydrofuroquinoline type: Skimmianine, dictamnin, γ-fagarine,
- Acridone-type: Arborinin, among others,
- Dihydrofuroacridin-type: Rutacridone, gravacridonediol acetate.
- Quinazoline alkaloids: Arborin, among others [34, 40, 42, Ü37].
- Flavonoids: Rutin as the main component (2 to 5%) [57].

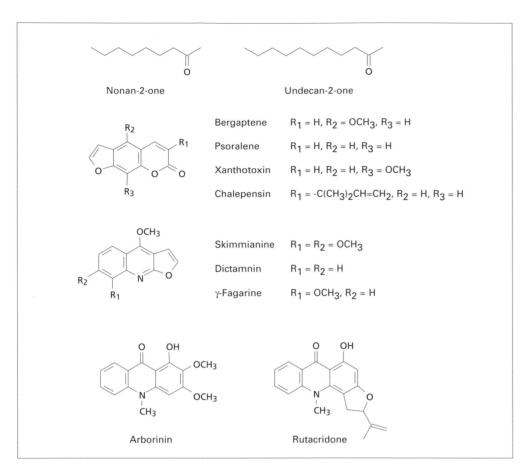

Nonan-2-one Undecan-2-one

Bergaptene	R_1 = H, R_2 = OCH_3, R_3 = H
Psoralene	R_1 = H, R_2 = H, R_3 = H
Xanthotoxin	R_1 = H, R_2 = H, R_3 = OCH_3
Chalepensin	R_1 = -$C(CH_3)_2CH=CH_2$, R_2 = H, R_3 = H

Skimmianine	R_1 = R_2 = OCH_3
Dictamnin	R_1 = R_2 = H
γ-Fagarine	R_1 = OCH_3, R_2 = H

Arborinin Rutacridone

Tests for Identity

Tests for Identity based on morphological and anatomical features of the herb as well as with TLC of the coumarins [Ü102] or the furoquinoline alkaloids, respectively [DAC 86].

Quantitative assay of the flavonoids, after hydrolysis and liquid/liquid extraction of the aglycones, with colorimetric method [DAC 86]; the contents of coumarins and furanocoumarins are determined with GC [10, 13, 21] or HPLC [6, 21] and the furoquinoline alkaloids are quantified with GC [21, 24, 39] or HPLC [24]. The components of the essential oil are assayed with GC [11], after steam distillation or extraction.

Adulterations, Misidentifications and Impurities: The leaves of tarragon, *Artemisia dracunculus* L., have been observed as an adulterant. They are smaller, with a revolute margin and usually bear hairs with split terminal cells as well as composite glandular trichomes [DAC 86].

Actions and Uses

Actions: Due to their aromatic taste, rue leaves are appetite stimulating and digestion promoting.

In isolated rabbit intestine, dry extracts of rue leaves and rue essential oil counteracted the spasm-inducing effects of $BaCl_2$, histamine or acetylcholine. The antispasmodic active constituents are mainly the furanocoumarins and the furoquinoline alkaloids (ED_{50} 6 to 20 µg/ml), but also some components of the essential oil [35].

In animal tests (mice), ethanolic dry extracts of rue leaves (200 mg/kg body weight, p.o.) showed antiphlogistic (granuloma test) and anti-nociceptive (hot plate- and writhing-tests following i.p. injection of diluted acetic acid) [1].

Rue oil kills helminth in vitro (ED_{50} for roundworms 6 to 120 mg/100 ml) [37, 58]. The furoquinoline derivatives have a phototoxic effect on some bacteria and yeasts [61].

Toxicology: There is probably no acute or chronic toxicity with the use of rue as a spice at usual doses. Rue leaves, however, should only be used very sparingly and avoided altogether during pregnancy.

In animal tests (with rats), fertilization-inhibiting effects were observed after the administration of rue leaf infusions (1 ml/kg body weight, p.o.): the implantation rate was reduced, the rate of resorption was increased [19]. Doses of 4 to 8 g rue herb powder/kg body weight, p.o., or 4 ml herb infusion/kg body weight, p.o, corresponding to 8 to 12 g dried herb, over a period of 10 days, reduced gestation by 40 to 80%. In golden (Syrian) hamsters there were no antifertility effects [14]. The effect is attributed to chalepensin, which, in a dose of 0.36 g/kg body weight, reduced fertility by 80% [29]. The fertilization-inhibiting doses used for animal tests are much larger in magnitude when compared to the amounts used as a spice.

The juice of fresh leaves can lead to painful stomach- and gastrointestinal irritations, swelling of the tongue, somnolence, loss of consciousness and abortion [Ü58]. The intake of therapeutic doses of the drug can sometimes lead to a melancholic mood, dizziness, convulsions and sleep disturbances, as well as fatigue [28]. The use of large amounts of the plant extract as an abortive led to vomiting, pain in the upper abdomen, delirium, tremor and even death [29].

Skin contact with the fresh plant leads to photosensitization due to the content of furanocoumarins and to a lesser extent the furoquinoline alkaloids. Upon exposure to the sun, erythema and edema develop in the sensitized areas of the skin [16, 20, 41, 52, 65, 69, Ü58]. These constituents also have photomutagenic effects [53, 54].

After the intake of large doses of rue essential oil, nausea, stomach pains, vomiting, diarrhea, hematemesis, hemorrhage as well as liver- and kidney damage have been observed. With the use of very high doses (in abortion attempts), loss of consciousness, delirium and collapse were observed [37, Ü84].

Culinary use: Rue should only be used extremely sparingly (1 to 2 leaves) due to the unpleasant aroma and bitterness as well as its toxicity when used in larger quantities. Rue should definitely not be used during pregnancy. Rue leaves are added to cooked dishes shortly before the finish of the cooking process.

The small chopped leaves or shoot tips are used as a seasoning of salads, sauces, vegetable soups, marinades, herb vinegar, herb butter, meat dishes, especially of lamb or mutton, poultry and game, herb fillings, fish- and egg dishes, legumes, spinach, mushrooms, quark dishes and cream cheese. Combined with other herbs, it serves also as a bread spread. For the preserving of pickling gherkins or tomatoes, the leaves can also be added. They are an ingredient of Hamburger eel soup [Ü1, Ü2, Ü13, Ü30, Ü45, Ü51, Ü59, Ü65, Ü74, Ü92].

In Ethiopian cooking, it is often added to coffee, tea and other beverages [27].

In the liqueur industry, rue oil serves as an ingredient of the Italian grape schnapps 'Grappa', among others [Ü51].

Combines well with: Bay leaves, juniper berries, sage, and thyme.

As a component of spice mixes: Used as a salt substitute combined with basil, mint, oregano, parsley, summer savory, and thyme.

Other uses: The dried infructescences are also used for decorative purposes, for example in dried flower arrangements, or, sprayed with gold color, as a Christmas ornament.

Medicinal herb

Herbal drug: Rutae herba, Rue herb, contains minimum 0.5% flavonoids, calculated as hyperoside [DAC 86].

Indications: In folk medicine it was formerly used internally for, among other conditions, loss of appetite and dyspeptic complaints, nervousness, hysteria, fever, headaches, neuralgia, circulatory disorders, helminthic infections, eye problems, high blood pressure, menstrual disorders (max. daily dose 1 g), as well as misused to prevent pregnancy or as an abortifacient. Externally it was used for the treatment of rheumatic pains, sprains, skin diseases and inflammations (tincture 1:10 diluted). The essential oil (2 to 6 drops) was used for menstrual complaints and cramps [2, 18, 62, Ü37, Ü66]. In South America, rue is used for symptomatic treatment of multiple sclerosis [2]. Due to the high risk of undesired side effects and the insufficiently substantiated efficacy, the therapeutic use of rue should be avoided [28].

Similarly used leaf herbs

Fringed-rue, *Ruta chalepensis* L. (Rutaceae), native to the entire Mediterranean region, cultivated in the islands of the West Indies, in Mexico, Central- and South America [Ü61]. The constituents include essential oil, of which the main components are undecan-2-one (methylnonyl ketone, comprising 40 to 60%) and nonan-2-one (methylheptyl ketone, 26 to 63%) [31]. Furoquinoline alkaloids (main alkaloids are kokusaginine, skimmianine, γ-fagarine), acridone alkaloids (among others, 1-hydroxy-*n*-methylacridone, chaloridone), quinoline alkaloids, hydroxycoumarins (mainly bergaptene) and furanocoumarins (chalepensin, rutalpinin, among others) [7, 12, 63]. In studies with pregnant mice, it was shown to be embryotoxic (0.16 to 1.6 g/kg body weight, p.o.) [70].

Mountain-rue, *Ruta montana* L. (Rutaceae), native to Southern Europe, Northern Africa, cultivated in Northern Africa, used the same as rue [Ü61].

Curry leaves (murraya, daun salam, curry patte, leaves of the cinnamon tree, see → Cinnamon, are sometimes also referred to as curry leaves), of *Murraya koenigii* (L.) SPRENG. (Rutaceae), native to Central- and Southeastern Asia, cultivated in India (also as an ornamental tree), in Zanzibar and Pemba [Ü61]. The leaves of Indian origin contain 0.2 to 0.8% essential oil, of which the main components are sabinene (32 to 45%), α-pinene (19 to 20%), β-phellandrene (6 to 8%), terpinenol-4 (5 to 10%), β-pinene (about 5%), γ-terpinene (4 to 7%) and α-terpinene (1 to 4%), furthermore, among others, myrcene, linalool, β-caryophyllene, kongol (11-selinene-4α,5α,7β,10β-4-ol) and globulol (10-aromadendranol) [32, 64]. In material of other origins, the essential oil is dominated by β-phellandrene (about 50%), α-pinene (about 9%), (*E*)-β-ocimene (about 7%), α-phellandrene (about 6%) and β-caryophyllene (about 5%) (Sri Lanka, India), α-pinene, β-pinene, β-caryophyllene and γ-elemene (China) or β-phellandrene (about 25%), α-pinene (about 18%), limonene (about 5%) and β-caryophyllene (about 7%) (Malaysia) [32, 33, 67]. The leaves, which, just like other organs of the plant, also contain carbazole alkaloids including, among others, mahanimbine, mahanimbicine, isomahanine, murrayanol and girinimbine, furthermore a significant amount of scopolin (hydroxycoumarin derivate, scopoletin glucoside) [5, 49]. In animal tests, it has shown hypoglycemic [25] and antilipidemic [26] action. In humans these effects occur only transiently [23]. Fresh leaves, rarely also the dried leaves, are used in the cooking of Southern India and Sri Lanka in the same way as bay leaves as a seasoning for meat- and rice dishes. They are cooked with the dish and removed before serving. In chopped form, they also serve as an ingredient of chutneys as well as dried and ground sometimes as a components of → Curry powder [Ü61, Ü92].

Clausena leaves, from *Clausena anisata* J.D. HOOK. (Rutaceae), native to tropical Africa, cultivated also in Indonesia, constituents include 3.5 to 8% essential oil, of which the main component is *trans*-anethole (75 to 90%), as well as, among others, anisaldehyde, anisketone, estragole and α-elemene [15, Ü92]. In a chemotype from Western Africa, which is also cultivated in Indonesia, the essential oil is dominated by estragole (comprising over 80%, hepatotoxic!) [15, 36]. (E)-Foeniculin (comprising over 78%), *trans*-anethole (57 to 67%) + (E)-foeniculin (38 to 29%) or sabinene occur as main components of the essential oil of other West African strains [15]. Carbazole alkaloids, e.g. clausanitin, clausamine-A, -B, and -C, clausenol and clausenine, isolated from the root, bark and branches have shown strong antimicrobial action [22, 50]. Extracts of the leaves and the essential oil are used in the bakery and confectionary industries and are used as a flavoring of anisados, a typical alcoholic drink of the Philippines [Ü31, Ü92].

Buchu leaves, of *Barosma betulina* (BERGIUS) BARTL. et WENDL. (Rutaceae), native to and cultivated in South Africa [Ü61]. The leaves contain 1.5 to 2.5% essential oil, of which the main components are (–)-isomenthone (about 35%), diosphenol (about 12%), ψ-diosphenol (about 8%, a mixture of diosphenols referred to as buchu camphor), pulegone (about 11%) and (+)-limonene (about 10%) [Ü37]. It is used as a seasoning and as a flavor corrective in herbal tea blends [Ü61, Ü37].

Curry plant, the herb from *Helichrysum italicum* (ROTH) GUSS. (Asteraceae), native to the Eastern Mediterranean region, and cultivation in Central Europe is possible. Constituents include 0.1 to 0.2% essential oil, of which the main components of herb from Greek origin are geraniol (about 36%), geranyl acetate (about 15%), (E)-nerolidol (about 12%), and neryl acetate (about 7%) [8], and of Yugoslavian origin α-pinene, γ-curcumene and α-curcumene (*ar*-curcumene) [66], also occurring in the herb is helipyrone (a methylene-bis-triacetic acid lactone derivative) [8, 38]. Fresh branches of curry plant serve as a complement of stews with vegetables, lamb or pork (removed before serving!) [Ü74].

Literature

[1] Atta A.H., A. Alkofahi, J. Ethnopharmacol. 60(2):117–124 (1998).

[2] Bautz C. et al. in: H. Albrecht, G. Franz (Hrsg.): Naturheilverfahren, Springer-Verlag Berlin, Heidelberg 1990, p. 87–114.

[3] Becela-Deller C., Dtsch. Apoth. Ztg. 131(51/52):2705–2709 (1991).

[4] Becela-Deller C., Z. Phytother. 16(5):275–281 (1995).

[5] Begley M.J. et al., Chem. Industr. 1970: 958 (1970).

[6] Beier R.C. et al., Food Chem. Toxicol. 21: 163–165 (1983).

[7] Brooker R.M., Lloydia 30:73–77 (1967).

[8] Chinou I.B. et al., Planta Med. 62(4):377–379 (1996).

[9] Claßen B., K. Knobloch, Z. Lebensm. Untersuch. Forsch. 181:28–31 (1985).

[10] De Vries J.N. et al., Biomed. Environ. Mass Spectrom. 15:413–417 (1988), ref. in Ü37.

[11] Drawert F. et al., Z. Naturforsch. 39c: 525–530 (1984).

[12] El Sayed Kh. et al., J. Nat. Prod. 63: 995–997 (2000).

[13] Elliot S., J. Brimacombe, J. Ethnopharmacol. 19:310–317 (1987).

[14] Gandhi M. et al., J. Ethnopharmacol. 34: 49–59 (1991).

[15] Garneau F.X. et al., J. Ess. Oil Res. 12: 757–762 (2000).

[16] Girard J. et al., Dermatologia 158:229 (1979), ref. in Ü39 (1979).

[17] Gray A.I. et al., Phytochemistry 17:845–864 (1978).

[18] Guarrera P.M., J. Ethnopharmacol. 68(1/3):183–192 (1999).

[19] Guerra M.O., A.T.L. Andrade, Contraception 18:191–199 (1978).

[20] Harber L.C. et al., Arch. Derm. 90:572 (1964), ref. in Ü39.

[21] Heath-Paglioso S. et al., Phytochemistry 31:2683–2688 (1992).

[22] Ito C. et al., Chem. Pharm. Bull. 46 (2): 344–346 (1998).

[23] Iyer U.M., U.V. Mani, Plant Foods Hum. Nutr. 40(4):275–282 (1990).

[24] Kanamori H. et al., Chem. Pharm. Bull. 34:1826–1829 (1986).

[25] Khan B.A. et al., Indian J. Biochem. Biophys. 32(2):106–108 (1995).

[26] Khan B.A. et al., Plant Foods Hum. Nutr. 49(4):295–299 (1996).

[27] Kloos H., Ethnomed. 4:63–103 (1977).

[28] Kommission E beim BfArM., BAnz-Nr. 43 vom 02.03.89.

[29] Kong Y.C. et al., Planta Med. 55(2): 176–178 (1989).

[30] Kubeczka K.H., Flora Abt. A. 158: 519–544 (1967).

[31] Kubeczka K.H., Herba Hung. 10: 109–117 (1971).

[32] Mallavarapu G.R. et al., J. Ess. Oil Res. 11:176–178 (1999).

[33] Mallavarapu G.R. et al., J. Ess. Oil Res. 12:766–768 (2000).

[34] Novák I. et al., Tr. Vses S'ezda Farmatsevtov, 1st 1967:343–350 (1970).

[35] Novák I. et al., Planta Med. 13:226–233 (1966).

[36] Okunade A.L., J.I. Olaifa, J. Nat. Prod. 50(5):990–991 (1987).

[37] Opdyke D.L.J., Food Chem. Toxicol. 13: 455–456 (1975).

[38] Opitz L, R. Hänsel, Tetrahedron. Lett. 1970, 3369 (1970), ref. Ü43.

[39] Paulini H. et al., Mutagenesis 2:217–273 (1987).

[40] Paulini H., et al. Planta Med. 57:82 (1991).

[41] Pether J.V.S., Lancet 26:957 (1985), ref. Ü37.

[42] Petit-Paly et al., Plant Med. Phytothérapie 16(1):55–72 (1982).

[43] Pino J.A. et al., J. Ess. Oil Res. 9(3): 365–366 (1997).

[44] Reisch J., Tetrahedron. Lett. 4395–4396 (1968).

[45] Reisch J. et al., Tetrahedron. Lett. 4305–4308 (1970).

[46] Reisch J. et al., Planta Med. 16:372–376 (1968).

[47] Reisch J. et al., Acta pharmac. suecica. 4: 179–181 (1967).

[48] Reisch J. et al., Planta Med. 17:116–119 (1969).

[49] Reisch J. et al., Phytochemistry 31:2877–2879 (1992).

[50] Reisch J. et al., Sci. Pharm. (Wien) 53: 153 (1985), ref. Ü43.

[51] Rhodighiero G. et al., Gazzetta Chim. Ital. 84:874–878 (1954), zit. Ü37.

[52] Schempp C.M. et al., Hautarzt 50(6): 432–434 (1999).

[53] Schimmer O., Z. Phytother. 12(5): 151–156 (1991).

[54] Schimmer O., I. Kühne, Mutat. Res. 243: 57–62 (1990).

[55] Schmidt L, Drogenreport 6(9):39–40 (1993).

[56] Schneider G. et al., Arch. Pharm. 300: 73–81, 913–916 (1967).

[57] Sprecher E., Pharmazie 13:151–153 (1958).

[58] Srepel B., B. Acacic, Acta Pharm. Jug 12:79–87 (1962).

[59] Tattje D.H., Pharm. Weekblad 105:1242–1260 (1970).

[60] Tattje D.H., R. Bos, Pharm. Weekblad 107:261–265 (1972).

[61] Towers G.H.N. et al., Planta Med. 41(2):136–142 (1981).

[62] Tyler V.E., S. Foster, Tyler's Honest Herbal, Haworth Press, Inc., Binghampton, NY 1999, p. 325–326.

[63] Ulubelen A. et al., Phytochemistry 25: 2692–2693 (1986).

[64] Waßmuth-Wagner I. et al., Planta Med. 61(2):196–197 (1995).

[65] Wessner D. et al., Contact Dermatitis 41(4):232 (1999).

[66] Weyerstahl P. et al., Progr Ess. Oil Res. 177–195 (1986).

[67] Wong K.C., D.Y. Tie, J. Ess. Oil Res. 5:371–374 (1991).

[68] Yaacob K.B. et al., J. Ess. Oil Res. 1:203–207 (1989).

[69] Zaynoun S.T. et al., Contact Dermatitis 3:225 (1977), ref. Ü39.

[70] Zeichen de Sa R. et al., J. Ethnopharmacol. 69(2):93–98 (2000).

Literature references identified by Ü can be found in the general listing of books and monographs at the back of this book.6

Saffron

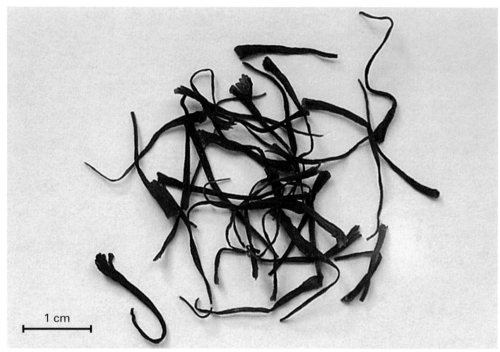

Fig. 1: Saffron

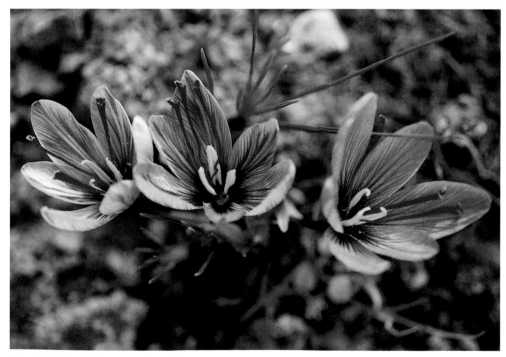

Fig. 2: Saffron (*Crocus sativus* L.)

Plant source: *Crocus sativus* L.

Synonym: *Crocus autumnalis* SM.

Taxonomic classification: The species can be subdivided into several varieties, which are differentiated by the lengths of their pistils and color of their flowers.

Family: Iris family (Iridaceae).

Common names: Engl.: saffron, crocus; Fr.: safron, safran; Ger.: Safran, Echter Safran, Gewürz-Safran, Safrankrokus, Suppengelb.

Description: A tuberous, triploid, therefore sterile, perennial plant with 6 to 9 narrow leaves up to 30 cm in length, directly emerging from the tuber. The flower bears 2 bracts, 6 lilac, violet-veined perigone leaves with a long tubular base, 3 yellow stamina and a thin yellow stylus, up to 10 cm long, with 3, up to 3.5 cm long, orangered, funnel-shaped stigmata. Flowering period is from September to the beginning of November [Ü42].

Native origin: Only known in cultivation. Related wild species occur in the Eastern Mediterranean region. The wild form is possibly *Crocus cartwrightianus* HERB., a native of Greece.

Main cultivation areas: Iran (Khorassan Province), Greece, Spain (Albacete, Alicante, La Mancha, Murcia), India (highlands of Kashmir), and to a lesser extent in France (Gâtinais), Switzerland (Mund/ Wallis), Italy, Turkey, southern parts of the Russian Federation (Azerbaijan), Morocco (Taliouine), Pakistan (Baluchistan Province), China, Japan, in the USA (Pennsylvania), in Germany experimental planting only in Ilbesheim, Landau/Pfalz [6, 30].

Main exporting countries: Iran, furthermore India, Spain, and Greece.

Cultivation: Saffron prefers light loam- or sandy soils in sunny positions in regions with a warm summer climate. Because it is sterile it can only be propagated vegetatively. Tubers are planted out in spacing of 8 to 10 × 20 cm. The crop needs to be replanted annually or after 3 to 4 years in order to prevent the tubers from creeping deeper into the soil [25, Ü38, Ü89].

Culinary herb

Commercial forms: Saffron: Saffron tips (Saffron stigma, Crocus electus, style remains are removed) and Natural saffron (Crocus naturalis, stigmata attached to part of style, up to 10% style remains are allowed). Spanish saffron is classified according to the growing region and purity (e.g. Coupé – best quality, only 5% floral remains, other varieties include Mancha, Rio and Sierra). Grading according to ISO 3632-1 includes the types Mancha (with up to 7% floral waste), Rio (13 to 15% floral waste) and Sierra (17 to 20% floral waste). Ground saffron is also commercially traded.

Production: The style tips with the stigmata are removed from the freshly picked, just opened flowers by pinching with the fingers, and then sun- or artificially dried.

Forms used: Saffron or saffron powder [38].

Storage: Saffron is hygroscopic and light-sensitive; it must be stored as cool as possible, in tightly closed porcelain-, glass- or suitable metal containers protected from light and moisture. It is recommended that whole saffron is purchased (saffron powders can be easily adulterated) and only in small amounts (the spicy aroma quickly dissipates). However, even under the correct storage condition, the aroma is rapidly lost.

Description. Whole stigma (Fig. 1 and 3)**:** The dried, brick-red stigmata are 20 to 40 mm long and are mostly held together by a not more than 5 mm long, pale-yellow part of the style. The tubular stigmas, with a slit on the side, have an infundibular expansion at the top. The upper margin is finely serrate. When moistened with water and flattened, they show a spatulate outline (Fig. 3) [DAC].

Powdered stigma: Saffron powder is dark orange-red and colors the entire liquid of the water or chloral hydrate preparation yellow. It is characterized by delicate, elongated parenchyma cells with fine spiral vessels in between, epidermis cells with papillose protuberances, very large, spherical and smooth pollen grains (up to 100 μm in diameter) without visible pores, as well as the finger-like papillae of the stigmata, which occur rarely in the powder [DAC]. If a few drops of sulfuric acid are added to the dry powder, all particles become surrounded by a deep blue zone, which soon turns violet and then brown-red [DAB 6]. This color reaction merely detects the carotenoids and hence also develops with carotenoid-containing flower parts from other plants.

Odor: Characteristic, reminiscent of iodoform, **Taste:** Spicy, slightly bitter, somewhat pungent, colors the saliva orange-yellow when chewed.

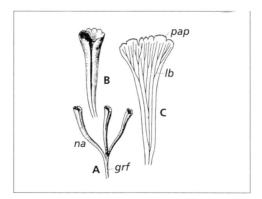

Fig. 3: Saffron. **A** Style (grf) with the 3 stigmata (na), **B** Tubular stigma, **C** Flattened stigma, lb vascular bundle, pap papillae. From Ü50.

History: Saffron was already described in the Papyrus Ebers and in the Bible, as well as in numerous texts from ancient Greece and Rome. In the 7th century, it was also known in China. In the 10th century, it was brought to Spain by the Arabs and in the 11th century, it reached France and in the 14th century England [Ü42, Ü73, for an overview of its history and mythology, see 11, 30, 33, Ü97].

Constituents and Analysis

DIN- and ISO-Standards. ISO 3632-1 (Saffron — Specification), ISO 3632-2 (Saffron — Test methods), DIN Standard 10221-2 (Determination of moisture content and volatile components, oven-drying method for mustard seeds and saffron).

- Essential oil: 0.4 to 1.3%, the main component is safranal (4,5-dehydro-β-cyclocitral, about 47% of the volatile substances). The fresh stigmata only contain small amounts of essential oil. During drying and storage, the picrocrocin contained in the stigmata is transformed to safranal by cleavage of the glucose moiety. Other breakdown products of picrocrocin, which significantly contribute to the odor, are 4-hydroxy-β-cyclocitral (possibly an intermediate in the formation of safranal), isophorone, 4-oxoisophorone, 2,2,6-trimethylcyclohexa-1,4-dione and 2-hydroxy-4,4,6-trimethylcyclohexa-2,5-diene-1-one, among others. Additionally, 100 other volatile constituents have been detected in saffron [24, 35, 46, 47, Ü83]
- Picrocrocin (bitter principle of saffron): 3 to 13% [47].
- Crocins: 10 to 25%, water-soluble mono- or di-esters of the non-water-soluble, brick-red crocetin (8,8´-diapo-Ψ,Ψ´-carotenoiddicarboxylic acid) with β-D-glucose, β-D-gentiobiose (disaccharide) or β-D-neapolitanose (trisaccharide). The main component is crocetin-di-(β-D-gentiobiosyl)-ester (crocin A); also present are, among other constituents, crocetin-mono-di-(β-D-gluco-

syl)-ester, crocetin-di-(β-ᴅ-glucosyl)-ester, crocetin-mono-(β-ᴅ-gentiobiosyl)-ester, crocetin-(β-ᴅ-gentiobiosyl)-(β-ᴅ-neopolitanosyl)-ester and crocetin-di-(β-ᴅ-neopolitanosyl)-ester as well as traces of free crocetin (α-crocetin), methylcrocetin (β-crocetin, monomethylesters of α-crocetin) and *trans*-dimethylcrocetin (γ-crocetin). It is suspected that picrocrocin and the crocins develop from the hypothetical precursor protocrocin, a C_{40}-carotenoid [12, 24, 32, 47].

- Carotenoids: α- (?), β- and γ-carotene, lycopene, zeaxanthin, among others [30, 32, 47].
- Flavonoids: Kaempferol-7-*O*-sophoroside, kaempferol-7-*O*-glucoside-3-*O*-sophoroside [46].
- Mangicrocin, a xanthone-carotenoid glycoside conjugate [17].
- Fatty oil: 7 to 10% [30].

Tests for Identity: Based on morphological and anatomical characteristics as well as TLC [39–41, Ü102, ISO-3632, DAC], GC/MS [4], HPLC [41] or HS/GC-MS [24].

Quantitative assay: Through determination of the dye strength [DAC, ISO 3632] or HPLC determination of the crocetin glycosides, picrocrocin, safranal and flavonoids with HPLC [9, 44], as well as GC analysis of safranal [5, 41] or, after extraction with supercritical CO_2, with HPLC or GC [21].

Adulterations, Misidentifications and Impurities: Saffron is often adulterated due to its very high price. Observed adulterations are, among others, filiform saffron styles (yellow, without the funnel-shaped stigmata!), saffron filaments (high amount of pollen grains!), spent saffron, already extracted, which has been colored with synthetic dyes afterwards (TLC!), stigmata of other Crocus-species (no or little dye strength, assay according DAC or ISO-3632, bitter taste is absent!), artificially colored ligulate flowers from calendula, *Calendula officinalis* L. (if soaked in water, the ovary and style become visible!) or single florets of safflower, *Carthamus tincto-rius* L. (with style filaments and small, coarsely granular pollen grains with distinct pores!). In UV, saffron does not exhibit fluorescence, in contrast to many adulterants (turmeric, stigmata of *Crocus vernus*, flowers of *Calendula officinalis* and *Carthamus tinctorius* with conspicuous fluorescence). In order to increase the weight, saffron powders in the past, were occasionally mixed with soluble or insoluble mineral salts (to detect high ash contents, see assays according to DAC or ISO 928 and 930, respectively) [30, Ü37].

Actions and Uses

Actions: Due to its aromatic and slightly bitter taste, saffron is an appetite stimulant and digestion promoter.

In animal tests, crocetin applied intramuscularly showed antiarteriosclerotic action [34]. In rabbits fed a high cholesterol diet it inhibited the occurrence of hypercholesterolemia, caused a decrease in serum cholesterol levels of about 30% and an approximately 80% increased diffusion of oxygen in blood plasma [15]. Moreover saffron also contains a macromolecular substance, which is a thrombocyte aggregation inhibitor [20].

Saffron extracts have shown antitumor action in animal experiments [1, 2, 26, 27, 29, 34]. For example, with transplantation of tumors (Sarcoma-180, Ehrlich-, Ascites- and Dalton-lymphoma cells) in mice the tumor initiation rate was decreased, tumor growth was slowed down and the survival time of the animals was extended by 2 to 3 times [28]. A prolongation of survival time was also demonstrated in female mice (but not in males) with adenocarcinoma of the colon following application of crocin A (400 mg/kg body weight, subcutaneously, over 13 weeks) [16]. Tumor induction by the carcinogens dimethylbenzanthracene/croton oil or methylcholanthrene was also inhibited [37].

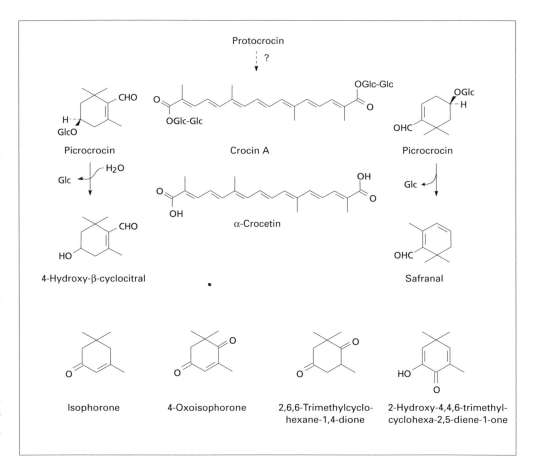

Protocrocin

Picrocrocin

Crocin A

Picrocrocin

4-Hydroxy-β-cyclocitral

α-Crocetin

Safranal

Isophorone

4-Oxoisophorone

2,6,6-Trimethylcyclo-hexane-1,4-dione

2-Hydroxy-4,4,6-trimethyl-cyclohexa-2,5-diene-1-one

In isolated uterus, saffron extracts caused rhythmic contraction [19]. In animal tests (mouse, rabbit, dog), they also stimulated in situ gravid and non-gravid uterus [10].

In animal tests, saffron extracts can mitigate ethanol-induced impairments of cerebral function. In mice pretreated with ethanol, but not in normal mice, the administration of saffron extracts (125 to 500 mg/kg body weight) improved memory functions compared to the animals that were given only ethanol [3, 48].

Due to the very low quantities of saffron that are used as a seasoning, the above-mentioned effects are not to be expected with the use of saffron as a spice.

Toxicology: Based on existing data, there is no acute or chronic toxicity with use of saffron as a spice at normal doses. Up to this point, there are no documented risks with a maximal daily intake of 1.5 g [18]. High doses, often used as an abortifacient, lead to lightheadedness, dizziness, vomiting, bloody diarrhea, hematuria, bleeding from the membranes of the nose and uterus as well as lips and eyelids. Sclerae, skin and mucous membranes turn yellow. Lethal cases have been described. The intake of 5 g saffron (in combination with estrogen-containing tablets, 20 tabl. Cyren B) by a pregnant 28 year old led to an abortion after a few hours; furthermore, thrombocytopenia and hypothrombinemia with severe purpura, as well as collapse with uremia were observed. After the intake of a sauce heavily seasoned with saffron, agitation, malaise, rapid, irregular pulse and restless sleep were noted. The symptoms subsided after about 15 h [Ü84]. The lethal dose for humans is 5 to 20 g saffron [14, 18, Ü58].

Culinary and colorant use: Saffron is used mainly in the Mediterranean countries, in Asia Minor and Southeastern Asia. It serves especially as a spice, but most of all as a food coloring, for southern European fish-, meat- and rice dishes, e.g. in France for bouillabaisse (Provençal fish soup with crabs or lobster and mussels), in Spain for paella (rice dish with seafood or also poultry or rabbit) and zarzuela (fish stew with garlic, onions and tomatoes), in Morocco for so-called tajine-sauce (combined with ginger, pepper + onions or paprika + cumin + ginger), in Italy for risotto alla Milanese and in India for pilaws. The traditional Jewish Sabbath bread challah is also colored with saffron. In England and in Northern countries it is used as an ingredient in cakes. In Central Europe it no longer plays a meaningful role as a spice. In the food industry, due to its very high price, it has been replaced by artificial food colors or other, less expensive natural colors (see below).

Saffron should be placed into lukewarm water prior to use. It should not be added to the meal until the end of preparation time. If it is only being used for its colorant value, it can be cooked with the dish. Only a few filaments are necessary for seasoning (about 0.1 g for a dish that serves 3 persons). Higher doses will cause the foods to taste iodoform-like ("like medicine").

In German cooking, saffron can be used as a flavoring and coloring for sauces (e.g. for fish, sea foods, poultry, lamb, mutton), soups (e.g. cauliflower soup, asparagus soup, broth), rice dishes, noodles, stewed vegetables and cream cheese [Ü1, Ü2, Ü45, Ü90, Ü111].

Saffron is also used in sweet dishes, e.g. semolina pudding, groats, milk pudding, sweet chestnut purée, desserts and ice cream [30, Ü1, Ü55, Ü68, Ü73].

Saffron powder is added mainly as a food coloring to bakery products (especially in England and in Northern Europe: Saffron rolls, Easter bread and saffron cake) and butter or cheese. Due to the high price of saffron in Germany, it is often substituted with less expensive carotenoids, → Annatto or safflower (see below) [Ü55, Ü73].

In the liqueur industry saffron is also used as a colorant, although rarely (e.g. in Abtei, Benedictine, Boonekamp, Chartreuse, Kartäuser). It is also sometimes used as a colorant in non-alcoholic beverages [30].

Only as an exception should Saffron be combined with other spices, e.g. with ginger, garlic, bay leaves, nutmeg or pepper.

As a component of spice mixes and preparations: → Cookie spices, → Ras en hanout, → Salsa comum, → Scappis spice mix.

Other uses: In the cosmetic industry, saffron was sometimes used as a colorant. Due to saffron's lipophilic character, saffron extract is used as a special stain in microscopy. In the textile industry, it is still applied to some extent as a dye, e.g. to stain Oriental rugs. The "saffron-colored" robes of Buddhist monks, however, are dyed with other plant-based colorants (e.g., in Thailand with extracts of the heartwood from *Artocarpus integer* (THUNB.) MERR., Moraceae).

Medicinal herb

Herbal drugs: Croci stigma, Saffron [DAC], Flos Croci, Saffron [ÖAB].

Indications: For nervousness, cramps and asthma. Efficacy for these uses has not been substantiated [18].

In folk medicine, saffron is used as a stomachic, for dysmenorrhea and for spastic coughs, among other uses. 0.5 to 1.5 g saffron powder is given as the daily dose. Due to the abortifacient action, the ingestion of therapeutic doses of saffron during pregnancy must be avoided [Ü37].

In Chinese medicine, saffron is used for the treatment of hematoma, amenorrhea, depression, cramps and nervousness [43]. Additional indications for use described in US patents include papilloma, hypertension, spinal cord injuries and cerebral edema [13].

Similar herbs used mainly as food coloring

Safflower (false saffron, bastard-saffron, Mexican saffron, Ger.: Saflor, Färbersaflor, Färberdistel, Falscher Safran, Bastard-Safran, Mexikanischer Safran), dried single florets of *Carthamus tinctorius* L. (Asteraceae), native to Anterior Asia, cultivated mainly in Mexico, in the Southern USA, India, China, and in the Middle

East, as well as in Northern Africa, South Africa, and in the Mediterranean countries. Safflower was already in use in ancient times as a dye- and oil-plant (25 to 37% fatty oil in the achenes). The fatty oil of safflower (safflower oil) is rich in unsaturated fatty acids (linoleic acid up to 80%) and a good vitamin E donor. The flowers are plucked by hand and rapidly dried at 50 to 60 °C. The constituents responsible for its coloring matter are monomeric or dimeric chalcone glycosides: carthamin (0.4% contained in the dried flowers, designated as safflower red, Spanish red, carthamus chalcone, a dimer that is easily oxidized to carthamone, the corresponding *p*-quinone and the actual fat-soluble coloring agent), the water-soluble constituents safflower yellow A and B, safflomins A, B and C, hydroxy-safflower yellow A and tinctormin [22, 31, 36, 42]. Safflower is also traded in its washed form, wherein the yellow safflower pigments have been removed by treatment with water. It is used the same as saffron, especially in the Mediterranean region and in India, for coloring dishes yellow, but it has no seasoning properties. Carthamus extracts are also used as textile colorants. Dye extracts from safflower petals are commercially traded as Carthamus Red and Carthamus Yellow [Ü36, Ü61, Ü73]. In Eastern Asia, safflower is still used today to treat many diseases, e.g. cardiac-circulatory-disorders, thrombosis, menstrual problems, post-natal uterine hemorrhage, hematomas, abdominal pains of uncertain origin, spastic constipation, chronic headaches, migraine and inflammations [7, 8].

Cape-saffron, *Sutera atropurpurea* (BANKS) HIERN. (*Lyperia atropurpurea* BENTH., Scrophulariaceae), its flowers are used as a saffron substitute.

Crocus-tritonia, *Tritonia crocata* (L.) KERGAWL. (*Crocosmia aurea* PLANCH., Iridaceae), native to South Africa, the flowers are used as a saffron substitute.

Feminell: A name used for various similar plant parts to that of saffron that are used

as saffron substitutes or saffron adulterants, usually saffron styles without stigmata, style pieces from *Crocus biflorus* MILL. or tubular florets of yellow Asteraceae, e.g. of calendula, *Calendula officinalis* L., or of safflower (see above) [Ü98].

Hollyhock flowers (Ger.: Stockrosenblüten), from *Alcea rosea* L. (Malvaceae), probably native to Asia Minor and Southeastern Europe, today widely distributed westward to the Eastern Mediterranean region, eastward to China, and also cultivated as a garden plant. It contains the water-soluble pigment constituent althaein (0.1 to 0.2%, mixture of anthocyans). Petals from black-red flowering varieties are used as a red food coloring for confectionaries, syrup, liqueur and wine [Ü37, Ü61].

Red beet juice, from *Beta vulgaris* L. ssp. *vulgaris* var. *conditiva* ALEF. (Chenopodiaceae), red beet, is only known in cultivation. Important water-soluble pigment constituents include betanin (beet red, 0.05 to 0.14% of fresh weight, 5-*O*-β-D-glucoside of betanidin, a betalain) and vulgaxanthine, in addition to other betanins and betaxanthines. The juice is used as a red food coloring for ice cream (raspberry ice cream) and mayonnaise [45, Ü36, Ü98].

Carrot extract, from *Daucus carota* L. (Apiaceae), carrot, only known in cultivation. Important colorant constituents include α- and β-carotene. The extract is used as a yellow food coloring for delicatessen and instant vegetable soups, as well as for confectionaries and beverages [Ü36].

Alkanet root, from *Alkanna tuberculata* (FORSSK.) MEIKLE (*A. tinctoria* (L.) TAUSCH, Boraginaceae), native to the Mediterranean region, cultivated in Southern France, Turkey, and Hungary. Pigment constituents include the fat-soluble alkanna red (about 5% contained in the dried root, being esters of alkannin, an isoprenylated naphthoquinone). Hepatotoxic and carcinogenic pyrrolizidine alkaloids also

occur in the root, including, among others, 7-angeloyl retronecine and triangularine. Extracts of alkanet root were formerly used as red coloring for liqueurs, sweets and baked goods. Due to its pyrrolizidine alkaloid content, its use is prohibited in many countries, including Germany, among others [Ü37].

Extracts of hibiscus calyx (*Hibiscus sabdariffa* L., Malvaceae), chokeberry fruit (*Aronia melanocarpa* (MICHX.) ELLIOT, Rosaceae), black currant fruit (*Ribes nigrum* L., Saxifragaceae), European black elder berry (*Sambucus nigra* L.,

---

Saffron risotto with zucchini-nut-vegetables

2 shallots, 4 teaspoons butter, 250 g risotto rice, 1/8 l white wine, 1/2 teaspoon of saffron, 3/4 l vegetable broth, 1 bundle of arugula, 2 garlic cloves, 20 g freshly grated parmesan, salt, cayenne pepper, 50 g coarsely chopped walnuts, 1 small zucchini squash, 1/2 of an eggplant fruit, 3 tablespoons olive oil, freshly ground pepper.

Peel and finely dice the shallot and sauté in butter. Add the rice and continue to sauté until the rice is opaque; add wine and let the liquid boil down. Mix in the saffron and add the broth while stirring. Let it simmer for 12 to 15 minutes, the rice should still be firm. Pluck the arugula leaves, wash, drain and finely mince them. Peel and finely mince 1 garlic clove. Mix the arugula herb, garlic and Parmesan into the cooked rice; season to taste with salt and pepper. Slightly brown the nuts in an ungreased pan. Dice the eggplant fruit and the zucchini squash and shortly sauté in butter with an unpeeled garlic clove; add salt and pepper. Mix in the chopped nuts. Serve the risotto on preheated plates with a small serving of vegetables placed in the middle of the dish [Ü90].

Caprifoliaceae), red wine grape (*Vitis vinifera* L. var. *vinifera*, Vitaceae) and the leaves of red cabbage (*Brassica oleracea* L. convar. *capitata* (L.) ALEF. var. *capitata* f. *rubra*, Brassicaceae) are used as red colorants for foods and beverages due to their anthocyan content.

Due to their chlorophyll content, the juice of spinach (*Spinacea oleracea* L., Chenopodiaceae) and nettle (*Urtica dioica* L., Urticaceae) serve as green colorants [Ü36].

Other herbs used as food colorings include → Paprika, → Annatto, and → Turmeric.

Literature

[1] Abdullaev F.I., BioFactors 4:83–86 (1993).

[2] Abdullaev F.I., E. Gonzales de Mejia, Arch. Latinoam. Nutr. 47(3):195–202 (1997), ref. CA 128:043322k.

[3] Abe K., H. Saito, Phytother. Res. 14(3):149–152 (2000).

[4] Alonso G.L. et al., J. Food Prot. 61(11):1525–1528 (1998).

[5] Alonso G.L., M.R. Salinas, J. Agric. Food Chem. 44:185–188 (1996).

[6] Anonym, Westfälischer Anzeiger Hamm 05.08.1999.

[7] Beal J.L., E. Reinhard, Natural Products as Medicinal Agents, Hippokrates Verlag Stuttgart 1988.

[8] Blaszczyk T., Pharm. Ztg. 145(15):30–33 (2000).

[9] Castellar M.R. et al., J. Chromatogr. A. 648:187–190 (1993).

[10] Chang P.Y. et al., Acta Pharm. Sin. 11(2):94–100 (1964), ref. CA 61(1964):& hs;2348b.

[11] Czygan C.F., Z. Phytother. 7:180 (1986).

[12] Dhingra V.K. et al., Indian J. Chem. 13:339 (1975), ref. CA (1975):5060t.

[13] Dufresne Ch. et al., Planta Med. 63(2):150–153 (1997).

[14] Frank A., Dtsch. Med. Wochenschr. 86:1618–1620 (1961).

[15] Gainer J., J. Jones, Experientia 31:548–549 (1978).

[16] Garcia-Olmo D.C. et al., Nutr. Cancer 35(2):120–126 (1999).

[17] Ghosal S. et al., J. Chem. Res. Synop.:70–71 (1989).

[18] Kommission E beim BfArM., BAnz. 76 vom 23.04.1987.

[19] Lewin L., Die Fruchtabtreibung durch Gifte und andere Mittel, Verlag Georg Stilke, Berlin 1925, p. 391–394.

[20] Liakopoulou-Kyriakides M., A.I. Skubas, Biochem. Intern. 22:103–110 (1980).

[21] Lozano F. et al., J. Biochem. Biophys. Methods 43(1/3):367–378 (2000).

[22] Meselhy M.R. et al., Chem. Pharm. Bull. 41(10):1796–1802 (1993).

[23] Morimoto S. et al., Planta Med. 60(5):438 (1994).

[24] Meyer P., Untersuchung der Aromastoffe und Carotinoide aus Safran (Crocus sativus L.), Dissertation Universität Bern 1995.

[25] Munshi A.M. et al., Indian Farming 39(3):27–30 (1989).

[26] Nair S.C. et al., Cancer Lett. 57:109–114 (1992).

[27] Nair S.C. et al., Cancer Biother. 10:257–264 (1995).

[28] Nair S.C. et al., Intern. J. Pharmacogn. 2:105–114 (1994).

[29] Nair S.C. et al., BioFactors 4:83–86 (1992).

[30] Oberdieck R., Dtsch. Lebensm. Rdsch. 87(8):246–251 (1991).

[31] Onodera J.I. et al., Chemistry Lett. 201:1327 (1979).

[32] Pfander W., F. Wittwer, Helv. Chim. Acta 58:1608, 2233 (1975).

[33] Rätsch Ch., Enzyklopädie der psychoaktiven Pflanzen – Botanik, Ethnopharmakologie und Anwendungen, AT-Verlag, Arau, Wiss. Verlagsges., Stuttgart 1998.

[34] Ríos J.L. et al., Phytother. Res. 10:189–193 (1996).

[35] Rödel W., M. Petrzika, High Resolut. Chromatogr. Chromatogr. Comm. 14:114–116 (1991).

[36] Saito K. et al., Z. Lebensm. Unters. Forsch. 189:418–421 (1989).

[37] Salomi M.J. et al., Nutr. Cancer 16:67–72 (1991).

[38] Sampathu S.R. et al., CRC Crit. Rev. Food Sci. Nutr. 20:123–157 (1984).

[39] Stahl E. (Hrsg.):Chromatographische und mikroskopische Analyse von Drogen, Fischer Verlag Stuttgart, New York 1978.

[40] Stahl E., C. Wagner, J. Chromatogr. 40:308 (1969).

[41] Sujata V. et al., J. Chromatogr. 624:497–502 (1992).

[42] Takahashi Y. et al., Tetrahedron Lett. 23:5163 (1982).

[43] Tang W., G. Eisenbrand, Chinese Drugs of Plant Origin, Springer-Verlag Berlin, Heidelberg 1992.

[44] Tarantilis P.A. et al., J. Chromatogr. A 664:55–61 (1994).

[45] Tyihak E., Herba Hung. 3:259 (1964), ref. Ü43.

[46] Winterhalter P., M. Straubinger, Food Rev. Int. 16(1):39–59 (2000).

[47] Zarghami N.S., D.E. Heinz, Phytochemistry 10(11):2755–2761 (1971).

[48] Zhang Y. et al., Biol. Pharm. Bull. 17:217–221 (1994).

Literature references identified by Ü can be found in the general listing of books and monographs at the back of this book.

Sage

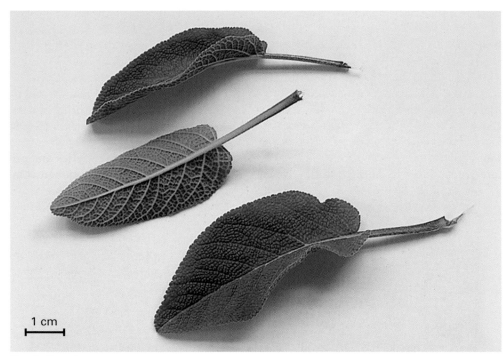

Fig. 1: Sage leaves

Plant source: *Salvia officinalis* L.

Taxonomic classification: *S. o.* is morphologically very diverse and can be subdivided into several subspecies, which are classified as separate species by modern authors.

Family: Mint family (Lamiaceae, synonym Labiatae).

Common names: Engl.: sage, common sage, garden sage; Fr.: grande sauge, sauge, sale, herb sacrée; Ger.: Salbei, (der or die) Echte(r) Salbei, Garten-Salbei, Edel-Salbei.

Description: Wintergreen subshrub, woody at the base and up to 80 cm tall, with characteristically aromatic leaves, opposite arranged, long petiolated, 3 to 10 cm in length, up to 3 cm in breadth, grayish green due to the velvety tomentum, having a distinctly crenulate margin, a net-like venation which is deeply depressed on the upper surface and very prominent on the lower surface and a lamina which is rounded and sometimes singly or doubly auriculate at the base. The flowers are about 2 cm long, mostly with a blue-violet corolla, and arranged in 6 to 8, multiflorous loose false whorls one upon the other [Ü106].

Native origin: Northern- and Central Spain, Southern France, Western Balkans, in Southern Europe, and naturalized in southern Central Europe, as well as in Asia Minor.

Main cultivation areas: Former Yugoslavia (Dalmatia), Albania, Hungary, Bulgaria, Romania, Spain, Italy, Turkey, Algeria, Czech Republic, Germany (Rhineland-Palatinate), Austria, Russian Federation, India, Indonesia, Tanzania, South Africa, Antilles, and the USA.

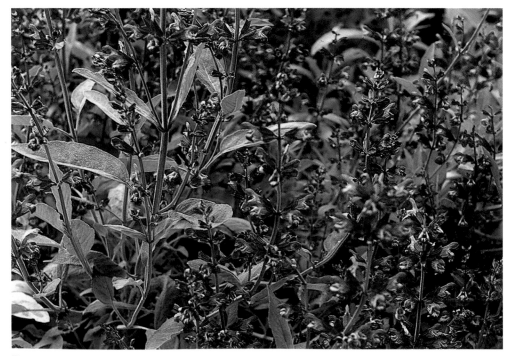

Fig. 2: Sage (*Salvia officinalis* L.)

Main suppliers: Regions of the former Yugoslavia (Dalmatia), Bulgaria, France, and Turkey.

Cultivation: Sage prefers dry soil with good lime status in warm, sunny, wind-protected locations. Stagnant moisture and humus soils are not tolerated. It has moderate frost susceptibility, and several days of temperatures below –15 °C can ruin the crop. Direct seeding at the end of April is possible, row width of 25 to 60 cm. It is safer to propagate after March under glass and plant out after the end of May or propagate with top cuttings (cut in May, plant out in June) or stock divisions. For growing sage in the garden, it is expedient to purchase a plant. It is usually cultivated as a perennial. Cultivated varieties include, among others, 'Bona', 'Extrakta', 'Krajova', and less often also the red-leaved varieties ('Purpurea') or varieties with golden yellow spotted leaves (Gold sage) [Ü14, Ü21]. For personal need, it is also possible to cultivate sage in a flower-pot.

Culinary herb

Commercial forms: Sage leaf: the dried, whole or cut leaves, sage essential oil, and sage oleoresin.

Production: Sage is harvested with cutter loaders on industrial farms in the first growing season at the end of August, and after the second growing season at the beginning of June and end of August. It must be dried rapidly at 45 °C. The stems are removed before or after drying. Some amount of the supply is obtained by collection from wild populations [Ü21]. For personal need of fresh leaves, they can be harvested continually from May to September. For drying, the young shoots harvested just before flowering are used.

Forms used: Fresh or dried leaves.

Storage: The fresh leaves can be kept fresh in plastic bags in the refrigerator for a few days. The dried leaves are stored in a cool place, in airtight porcelain-, glass- or suitable metal containers, protected from light and moisture. The dried material has relatively good stability for storage. Within 2 years, about 50% of the essential oil is lost

Description. Whole leaf (Fig. 1): For the leaves, see description of the whole plant.

Powdered leaf: Very prominent in the powder are the fragments of the epidermis with straight-walled epidermis cells, stout-walled, bent articulate trichomes with a strongly thickened basal cell, and labiate, glandular scales with 8 secretory cells (Fig. 3), fragments of the lower epidermis with wavy-sinuate cells having diacytic stomata; rarely, glandular trichomes with 1- to 2-celled heads are present [Ü49, Ph Eur].

Odor: Spicy, piney, **Taste:** Spicy, somewhat bitter and burning, camphor-like, astringent.

History: In Egypt, sage was probably used as early as 6000 BCE. It is likely that it was first cultivated in Greece. In Central Europe, sage was grown in cloister and country gardens since the 8th century. In the government decree "Capitulare de villis" (authored in about 795, see footnote → Anise), its cultivation was required [3, Ü56, Ü86].

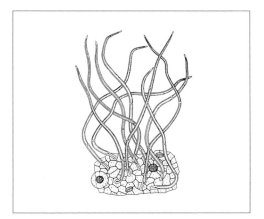

Fig. 3: Sage. Fragment of the epidermis from the upper leaf surface with articulate trichomes and labiate glandular scales. From Ü29.

Constituents and Analysis

DIN- and ISO-Standards: ISO Standard 11165 (Dried sage).

- Essential oil: 1.2 to 3.6%, the main components are thujone (30 to 70% in Dalmatian sage, high amounts present in the tops of the plant, increasing in fall, (–)-thujone up to 40% and (+)-thujone 4 to 28%), camphor (8 to 37%), 1,8-cineole (8 to 24%) and limonene (0.3 to 15%), also present are, among others, borneol, bornyl acetate, camphene, α- and β-caryophyllene, myrcene, α- and β-pinene, α-terpineol, viridiflorol and manool. In a few sage varieties and origins, respectively, other dominant components include camphor, 1,8-cineole or α-caryophyllene (humulene) [2, 3, 5, 7, 9, 16, 17, 20, 23, 32, 35, 38–40, 46, 49, 50–53, 67, 69, 71].
For Dalmatian sage, the following content limits are required by the German Drug Codex: cineole 6 to 16%, (–)-thujone + (+)-thujone at least 20%, camphor 14 to 37%, bornyl acetate not more than 5%, borneol not more than 5% [DAC].
- Diterpenephenols: In the fresh leaf, predominantly carnosolic acid (salvin, 0.2 to 0.4%), which transforms to carnosol (picrosalvin, bitter tasting, chemical structure, see → Rosemary) [3, 60, 64, 74].
- Hydroxycinnamic acid derivatives (known as labiate tannins) and phenol-carboxylic acids: Particularly rosmarinic acid (0.1 to 3.3%), furthermore, among others, caffeoyl- and p-hydroxybenzoyl-glycosides, p-hydroxybenzoic acid, caffeic acid and 1-O-(2,3,4-trihydroxy-3-methyl)-butyl-6-O-feruloyl-β-D-glucoside [3, 22, 25, 28, 30, 31, 41, 65, 72, 73].
- Jasmonic acid derivatives: (–)-Hydroxy-jasmonic acid and ethyl-β-D-glucosyl-tuberonate [73].
- Flavonoids: About 1%, apigenin-7-glucoside, luteolin-7-glucoside, luteolin-7 and –3′-glucuronide, 6-hydroxylutein, vicenin-2, among others; highly methoxylated aglycones such as genkwanin, genkwanin-6-methylether and salvi-

genin-5-methylether, among others [1, 3, 4, 42].

- Triterpenes: Particularly ursolic acid (2 to 5%) [3, 6].

Tests for identity: The identity of sage can be determined with sensory examination, macroscopic and microscopic analysis [37] and TLC of extracts [Ph Eur, DAB, PF X, Ph Helv, for a description and other methods, see Lit. 63, Ü37, Ü77, Ü102] or TLC [Ü106, Ph Helv, DAC] or GC, respectively, of the essential oil [Ü37, DAC].

Quantitative assay: The determination of the essential oil content can be carried out, volumetrically according to European Pharmacopoeia, with steam distillation and xylol in the graduated tube [Ph Eur]. The rosmarinic acid content is measured with HPLC [22], or, after silylation, with GC [54].

Adulterations, Misidentifications and Impurities have been described, with the leaves of three-lobed sage, *S. triloba* L. f. The detection of this adulterant is possible by microscopic analysis (e.g., the stiff, patulous hairs of the leaf surface [37]) or with TLC of the flavonoids [Ü37].

Actions and Uses

Actions: Due to their aromatic and bitter taste, sage leaves are appetizing and digestion promoting.

An antispasmodic effect in vitro in animal intestinal preparations has been demonstrated for aqueous-alcoholic extracts of sage, sage flavonoids and for saturated aqueous solutions of sage oil. Sage flavonoids also reduced $BaCl_2$-induced spasms in vitro in rat duodenum. Similar results were produced with guinea pig ileum (acetylcholine, histamine, and serotonin as spasmogens) [12, 33, 66].

Sage extracts suppress perspiration. This was demonstrated in 18 healthy subjects given a preparation of fresh sage leaves taken orally. The dermal water elimination was reduced by 18 to 52%. The effect commenced between the 1st and 4th day of treatment and subsided after 9 days. Clinical observations have also shown that sage extracts can inhibit excessive sweat secretion in patients suffering from tuberculosis [44, 59, Ü37].

Extracts of dried sage leaf and of the essential oil have antimicrobial action [2, 15, 21, 58, 62].

The observed antiviral action of sage extracts in vitro [24], which is predominantly dependent on the rosmarinic acid content, but possibly also on the diterpenediphenols, is probably only relevant for topical application.

Sage extracts, through their content of diterpenediphenols, rosmarinic acid and flavonoids, act by functioning as oxygen donators and radical scavengers, are strongly antioxidative, preventing the peroxidation of lipids. Therefore they are typically used to retard the occurrence of rancidity of fats in meat products [11, 28, 29].

Toxicology: Based on existing data, there is no acute or chronic toxicity with the use of sage leaves or its essential oil (up 15 drops/d) as a spice at normal doses.

Besides thujone's local irritant effect, it also has central exciting and psychotomimetic activity when absorbed. Chronic intake can lead to permanent damage of the CNS and to impairment of renal, hepatic and cardiac functions [55, Ü58, Ü100]. Due to the low amounts used in seasoning, any hazard to human health based on the thujone content can be ruled out. Very high amounts (exceeding 15 g/dose, dry weight), however, can lead to dry mouth, outbursts of sweating, racing heart and dizziness. Acute toxicity from sage oil has been documented after intake of large amounts (2 g and more). Regular use of sage, e.g. as a house tea, is not recommended [8, 57].

The sensitization potential of sage is very low. Up to this point, allergic reactions have been observed only rarely; the responsible allergen is probably carnosolic acid [18, 27, Ü37].

Culinary use: Sage is used mainly in Italian and Greek cooking. In Italy, sage is used to season, among others, focaccia (spiced leavened bread), polenta, veal (Saltimbocca alla Romana, see below) and calf liver. In France, it is used especially as a seasoning for pork and veal, and in Provençal cooking to season the garlic soup Aigo Boulido as well as in England for sausages and fish dishes.

Due to the dominating taste, dried sage leaves should be used sparingly. The fresh young, milder tasting leaves, which are preferable to the dried leaves when possible, can be dosed somewhat more liberally. The aroma of sage develops best when it is sautéed in butter or cooked with the meal. Powdered sage can also be sprinkled immediately before serving.

Fresh, chopped or whole leaves and powder of the dried leaves are used mainly as a seasoning of dishes with fatty meat (especially of pork and lamb, for fillings of goose and duck), meatballs, beef steaks, kidney dishes, liver (e.g. chicken liver) and fatty fishes (e.g. eel). Sage is however also well suited as a seasoning of sauces (e.g. with flour, onions, salt and pepper for pork), soups (e.g. of eel soup), stews (e.g. of peas and white beans), vegetable dishes (of carrots, kohlrabi and leeks), mushroom dishes (e.g. of mushroom omelets), noodle-, venison-, tomato- and egg dishes (e.g. of omelets and pancakes), of sausages and meats (e.g. of mortadella, salami and corned beef), fish (e.g. of fried herring, trout and anchovies), quark, cheese (of sage cheese and sage derby), salads (e.g. of fish-, poultry-, tomato-, potato- and bean salad), herb sauces (e.g. of butter and parmesan as noodle sauces, tomato-based sauces, salad sauces), gravy and cream sauces, hash browns, rice and polenta [Ü23, Ü30, Ü45, Ü71, Ü79, Ü90-Ü92, Ü107].

For the preparation of shish kebab, a few sage leaves can be placed in-between the meat-, bacon- and onion slices on the spear [Ü46, Ü59].

Sweet or salty baked goods are also seasoned with sage (e.g. breaded and fried sage leaves "Salbeimäuschen", sage beignets, sage bread, sage leaves baked in wine- or beer flour) [Ü23, Ü51, Ü59, Ü71, Ü95].

Powder of the dried leaves and extracts serve as preservatives to prevent spoilage of fats and meats [10, 19, 25, 61].

Sage oil is sometimes used for the production of spice essences.

Combines well with: Basil, bay, garlic, marjoram, onions, oregano, parsley, peppermint, rosemary, summer savory, and thyme, together with hyssop, parsley and peppermint, it is made into herb butter with an Italian note.

As a component of spice mixes and preparations: → Bouquet garni, → Bread spice, → Fines herbes, → Fish spice, → Hamburger meat spice, → Herb vinegar, → Herbes de Provence, → Parisian pepper, → Poultry spice, → Roast spice, → Venison spice.

Other uses: Sage oil is used in the perfume industry. Sage extracts are applied as antitranspirants, for skin cleansing and treatment of large pores as well as in bath products, mouthwashes and gargles [Ü24].

Medicinal herb

Herbal drugs: Salviae officinalis folium, Sage leaves, contains minimum 15 ml/kg essential oil, with TLC, the amounts of thujone and cineole comparable to the reference solution, must be detectable [Ph Eur], Salviae officinalis aetheroleum, Dalmatian sage oil [DAC], Salviae aetheroleum [Ph Helv]. Salviae lavandulifoliae aetheroleum, Spanish sage oil [DAC] is obtained from *S. lavandulaefolia* VAHL. Its main components are 1,8-cineole, camphor, linalool and borneol as well as less than 0.5% thujone.

Indications: Internally for dyspeptic pains and hyperhydrosis (daily dose 4 to 6 g of the leaves, 0.1 to 0.3 g of the essential oil) in the form of tea infusions (1 to 1.5 g sage leaves/150 ml water) or solutions of the essential oil (1 to 2 drops/150 ml water), externally for inflammations of or oral- and pharyngeal mucosa, such as stomatitis, gingivitis and pharyngitis, as a gargle in the form of tea infusions (2.5 g of sage leaves/100 ml water), of alcoholic extracts (5 g in a glass of water), of solutions of sage essential oil (2 to 3 drops/100 ml) or of paints (undiluted alcoholic extracts). Alcoholic extracts of sage leaves and sage oil should not be taken internally during pregnancy [34]. Due to the contribution of the non-volatile constituents to the efficacy (labiate tannins, diterpene diphenols), extracts of the dried leaf are preferable over the essential oil.

In folk medicine, sage is used for, among other conditions, headaches, nervous exhaustion, weak heart, coughs, menstrual problems and to facilitate weaning [Ü37, Ü106].

Other Salvia-species used as culinary herbs

Clary sage, *Salvia sclarea* L., native to Syria, cultivated in the Russian Federation, Kenya and in the Mediterranean region, and may also be grown in Central Europe (varieties 'Alkali', 'Trakiyska', 'Boiana'). The main components of its essential oil are linalyl acetate (up to 85%) and linalool (up to 35%), as well as, among others, β-pinene, 1,8-cineole, α-terpineol, nerol, geraniol, eugenol, β-caryophyllene and β-cubebene. The oleoresin obtained by extraction contains up to 50% of the heavy-volatile diterpene sclareol. In Sardinian races the oil is dominated by estragole (methyl chavicol, 35 to 56%) or α-terpineol (about 47%), α-terpinyl acetate (about 22%) and linalyl acetate (about 13%) [13, 26, 45, 47, 48, 68]. Other noteworthy constituents are the diterpenes, e.g. sclareol, manool, ferruginol and 7-oxoroyleanol [70]. The essential oil is used especially in the alcoholic beverage industry as a wine- and liqueur flavoring and in the cosmetics industry for perfuming of soaps. The dried leaf is suitable, dosed sparingly, as a spice for marmalades and fruit desserts as well as of soups and stews [14, Ü17].

Three-lobed sage (Greek sage)**,** *Salvia triloba* L. f. (Synonym: *S. fruticosa* MILL.), is cultivated in Italy, Albania, the former Yugoslavia, in Greece and Turkey. Its essential oil is rich in 1,8-cineole (30 to 85%) and low in thujone (below 10%) [3, 5, 32, 36, 56].

Pineapple sage, *Salvia elegans* VAHL, is native to Mexico and Guatemala, has a pineapple-like odor, and can be grown in Central Europe. The main components of its essential oil are *trans*-β-ocimene, linalool, β-caryophyllene, germacrene D, spathulenol, 2-propanol, 3-octanol, *trans*-hexenal, and, furthermore *cis*-jasmone [43]. Pineapple sage leaves are used as a seasoning and garnish for fish, salads, fruit juices, and sweet dishes [Ü47, Ü74].

Bengali sage, *Salvia bengalensis* KÖNIG ex ROXB. (Synonym: *Meriandra bengalensis* (KÖNIG ex ROXB.) BENTH) is cultivated in India and Pakistan. Its essential oil is rich in camphene and cineole. It is used as a seasoning for meat dishes, among others [Ü61].

Scarlet sage (bluebeard), *Salvia viridis* L. (Synonym: *S. hormium* L.), is native from Morocco to Tunisia and Southern Europe. The leaves were formerly used as a spice of wine and beer, but today serve mainly as an ornamental, edible accompaniment to salads [Ü47, Ü61].

Literature

[1] Adzet T. et al., J. Biochem. Syst. Ecol. 16:29–32 (1988).

[2] Baratta Z.M. et al., J. Ess. Oil Res. 10: 618–627 (1998).

[3] Brieskorn C.H., Z. Phytother. 12(2): 61–69 (1991).

[4] Brieskorn C.H., W. Biechele, Arch. Pharm. 304:557–561 (1971).

[5] Brieskorn C.H., S. Dalferth, Dtsch. Apoth. Ztg. 104:1388–1392 (1964).

[6] Brieskorn C.H., Z. Kapadia, Planta Med. 38:86–90 (1980).

[7] Brieskorn C.H., E. Wenger, Arch. Pharm. 293:21–26 (1960).

[8] Centini F. et al., Zacchia (Rom) 60:263–274 (1987).

[9] Chalchat J.C. et al., Flavour Fragrance J. 13(1):68–70 (1998).

[10] Cuvelier M.E. et al., J. Ess. Oil Chem. 73(5):645–652 (1996).

[11] Darmati Z. et al., Tehnol. Mesa 38(1): 15–19 (1997) ref. CA: 128:127249e.

Saltimbocca alla Romana
(Serves 4)
8 small thin veal cutlets, 8 slices of prosciutto, 8 large sage leaves, salt, ground white pepper, 4 teaspoons of butter or olive oil, 75 ml dry white wine.

Carefully pound the cutlets with a meat hammer until flat. Place a slice of ham and a sage leaf on each cutlet and attach them with toothpicks or metal skewers. Turn the cutlets and season with salt and pepper on the other side. The side of the cutlet with the ham and sage will absorb enough spice-flavor from these ingredients. In a large pan, melt but do not brown butter. Place the veal cutlets on the side with the ham and sauté for 2 minutes. Turn them around and sauté on the other side for 1/2 minute. Remove the cutlets from the pan and keep them warm on a preheated plate. Deglaze the pan, collecting meat drippings with white wine and bring to a boil shortly; pour the sauce over the cutlets [Ü88].

[12] Debelmas A.M., J. Rochat, Plant Méd. Phytothér. 1:23–27 (1967).

[13] Dzumayev Kh.K. et al., J. Ess. Oil Res. 7(6):597–604 (1995).

[14] Embong M.B. et al., Canad. Inst. Food Sci. Technol. J. 10:201–207 (1977).

[15] Farag R.S. et al., Fette, Seifen, Anstrichm. 88:69–72 (1986).

[16] Fehr D., Pharm. Ztg. 127:111–114 (1982).

[17] Formacek V., K.H. Kubeczka, Essential Oils Analysis by Capillary Gas Chromatography and Carbon – 13 NMR Spectroscopy, John Wiley & Sons. Chicester etc., 1982.

[18] Futrell J.M., R.L. Rietschel, Cutis 52(5): 288–290 (1993).

[19] Gerhardt U, T. Böhm, Fleischwirtschaft 60:1523–1526 (1980).

[20] Góra J. et al., Riv. Ital. EPPOS (Spec. Num, 15th Journees Internat Huiles Essentielles, 1996):761-766 (1997).

[21] Gottshall R.Y. et al., J. Clin. Invest. 28:920–923 (1949).

[22] Gracza L, P. Ruff, Arch. Pharmaz. 317: 339–345 (1984).

[23] Guillen M.D., M.L. Ibargoita, Chem. Mikrobiol. Technol. Lebensm. 17(5/6): 129–134 (1955).

[24] Herrmann E.C., L.S. Kucera, Proc. Soc. Exp. Biol. Med. 124:874–878 (1967).

[25] Herrmann K., Z. Lebensm. Unters. Forsch. 116:224–228 (1962).

[26] Hethelyi E. et al., Olaj, Szappan, Kozmet. 45(6):156–160 (1996), ref. CA:125: 284319h.

[27] Hjorther A.B. et al., Contact Dermatitis 37(3): 99–100 (1997).

[28] Hohmann J. et al., Planta Med. 65(6): 576–578 (1999).

[29] Hohmann J. et al., 46th Ann. Congress of the Soc. for Med. Plant Res. 1998 Vienna, Abstracts, J40 (1998).

[30] Jalsenjak V et al., Pharmazie 42(6):419–420 (1987).

[31] Janacsák G. et al., 46th Ann. Congress of the Soc. for Med. Plant Res. 1998 Vienna, Abstracts, B17 (1998).

[32] Kanias G.D. et al., J. Ess. Oil Res. 10(4): 395–403 (1998).

[33] Kantarev N., P. Peicev, Folia Med. (Plovdiv.) 19:41–45 (1977).

[34] Kommission E beim BfArM., BAnz. 90: 15.05.85, in der Fassung vom 13.03.1990.

[35] Kustrak D., Pharm. Acta Helv 63: 254–256 (1988).

[36] Kustrak D., Pharm. Acta Helv. 62:7–13 (1987).

[37] Länger R. et al., Sci. Pharm. 59:231 (1991).

[38] Länger R. et al., Phytochemical Analysis 7: 289–293 (1996).

[39] Länger R. et al., Planta Med. 59(7):A635 (1993).

[40] Lawrence B.M., Perfum. Flavorist 9:65–70 (1984/85), 11:79–80 (1986), 13:53–56 (1988) und 16:51–53 (1991).

[41] Litvinenko V.I. et al., Planta Med. 27: 372–380 (1975).

[42] Lu Y., L.Y. Foo, Phytochemistry 55(3): 263–267 (2000).

[43] Makino T., Foods Food Ingredients J. Jpn. 169:121–124 (1996), ref. CA 125: 140932e.

[44] Mayr J.K., Virchow's Arch. Path. Anat. Physiol. 287:297–308 (1933).

[45] Moretti M.D.L. et al., J. Ess. Oil Res. 9(2):199–204 (1997).

[46] Müller J., Planta Med. 58(7):A678 (1992).

[47] Peana A.T. et al., Planta Med. 65(8):753–754 (1999).

[48] Pecorari P. et al., Boll. Chim. Farm. 119: 584–590 (1980).

[49] Petricic J. et al., Planta Med. 45:139–140 (1982).

[50] Piccaglia R. et al., J. Ess. Oil Res. 9(2): 187–191 (1997).

[51] Pino J.A. et al., J. Ess. Oil Res. 9(2):221–222 (1997).

[52] Pitarevic I. et al., J. Nat. Prod. 47:409–412 (1984).

[53] Raic D. et al., Acta Pharm. Jugosl. 35:121 (1985).

[54] Reschke A., Z. Lebensm. Unters. Forsch. 176:116–119 (1983).

[55] Rice KC., R.S. Wilson, J. Med. Chem. 19:1054 (1976).

[56] Ronyal E. et al., J. Ess. Oil Res. 11:69–71 (1999).

[57] Saller R., J. Reichling, Drogenreport 9(14): 3–5 (1996).

[58] Sattar A.A. et al., Pharmazie 50(1):62–65 (1995).

[59] Schlegel B., H. Böttner, Z. Ges. Expt. Med. 107:267–274 (1940).

[60] Schwarz K., W. Ternes, Z. Lebensm. Unters. Forsch. 195:95–98, 99–103, 104–107 (1992).

[61] Shahidi F. et al., J. Food Lipids 2(3):145–153 (1995).

[62] Shelef L.A. et al., J. Food Sci. 49:737–740 (1984).

[63] Stahl E. (Hrsg.): Chromatographische und mikroskopische Analyse von Drogen, Fischer Verlag Stuttgart, New York 1978.

[64] Tada M. et al., Phytochemistry 35(2):539 (1994).

[65] Tada M. et al., Phytochemistry 45:1475–1477 (1997).

[66] Taddei I. et al., Fitoterapia 59:463–468 (1988).

[67] Telekova D. et al., Pharmazie 49:299–300 (1994).

[68] Torres M.E. et al., J. Ess. Oil Res. 9:27–33 (1997).

[69] Tucker A.O., M.J. Maciarello, J. Ess. Oil Res. 2:139–144 (1990).

[70] Ulubelen A. et al., Phytochemistry 44: 1297 (1996).

[71] Vernin G., J. Metzger, Perfum. Flavorist 11:79–84 (1986).

[72] Wang M. et al., J. Nat. Prod. 62(3):454–456 (1999).

[73] Wang M. et al., J. Agric. Food Chem. 48(2):235–238 (2000).

[74] Wenkert E. et al., J. Org. Chem. 30:2931–2934 (1965).

[75] Weymar H, Buch der Lippenblütler und Rauhblattgewächse, Neumann Verlag, Radebeul 1961.

Literature references identified by Ü can be found in the general listing of books and monographs at the back of this book.

Salad burnet

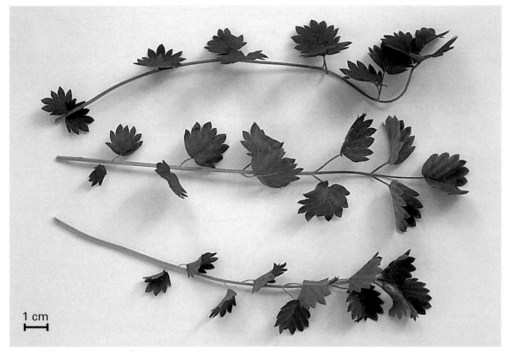

Fig. 1: Salad burnet leaf

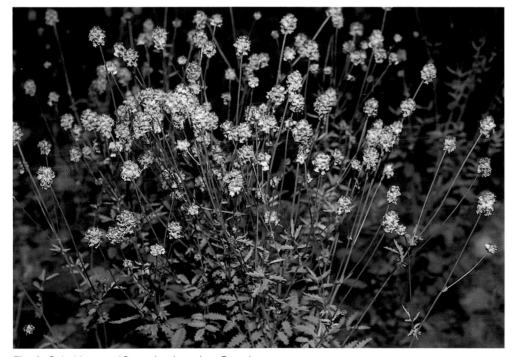

Fig. 2: Salad burnet (*Sanguisorba minor* SCOP.)

Plant source: *Sanguisorba minor* SCOP.

Synonyms: *Pimpinella minor* (SCOP.) LAM., *Poterium sanguisorba* L.

Taxonomic classification: The species is morphologically very diverse and can be subdivided in up to 5 subspecies including, among others:
S. minor SCOP. ssp. *minor*,
S. minor SCOP. ssp. *muricata* (SPACH) BRIQ. (Also considered to be a separate species *S. muricata* (SPACH) GREMLI), cultivated in a few countries as forage. *S. minor* ssp. *minor* serves predominantly as a culinary herb.

Family: Rose family (Rosaceae).

Common names: Engl.: salad burnet, sheep's burnet; Fr.: petite pimprenelle; Ger.: Pimpinelle, Bibernell(e), Kleine Bibernelle, Pimpernell, Pimpernelle (not to be confused with *Pimpinella saxifraga* L., Apiaceae, which is also called Kleine Bibernelle or Kleine Pimpinelle), Gartenpimpernelle, Kleiner Wiesenknopf, Steinpilzpetersilie, Bockspetersilie, Rotkopf, Hosenknopf, Nagelkraut, Becherblume.

Description: Perennial plant, up to 1 m tall. Leaves imparipinnate, length 10 to 30 cm, pinnules egg-shaped, dentate, short-stalked, up to 5 cm long. The unisexual or bisexual flowers are arranged in greenish-red, globular to elliptic, up to 3 cm long terminal capitula, they have numerous down-hanging filaments and 2 styli with penicillate scarlet-red stigmata, petals are absent, the calyx is often reddish-colored. The fruit is net-like rugose and winged (*S. minor* ssp. *minor*) or unwinged (*S. minor* ssp. *muricata*). Flowering period is from May to August [Ü42].

Native origin: Europe, from Southern France and Italy up to the Caucasus, Western Siberia up to the Himalayas, Northern Africa.

Main cultivation areas: England, Germany, France, North America, far eastern Russian Federation, Java, also used as forage.

Main exporting countries: No commercial trade.

Cultivation: The plant prefers dry, permeable, preferably calcareous soil. Propagation is carried out by sowing from March to April or in August in seed bowls or direct in the open field. Row width of 20 cm, after sprouting separate to 20×20 cm apart. Propagation by stock division is also possible. For one household 1 to 2 plants are sufficient. Every 2 to 3 years sow new seeds because the plants become stunted with aging. The flowers should be removed and the herb cut back to a height of about 15 cm, thereby increasing the formation of young leaves [Ü66, Ü96].

Culinary herb

Commercial forms: Not in commerce.

Production: The tender young leaves can be harvested at any time, older leaves are tough and taste bitter.

Forms used: Fresh or deep frozen, young leaves.

Description. Whole leaf (Fig. 1): See description of the plant.

Storage: The fresh leaves can be kept in plastic bags refrigerated for a few days, or stored for a longer periods, finely chopped and deep frozen in water in the ice-tray or frozen in freezer bags in the deep freezer. Drying is not suitable due to aroma loss.

Odor: Cucumber-like, **Taste:** Somewhat cucumber- and nut-like; young leaves are slightly astringent and older ones more strongly astringent.

History: Salad burnet was already cultivated in medieval herb gardens as a medicinal plant; it was applied as a remedy for the prophylaxis of plague infections. In England, it was used as a popular spice during the reign of Queen Elisabeth [Ü59, Ü70, Ü95].

Constituents and Analysis

Constituents

- Hydroxycinnamic acid derivatives: Caffeic acid, *p*-coumaric acid, among others [5].
- Phenolcarboxylic acids: *p*-Hydroxybenzoic acid, vanillic acid, gallic acid, among others [5].
- Tannins: About 10% [2].
- Flavonoids: About 3%, including isoquercitrin, avicularin, kaempferol-3-glucoside, flavonoid sulfates, among others [1, Ü37].
- Triterpenes: Ursolic acid, tormentillic acid, tormentoside (tormentillic acid-28-*O*-esterglucoside), 23-hydroxytormentillic acid, nigaichigoside F1 (23-hydroxytormentillic acid-28-*O*-esterglucoside) [3, 4].
- Saponins: Sanguisorbin (?) [Ü30].

There are no data with regard to its aroma compounds.

Tests for Identity with morphological characteristics of the plant or the leaves, respectively.

Quantitative analysis: Determination of the hide powder precipitable tannins [2].

Adulterations, Misidentifications and Impurities are possible with the leaves of *Sanguisorba officinalis* L.; the pinnules of this species have a cordate lamina.

Actions and Uses

Actions: No studies of its pharmacological actions exist.

Toxicology: Based on existing data, there is no acute or chronic toxicity if salad burnet is used as a spice in normal amounts. Because they have high tannin content, after intake of larger quantities of leaves it is probable that a feeling of fullness, indigestion and constipation may occur.

Culinary use: Salad burnet is favored today in French and Italian cooking. Its use in German cooking is on the rise. Salad burnet is one of the seven classic spice herbs used in "Frankfurter green sauce".
Before chopping, one should drip lemon juice on the leaves in order to prevent them from turning brown. They are added only to the finished dish.
The fresh plucked or deep-frozen, young, chopped leaves, rarely also the young, fresh sprout tips serve as a side dish to sauces, dips, dressings, salads (e.g. to leaf-, tomato-, radish- or potato salad), cold and warm soups (e.g. potato- or asparagus soup), to cold cuts, potatoes, egg dishes, cream cheese, quark, sea foods, poached fish, poultry dishes, marinated mushrooms, and as a flavoring of herb vinegar, herb butter, cold beverages or white wine punches. They also can be used to refine the taste of sorbets with strawberries and peaches [1, Ü30, Ü47, Ü51, Ü55, Ü59, Ü70, Ü71, Ü74, Ü79, Ü96].
Salad burnet leaves are also used with other herbs in the pickling of cucumbers [Ü98].
Likewise it can be enjoyed as a wild salad or cooked as a vegetable [Ü98].

Combines well with: Borage, chervil, dill, lemon balm, rosemary, and tarragon.

As a component of spice mixes and preparations: → Fines herbes, → Frankfurter green sauce, → Herb butter, → Salad spice.

Medicinal herb

Herbal drug: Sanguisorbae minoris herba, Salad burnet herb, formerly referred to as Pimpinellae italicae minoris herba.

Indications: In folk medicine it is taken internally in the form of aqueous infusions for diarrhea and externally it is applied for the treatment of wounds and hemorrhoids (tannins) [Ü37].

Similar culinary herbs

Great burnet, *Sanguisorba officinalis* L. (Synonym: *S. major* GILIB.), native to temperate regions of Europe, Asia, and North America, cultivated especially in Central Asia and Japan, its constituents and uses are similar to those of salad burnet, the leaves are however somewhat tough; cooked leaves are also used as a vegetable [Ü61].

Literature

[1] Harborne J.B., Phytochemistry 14:1147 (1975).

[2] Lamaison J.L. et al., Ann. Pharm. Fr. 48(6):335–3340 (1990).

[3] Reher G. et al., Phytochemistry 31:3909–3914 (1992).

[4] Reher G. et al., Planta Med. 57:506 (1991).

[5] Rodriguez M.J., P. Bermejo, Fitoterapia 57:446–44 (1986).

Literature references identified by Ü can be found in the general listing of books and monographs at the back of this book.

Sarepta mustard

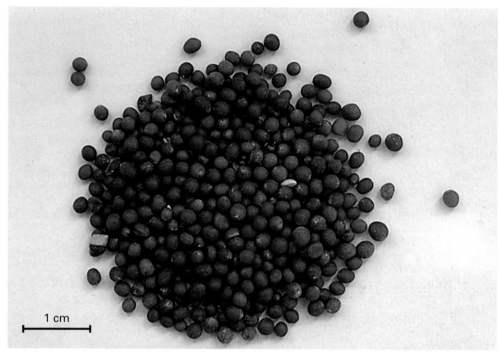

Fig. 1: Brown mustard seeds

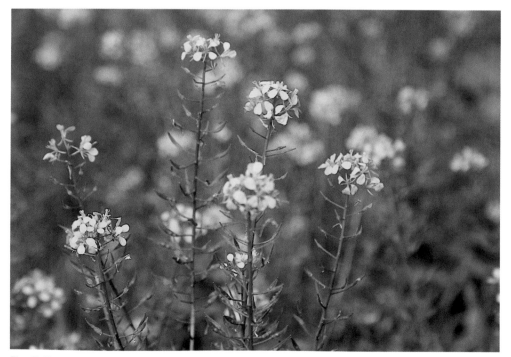

Fig. 2: Sarepta mustard (*Brassica juncea* (L.) CZERN.)

Plant source: *Brassica juncea* (L.) CZERN.

Synonym: *Sinapis juncea* L.

Taxonomic classification: Probably a hybrid of *Brassica nigra* (L.) KOCH × *Brassica campestris* L. (according to other authors of *B. rapa* L. emend. METZG. × *B. nigra* (L.) KOCH). A very morphologically diverse taxon, particularly in China there are numerous varieties used as vegetables (with thickened stems, fleshy inflorescence axis, thickened petioles, turnip-like roots, various leaf shapes – rosulate, crispate, laevigate). A generally accepted sub-classification in infraspecific taxa however does not exist.

Family: Mustard family (Brassicaceae, synonym Cruciferae).

Common names: Engl.: Sarepta mustard, brown mustard, Chinese mustard, Indian mustard, leaf mustard cabbage; Fr.: moutarde de Chine, moutarde de Sarepte, moutarde joniciforme; Ger.: Sareptasenf, Brauner Senf (sometimes also the name used for *Brassica nigra*), Indischer Senf, Russischer Senf, Chinesischer Senf, Rutenkohl.

Description: Annual plant, up to 1 m tall, stem bluish-pruinose, at the ground hairy, in the upper part ramified. The stalked, bluish-pruinose leaves are entire or oblong, lyrate-pinnatifid with a large terminal lobe; the lower surface bares fine bristles. The inflorescences are terminal or axial corymbs. The typical cruciform flower has 4 horizontal spreading sepals, 4 bright-yellow unguiculate petals, 2 short and 4 longer stamina. From the superior ovary develops a rostrate, glabrous pod with 16 to 24 seeds. The seeds are light brown or brown, nearly globular, pitted, with diameters of 1.5 to 2 mm. Flowering period is from June to September [35, Ü37].

Native origin: Native to Southeastern section of the European parts of the Russian Federation, the Caucasus region, Central Asia, Southern Siberia, and partially introduced in Central Europe.

Main cultivation areas: India, Pakistan, China, Canada, furthermore Northern Africa, Romania, Hungary, Holland, France, Southeastern section of the European parts of the Russian Federation, England, Germany, Poland, and North America. Cultivation of black mustard, *Brassica nigra* (L.) KOCH, is increasingly being replaced by Sarepta mustard.

Main exporting countries: For the production of table mustard, Canada and Hungary.

Cultivation: The same as → White mustard, but it prefers lighter soils. Cultivated varieties include, among others 'Budakalaszifekete', 'Divia', 'Domo', 'Forge', 'Ficita', 'Lethbridge 22A', 'Malopolska', 'Musta', 'Negro caballo', 'Serub', 'Sutton', 'Vulkan' 'Vitasso' and 'Aurea' (the latter two varieties are permitted in Germany for mustard production) [10, Ü21, Ü98]. For oil production, glucosinolate-free varieties are selected [3].

Culinary herb

Commercial forms: Brown mustard seed: dried, ripe seeds, brown (brown mustard, Indian mustard) or yellow (Oriental mustard), powdered seed, usually with oil removed in order to prevent rancidity during storage, thereby removing a negative influence on taste.

Production: → White mustard.

Forms used: Ripe, dried seeds (grain mustard, mustard seed), and powdered seeds (mustard flour).

Storage: The seeds are kept as cool as possible in well-closed containers, protected from light and moisture. They can be stored for several years. The leaves can only be used fresh.

Description. Whole seed (Fig. 1): See plant description (for details to differentiate the seeds of Brassica-species, see [Ph Helv]).

Powdered seed: The powder is characterized by the surface view of testa fragments with polygonal, 8 to 25 µm wide, narrow-lumenal cells, and above or below, a coarsely reticulate, rounded polygonal reticulum with broad, darker-shaded mesh boundaries (Fig. 3). Also present are fragments of the cross section from the testa. The cells of the embryo fragments contain aleuron grains and oil droplets [Ü55, Ph Helv].

Odor: Odorless; pungent after moistening of the powdered or crushed seeds, **Taste:** First weakly mucilaginous, somewhat bitter, then burning and pungent.

History: Sarepta mustard has been cultivated since end of the 18th century in the southeastern part of the European parts of the Russian Federation (Sarepta is a city near the Volga). In 1950, it increasingly started to replace the cultivation of black mustard [Ü61].

Constituents and Analysis

Constituents
- Glucosinolates: In the seeds, the main components are sinigrin (about 1 to 4%), besides gluconapin, glucoiberverin, glucobrassicanapin, gluconasturtiin, glucotropaeolin and 4-hydroxyglucobrassicin, among others; in the leaves sinigrin (about 0.1%) and also glucobrassicin, 4-hydroxy- and 4-methoxy-glucobrassicin, among others [8].
- Mustard oils: Upon injury of plant tissue in the dried seeds, and after moistening, the glucosinolates come into contact with the enzyme myrosinase, which is located in the so-called myrosine-cells, thereby, mustard oils (alk(en)yl- or alkarylisothiocyanates) are formed (Fig. 12, → General Section). Sinigrin transforms to the easily volatilized, pungent smelling and tasting allyl mustard oil (allylisothio-

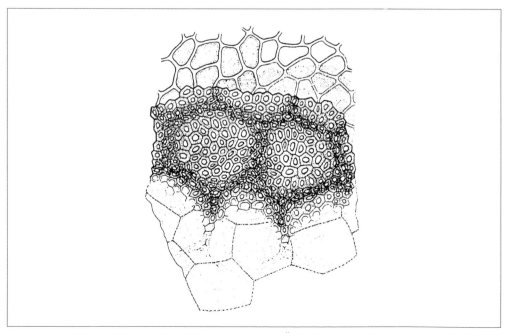

Fig. 3: Sarepta mustard. Fragment of the testa. From Ü29

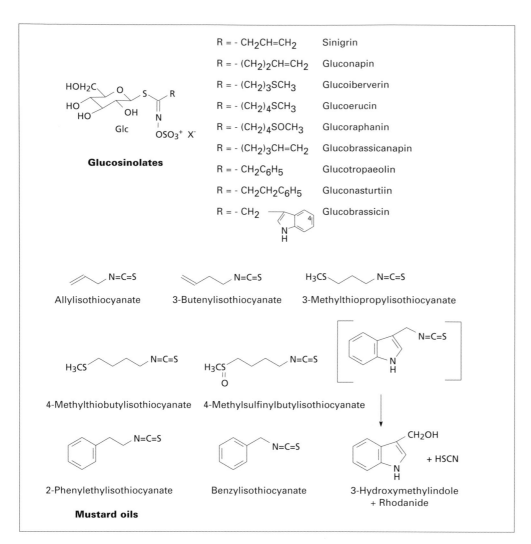

Glucosinolates

R = - CH₂CH=CH₂   Sinigrin
R = - (CH₂)₂CH=CH₂   Gluconapin
R = - (CH₂)₃SCH₃   Glucoiberverin
R = - (CH₂)₄SCH₃   Glucoerucin
R = - (CH₂)₄SOCH₃   Glucoraphanin
R = - (CH₂)₃CH=CH₂   Glucobrassicanapin
R = - CH₂C₆H₅   Glucotropaeolin
R = - CH₂CH₂C₆H₅   Gluconasturtiin
R = - CH₂ [indole]   Glucobrassicin

Allylisothiocyanate   3-Butenylisothiocyanate   3-Methylthiopropylisothiocyanate

4-Methylthiobutylisothiocyanate   4-Methylsulfinylbutylisothiocyanate

2-Phenylethylisothiocyanate   Benzylisothiocyanate   3-Hydroxymethylindole + Rhodanide

Mustard oils

cyanate), gluconapin converts to 3-butenylisothiocyanate, glucoiberverin to 3-methylthiopropylisothiocyanate, glucoerucin to 4-methylthiobutylisothiocyanate, glucoraphanin to 4-methylsulfinylbutylisothiocyanate, glucobrassicanapin to 4-pentenylisothiocyanate, gluconasturtiin to 2-phenylethylisothiocyanate and glucotropaeolin to benzylisothiocyanate. The glucobrassicins generate, with the instable 3-indolylmethyl mustard oil as intermediate, the corresponding 3-hydroxymethylindole derivatives and rhodanide [7, 11, 13, 36, Ü100].

A group of French authors detected the main component sinalbin (see chemical structure → White mustard) besides small amounts of 9-(methyl-sulfonyl)-nonylglucosinolate, 8-(methylsulfonyl)-octylglucosinolate and only traces of sinigrin (?) [7].

As with rape, practically glucosinolate-free varieties of Sarepta mustard also exist [3].

■ Fatty oil: 30 to 45%; the content of erucic acid depends on the variety. For obtaining the fatty oil, varieties which are almost free of erucic acid are cultivated [19].

Tests for Identity: The identity of Sarepta mustard can be determined with sensoric examination as well as with macroscopic and microscopic analysis. TLC of the glucosinolates [Ü101], RP-HPLC of the glucosinolates [1, 36], HPLC or GC of the TMS derivatives of the desulfoglucosino-lates [12, 32, 37] or after fermentation, by detection of the allylisothiocyanates with GC, respectively [27].

Quantitative assay: The content of sinigrin is determined iodometrically in ammonia solution after fermentation and distillation of the obtained allylmustard oil by measuring the formed allyl thiourea [Ph Helv]. Acidimetric determination after reaction of the allyl mustard oil with piperidine or pyrrolidine [2], or quantification with RP-HPLC [25] is also possible. The volatile isothiocyanates can be determined quantitatively with GC/MS or liquid chromatography after enzymatic hydrolysis and steam distillation [15, DAC]. The quantification of the glucosinolates can be carried out with RP-HPLC [Ü83] and GC after derivatization with TMS [34], or, after reaction to desulfoglucosinolates, with HPLC [26] as well as colorimetrically after reaction with palladium dichloride [33].

Adulterations, Misidentifications and Impurities are possible with seeds from other Brassica species, e.g. rape, wild turnip or field mustard. A differentiation is based on the morphological and anatomical characteristics of the seeds and analysis (see above) of the constituents (sinigrin is absent).

Actions and Uses

Actions: Due to its pungent taste, it is appetite stimulating and digestion promoting. Local application of extracts made from the ground, fermented mustard seeds or mustard flour stirred with water has skin irritant action, and therefore cause hyperemia and promotes peripheral blood flow [5]. Mustard footbaths (80 g fresh ground seeds of black mustard in 10 l water, temperature 40 °C, duration of use 10 minutes) reduce, compared to pure water baths, the blood flow rate in the brain [5].

Sarepta mustard has shown a hypoglycemic effect in rats, which has been attributed to an elevation of the glycogen synthesis and an inhibition of glycogenolysis in the liver [17].

Supplementation of very high doses of Sarepta mustard seeds (10% in feed) in rats, which were given an additional 20% coconut oil in their feed, reduced, compared to the control group, the total cholesterol content of the blood as well as the level of LDL + VLDL and elevated the level of HDL [18].

The urine of rats that were fed with black mustard seeds and were injected with the carcinogen benzo[a]pyrene, showed reduced mutagenic activity in the AMES-Test compared to the control group (with only the benzo[a]pyrene injection) [29].

The seeds of Sarepta mustard and black mustard both have good bacteriostatic and low fungistatic properties.

Toxicology: Based on existing data, there is no acute or chronic toxicity with the use of normal doses of the seeds as a salad or salad ingredient by healthy individuals. The intake of higher doses, e.g. in the form of table mustard, can lead to vomiting, abdominal pain, diarrhea, and, in sensitive people, to irritation of the kidneys. Sarepta mustard and black mustard irritate the skin and mucous membranes more strongly than → White Mustard. Mustard cataplasms and plasters, which have been left on the skin for an extended period of time (they should be removed after 15 minutes), lead to vesication and suppurating, poorly healing wounds and necrosis. Due to the volatility of the strongly irritating allyl mustard oil, eye protection is recommended during such procedures. Inhalation of the volatilized allyl mustard oil can lead to sneezing, coughing and even to asthmatic symptoms. In serious circulatory insufficiency, varicose veins and other venous complaints, Sarepta and black mustard should not be used. The internal use of therapeutic doses (10 g mustard powder in warm water, e.g. for constipation, bronchitis and amenorrhea) is not recommended due to possible irritation and damage to the mucous membranes of the gastrointestinal tract [Ü58, Ü100].

Allergic reactions after the intake of the seeds from *Brassica nigra*, *B. juncea* or *Eruca sativa*, respectively, as well as con-

tact dermatitis after the use of mustard cataplasms or inhalation of vapors, have been observed. The allergen, a low molecular weight protein with 2 chains (Bra j IE), was isolated from the seeds of *B. juncea* [4, 6, 16, 20–24, 28, 30].

Culinary use: In order to not prevent the enzymatic release of the flavor-determining mustard oils, the mustard seed must not be heated over 55 ºC in the preparation of meals. In India, mustard seeds are roasted in hot oil prior to use. Thus, mustard oil cannot be formed if the thioglucosidase (enzyme, heat labile!) is destroyed. Seeds treated in this way taste nutlike. In Japan, boiling water is poured over the powder; also no mustard oil is formed [Ü73, Ü74].

The crushed seed can be used together with herb oil and vinegar for salad sauces. The milder → White mustard is usually used, however, its flavor-determining mustard oil is not volatile and it has a more pleasing appearance especially in light sauces and dishes. Sarepta mustard is used, just like black mustard, mainly for the manufacture of → Table mustard.

Powdered mustard seeds, stirred with cold(!) water and left to stand for 15 minutes, are used for example as a seasoning of soups and stews. In order to prevent the escape of volatile mustard oils, Sarepta mustard and black mustard should not be added to the dish until the end of the cooking process [Ü55].

The fresh leaves and the seedlings are used in the same way as → White mustard, for example as a supplement of tomato- or potato salad and of steamed vegetables in the wok as well as to season ham or roast beef sandwiches [Ü74].

Leaves, stems and roots of different varieties of Sarepta mustard serve as salads or vegetables, especially in China.

As a component of spice mixes and preparations: → Table mustard.

Other uses: Ground mustard whose myrosinase has been inactivated and therefore no longer has a pungent taste, is used in the food industry as a filler, e.g. in

the manufacture of meat products, due to its mucilage content and antioxidative activity.

Medicinal herb

Herbal drugs: Sinapis nigrae semen, Black mustard seed, minimum 0.7% glycosidically bound essential oil [Ph Helv, ÖAB] or minimum 0.4% allylisothiocyanate [DAC], plant sources include suitable species of the genus Brassica. In addition to *B. j.*, among others, *B. nigra* (L.) KOCH is permitted in Switzerland [Ph Helv] or only *B. nigra* in Austria and Germany [DAB and ÖAB].

Indications: In the form of cataplasms or mustard plasters for acute bronchitis, bronchopneumonia and for segmental therapy of chronic joint diseases and soft tissue rheumatism. For the listed indications, a less aggressive cataplasm made from the powdered seeds of → White mustard is preferable because the use of Sarepta mustard and black mustard, due to the rapid penetration of their allyl mustard oils into deep skin layers and due to possible inhalation, can lead to a long-lasting irritation of the skin (up to 48 hours) and bronchial as well as skin inflammations.

Similar Brassicaceae used as culinary herbs

Black mustard (just like Sarepta mustard it is also referred to as brown mustard, true mustard, Fr.: moutarde noire, sénevé noire, Ger.: Schwarzer Senf), *Brassica nigra* (L.) KOCH, native from Southern Europe to Northern Africa and from Hindustan to Western India, and naturalized in North America, formerly cultivated in many European countries, only the cultivar 'Giebra' is known, today for the most part it has been replaced due to the non-synchronous dehiscence of its pods by Sarepta mustard, *Brassica juncea* (L.) CZERN. (See above), which is better suited for mechanical harvesting methods. Cultivation is limited to those countries where hand harvest is economically feasible because of low labor costs (Ethiopia, Morocco, India, China). The essential constituents of the seeds are glucosinolates, of which the main components are sinigrin (1 to 5%) in addition to a small amount of gluconasturtein [11]. With regard to analytics, actions, toxicology and therapeutic indications, Sarepta mustard and black mustard are comparable. The seeds are used in the same way as → White mustard as a seasoning of mixed pickles and also for the production of mustard or fatty oil [Ü61].

Roman rocket (arugula, Persian mustard, rocket salad, Italian cress Fr.: roquette, Ger.: Rukola), *Eruca sativa* MILL. (Synonym: *Eruca vesicaria* (L.) CAV. ssp. *sativa* (MILL.) THELL.), native to the Mediterranean region, Northeastern Africa, Balkan Peninsula, and Western- and Central Asia to Afghanistan, cultivated in Southern Europe, Northern- and Northeastern Africa, Western- and Central Africa, and India, predominantly as an oil plant, recently also cultivated in Europe as a spice- and salad plant. Glucosinolates are essential constituents, the main components of the seeds are glucoerucin (4-methylthiobutylglucosinolate, yielding 4-methylthiobutylisothiocyanate) [9, 31]. The seeds are also used for the production of fatty oil and table mustard and, same as the leaves, as a seasoning of sauces and vegetable dishes. The leaves are also used as a salad or salad component. In Northern Africa, *E. pinnatifida* (DESF.) POMEL is cultivated as a salad plant [Ü61, Ü66, Ü98].

Hoary cress (whitetop, pepperwort), *Cardaria draba* (L.) DESV., native to Europe, only rarely is it cultivated. The main components in the seeds are glucoerysolin (yields 4-methylsulfonylbutylisothiocya-nate = erysolin) and glucoraphanin (4-methylsulfinylbutylglucosinolate, yields sulforaphane = 4-methylsulfinylbutylisothiocyanate, possibly responsible for anticarcinogenic action) [7, 14]. The seeds are used in the same way as mustard seeds and the leaves as salad [Ü61].

For other herbs with glucosinolates that are used as salads or as salad ingredients → Garden cress.

Literature

[1] Björnquist B., A. Hase, J. Chromatogr. 435:501–507 (1988).
[2] Chikkaputtaiah K.S. et al., Flavour Ind. 2:591–593 (1971).
[3] Cohen D.B. et al., Z. Pflanzenzüchtg. 91: 169–172 (1983).
[4] Dannaker C.J., I.R. White, Contact Dermatitis 16(4):212–214 (1987).
[5] Doering Th.J. et al., Forsch. Komplementärmedizin 5:279–282 (1998).
[6] Dominguez J. et al., Ann. Allergy 64(4): 352–357 (1990).
[7] Dornberger K. et al., Pharmazie 30(12): 792–796 (1975).
[8] Fabre N. et al., Phytochemistry 45(3): 525–527 (1997).
[9] Gmelin R., M. Schlüter, Arch. Pharmaz. 303(4):330–334 (1970).
[10] Hackl G., Arznei- und Gewürzpflanzen 1(2):48–54 (1996).
[11] Hälva S. et al., J. Agric. Sc. Finland 58(4): 157–162 (1986).
[12] Heaney R.K. et al., J. Sci. Food Agric. 31:593–599 (1980).
[13] Hill C.B. et al., J. Am. Soc. Hort. Sci. 112(2):309 (1987).
[14] Iori R. et al., Bioorg. Med. Chem. Lett. 9(7):1047–1048 (1999).
[15] Jiang Z.-T. et al., J. Ess. Oil Res. 11:505–506 (1999).
[16] Jorro G. et al., J. Invest. Allergol. Clin. Immunol. 5(1):54–56 (1995).
[17] Khan B.A. et al., Indian J. Biochem. Biophys. 32(2):106–108 (1995).
[18] Khan B.A. et al., Plant Foods Hum. Nutr. 49(4):295–299 (1996).
[19] Kirk J.T.O., R.N. Oram, J. Austr. Inst. Agr. Sci. 61:51–52 (1981).
[20] Kohl P.K., P.J. Frosch, Contact Dermatitis 23(3):189–190 (1990).
[21] Leanizbarrutia I. et al., Contact Dermatitis 17(4):262–263 (1987).
[22] Liccardi G. et al., J. Allergy Clin. Immunol. 101(4 Pt):559–560 (1998).
[23] Malet A. et al., Allergy 48(1):62–63 (1993).
[24] Monsalve R.I. et al., Biochem. J. 293(Pt 3):625–632 (1993).
[25] Murthy T.N., V.D. Devdhara, J. Oil Technol. Assoc. India (Bombay):20:12–13 (1988), zit. Ü37.
[26] Muuse B.G., H.J. van der Kamp, World Crops: Prod. Util. Descr. 13 (Glucosinolates, Rapeseed):38–49 (1987).
[27] Muuse G.B., H.J. van der Kamp, in J.P. Whatelet (Ed.): Glucosinolates in Rapeseeds: Analytical Aspects, Martinius Nijhoff Publ., Dordrecht 1987, p. 38–49 (1987).
[28] Pigatto P.D. et al., Contact Dermatitis 25(3):191–192 (1991).
[29] Polasa K. et al., Food Chem. Toxicol. 32(8):777–781 (1994).
[30] Rance F. et al., Allergy 55(5):496–500 (2000).
[31] Schlüter M., R. Gmelin, Phytochemistry 11:3427 (1972), ref. in Ü43 (1972).
[32] Thies W., Naturwissenschaften 66:364–365 (1979).
[33] Thies W., Fette, Seifen, Anstrichm. 84:89–95 (1982).
[34] Underhill E.W., D.F. Kirkland, J. Chromatogr. 57:47–54 (1971).
[35] Weymar H., Buch der Kreuzblütler, Neumann Verlag, Leipzig-Radebeul 1988.
[36] Zrybko C. et al., J. Chromatogr. A 767(1/2):43–52 (1997).
[37] Zukalova H., I. Vasak, Rostl. Vyroba 24(10):1009–1017 (1978).

Literature references identified by Ü can be found in the general listing of books and monographs at the back of this book.

Sassafras

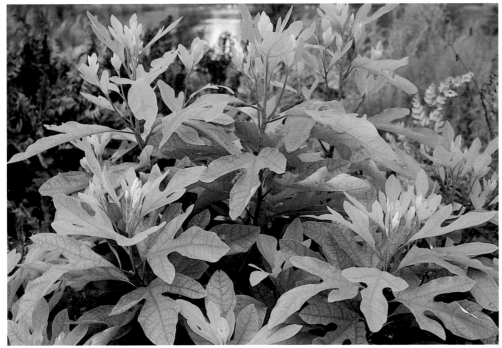

Fig. 1: Sassafras (*Sassafras albidum* (NUTT.) NEES var. *molle* (RAF.) FERN.)

Plant source: *Sassafras albidum* (NUTT.) NEES var. *molle* (RAF.) FERN.

Synonym: *Sassafras officinale* NEES et EBERM.

Taxonomic classification: This species is classified in 2 varieties: *S. albidum* (NUTT.) NEES var. *albidum* and *S. albidum* (NUTT.) NEES var. *molle* (RAF.) FERN.

Family: Laurel (Lauraceae).

Common names: Engl.: sassafras, ague tree, cinnamom wood, saloop; Fr.: bois de sassafras; Ger: Sassafras, Fenchelholzbaum.

Description: A deciduous shrub or an up to 30 m tall, dioecious tree, with alternate and very variable petiolated leaves (from ovate to 2- or 3-lobed), up to 18 cm long and up to 9 cm wide. The small, ternate flowers are arranged in corymbs and appear before the leaves, their yellowish perigone is hexaphyllous, male flowers have 9 stamina, female flowers an ovoid ovary and 6 stunted stamina. The oval, pea-shaped, dark-blue drupes are sitting in a cup-like enlarged axis [Ü60].

Native origin: The Atlantic coast of North America, from Canada to Florida.

Main cultivation areas: Atlantic North America, Northern Mexico, Brazil, and Taiwan.

Main exporting countries: Canada, Atlantic North America, and Brazil.

Cultivation: The tree prefers sunny, protected locations. There are no special soil requirements. In Central Europe it needs, especially the young trees, winter protection (straw collars). Propagation can be done by seed, root cutting or cuttings cut from the young shoots [Ü5].

Culinary herb

Commercial forms: Sassafras leaf: dried leaves, whole or as filé powder (gumbo filé): dried, ground leaves.

Production: The young leaves are harvested in the spring.

Forms used: Gumbo filé: the ground, dried leaves.

Storage: Protect the filé-powder from light and moisture in sealed, airtight porcelain-, glass- or suitable metal containers.

Description. Whole leaf: See description of the whole plant.

Powdered leaf: Green or yellow powder.

Odor: The filé-powder smells acidulous, lemon-like, **Taste:** Acidulous.

History: Parts of the sassafras tree were first used by the Choctaw-Indians in Louisiana as a fever remedy, masticatory and beverage ingredient. The Spaniards brought the root bark and root wood to Europe where it was used as an antisyphilitic remedy, among other uses [Ü55].

Constituents and Analysis

Constituents

- Essential oil: The main components are safrole (about 45%, approximately 150 to 200 mg/100 g leaves), camphor (30%), limonene (5%), furthermore, among others, 1,8-cineole, α-pinene, citral and phellandrene [6, 13].
  The filé-powder is mostly free of essential oil and therefore free of safrole [Ü74].
  In the wood from the roots, 1 to 2% essential oil, in the root bark, 6 to 9%; safrole is the main component (about 80 to 90%); also present are, among others, 5-methoxyeugenol, asarone, methyl eugenol (eugenol methyl ether) and camphor [10, Ü37].
- Mucilage.

Tests for Identity: Sassafras can be identified with sensoric examination as well as with macroscopic and microscopic analysis; safrole is detected with TLC [Ü101].

Quantitative assay of safrole with LC [4], or after SFE, with GC/MS [9].

Actions and Uses

Actions: Due to the rapid loss of aromatic compounds, the appetite stimulant and digestion promoting action of filé powder is probably low. Proof of therapeutic actions of sassafras leaves and of safrole are not available [3].

Toxicology: In animal tests, safrole showed hepatotoxic and hepatocarcinogenic activities [3, 8, 7, 15]. For example, in rats that were fed large doses of safrole (5 g safrole/kg feed), pathological changes of the liver and liver tumors were observed. With lower doses (0.5 and 0.1 g/kg feed), the tumor rate was not elevated [12]. Male mice whose lactating mothers received safrole (120 mg/kg body weight), also showed a higher incidence of tumors in later life [14]. In mice and rats, safrole is metabolized to 1-hydroxysafrole, which, after metabolic activation (by conjugation with

acetic or sulfuric acid or epoxidation), is able to alkylate DNA, RNA and/or proteins. In dogs, 40 to 80 mg safrole/kg body weight led to liver damage but not to tumors [1]. In an animal test with safrole-free essential sassafras oil, an elevated tumor rate was observed as well [11]. Even though carcinogenic effects have not been substantiated in humans, safrole-containing preparations are not to be used as drugs and spices. Since the filé-powder is practically free of essential oil and thus contains no or only traces of safrole, its use as a normally-dosed seasoning (1 tsp/dish for a single person) is without risk.

Food regulatory status: In Europe, the allowable limits for safrole content in foods and beverages are: maximum 1 mg/kg in beverages and foods, maximum 5 mg/kg in alcoholic beverages with more than 25% alcohol content, maximum 15 mg in foods that contain mace or → Nutmeg [5].

Culinary use: The powdered leaf (filé powder) is a very popular flavor ingredient in the southern states of the USA; above all it is used mainly to thicken stews, so-called gumbos (made from okra, pepper pods, chillies, onions and tomatoes, served with rice). It is added after cooking when the dish is still hot, but no longer boiling. Dishes cooked with filé powder are stringy [Ü13, Ü55, Ü74, Ü93].
Filé powder can be used as a thickener and seasoning for fish, seafoods, poultry, and venison, as well as for strongly spiced meat and vegetable stews [Ü55].
Young fresh sassafras leaves are used as accompaniments to green salads. Due to the possible carcinogenicity of safrole, there are objections to this use [Ü55].
In addition to dried, powdered sassafras leaves, filé powder often contains dried powdered leaves of thyme, oregano or bay [Ü74].

Note: Safrole serves as a starting material for designer drugs. Safrole and sassafras oil are subject to the controlled substance regulation (GÜG) in Germany. They may only be dispensed by persons in pharmacies that have a permit as per §7 GÜG [2].

Medicinal herb

Herbal drugs: The dried leaf is not official. Sassafras cortex, Sassafras root bark [EB 6, Ph Helv V], Sassafras lignum, Sassafras root wood [DAB 6, ÖAB] and Sassafras aetheroleum, Sassafras wood oil [EB 6] are no longer used today due to their high essential oil content, which have shown hepatotoxic and hepatocarcinogenic effects in animal tests.

Indications: There are no justified therapeutic uses for sassafras leaves. Market authorization for safrole-containing medicines has been revoked (with the exception of homeopathic medicines with a final potency of D3) [2].

Gumbo with shrimp and crab meat
(Serves 6 persons)
500 g cooked shrimp, 500 g cooked crab meat, 1/2 teaspoon chili sauce, 4 tablespoons vegetable oil, 1 onion (finely minced), 4 green onions (finely minced), 4 stalks of blanched celery (minced), 1 green pepper (seeds removed, minced), 4 teaspoons of flat-leaf parsley (minced), 3 tablespoons of wheat flower, 1 teaspoon of filé powder, salt.

Combine the oil, onions, celery and the green pepper in a large saucepan and sauté the ingredients until soft. Add the sieved flour and let the mixture boil for 2 to 3 minutes. Add 2 l water, bit by bit, under constant stirring and season to taste with salt. Bring to a boil and let it simmer while covered. Add the crabmeat and shrimps and cook them well. Mix in the chili sauce and parsley. Remove the pan from the heat and thoroughly stir in the filé powder. Serve with cooked grain rice [Ü55].

Literature

[1] Abel G. in De Smet PAGM et al. (Eds.): Adverse Effects of Herbal Drugs, Vol. 3, Springer-Verlag, Berlin, Heidelberg 1997, p. 105–122, 123–128 (1997).

[2] Albert K., Pharm. Ztg. 142(11):878 (1997).

[3] Bundesinstitut für Arzneimittel und Medizintechnik (BfArM), Dtsch. Apoth. Ztg. 135(5):366–368 (1995).

[4] Carlson M., R.D. Thompson, J. Am. Off. Anal. Chem. Int. 80(5):1023–1028 (1997).

[5] Council of Europe, Partial Agreement in the Social and Public Health Field, Strasbourg, in: Lebensmittelrecht, Bd. 2, S.145, C.H. Becksche Verlagsbuchhandlung, München 1993.

[6] De Assis Brasil e Silva G.A. et al., Trib. Farmaceut. 47(1):3–6 (1979), zit. in Ü30.

[7] Eisenbrand G., W. Tang, Z. Phytother. 19(1):39–42 (1998).

[8] Fiedler H.P., Pharm. Industrie 42:532–535 (1980).

[9] Heikes D.L., J. Chromatogr. Sci. 32(7): 253–258 (1994).

[10] Kamdem D.P. et al., Planta Med. 61(6): 574–575 (1995).

[11] Kapadia G.J. et al., J. Nat. Cancer Inst. 60:683–686 (1978).

[12] Long E.L. et al., Arch. Pathol. 75:595–604 (1963).

[13] Sultatos L.G. et al., Fed. Proc. 45:343 (1986).

[14] Vesselinovitch S.D. et al., Cancer Res. 39:4378–4380 (1979).

[15] Wiseman R.W. et al., Cancer Res. 47: 2275–2283 (1987).

Literature references identified by Ü can be found in the general listing of books and monographs at the back of this book.

Scallion

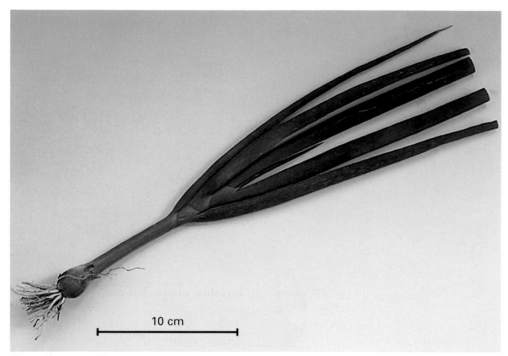

Fig. 1: Young scallion

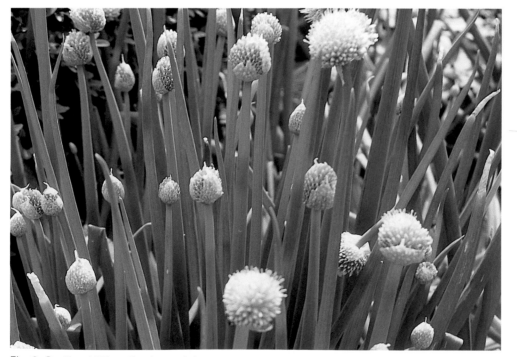

Fig. 2: Scallion (*Allium fistulosum* L.)

Plant source: *Allium fistulosum* L.

Taxonomic classification: The species *Allium fistulosum* L. can be subdivided into the varieties *A. fistulosum* var. *caespitosum* MAKINO and *A. fistulosum* var. *giganteum* MAKINO. It is also considered to be a subspecies of *A. cepa* (→ Onion).

Family: Allium plants (Alliaceae; in older literature this species was placed in the lily family, Liliaceae).

Common names: Engl.: scallion, Welsh onion, spring onion, Japanese bunching onion, negi; Fr.: ciboule, ail fistuleux, oignon d'hiver; Ger.: Winterzwiebel, Winterhecken-Zwiebel, Winter-Heckzwiebel, Hecken-Zwiebel, Welsch-Zwiebel, Röhren-Zwiebel, Röhrenlauch, Winterlauch, Hohllauch, Klöwen.

Description: Perennial, tufted, very variable plant, 0.3 to 1 m tall. The slightly distinct bulb is oblong, cylindrical, bears thin white, later brown skins and many offset bulbs. The basal unifacial leaves are tubiform-inflated, glabrous, shorter than or as long as the inflorescence axis, which is inflated below the middle and compressed at the base. The inflorescence is a globose pseudoumbel; its coat is 2-valvate. The 6 perigone leaves are greenish-white or greenish-yellow, the 6 stamina are much taller than the perigone. The ovary is three chambered. The fruit is a globose capsule with trigonous seeds. Flowering period is from June to August [Ü42, Ü85].

Native origin: Not known in the wild, its domestication center of origin is probably Central- and Western China.

Main cultivation areas: China, Japan, Southeastern Asia, Russian Federation, there it is the most important cultivated species of the genus Allium, and cultivated to a lesser extent also in Europe, and North America.

Main exporting countries: No significant world trade.

Cultivation: Scallions prefer deep, humus soil in sunny, protected locations. Propagation is carried out by direct drilling in March or April or in August, respectively. The seedlings, when they become large enough, are transplanted in small clusters spaced at 20 × 40 cm. In order to assure better leaf development, the flowers should be removed. The plant is extremely winter hardy. It is possible to use the stock for 3 to 4 years. After that they should be transplanted. Varieties that are harvested as whole plants include the so-called bunching- or bundling onion, which is planted in June. In Eastern Asia, soil is mounded up over the basal plant parts in order to attain a bleaching (white negi) [7, Ü96].

Culinary Herb

Commercial forms: In the vegetable trade scallion: fresh whole plants, fresh whole plants with the lower parts bleached, fresh leaves.

Production: The leaves can be harvested throughout the year. The bundled onions are harvested as whole plants in March.

Forms used: Fresh leaves, fresh plants, in Eastern Asia also the chlorophyll-free lower parts of the plants.

Storage: The leaves or the whole plant should be used as fresh as possible. In plastic bags, they can be stored in the refrigerator for 1 to 2 weeks. Longer storage is possible by deep-freezing in plastic bags or the leaves can be chopped and frozen with water in the ice-tray. Drying leads to aroma loss.

Description. Whole plant: See description of the plant.

Odor: Almost odorless if not bruised, alliaceous upon bruising, **Taste:** Cepaceous, with little pungency.

History: The scallion was already cultivated in China 2000 years ago. Its cultivation spread to Europe in the 16th and 17th century [Ü92].

Constituents and Analysis

Constituents

- Alliins (*S*-alk(en)ylcysteine sulfoxides) in the unbruised plant: *S*-methyl-L-cysteine sulfoxide, *S*-propyl-L-cysteine sulfoxide, *S*-allyl-L-cysteine sulfoxide and *S*-prop-1-enyl-L-cysteine sulfoxide (see chemical structures → Garlic and → Onion) [10, Ü43].
- Alliaceous oils: The non-volatile alliins come into contact with the enzyme alliinase upon tissue injury, and are then transformed to the volatile alk(en)ylsulfenic acids, which spontaneously convert to the odor-determining reaction products, the alk(en)yl-alkane/alkene thiosulfinates (Fig. 10, → General Section). Also detected were propylpropane thiosulfinate (35%), (*E,Z*)-prop-1-enyl-propane thiosulfinate (25%), prop-1-enyl-methane thiosulfinate (18%), methylmethane thiosulfinate (about 8%) and propylmethane thiosulfinate (about 8%) [1]. Breakdown products of these constituents form upon heating; the main compounds identified were dipropyldisulfide (in the steam distillate 31%), methylpropyltrisulfide (in the steam distillate 12%), dipropyltrisulfide (in the steam distillate 12%, see chemical structures → Onion), dimethyltrisulfide (in the steam distillate 6%), and, among others, dimethylthiophene [9, 10, 13, Ü83].
- Steroid saponins: Fistulosides A, B and C (yuccageninglycosides), dioscin, saponin P-d [4].
- Poly-, oligo- and monosaccharides: Fructosans (about 10 to 40%), mucous-like heteropolysaccharides, oligofructosides, saccharose (5 to 8%), glucose and fructose [11].

- Sterols: Cholesterol, cycloartenol, lophenol, β-sitosterol [8].

Tests for Identity based on the detection of the volatile constituents in the steam distillate with GC/MS [10], → Onion.

Quantitative assay of the volatile constituents in the steam distillate with GC/MS [10], → Onion.

Adulterations, Misidentifications and Impurities are possible with shallots; they lack the typically inflated, hollow leaves of the scallion.

Actions and Uses

Actions: Due to the pungent taste of scallions as well as the irritant effect of the alliaceous oils on the gastric mucosa, they are appetite stimulating and digestion promoting.

Ingestion of raw, however not cooked scallions in rats (2 g/kg body weight for 4 weeks), lowered systolic resting blood pressure, increased the plasma level of 6-keto-$PGF_{1\alpha}$, diminished blood platelet aggregation and –adhesion and thereby prolonged bleeding time [2]. In vitro, extracts of fresh scallion caused relaxation of precontracted aortae rings of rats by stimulating the formation of nitric oxide derived from the endothelial cells of the blood vessels. High doses induced endothelium-independent vasorelaxation [3].

Epidemiological studies in China have shown, that the frequent ingestion of scallions (same as for garlic, onions, Chinese chives) lowers the risk of developing esophagus- or gastric cancer [6].

Similar to extracts of other plants that contain alliaceous oils, scallion also has antimicrobial action. The fungicidal activity extends also to mycotoxigenic fungi [5, 14]. Additionally, its effects may be similar to those of → Onion.

Toxicology: Based on existing data, there is no acute or chronic toxicity with the use of normal amounts of scallion by healthy individuals.

Culinary use: Scallion is indispensable for Asian cooking.

Chopped leaves or the chopped whole plants serve (similar to chives, added at the end of cooking time) as a seasoning of soups, sauces, marinades, meat-, fish-, legume- as well as egg dishes and vegetables. They are also used for improving the taste of salads and potatoes [Ü74, Ü92].

Similar culinary herbs: → Chives.

Medicinal herb

Herbal drug: Allium-fistulosum, whole plant.

Indications: In China it us used for the treatment of colic, diarrhea, headaches, feverish diseases and eye diseases [12]. The seeds are used as a tonic [Ü60].

Literature

[1] Block E. et al., J. Agric. Food Chem. 40: 2431–2438 (1992).
[2] Chen J.H., J. Nutr. 130(1):34–37 (2000).
[3] Chen J.h. et al., J. Cardiovas. Pharmacol. 33(4):515–520 (1999).
[4] Do J.Ch., K.Y. Jung, J. Nat. Prod. 55: 168–173 (1992).
[5] Fan J.J., J.H. Chen, J. Food Prot. 62(4): 414–417 (1999).
[6] Gao C.M. et al., Jpn. J. Cancer Res. 90(6): 614–621 (1999).
[7] Hanelt P., Drogenreport 7(11):17–25 (1994).
[8] Itoh T. et al., Phytochemistry 16:140 (1977), ref. in Ü43.
[9] Kameoka H. et al., Phytochemistry 23: 155–158 (1984).
[10] Pino J.A. et al., J. Ess. Oil Res. 12:553–555 (2000).
[11] Rubat de Mérac M.L., Recherches sur le métabolisme glucidique du genre Allium et en particulier d'Allium ursinum L., Theses (Sci. nat) Univ. Paris 1949, ref. in Ü43.
[12] Shougakukan, The Dictionary of Chinese Drugs, Shanghai Science and Technologic Publ. and Shougakukan, Tokyo III 1985, Vol. III p. 1599–1600, zit. in Lit. 4 (s.o.).
[13] Tsai Sh.J. et al., Shipin Kexue (Taipei) 22(2): 185–194 (1995), zit.: CA:123: 312568t.
[14] Yin M.C., S.M. Tsao, Int. J. Food Microbiol. 49(1/2):49–56 (1999).

Literature references identified by Ü can be found in the general listing of books and monographs at the back of this book.

Sesame

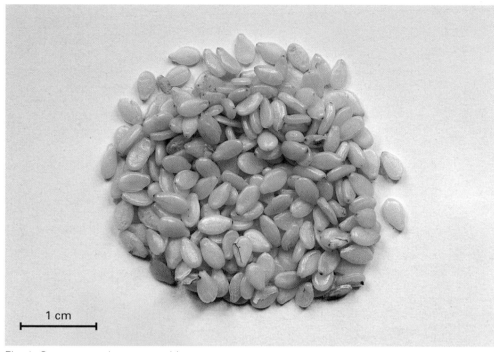

Fig. 1: Sesame seeds, cream white

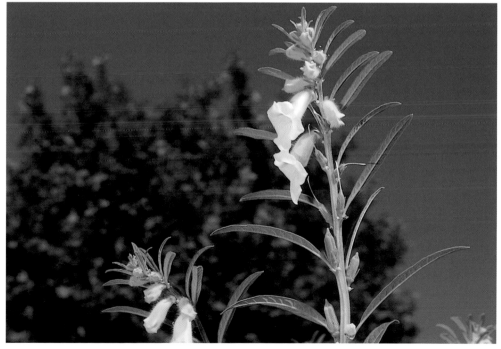

Fig. 2: Sesame (*Sesamum orientale* L.)

Plant source: *Sesamum orientale* L.

Synonym: *Sesamum indicum* L.

Taxonomic classification: The species is subdivided into numerous varieties [1], the subdivision, however, plays no role in the chemistry, pharmacology and use of the plant as described in the literature.

Family: Sesame family (Pedaliaceae).

Common names: Engl.: sesame, beniseed, gingelly, oriental sesam; Fr.: sésame; Ger.: Sesam.

Description: Annual plant, 1 to 1.2 m tall, seldom up to 3 m, stalk rarely ramified, completely or only in the upper part hairy. Leaves 3 to 17 cm long, 1 to 7 mm wide, in the lower part of the stalk opposite arranged, oblong ovate, with a complete margin or 3- to 5-lobed and dentate, in the lower part alternate arranged and lanceolate. The white or reddish flowers with a foxglove-like, 5-lobed corolla are located singly or up to 3 in clusters in the upper leaf axils. The fruits are 2 to 3 cm long and 0.5 to 1 cm wide, 4- to 10-chambered capsules [Ü26, Ü37].

Native origin: Probably native to the Ethiopian region or India, today only known in cultivation.

Main cultivation areas: India, China, and Myanmar, furthermore Mexico, Nigeria, Sudan, Bangladesh, Somalia, Uganda, Turkey, Vietnam, Cambodia, Japan, southern Russian Federation, Costa Rica, Nicaragua, Guatemala, Venezuela, southeastern states of the USA, Greece, former Yugoslavia, and Pakistan.

Main exporting countries: India, China, Myanmar, Mexico, Sudan, Nigeria, and Guatemala.

Cultivation: Sesame prefers well-drained, sandy loam soil with neutral reaction in regions with constant high temperature (optimum 25 °C). The plant is very susceptible to frost. The crop margin lies between latitudes 42° north and 35° south, in which the main growing regions fall between 25° north and 25° south latitude. Seeds are sown 1 to 3 cm deep in row widths of 30 to 100 cm. Due to the short growing period of this plant (3 to 4 months), 2 harvests per season are possible [Ü26, Ü82].

Culinary herb

Commercial forms: Sesame seed: whole, hulled or ground, sesame paste (→ Tahini paste).

Production: Sesame is harvested by cutting or pulling out the plants before the lower capsules fully ripen. After storage for post-harvest maturation the plants are cleaned by beating them on a suitable pad. Mechanical harvest is only possible for varieties with indehiscent capsules [Ü26].

Forms used: The seeds are used unhulled, hulled, unroasted or roasted (15 minutes at about 220 °C), whole or ground.

Storage: In sealed, airtight containers, in a cool and dark location.

Description. Whole seed (Figs. 1 and 3): The seeds have a pyriform outline, 1.5 to 4 mm long, 1 to 2 mm wide, 0.5 to 1 mm thick, cream-white, brownish, reddish, brown or black, smooth or finely veined [Ü26].

Microscopic description: The testa shows the palisade epidermal cells, which contain at the upper end, large spherical calcium oxalate masses; only the more elongated, arched cells of the skin surface at the thin ribs of the seeds are free of oxalate (Fig. 4). Below the epidermis are two indistinct-

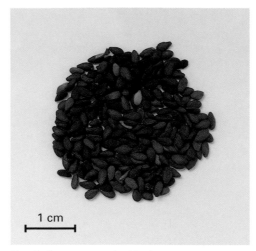

1 cm

Fig. 3: Sesame seeds, black

ly visible cell layers, of which the inner one shows thickened, yellowish walls. The endosperm consists of 2 to 5 layers of thin-walled cells and the cell content is made of fatty oil droplets and aleuron grains. The cotyledon cells also contain fatty oil [Ü29].

Powdered seed: The chloral hydrate preparation shows the typical fragments of the testa (see above) [Ü29].

Odor: None, **Taste:** Mild, sweet, nut-like, during the roasting process, the nut-like aroma component is intensified.

History: About 3000 years ago, sesame was introduced from Africa as a cultivated plant to Sumer and Mesopotamia, and

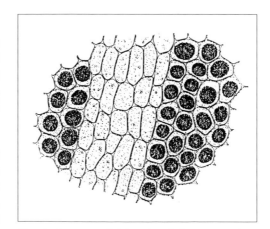

Fig. 4: Sesame. Epidermis of the testa, view from the top. From Ü29.

from there, it was later brought to China, Vietnam, Cambodia, Malaysia, and Japan, and via Afghanistan to Asia Minor, as well as to the southern regions of the Russian Federation, and Mediterranean countries. In the Papyrus Ebers (1150 BCE), sesame is mentioned. Excavations in Turkey have shown that sesame oil was already produced in 700 BCE. In China, sesame has been known for about 2000 years. Sesame was brought to America in the 17th or 18th century by African slaves [Ü61, Ü73].

Constituents and Analysis

Constituents

- Fatty oil: 40 to 60% (high oil content in the black seeds); the main fatty acids are 35 to 57% oleic acid, 35 to 57% linoleic acid, 7 to 12% palmitic acid and 3 to 6% stearic acid [15, 23, Ü8].
- Lignans: About 1%, the bisepoxylignan sesamin (0.2 to 0.5%), sesamolin (0.1 to 0.3%, transforming to sesamol), sesamolinol, sesaminol, pinoresinol, simplexoside aglycone and (+)-episesaminone, furthermore lignan glycosides, e.g. glucosides, diglucosides and triglucosides of pinoresinol and sesaminol [2, 3, 10, 12, 18, 24]. The lignans pass into the fatty oil: in sesame oil, about 0.3 to 2.5% sesamin and 0.1 to 0.6 sesamolin, among others [3, 25, 27].
- Proteins: About 25% [Ü60].
- Starch: 15 to 20% [Ü60].
- Hydroxycinnamic acid derivatives: Ester of *p*-coumaric acid, ferulic acid and caffeic acid [4].
- Oligosaccharides: Planteose (trisaccharide), lychnose and sesamose (tetrasaccharides), among others [6, 28].

The following flavor- and odor- determining constituents of the roasted seeds have been identified: 2-furfurylthiol (coffee-like aroma), 2-phenylethylthiol (rubber-like odor), 4-hydroxy-2,5-dimethyl-3(2H)-furanone (caramel-like odor), 2-acetyl-1-pyrroline (roasting aroma), 2-methoxyphenol, 2-pentylpyridine, 2-ethyl-3,5-dimethylpyrazine, acetylpyrazine, deca-2(*E*),4(*E*)-dienal and 4-vinyl-2-methoxyphenol [14, 22].

Sesamin

Sesamol

Sesamolin $R_1 + R_2 = $ -CH$_2$-O-CH$_2$-
Sesamolinol $R_1 = $ OCH$_3$, $R_2 = $ OH

Tests for Identity: Sesame oil is analyzed using the Baudouin reaction: 2 drops sesame oil + 3 drops ethanolic furfurol solution (2%) mixed with 10 ml fuming hydrochloric acid produce a red coloration [Ü49]; after shaking sesame oil with a hydrochloric saccharose solution, the aqueous layer takes on a pink color and turns red after some time [USP XXII]. The identity can also be determined with TLC [Ü77].

Quantitative assay: For determining sesamin, sesamolin and sesamol levels, see Lit. [3]; determination of the quantitative composition of the triacylglycerols with liquid chromatography [Ph Eur].

Adulterations, Misidentifications and Impurities are not known.

Actions and Uses

Actions: Due to its nutlike taste, sesame seeds are appetite stimulating. The roasted seeds may possibly limit the rate of digestion.

Supplementation of cholesterol free and cholesterol containing diet of rats with a globulin fraction of sesame seed protein with a lysine : arginine ratio 0.67 lowered concentrations of cholesterol in both HDL and LDL + VLDL fractions though increased cholesterol synthesis in the liver. The reasons were promotion of the increase of conversion of cholesterol to bile acids and their increased fecal excretion [21]. Sesamin and episesamin administered to rats on a normal diet led to an increase of HDL-cholesterol, in contrast to a decrease of VLDL-cholesterol concentration. In rats given a fat- and cholesterol-rich diet, only episesamin showed this positive effect [16]. Sesamin has been shown to lower the blood concentration of cholesterol in humans, especially LDL-cholesterol [7].

The lignans, especially the pinoresinol glucosides, have strong antioxidative activity. For example, they can protect lipids of the erythrocyte membrane in vitro from oxidative attack and thereby preventing the lipid hydroperoxides, formed by oxidative stress, reacting with nucleophilic components of the cells, e.g. proteins and phospholipids, resulting in cell damage. Supplementation with sesame seeds (5% in feed) and their lignans (sesamin, sesaminol) could also be shown in vivo in rats fed a low alpha-tocopherol diet to suppress lipid peroxidation in the liver and the hemolysis of erythrocytes. There was a significant increase of tocopherol content in the liver and blood plasma [29]. Sesame lignans should also improve liver function, e.g. by accelerating catabolism of ethanol. The lignans are responsible for the very good shelf life of sesame oil [5, 8, 11, 17, 24]. Sesame lignans should also have antihypertensive activity [26].

Sesamolin and to a lesser extent sesamin potentiate the insecticidal activity of pyrethrine [3].

Toxicology: Based on existing data, there is no acute or chronic toxicity with the use of sesame seeds as a seasoning, garnish or food ingredient at usual doses.

Based on the sesamin and sesamolin content, sesame seeds and oil do have a sensitization potential, even though the risk is small. Allergic reactions after skin contact with sesame oil were urticaria, burning and inflammation of the skin [9, Ü39].

Culinary use: In the countries where sesame seeds are grown, especially in the Anterior Asia and Egypt, the roasted or unroasted seeds are used as a seasoning (same as caraway) of bread and cakes. In Japan, Korea and China they are roasted and sprinkled over rice-, poultry- and beef dishes. There they are also used in ground form as a binder of sauces. In the Middle East, the ground seeds are used to make tahina sesame paste (→ Tahini paste) or similarly, in Asia, the roasted seeds are used to prepare pastes, which serve as seasoning for noodle-, vegetable- and rice dishes, but also of fruit dishes. Tahini paste is also an important component of Turkish garbanzo bean soup (humus, hummus bi tahina). It is also used as a salad sauce or as a dip, e.g. for oriental meat dishes (kebabs) and for sandwiches. Seasoned with garlic and lemon juice, it is consumed with bread as an appetizer. In Asian countries, the hulled seeds are frequently used as components of foods and snacks, e.g. as a paste for flat bread, as a component of the Jewish Sabbath bread challah (made from sesame seeds, candied lemon peel and honey), of Turkish honey (a sticky glutinous foam mass made from sugar, honey, glucose syrup, egg whites and gelatin, as well as nuts, almonds and/or sesame seeds) or of halva (halwa, chalva, a confectionary made from thoroughly roasted egg white foam mass with addition of nut-, almond- or sesame kernels). North Americans use sesame seed as a fish spice [Ü13, Ü53, Ü55, Ü73, Ü92, Ü98].

When using sesame seeds as a seasoning, they should be dry roasted shortly before use. As a decorative spice, they are added whole, as a supplement to meals they are sometimes ground in a spice mill or crushed in a mortar prior to use.

In Central Europe, sesame seeds serve primarily as a decorative spice for bread, rolls, bakery goods and confectionaries.

For these applications, they are sprinkled on the bakery products before baking [Ü2].

Sesame seeds can also be used as a seasoning for cauliflower, broccoli, spinach, asparagus, green beans and poultry [Ü13, Ü45]. The roasted seeds serve as an accompaniment to quark [Ü30, Ü73]. Sesame oil made from roasted sesame seeds tastes nutlike and is added to dishes as a flavor component before preparation [Ü73].

Combines well with: Caraway, garlic, and paprika.

As a component of spice mixes and preparations: → Dukkah, → Gomasio, → Shichimi tograrashi, → Tahini paste, → Tofu spice, → Zahtar.

Other uses: Sesame oil is a very good cooking oil with a long shelf life due to the antioxidative effects of the lignans. It is used for the manufacture of baked goods, margarine, baking oils, cosmetics and insecticides. Because it is easily detected (Baudouin reaction), it is added as an indicator to margarine in some countries in order to distinguish margarine from butter. Due to its content of L-methionine and L-tryptophan, defatted sesame flour is added to grain and legume products in order to improve their amino acid profiles. Sesame bread must be made from flour containing not less than 8% sesame flour [Ü98]. The expressed residue from sesame oil production is used for the manufacture of oriental sauces and as an ingredient for confectionaries, baked goods and concentrated feed for pets [Ü45]. The shoots from the young leaves are used in West Africa as a vegetable [Ü82].

Medicinal herb

Herbal drug: Sesami semen, Sesame seed.

Indications: In the folk medicine of the countries where it is cultivated, it is used internally for menstrual problems, as an aphrodisiac, diuretic, laxative and antirheumatic, and applied externally in the form of cataplasms for ulcers and burns [Ü60].

Similar culinary herbs

Poppy, seeds of *Papaver somniferum* L. ssp. *somniferum*, garden poppy, opium poppy (Papaveraceae). Poppy is an economic plant, which has been domesticated in the western Mediterranean region and was already cultivated in ancient times in Asia Minor. There are strains with white, brown or blue-gray seeds. The seeds have a slightly nut-like aroma. They contain 40 to 55% fatty oil (high levels in the white seed varieties), of which the main fatty acids are 65 to 75% linoleic acid, about 30% oleic acid and about 10% linolenic acid [Ü26], furthermore 20 to 25% proteins and small amounts of isoquinoline alkaloids (0.009%, including, among others, morphine, codeine, narcotine, papaverine, thebaine) [19, 20]. The seeds become bitter during long storage through the oxidation products of linoleic acid [13]. Poppy seeds are sprinkled as a decorative spice onto bakery goods (e.g. on rolls, poppy (twisted) buns), worked into cake dough or made into poppy paste (poppy filling), in which ground (e.g. in the coffee grinder) blue-gray poppy seeds are treated with boiling milk and mixed with fat, sugar and eggs. Poppy paste is used either alone

Bulgogi

500 g rump- or beefsteak, from the top side of the hind leg, cut into thin strips, 3 teaspoons brown sugar, 125 ml soy sauce, 3 teaspoons sesame oil, 2 garlic cloves (minced), 3 spring onions (finely minced), 2 tablespoons sesame seeds (lightly roasted).

Marinate the beef with the other ingredients (without the sesame seeds) for 2 to 4 h; turn the meat pieces over from time to time. Heat up a frying pan, remove the meat from the marinade and quickly sauté on high heat so it turns brown and is almost done. Place the cooked meat strips on a preheated serving plate. Reduce the heat of the pan and add 45 to 60 ml marinade; bring to a boil and let it thicken. Before serving, pour the sauce over the beef and sprinkle with sesame seeds [Ü2].

(poppy seed cake, poppy seed torte) or combined with fruit or quark spread onto the dough (poppy-quark-cake, poppy-apple-cake), rolled into the dough (poppy seed rolls) or used as a filling [Ü98]. In Turkey, poppy seeds serve as an ingredient for preparing desserts (e.g. mixed with grape syrup and nuts) and halva (see below) [Ü73, Ü92]. Poppy seeds can also be used in cooking, e.g. for curry dishes, meat- and fish sauces, salad dressing with cream, egg noodles and for sprinkling on vegetables [Ü55]. The full flavor of the seeds is attained by roasting. Roasted poppy seeds are suitable especially for dressings, for example for potato-, tomato-, egg-, noodle- or herb salad [Ü68].

Literature

[1] Bedigian D. et al., Econ. Bot. 40:353–365 (1986).

[2] Bedigian D. et al., Biochem. Syst. Ecol. 13:133–139 (1985).

[3] Beroza M., M.L. Kinman, J. Am. Oil Chemists' Soc. 32:348 (1955).

[4] Dabrowski K.J., F.W. Sosulski, J. Agric. Food Chem. 32:128–130 (1984).

[5] Fukuda Y. et al., J. Am. Oil Chemist's Soc. 63:1027 (1986).

[6] Hatanaka S.I., Arch. Biochem. 82:188 (1959), ref. in Ü37.

[7] Hirata F. et al., Atherosclerosis (Shannon, Israel.):122(1):135–136 (1996), ref. CA 125:001064k.

[8] Kamal-Eldin A. et al., in: Spec. Publ. R. Soc. Chem. 1996, 181 (Natural Antioxidants and Food Quality in Atherosclerosis and Cancer Prevention), p. 230–235 (1996), ref. in CA 125:274567y.

[9] Kanny G. et al., Allergy (Copenhagen):51(12):952–957 (1996).

[10] Katsuzaki H. et al., Phytochemistry 35(3): 773–776 (1994).

[11] Kuriyama K., T. Murai, Nippon Nogei Kagaku Kaishi 70(2):161–167 (1996), ref. CA 124:259103e.

[12] Marchand P.A. et al., J. Nat. Prod. 60(11):1189–1192 (1997).

[13] Meshdani T. et al., Nahrung 34:769–772 (1990).

[14] Nakamura S. et al., Agric. Biol. Chem. 53:1891–1897 (1989).

[15] Oezcan M., A. Akguel, Turk. Agric. For. 19(1):59–65 (1995), ref. CA 123: 052372a.

[16] Ogawa H. et al., Clin. Exp. Pharmacol. Physiol. 22(Suppl.1): S310–S312 (1995), ref. CA 124:220151u.

[17] Osawa T., Shipin Kexue (Taipei) 24(6): 679–689 (1997), ref. CA 128:179745h.

[18] Osawa T., Agric. Biol. Chem. 49: 3351–3352 (1985).

[19] Paul B.D. et al., Planta Med. 62(6): 544–547 (1996).

[20] Preininger V. et al., Pharmazie (20): 439–441 (1965).

[21] Rajamohan T., P.A. Kurup, Indian J. Exp. Biol. 35(11):1218–1223 (1997).

[22] Schieberle P., Food Chem. 55(2):145–152 (1996).

[23] Sengupta A., S.K. Roychoudhury, J. Sci. Food Agric. 27(2):165–169 (1976).

[24] Shukla V.K.S. et al., Nat. Antioxid. 1997:97–132 (1997).

[25] Soliman M.M. et al., Agric. Biol. Chem. (Tokyo) 39:973–977 (1975), zit. in Ü30.

[26] Sugano M., Shoku no Kagaku 218:39–43 (1996), ref. CA 125:009270v.

[27] Tashiro T. et al., J. Am. Oil Chemists' Soc. 67:508–511 (1990).

[28] Wankhede D.B., R.N. Tharanathan, J. Agric. Food Chem. 24(3):655–659 (1976).

[29] Yamashita K. et al., Lipids 30(11): 1019–1028 (1995).

Literature references identified by Ü can be found in the general listing of books and monographs at the back of this book.

Shallot

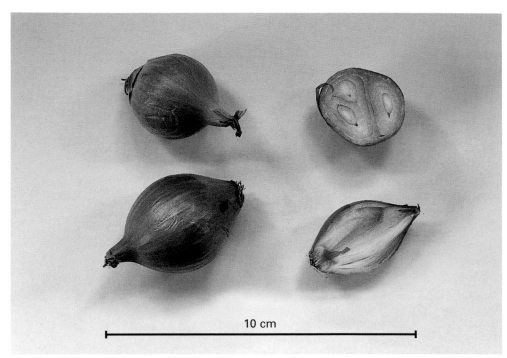

Fig. 1: Shallots

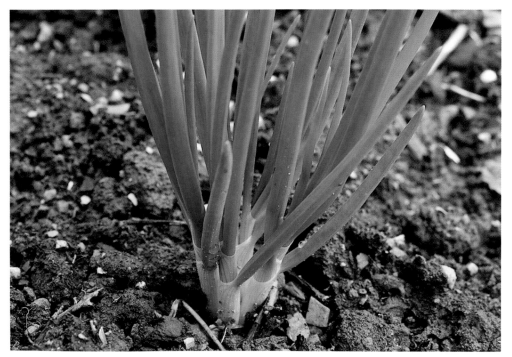

Fig. 2: Shallot (*Allium cepa* L. var. *ascalonicum* BACKER)

Plant source: *Allium cepa* L. var. *ascalonicum* BACKER.

Synonym: *Allium ascalonicum* auct. non L.

Taxonomic classification: According to the opinion of a few authors, shallot and potato onion, *Allium cepa* var. *aggregatum* G. DON, are identical [Ü61]. Sometimes the varieties are articulated into provarieties: *A. cepa* var. *ascalonicum* provar. *ascalonicum* (an approximately walnut-sized bulb), *A. cepa* var. *ascalonicum* provar. *chinense* (with filbert-sized bulbs), *A. cepa* var. *ascalonicum* provar. *majus* (a larger than walnut-sized bulb). See also → Onion.

Family: Allium plants (Alliaceae; in older literature this species was placed in the lily family, Liliaceae).

Common names: Engl.: shallot (→ Welsh onion is sometimes also referred to by the same name), eschalot; Fr.: échalotte, ail stérile, ciboule; Ger.: Schalotte, Charlotte, Aschlauch, Eschlauch, Esslauch, Levantelauch, Syrische Zwiebel, Ascalonzwiebel, Klöben, Batatenzwiebel, Schlotte.

Description: Perennial plant, 0.2 to 1 m tall. Shape, size and color of the bulb depend on cultivar. The bulbs of *A. ascalonicum* var. *ascalonicum* provar. *ascalonicum* are up to 1.5 cm long and have a diameter of 0.2 to 2.0 cm. Numerous offset bulbs and the main bulb are arranged nest-like together. The basal unifacial, glabrous leaves are tubiform but not inflated; they are shorter than the inflorescence axis. The inflorescence is a globose pseudoumbel; its coat is 3-valvate, bulbils are usually present. The 6 perigone leaves are bluish, whitish or pink with a dark-blue ribbon in the middle, the 6 stamina are as long as or a little longer than the perigone.

The ovary is three chambered. The fruit is a globose capsule with trigonous seeds. Shallot seldom flowers in temperate latitudes [Ü42, Ü85].

Native origin: Probably native to Central Asia, occurs wild in Anterior Asia, and in the Orient.

Main cultivation areas: Due to its bolting-resistance and disease resistance it is preferred over onions, especially in tropical and subtropical regions (West Africa, Caribbean, Southeastern Asia). In the Orient, Europe and in North America, it is mainly cultivated in gardens.

Main exporting countries: Fresh shallots are mainly traded locally. Producers of dry product include especially China, India, Egypt, and Syria.

Cultivation: Shallots prefer loose humus soil in sunny, warm locations. It must be well watered and hoed flat. Propagation is carried out in March or April either by sowing, about 1 cm deep, with row spacing of about 20 cm, later the seedlings are separated to a spacing of about 15 cm, or through propagation bulbs (spacing of 15×20 cm). The cultivar "Creation" (F_1-hybrid) is suitable for sowing, among other varieties. In regions with mild climates, propagation bulbs can also be planted in the autumn. Around the main bulb, a nest of small bulblets fused at the base, develops rapidly [Ü96].

Culinary Herb

Commercial forms: Shallots: young fresh bulbs with leaves, and mature fresh bulbs.

Production: The harvest of bulbs with foliage is possible in July when sowing, in June when propagation with propagation bulbs is carried out. The ripe bulbs can be harvested in August, when the foliage is dried up. [Ü96].

Forms used: Young fresh bulbs with leaves, mature fresh bulbs.

Storage: The fresh baby bulbs and leaves are suitable for immediate consumption. The ripe bulbs should be kept in a cool and dry place, hung up with the dried leaves, in nets or in wide meshed bags. Shallots have a longer shelf life than → Onions.

Description. Whole bulb (Fig. 1): The individual bulb of the shallot consists of the fleshy, helically arranged and fused scales, which are attached to a disk-like axis (basal plate). The outer bulb scales (tunic) are paper-thin, yellow-brown or red. The shape of the shallot bulb is oblong-ovate to pyriform. Mostly the main bulb and bulbils are attached to a single basal plate and are all surrounded by a common outer wall [Ü37].

Odor: Odorless if unbruised, after bruising with a pungent, burning odor, causing tearing of the eyes, **Taste:** Sweet, pungent, spicy, milder than onion.

History: Shallots were already used during antiquity (named after the city Askalon in Southern Israel, destroyed in 1192 and 1270, near the present Aschkelon). In the 12th century, it was brought to Europe by the crusaders [Ü92].

Constituents and Analysis

Constituents

▢ Alliins (*S*-alk(en)ylcysteine sulfoxides) in the unbruised plant. The spectrum of constituents is comparable to that of → Onion. Detected were *trans*-(+)-*S*-(prop-1-enyl)-L-cysteine sulfoxide (about 0.9% of the fresh bulb, see chemical structures → Onion) [4]. From the composition of the alliaceous oils, it can be concluded that methyl-L-cysteine sulfoxide and n-propyl-L-cysteine sulfoxide should be present.

▢ Alliaceous oils: The non-volatile alliins come into contact with the enzyme allinase upon tissue injury and are then transformed to volatile alk(en)yl sulfenic acids, which spontaneously convert to their alliaceous smelling odor-determining breakdown products,

the alk(en)ylalkane/alkenethiosulfinates (Fig. 10, → General section). A number of constituents were identified, including, among others, propyl-propanethiosulfinate (about 26%), (*E,Z*)-prop-1-enyl-propanethiosulfinate (21%), (*E,Z*)-prop-1-enyl-methanethiosulfinate (15%), (*E*)-methyl-prop-1-enethiosulfinate (8%), methyl-methanethiosulfinate (7%), methyl-propanethiosulfinate (6%) and *cis*- as well as *trans*-zwiebelanes (17 and 12%, respectively, see chemical structures → Onion) [1]. Upon heating, methylpropyltrisulfide, dipropyltrisulfide, dimethyltrisulfide, dipropyldisulfide, dimethylthiophene, among others, are formed, as well as sulfur-free compounds, e.g. dimethylpyrazines, trimethylpyrazines and ethyldimethylpyrazines [Ü83].

▢ γ-Glutamyl-*S*-trans-1-propenylcysteine (0.18% of the fresh bulb) [4].

▢ Flavonoids: Quercetin glycosides, such as quercetin-4´-glucoside (spiraeoside), quercetin-3,4´-diglucoside, quercetin-7,4´-diglucoside and querectin-3-glucoside (isoquercitrin), among others [2, Ü43].

▢ Carbohydrates: Saccharose (about 4%), fructosanes (30 to 65%) [5].

Tests for Identity: → Onion.

Quantitative assay: → Onion.

Adulterations, Misidentifications and Impurities: Occasionally, small onions are traded as shallots.

Actions and Uses

Actions: Due to the pungent taste of raw shallots as well as the irritant effect of the alliaceous oils on the gastric mucosa and the aromatic odor and taste of cooked or fried shallots, they have appetite stimulating and digestion promoting action.
In rabbits with hypercholesterolemia induced by feeding of egg yolks, extracts of shallots were able to prevent membrane damage of erythrocytes (crenate shape),

caused through this diet, without a significant decrease in blood lipid levels [6]. The pressed juice of shallots inhibited the growth of gram-positive bacteria [3] and has fungicide action [7].

Due to the spectrum of constituents of the shallot, which is very closely comparable to that of → Onion, the same effects produced by onions can also be expected for shallots.

Toxicology: Based on existing data, there is no acute or chronic toxicity in healthy individuals with the use of shallots at normal doses. In other respects, the toxicology of shallots is similar to → Onions.

Culinary use: Shallots play an important role in French, Chinese, and Japanese, but also in Russian, and North American cooking. In French cuisine, they are used especially as a seasoning of roast mutton and snipe as well as of Entrecôte à la bordelaise (steak with red wine and butter), béarnaise sauce, sauce bercy, sauce à la bordelaise, and sauce marchand.

Raw or cooked shallots serve as seasoning of sauces, salads, ragouts, cheese and quark. It can also be used as an added component for pickling of mixed pickles. Finely chopped, mixed with wine vinegar and spices, it is served with raw seafoods such as oysters and mussels [Ü2, Ü92, Ü59].

Roasted shallots are a popular side dish with fried meat or poultry [Ü55].

Shallot leaves are used in the same way as → Chive, → Onion or → Welsh Onion.

Combines well with: → Onion.

As a component of spice mixes and preparations: → Nam prik, → Worcestershire sauce.

Medicinal herb

Herbal drug: Allii ascalonici bulbus, Shallot bulb.

Indication: Digestive problems. The indications for use for shallot correspond to those of → Onion.

Similar culinary herbs

African onion, *Allium angolense* BAKER, cultivated in Angola, Congo, Zaire, Gabon, it used in the same manner as shallots [Ü61].

Triploid viviparous onion (Egyptian onion, Catawissa onion), *Allium cepa* L. var. *viviparum* (METZG.) ALEF. (*A.* × *proliferum* (MOENCH) SCHRAD. ex. WILLD., hybrid of *A. fistulosum* L. × *A. cepa* L.),

cultivated in gardens in Europe, Siberia, Eastern Asia, and North America, distinguished by its formation of bulbils 1 to 2 cm in size, often established in several stages. The bulbs and bulbils are used in the same manner as onions, and the leaves are used the same as shallots [Ü61].

Literature

[1] Block E. et al., J. Agric. Food Chem. 40: 2431–2438 (1992).
[2] Brandwein B.J., J. Food Sci. 30:680 (1965), ref. in Ü43.
[3] Dankert J. et al., Zentralbl. Bakteriol (Orig. A) 245(1/2):229–239 (1979).
[4] Fenwick G.R. et al., CRC Crit. Rev. Food Sci. Nutr. 22:199–377 (1985).
[5] Rubat de Mérac M.L.: Recherches sur le métabolisme glucidique du genre Allium et en particulier Allium ursinum L., Theses (Sci. nat.) Univ. Paris 1949, ref. in Ü43.
[6] Tappayuthpijarn P. et al., J. Med. Assoc. Thai 72(8):448–451 (1989).
[7] Yin M.C., S.M. Tsao, Int. J. Food Microbiol. 49(1/2):49–56 (1999).

Literature references identified by Ü can be found in the general listing of books and monographs at the back of this book.

Sichuan pepper

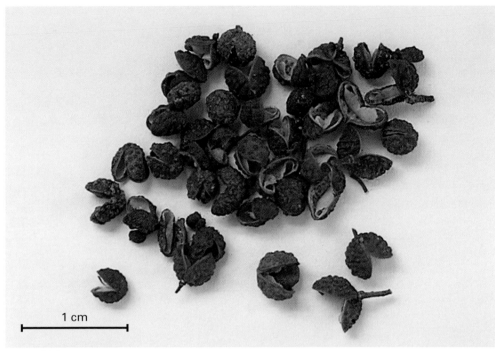

Fig. 1: Sichuan pepper

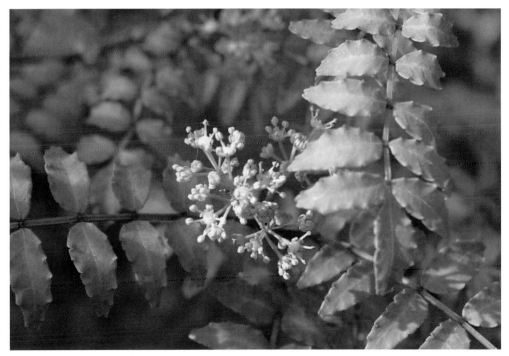

Fig. 2: Sichuan pepper (*Zanthoxylum piperitum* DC.)

Plant source: *Zanthoxylum piperitum* DC.

Synonyms: *Xanthoxylum piperitum* (L.) DC., *Fagara piperita* L.

Taxonomic classification: The genera Zanthoxylum and Fagara are difficult to differentiate and are integrated within the genus Zanthoxylum by many botanical authorities.

Family: Rue family (Rutaceae).

Common names: Engl.: Sichuan pepper, Japan pepper, *san sho*, Japanese prickly ash; Ger.: Japanischer Pfeffer, Pfefferbaum, Sanshopfefferbaum, Sansho, Chinesischer Gelbholzbaum, Pfeffergelbholz, Anispfeffer.

Description: Dioecious shrub or tree, leaves imparipinnate, 5 to 15 cm long, pinnate leaflets slightly crenate; at the base two 5 to 15 cm long thorns. Inflorescences with many flowers having greenish-yellow single perigones. Fruits are red capsules, opening with 2 valves and having a warty and granular surface and only one seed [Ü42, Ü60].

Native origin: Northern China, Korea, and Japan.

Main cultivation areas: Occurs in Japan, Korea, Northern China, and Mongolia, and is only rarely cultivated.

Main exporting countries: Japan.

Cultivation: The harvest of the fruits and leaves takes place for the most part from wild populations.

Culinary herb

Commercial forms: Sichuan pepper (sansho, Japanese pepper): pericarps of the ripe fruits, whole or ground, and Japanese oil (sansho oil).

Production: The fruits are harvested in the autumn and dried in the sun until they burst open. The seeds are mostly sieved out [Ü73].

Forms used: The dried pericarp of the fruits (the seeds are bitter and to a large extent are removed), young fresh leaves, fresh twigs (kinome-twigs), and dried leaves (sansho).

Storage: The twigs only stay fresh for a few days in the refrigerator. The dried pericarps are stored in a cool place, protected from light and moisture, in airtight porcelain-, glass- or suitable metal containers.

Description. Whole pericarp: For a description of the twigs and leaves, see description of the whole plant. Dried pericarps (Fig. 1): consisting of two, beak-like spreaded carpels, red-brown on the outside and warty, yellowish-white and smooth on the inner side, 4 to 5 mm long, sometimes with stem fragments; partially present are globular, black-brown seeds, diameter 3 to 4 mm. The seeds are brittle and splinter upon chewing [Ü60].

Powdered pericarp: Characteristic of the powder are the dark brown, about 500 μm wide secretory cavities, vascular bundles, stone cells with 2.5 μm thick walls and essential oil drops [Ü60].

Leaves. Odor: Mild and somewhat minty, grass-like, **Taste:** Slightly burning. **Pericarp. Odor:** Aromatic, **Taste:** Pine-like, produces a tickling sensation on the tongue, faintly pepper like.

History: Sichuan pepper is one of the oldest spices in Southeast Asia.

Constituents and Analysis

Constituents of the fruit

- Essential oil: About 2 to 7%, occurring in large quantities depending on the chemical races are citral, citronellal, (+)-limonene, 1,8-cineole, geraniol, linalool, citronellyl acetate as well as γ-terpineol, citronellol, isopulegol, piperitone, geranyl acetate and methoxy-citronellal [8, 11, Ü31, Ü60].
- Alkamides: Isobutylamides (2 to 3%, pungent taste, weakly anesthetizing), including α-sanshool (neoherculin), hydroxy-α-sanshool, γ-sanshool and sanshoamide [5].
- Tannins.
- Isoquinoline alkaloids: Magnoflorin [Ü60].

Constituents of the leaf

- Essential oil: (Z)-3-Hexenol and other C_6-compounds are responsible for the grass-like aroma; other components include, depending on the chemical race, linalool, isopulegol, citronellol, citronellal, benzyl alcohol, 2-phenylethanol, geraniol, geranyl acetate and piperitone, the alcohols that occur in the intact leaf are, in part, glycosidically bound [6, 11].
- Lignans: (+)-Sesamin, (+)-asarinin [Ü43].

The literature reports the presence of isoquinoline alkaloids in the root and trunk bark of *Z. piperitum*, but there are no findings for their occurrence in the fruits and leaves. Since such type of alkaloids have been detected in the leaves and pericarps of other Zanthoxylum species (e.g. in *Z. schinifolium* Sieb. et Zucc and *Z. simulans* Hance [4]), it can be assumed that they also occur in the same plant parts of *Z. piperitum*.

Tests for Identity: Organoleptic as well as macroscopic and microscopic analysis.

Quantitative assay: Volumetric determination of the essential oil by steam distillation and xylol in the graduated tube [Ph Eur].

Adulterations, Misidentifications and Impurities: None known.

Actions and Uses

Actions: Due to their pungent-aromatic taste, the pericarps and leaves of Sichuan pepper are appetite stimulating and digestion promoting. Pharmacological studies on the efficacy of the fruits and leaves, which certainly must be described in the Chinese and Japanese literature, are not known to this author.

Toxicology: Based on existing data, there is no chronic or acute toxicity with the normal use of Sichuan pepper pericarps or leaves.

α-Sanshool   R=H

Hydroxy-α-sanshool   R=OH

γ-Sanshool

Culinary use: In China and Japan, Sichuan pepper is an indispensable spice. It is especially suitable for fowl-, meat- and fish dishes. In China, it is necessary for the preparation of Szechuan duck or pang-pang chicken. It is also used as a spice for cakes and pastries (compotes, jams, puddings). The pericarps are frequently roasted in order to remove the essential oil [Ü73, Ü81].

In Europe and USA it is used mainly as a flavor component of seafood and sauces for fish salads. It is also suitable as a spice for pork, chicken and duck as well as rice and noodles. Likewise, it is used in green tea as a flavor enhancer [Ü13, Ü81].

Fresh young or dried, crumbled leaves serve as a spice for sauces, salads (especially raw root vegetable salads), soups and fish dishes [Ü2, Ü74]. The fresh leaves can also be cooked with sugar and soy sauce or eaten deep-fried coated in batter [Ü20].

The twigs are also used as a garnish for soups, tofu, seafood and grilled meat [Ü74].

Combines well with cinnamon and ginger.

As a component of spice mixes and preparations: → Five-spice-mix, → Gomasio, → Shichimi tograrashi.

Medicinal herb

Herbal drugs: Zanthoxyli piperiti pericarpium, Zanthoxyli fructus.

Indications: Used as a stomachic for digestive problems, and as an anthelmintic, especially for roundworms [Ü60].

Similar culinary herbs

Zanthoxylum acanthopodium DC. (Watara, Rutaceae), native to India and China, and used the same as Sichuan pepper [3]. The main component of the essential oil of the fruit is linalool, in addition to, among others, citral, methyl cinnamate, dipentene and phellandrene [2]. The fruit also contains isobutylamides.

Zanthoxylum alatum ROXB. (winged prickly ash, *Z. armatum* DC., *Z. bungeanum* MAXIM., Rutaceae), native to India and China, and used the same as Sichuan pepper [1, 7, 10, 12]. The fruits contain 1.5% essential oil, with the main components race-specific linalool (about 55%), limonene (ca. 23%) and methyl cinnamate (ca. 9%) or limonene (ca. 27%), β-myrcene (ca. 17%), β-ocimene (ca. 10%), thujan-3-ol (ca. 5%) and 2-phenyl-2-propanol (ca. 5%). Furthermore, it contains isobutylamides, and among others, hydroxy-α-, hydroxy-β- and hydroxy-γ-sanshool.

Zanthoxylum simulans HANCE (Chinese pepper, wild Sichuan pepper, *Z. bungeanum* MAXIM., Rutaceae), native to China, cultivated in China, and the Russian Federation, and used the same as Sichuan pepper [Ü61]. The fruits contain 0.7 to 0.9% essential oil, which is composed of, among others, linalool, 1,8-cineole, terpinenol-4, α-terpineol, 4-terpinylacetate, as well as piperitone. The fruit also contains isobutylamides [1, 7].

Fagara rhetsa ROXB. (Cabrit, *Zanthoxylum rhetsa* (ROXB.) DC., *Z. budrunga* WALL., Rutaceae), also described as false cubeb, native to India and Java, and cultivated in Sri Lanka. The essential oil (mullillam oil) of the fruits contains, among others, dihydrocarveol, terpinenol-4 and carvotanacetone [9]. The unripe fruits serve as a sauce- and meat spice [Ü61].

Fagara tessmannii ENGL. (*Zanthoxylum tessmannii*, Rutaceae), native to Cameroon and Equatorial Guinea, where it is also cultivated. The fruits are used as a sauce- and meat spice [Ü61].

Fagara xanthoxyloides LAM. (Senegal yellow wood, Rutaceae), native to West Africa, where it is also cultivated. The seeds and leaves are used as spices [Ü61].

Literature

[1] Ahmad A. et al., J. Nat. Prod. 56(4):456–460 (1993).

[2] Arthur H.R. et al., J. Chem. Soc. 1956:632 (1956), ref. in Ü43.

[3] Bowden K., W.J. Ross, J. Chem. Soc. 1963:3503 (1963), ref. in Ü43.

[4] Brader G. et al., Planta Med. 58(7):A692 (1992).

[5] Crombie L., J.D. Shah, J. Chem. Soc. 1955:4244 (1955), ref. in Ü43.

[6] Kojima H. et al., Biosc. Biotechnol. Biochem. 61(3):491–494 (1997).

[7] Mizutani K. et al., Chem. Pharm. Bull. 36:2362–2365 (1988).

[8] Pfänder H.F., D. Frohne, Dtsch. Apoth. Ztg. 127:2381–2384 (1987).

[9] Rao K.M., V.M. Bhave, CA: 55:21490 (1961), zit. in Ü43.

[10] Sharma M.L. et al., Indian Oil Soap J. 31:303 (1966).

[11] Shimoda M. et al., J. Agric. Food Chem. 45(4):1325–1328 (1997).

[12] Tirillini B. et al., Planta Med. 57:90 (1991).

Literature references identified by Ü can be found in the general listing of books and monographs at the back of this book.

Sicilian sumac

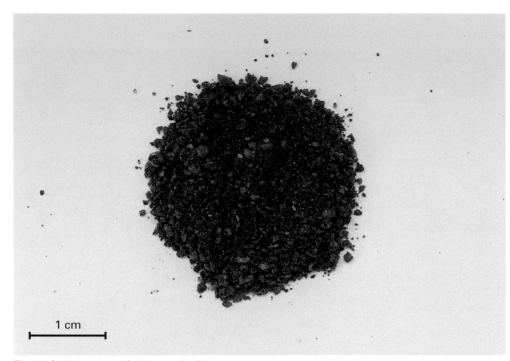

Fig. 1: Sicilian sumac fruits, crushed

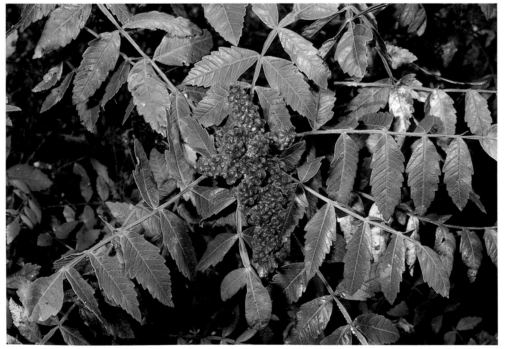

Fig. 2: Sicilian sumac (*Rhus coraria* L.)

Plant source: *Rhus coraria* L.

Synonym: *Toxicodendron coraria* KUNTZE.

Taxonomic classification: A few authors classify the genus Rhus (sensu lato) in the genera Rhus (sensu stricto) and Toxicodendron. This separation is however not generally accepted.

Family: Sumac family (Anacardiaceae).

Common names: Engl.: Sicilian sumac(h), Tanner's sumac, sumac(h); Fr.: sumac des corroyeurs; Ger.: Sumach, Gerber-Sumach, Italienischer Sumach, Sizilianischer Sumach, Sizilianischer Zucker, Färberbaum.

Description: Evergreen small tree, up to 3 m tall, with yellow-green hairy branches. The up to 18 cm long, imparipinnate leaves have up to 15 ovate, about 6 cm long, runcinate pinnules, sparsely pubescent on the upper side and abundantly pubescent on the lower side. The greenish-white, quinate flowers are arranged in terminal or lateral, up to 25 long, dense, paniculate inflorescences; the calyx is densely hairy. The globose stone-fruits with a diameter of 4 to 7 mm bear red, regular or glandular hairs [Ü42].

Native origin: Canary Islands, Mediterranean region, particularly Sicily and plateaus of Turkey to the Caspian Sea, and through the Arab countries.

Main cultivation areas: Southern India, Italy, Spain, Turkey, Afghanistan, Lebanon, Syria, Iran, and Iraq, predominantly for the extraction of tannins.

Main exporting countries: Turkey, and also Italy, Northern Africa, Greece, Iran, Canary Islands, and Afghanistan.

Cultivation: Tanning sumac prefers calcareous, relatively dry soil. Propagation is carried out through root cuttings or by seeds, which must be sown immediately or stored damp up until planting. In Central Europe, tanning sumac is not winter hardy. In freezing weather, it often dies off, all the way to the ground [Ü5, Ü42].

Culinary herb

Commercial forms: Sicilian sumac fruits: dried fruits, usually crushed (sometimes mixed with common salt).

Production: The fruits are plucked and dried before reaching maturity [Ü68].

Forms used: Fruits or fruit pulp with the seeds removed.

Storage: The dried fruits can be stored for a long time in well-closed metal- or glass containers, protected from light and moisture. The aroma of the comminuted fruits is quickly lost [Ü55, Ü68].

Description. Whole fruit: Fruits with bright red-brown color, dark brown to dark violet, roundish to lenticular. Diameter 4 to 7 mm, with regular or glandular hairs and reniform, very hard seeds, forming a brown powder when crushed (Fig. 1) [Ü92].

Odor: Almost odorless, **Taste:** Sour, fruity, slightly astringent.

History: Sicilian sumac was already used in antiquity by the Greeks and Romans as an acidifying agent [Ü68, Ü92].

Constituents and Analysis

Constituents
- Essential oil: 0.02 to 0.03%, very complex composition (120 constituents identified); the main components are dec-2(*E*)enal (4 to 22%), β-caryophyllene (4 to 14%), nonanal (2 to 12%), cembrene (diterpene hydrocarbons with 14-sided ring structure, 1.5 to 15%), deca-2(*E*),4(*E*)-dienal (1 to 6%), hept-2(*E*)-enal (0.5 to 4%) and carvacrol (0.3 to 10%) [2, 3].
- Fruit acids: Particularly malic, citric and tartaric acid, as well as succinic, maleic and fumaric acid [2, 7].
- Anthocyans: Chrysanthemin, myrtillin and delphinidin [7].
- Tannins: About 4%, probably gallotannins [4].
- Fatty oil: About 15% [1].

Tests for Identity: Analysis of the essential oil, see Lit. [2, 3].

Adulterations, Misidentifications and Impurities are not known. The fruits of the strongly sensitizing Toxicodendron-species (*T. quercifolium* (Michx.) Greene, *T. radicans* (L.) O. Kuntze, *T. verniciflua* (Stokes) Barkl.) are white or yellow.

Actions and Uses

Actions: Due to the acidic taste of Sicilian sumac fruits, they have appetite stimulating and digestion promoting action

Toxicology: Based on existing data, there is no acute or chronic toxicity with the use of Sicilian sumac as a spice at normal doses. In older literature, serious poisonings after the intake of large amounts of the fruits have been documented [Ü42]. In newer literature, such cases have not been confirmed.

Culinary use: Sicilian sumac is frequently used in the cuisine of Lebanon, Syria, Turkey, Afghanistan, and Iran. In Lebanese and Syrian cooking, coarsely ground Sicilian sumac is sprinkled on fish and meat; in Iraq and Georgia it is a seasoning for kebab. It is also used as a seasoning in fish-, meat- and vegetable stews [Ü68, Ü73]. In Central Europe, Sicilian sumac is rarely used.
The bruised, dried fruits and the fruit pulp alone or combined with salt serve as seasonings. An extract obtained from an about 20- to 30-minute infusion of 100 g of crushed fruits in 350 ml water can be used as a marinade or, similar to lemon juice, for acidifying foods. The extract is added at the end of meal preparation.
The coarsely ground fruits are suitable for rubbing onto grilled meat, for preparation of marinades to soak grill meat in, fish and poultry as well as seasoning of dishes made from meat, rice, fish, sea foods and poultry, vegetable salads, yogurt sauces and vinegar [Ü2, Ü13, Ü30, Ü73, Ü92].
The extract of the fruits can be used as an acidifier of foods, e.g. green beans, eggplant, marinades, salad dressing and beverages, as well as for rubbing onto grill meat [Ü13, Ü30, Ü68].

Combines well with: Onions.

As a component of spice mixes and preparations: → Zahtar.

Other uses: The leaves and shoots are still used for the tanning of Corduan-, Maroquin- and Saffian-leathers; roots and fruits serve as a red dye, and the bark is used as a yellow dye [Ü37, Ü61].

Medicinal herb

Herbal drug: Rhois corariae fructus, Sicilian sumac fruit.

Indications: In the Middle East, sour drinks made from the fruits are used for mild stomach- and intestinal complaints [Ü73].

Similar culinary herbs

Smooth sumac fruit, from *Rhus glabra* L., scarlet sumac (upland sumac), native to the USA and Canada, constituents include fruit acids, particularly malic acid, and tannins [Ü37]. They are used by the Native North Americans for making sour beverages [Ü73].

Stag's-horn sumac fruit, from *Rhus typhina* L., stag's-horn sumac, native to Eastern North America, often planted in Central Europe as an ornamental shrub, the fruits contain fruit acids, particularly malic acid (about 6%), tannins (gallotannins, about 14%) and anthocyans [6]. The fruits are used in the USA for the production of refreshing beverages (Indian lemonade) [Ü61].

Sweet sumac fruit, from *Rhus aromatica* AIT., sweet sumac (fragrant sumac, lemon sumac, skunkbush), native to Atlantic North America, the fruits contain malic acid (6.5 to 18%) and citric acid, among others. They can be used in the same way as Sicilian sumac fruit [5].

Literature

[1] Al-Hamdany R., F. Osman, J. Iraqi. Chem. Soc. 2:87–93 (1977), ref. in Ü37.

[2] Brunke E. et al., Flavor & Fragrance 8:209–214 (1993).

[3] Brunke E.J. et al., Dragoco Bericht 38:81–95 (1993).

[4] Buziashvili J.I. et al., Khim. Prir. Soedin. (6):789–793 (1973).

[5] Effenberg S., Phytochemische und andere Untersuchungen von Gewürz-sumachrinde – Cortex Rhois aromaticae Radicis (Erg. B 6) – (Rhus aromatica ATTON., Anacardiaceae), Dissertation, FU Berlin 1990.

[6] Fischer J., Pharmazie 15:83–89 (1960).

[7] Mavlyanov S.M. et al., Chem. Nat. Compd. (Transl. of Khim. Prir. Soedin.) 33(2):209 (1997), ref. CA: 128:099845q.

Literature references identified by Ü can be found in the general listing of books and monographs at the back of this book.

Southernwood

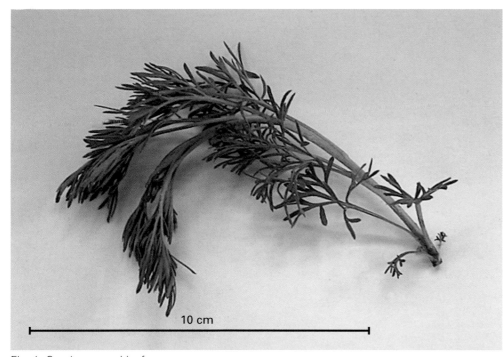

Fig. 1: Southernwood leaf

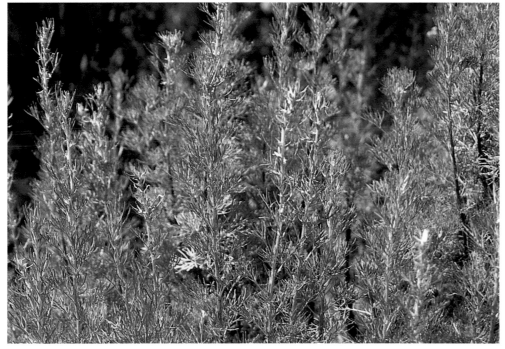

Fig. 2: Southernwood (*Artemisia abrotanum* L.)

Plant source: *Artemisia abrotanum* L.

Synonym: *Artemisia procera* WILLD.

Family: Composite plants (Asteraceae, synonym Compositae).

Common names: Engl.: southernwood, slovenwood, old man, ladies love; Fr.: armoise, aurone des jardins, abrotone, citronelle, ivrogne; Ger: Eberraute, Eberreis, Eberwurz(el), Gartenheil, Stabwurz(el), Stangenkraut, Zitronenkraut.

Description: Subshrub with erect stem, glabrous, often reddish pruinose, up to 1 m tall (rarely 2 m), with panicle-like branching at the top, often forming spherical bushes, the upper leaves are mostly trifid or undivided, the ones in the lower and middle section are bipinnate with nearly filiform, pinnatisect tips with glandular punctuation, upper surface glabrous, the underside more or less grayish pubescent. The anthodia are arranged in erect panicles, diameter 3 to 4 mm, quasi-spherical, drooping, outer involucral bracts lanceolate with short hairs, the inner ones obovate, blunt, with a wide skin-like margin, whitish, receptacle glabrous, corolla pale yellowish; the outer florets are female, the inner ones are hermaphrodite. Plants growing in Central Europe mostly do not bear flowers or fruits. Flowering period is from July to October [11, Ü37].

Native origin: Not known. Introduced to Southern- and Southeastern Europe, and from the Near East to Siberia.

Main cultivation areas: Cultivated in Southern-, Central- and Eastern Europe, mostly in gardens.

Main exporting countries: There is no significant commercial trade of this herb.

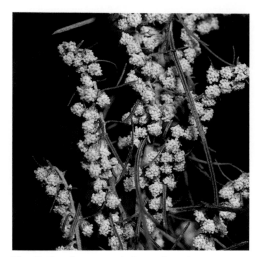

Fig. 3: Southernwood, flowering shoots

Cultivation: The plant prefers chalky, sandy to stony, permeable soil in a sunny, protected habitat. It is drought tolerant. Southernwood is propagated mostly by cuttings or root division. In the spring, the plant should be cut back somewhat. For personal use, one shrub is sufficient. Varieties include, among others, 'Oberlausitzer large-leaved southernwood' and 'Erfurter large-leaved southernwood' [Ü41, Ü45, Ü96].

Culinary herb

Commercial forms: Southernwood: the dried herb, and, in the vegetable trade, the fresh herb.

Production: Harvests take place in June/July and August/September. After drying, the herb is usually rubbed. For personal use the shoot tips can be plucked through the entire summer [Ü96].

Forms used: The fresh shoot tips, and less often the dried, cut or rubbed herb.

Storage: The fresh shoots, wrapped in plastic, stay fresh in the refrigerator for a few days. They can also be stored in freezer bags or chopped and frozen with water in the ice tray. The dried herb should be stored in a cool location, protected from humidity and light, in porcelain-, glass- or other suitable metallic containers.

Description. Whole herb (Fig. 1): See description of the whole plant.

Odor: Aromatic, faintly lemon-like, **Taste:** Spicy, bitter, slightly burning, reminiscent of mugwort.

History: Southernwood was already used during antiquity. By the 9th century, it was already employed in Central Europe. In a government decree of Karl the Great ("Capitulare de villis", authored in about 795 CE, see footnote under → Anise), the cultivation of Southernwood was called for [Ü23].

Constituents and Analysis

Constituents

- Essential oil: 0.6 to 1.4%, the main components are race-specific and include 1,8-cineole (20 to 60%) or thujone (up to 72%), furthermore fenchene, sabinene, α-caryophyllene (humulene), β-caryophyllene and hydroxydavanone were isolated [1, 2, 6, 10].
- Hydroxycoumarins: Isofraxidin, scopoletin, umbelliferone, drimartol A (sesquiterpene ether, drimenylisofraxidin) [3, 5, 8, 9].
- Flavonoids: Rutin and free methoxylated flavonols including quercetin-3,4′-dimethylether, quercetin-3,7-dimethylether, casticin and centaureidin [2, 7–9].
- Hydroxycinnamic acid derivates: Chlorogenic acid [8,9].

Tests for Identity: Macroscopic and microscopic analysis of the herb or TLC of the extract, according to [4, Ü102].

Quantitative assay: The content of essential oil can be determined volumetrically with steam distillation and xylol in the graduated tube [Ph Eur].

Adulterations, Misidentifications and Impurities: Not known.

Actions and Uses

Actions: Due to its aromatic and slightly bitter taste, southernwood has appetite stimulating and digestion promoting effects. Extracts of the herb have shown in vitro, predominantly due to their content of methoxylated flavonols, an antispasmodic activity on carbachol-induced contraction of guinea-pig trachea [EC_{50} values for casticin, centaureidin and quercetin-3,4′-dimethylether were 20 to 30 µmol/l] [2].

Toxicology: Based on existing data, there is no acute or chronic toxicity with the normal use of this herb as a spice [2, Ü37]. The essential oil constituent thujone is considered toxic (→ Sage), but due the low amount of herb used for seasoning, harmful effects on human health should not be expected.

Culinary use: The fresh leaves, and less often also the dried leaves of southernwood, which due to their slightly bitter taste should be dosed carefully, are used to spice fatty meats, especially roast goose and roast duck, mutton or pork, poultry fillings, fish dishes (eel, mackerel, salmon), quark, mayonnaise, raw fruit and vegetables and salads as well as for making herb vinegar. Occasionally, it is also used as a baking spice [Ü45, Ü63, Ü71, Ü74, Ü92].

Combines well with: Lemon balm, lemon thyme, and mugwort, in a → Bouquet garni together with hyssop, lovage and oregano for gravy spice [Ü46].

As a component of spice mixes and preparations: → Bouquet garni, → Herb vinegar.

Other uses: In the past, bunches of the plant or small bags filled with the leaves were hung up in closets to keep moths out. Rubbing the herb on the skin should repel mosquitoes [Ü66]. Due to the decorative appearance of its filigree leaves, southernwood is also used as a hedgerow plant or as a component of bouquets [Ü47].

Other Artemisia species used as culinary spices: → Mugwort.

Medicinal herb

Herbal drug: Abrotani herba, Southernwood herb.

Indications: Southernwood is used in folk medicine as an appetite stimulant and digestive aid, for the treatment of menstrual pains and as an anthelmintic [BHP 83].

Literature

[1] Banthorpe D.V. et al., Planta Med. 20(2): 147–152 (1971).

[2] Bergendorf O. et al., Planta Med. 61(4): 370–371 (1995).

[3] Cubukcu B. et al., Phytother. Res. 4:203–204 (1990).

[4] Gocan S. et al., J. Pharm. Biomed. Anal. 14(8/10):1221–1227 (1996).

[5] Greger H. et al., J. Nat. Prod. 45:455–461 (1982).

[6] Heeger E.F., C. Rosenthal, Pharmazie 4:381–390 (1949).

[7] Kranen-Fiedler U., Arzneim. Forsch. 6:475 (1956).

[8] Schmersahl P., Naturwissenschaften 17: 498 (1965).

[9] Schmersahl P., Planta Med. 14:179–183 (1966).

[10] Vostrowski O. et al., Z. Lebensm. Unters. Forsch. 179:125–129 (1984).

[11] Weymar H: Buch der Korbblütler, Neumann Verlag, Radebeul 1957.

Literature references identified by Ü can be found in the general listing of books and monographs at the back of this book.

Soybean

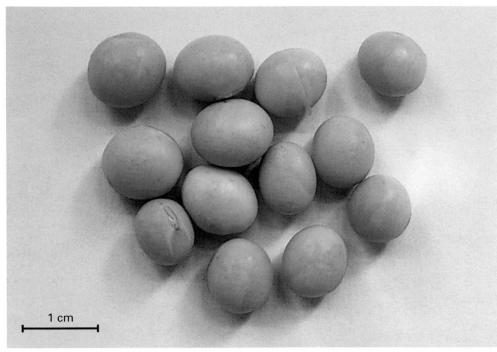

Fig. 1: Soybeans

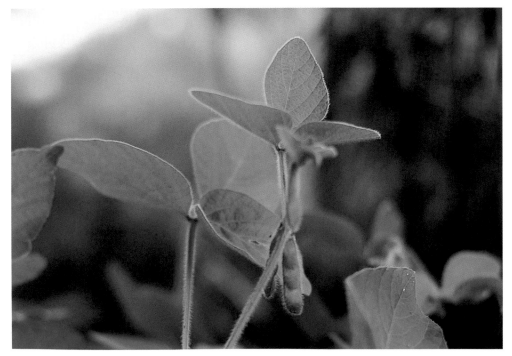

Fig. 2: Soybean (*Glycine max* (L.) MERR.).

Plant source: *Glycine max* (L.) MERR.

Synonyms: *Phaseolus max* L., *Soja hispida* MOENCH, *Glycine hispida* (MOENCH) MAXIM.

Taxonomic classification: This morphologically very diverse species can be divided in 6 convarieties and over 100 varieties [Ü26].

Family: Pea family (Fabaceae, synonym Papilionaceae; some authors also place it with Caesalpiniaceae and Mimosaceae in the legume family, Leguminosae).

Common names: Br. Engl.: soya bean, soya plant; Am. Engl.: soybean; Fr.: soya; Ger.: Sojabohne, Sojapflanze, Fettbohne.

Description: Annual plant, 20 to 90 cm tall (seldom up to 1.8 m), similar to a dwarf bean. The erect stalk is branched and usually villous-hairy. The long-stalked, ternate-pinnate leaves are 3 to 10 cm long; the entire pinnules are ovate, hairy at the border and on the veins of the lower side. 3 to 20 flowers respectively are arranged together in bunches mostly in the leaf axils; the flowers are small, short-stalked, sitting in the axils of small bracts, the calyx is bell-shaped and a little shorter than the corolla, the petals are violet to whitish, the vexillum is barely longer than wings and carina; the 10 stamina are synanthous. The hirsute pod is 2 to 10 cm long, about 1 cm wide, straw-colored, gray, black-brown or violet, and swollen around the 1 to 5 seeds [Ü26].

Native origin: A cultivated plant, not occurring in the wild. The wild form is probably *G. soja* SIEB. et ZUCC.

Main cultivation areas: USA, Brazil, China, and Argentina, and to a lesser extent the Russian Federation, Indonesia, Korea, Japan, Mongolia, India, Eastern Africa, Canada, and Southeastern Europe.

Main exporting countries: USA (soybeans), as well as China, Brazil, and Argentina (soybeans and soy products).

Cultivation: Soybeans prefer neutral, deep, loose, clay- or loam soils with sufficient humus and lime content in sunny, protected, warm locations. The optimal growing temperature lies between 24 to 25 °C, and the optimal length of daylight prior to flowering is 13 hours. During the germination stage the soil should be warm (minimum 10 °C) and damp, and during the growing period warm and relatively dry. After the flowering period up until maturation abundant rainfall is necessary. Sowing is carried out in Central European latitudes in May, row widths of 45 to 65 cm with 3 to 10 cm in the row spacing and 4 to 6 cm deep. When planting in soils, in which soybeans have never been planted before, the soil must be inoculated with suitable variety-specific *Bradyrhizobium* (*Rhizobium*)-strains, in order to assure sufficient nodulation and nitrogen uptake. Varieties are differentiated by early-maturing (vegetation period 85 to 95 days), average- (95 to 110 days) and late-maturing varieties (100 to 125 days). In genetically modified soybeans, a bacterial gene for the enzyme 3-phosphoshikimate-1-carboxyvinyltransferase is inserted (EC 2.5.1.19, participated in the biosynthesis of the phenylalanine and tyrosine basic structure, obtained from *Agrobacterium ssp.*), which, in contrast to the same enzyme in soybeans, is not inhibited by the herbicide glyphosate (Roundup®). Thus, genetically engineered soy (Roundup Ready® Soybeans) is resistant to herbicides whose active ingredient is glyphosate. There are labeling requirements for genetically engineered soybeans and their protein-containing products (EU Novel-Foods Regulation of 15.05.1997) [4, 5, Ü26, Ü82, Ü98, overview in Lit. 36].

Culinary herb

Commercial forms: Soybeans (differentiated by colors yellow, green or black), extracted soybean meal, full-fat soy flour (soy flakes, natural soy flour with about 40% protein and 20% fat), defatted soy flour (with 40 to 50% protein and 0.5% to 1% fat), soy protein concentrate (with 60 to 70% protein), soy protein isolate (contains about 95% protein), soy oil, soy lecithin (resulted from the refining of soy oil), soy sauce (see below), soy sprouts (heat preserved, canned in liquid) [Ü26].

Production. Soybeans: Harvest should take place in low rainfall periods. The harvest is carried out when the grains begin to become hard, which in Central European latitudes is in August or September, either manually by pulling out or cutting the plants and threshing them after drying or they are harvested with a combine harvester. In cultivation for domestic use, if the plants have not yet entirely matured before the first frost comes, they must be pulled out and stored frost-free; the beans then mature post-harvest [Ü5, Ü26].

Soy sauce (soyu, shoyu, shoya, schoyu, chiangyu, tsing-yeou, kecap, ketjap manis, kanjang, toyo, tao-yu, toung): A more or less inviscid black, red-brown or pale-yellow, liquid made from fermentation of cooked soybeans or defatted soybean meal and cooked or roasted, rolled wheat with Aspergillus-strains. The fermentation is introduced in a salt-containing fermentation yeast-mold starter (koji) with cultures of *Aspergillus oryzae* and/or *A. soyae*. After a few days, a concentrated saline solution is added to the starter in order stop the fungal growth. Subsequently a lactic fermentation step follows initiated through *Zygosaccharomyces rouxii, Torulopsis spec., Pediococcus halophilus* and/or *Lactobacillus delbrueckii*, which can last for several months. The resultant preparation is aged for up to 2 years at room temperature in wooden casks. Finally the solid components are removed by filtration and the liquid is pasteurized at 80 °C. For pur-

poses of export it is also preserved with sodium benzoate.

There is also industrial manufacture of soy sauces using accelerated methods by acid hydrolysis of defatted soybean meal and roasted wheat in bioreactors with frequent extrusion of the mash. This type of soy sauce has very little aroma and is enhanced by the addition of traditionally fermented soy sauces (in Japan, "koikuchi" contains 50% hydrolysate, and "usukuchi" of lower quality due to its higher proportion of hydrolysate).

Typical types of Japanese soy sauces are koikuchi and usukuchi (see above), tamari, saishhikomi and shiro. In China, mainly the tamari-type sauces are produced.

High value soy sauces contain about 18% sodium chloride (minimum 13% for shelf stability!) and have a pH-value of 4.6 to 4.8. They contain 1.5 to 1.8% total nitrogen (short chain peptides and amino acids, of which 20% is glutamic acid), 2 to 5% monosaccharides (mainly glucose), 1 to 2% ethanol and 1 to 2% organic acids (mainly lactic acid). Relevant aromatic components include, among others, 4-ethylguajacol, 4-hydroxy-2(or 5)-ethyl-5(or 2)-methyl-3(2H)-furanone, 3-hydroxy-2-ethyl-5-methyl-3(2H)-furanone, furaneol and sotolone [27, Ü8, Ü23, Ü92, Ü98].

Miso (misho, chiang, jang, doenjang, tauco, tauchao, tao-tjo, tao-chieo, taosi): Creamy to solid, produced similarly as soy sauce in the household, but also produced industrially. Cooked soybeans are mixed with sea-salt-containing koji (see above), or other osmophilic yeast- or bacteria cultures, often with the addition of rice (rice miso) or barley (barley miso), and rarely with buckwheat, the mixture is left in cedar wooden casks to cure for 1 to 2 years. The aroma can be strengthened by the addition of 3-hydroxy-2-ethyl-5-methyl-3(2H)furanone. Sometimes lower fermentation duration (5 to 20 days) is practiced for commercially produced miso-types. Miso types are differentiated according to the portion of soybeans in the starter. In Europe, miso is traded in glass jars or polyethylene bags. Varieties:

Hatcho-miso, mugi-miso, kome-miso, shiro-miso, genmai-miso, soba-miso, and natto-miso [Ü8, Ü92, Ü98].

Natto (soy cheese, toushih, tusi, tusu, taotjo, taosi): A seasoning paste made from fermented soybeans. Varieties of natto are differentiated by the microorganisms used to make it and the fermentation time. Japanese varieties include, among others, itohiki-natto (main bacteria *Bacillus natto*, fermentation time 16 hours at 42 °C), yukiwari-natto (main bacteria *Aspergillus oryzae*, fermentation time about 14 days), hama-natto (toushik, taotjo, touco, with addition of corn flour, main bacteria *Aspergillus oryzae*, fermentation time 12 days, seasoned with salt and ginger, cured under pressure for 6 to 12 months). The main aromatic components of natto are 2,5-dimethylpyrazine, trimethylpyrazine and 2,6-bis(1,1-dimethylethyl)phenol [28, Ü98].

Meju: Paste form seasoning made from fermented soybeans, produced in Korea [Ü98].

Forms used: See above.

Storage: Soybeans: dry, soy oil and soy lecithin: in tightly sealed containers with little headspace, cool (below 25 °C), protected from light. Upon exposure to light, a bean- and straw-like odor develops within a couple of hours (reversion-odor, formation of 3-methylnona-2,4-dione from the furan fatty acids present) [Ü8].

Description. Whole seed (Fig. 1): Seeds elongated-ovate, somewhat flattened or almost globose, 4 to 10 mm long, 3 to 7 mm wide, 2 to 6 mm thick, mostly yellow, but also white, greenish, brown, black-brown or two-colored, smooth, somewhat shiny, hilum about 3 mm long, about half as long as the total length of the seed, surrounded by a brown, circular crista [Ü60].

Microscopic description: The cross-section of the testa shows a stout, about 50 μm high palisade layer whose cells have strongly thickened walls in the upper part and a wide lumen at the base, hence the microscopic image of the cross-section changes depending on the focusing (Fig. 3). Adjacent to it is a layer of dumbbell-shaped support cells. Below, a layer of compressed cells is visible. The inner part of the seed encloses the large cotyledons with elongated, indistinctly punctate cells, aleuron grains and prisms of calcium oxalate. Small, spherical starch grains occur scarcely [Ü29].

Powdered seed: In the whitish-yellow powder from colored seeds with brown or greenish particles, the characteristic, dumbbell-shaped support cells (see above), cells with aleuron grains and calcium oxalate prisms are particularly prominent [Ü29].

Odor: Weak, characteristic, **Taste:** Somewhat bitter at first, then oily, nut-like.

History: Soybeans were probably first cultivated in China during the Shang-Dynasty (about 1700–1100 BCE). The today very popular soy sauce, prepared from soybeans and wheat, was developed in China in the 6th century. It originally served as a preservative for foods during winter storage. Since the beginning of the 20th century, soybean cultivation spread to the tropics, subtropics and temperate zones (between 50° northern and 40° southern latitude). At the start of the previous century, its use as a good source for cooking oil and as a raw material for margarine production gained importance in the West. After the 2nd world war, soybean and its products became popular seasonings in European and North American cuisine. Today, soy products are mainly produced in Eastern Asia and from there they are exported worldwide [Ü2, Ü55, Ü61].

Constituents and Analysis

Constituents

- Protein: About 35 to 50% (high values in small-seeded varieties), particularly globulins; the main components are glycinin, β- and γ-conglycinin (40, 28, or 3%, respectively), rich in essential amino acids (L-histidine about 2.3%, L-leucine about 7.5%, L-isoleucine about 4.5%, L-lysine about 6%, L-methionine about 2%, L-phenylalanine about 5.0%, L-tyrosine about 3%, L-threonine about 4%, L-tryptophan about 1.2%, L-valine about 4.5%) [19, Ü8].
- Protease inhibitors: Bowman-Birk inhibitors (with 2 active centers, due to the numerous disulfide bonds, it is difficult to denature, pepsin resistant) directed particularly against trypsin and chymotrypsin, as well as Kunitz-inhibitors (with one reactive center, inactivated by pepsin) [Ü8].
- Lectins: Soy lectins (D-GalNAc-specific) [18, 19, Ü8].
- Enzymes: Urease, lipoxygenase, monophosphatase, phosphodiesterase, α-galactosidase, β-amylase [19, Ü8].
- Fatty oil: About 12 to 25% (high levels in yellow-seeded varieties); the main components are linoleic acid (44 to

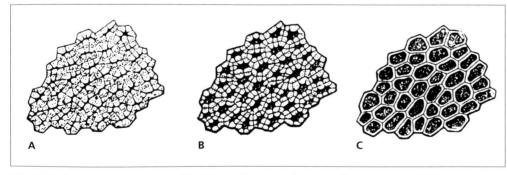

Fig. 3: Soybean. Palisade layer, with 3 focal distances; **A**, upper, **B**, medium, and **C** lowest level. From Ü29.

62%), oleic acid (19 to 30%), palmitic acid (7 to 14%) and α-linolenic acid (3 to 11%), small amounts of furan fatty acids (epoxy-compounds, about 0.02%) [37, Ü8, Ü82].

■ Phospholipids: About 25% so-called soy lecithin, particularly phosphatidylcholine, phosphatidylethanolamine, phosphatidylinositol and phosphatidic acid [19, 50].

■ Phytic acid: About 1 to 2% [19].

■ Tocopherols (vitamin E): In the seeds 14 to 20 mg/100 g, chiefly γ-tocopherol (49 to 74%), in soy oil about 60 mg/100 g γ-tocopherol, about 18 mg/100 g α-tocopherol [58, Ü8].

■ Sterols: Particularly β-sitosterol (60%) and campesterol (30%), furthermore stigmasterol, among others [Ü8].

■ Carbohydrates: 20 to 35%, particularly stachyose, raffinose, xylogalactomannans and arabinogalactans [19, Ü60].

■ Triterpene saponins: Monodesmosides with soyasaponins I, II, III, IV, V, VI and the bisdesmosides soyasaponins A_1 and A_2, bitter tasting; the aglycones are soyasapogenols A, B, C and E [30, 38, 57, Ü8].

■ Isoflavonoids: 0.8 to 1.6% (high values in varieties with green seeds), daidzin (daidzein-7-O-glucoside, about 0.3 to 1.0%), daidzein (0.01 to 0.03%), genistin (genistein-7-O-glucoside, 0.4 to 0.7%), genistein, glycitein, glycitin, (glycitein-7-O-glucoside), the 6″-O-malonyl conjugates of the glucosides (the main components of the intact soybean, upon heating they transform to the corresponding acetates by decarboxylation), formononetin, isoformononetin, 6,7,4′-trihydroxyisoflavone and cumestrol [15, 19, 45, 58, Ü8]

Tests for Identity: The identity of soybean is determined with macroscopic and microscopic analysis as well as with HPLC of the isoflavonoids [56].

Quantitative assay of the isoflavonoids with HPLC [19, 45, 56], of the proteins with RP-HPLC [19], of the mineral constituents with Atomic Absorption Spectroscopy [19] and of the phytates with RP-HPLC and GC [19].

Adulterations, Misidentifications and Impurities are not known.

Actions and Uses

Actions. Digestive promoting action: In rats, soybeans increased cholecystokinin-release and thereby pancreatic enzyme secretion. Soybeans induced pancreatic growth [21].

Antitumor action: Epidemiological studies show a connection between the use of soy products and the relatively low rate of occurrence of breast-, uterine-, intestinal- and prostate carcinomas in Japan and China [35, 61]. Conversely there are however other studies and opinions [2, 26, 40]. The postulated antitumor activity can be attributed to the isoflavonoids, functioning as inhibitors of tyrosine kinase and topoisomerase II, phytoestrogens (see below), protectors of DNA through antioxidative action, inhibitors of the growth of new blood vessels supplying tumors with blood (anti-angiogenic) and inductors of cellular differentiation [61], the antimutagenic action of the saponins [13], the Bowman-Birk-protease inhibitors [25, 59], and the ability of the microflora of fermented soy products, such as soy sauces, miso, natto or tofu, to bind with mutagens and carcinogens [Ü98].

There are numerous reports from in vitro and animal studies concerning the antitumor action of soy products [61]. The occurrence of liver- and bladder tumors was averted by supplementation of 30% ground soybeans in the feed of mice following administration of carcinogens (dibutylamine, sodium nitrite) in the drinking water [43]. Also supplementation of 10% soy protein or miso in the feed in rats significantly decreased N-nitroso-N-methylurea-induced rat mammary cancer [20]. Through supplementation of a protease inhibitor rich protein fraction from soybeans, a similar effect could be attained [12]. Tumor volumes were about 11 to 28% lower than in the control animals after implantation of human prostate car-

Daidzein R_1 = H R_2 = H
Daidzin R_1 = H R_2 = Glc
Genistein R_1 = OH R_2 = H
Genistin R_1 = OH R_2 = Glc

Soyasaponin III   R = CH_2OH
Soyasaponin IV   R = H

Soyasaponin I   R = CH_2OH
Soyasaponin II   R = H

cinoma cells in immune-deficient mice that were given soy protein (20% in feed) and/or a concentrate of micromolecular constituents of soybeans (0.2 to 1% in the feed) [63]. After injection of gonadal carcinoma cells in rats, genistein (50 mg/kg body weight, s.c.) was able to decrease the occurrence of tumors from 44% (control animals) to 11% and metastasis formation from 89% to 44% [54].

Antithrombotic action: Soyasaponins in rats (10 to 200 mg/kg body weight, p.o.) averted the occurrence of endotoxin- or thrombin-induced (both i.v.) thrombi in the kidneys and blood vessels [31].

Hepatoprotective action: Soyasaponins (50 mg/kg body weight, p.o.) reduced the increase of serum transaminases concentration (an indicator of liver damage) induced by the administration of liver-damaging peroxidized fats (25% in the feed) [47].

Antilipidemic action: Soybean proteins in rats (20% in feed) lowered the plasma cholesterol- and triacylglycerol level [24, 53]. Supplementation with soybean raw protein (20% in feed) in male and female rhesus monkeys given moderately atherogenic diets reduced LDL- and VLDL- cholesterol concentrations in the blood by about 30 to 40%, increased HDL-cholesterol concentrations by approximately 15% and lowered total plasma cholesterol levels, approximately by 20% for males and 50% for females, compared to the control animals that had received soy protein with the alcohol-soluble substances (isoflavonoids, saponins) removed [7]. Feeding a fat diet with 0.5% cholesterol in guinea pigs for 6 weeks led to hypercholesterolemia, additionally given doses of 7.5% soy lecithin in the feed lowered the cholesterol level by about 49% [46]. In healthy human subjects, administration of soybean protein reduced the LDL- but also the HDL- levels and caused an increased fecal excretion of neutral sterols [17]. A three-month daily dose of 36 g soy lecithin in patients with hypercholesterolemia (over 300 mg serum choles-

terol/100 ml) caused a reduction in blood cholesterol level by approximately 41 mg/100 ml [44]. The anticholesterolemic action possibly occurs through an interaction of soy proteins with soy isoflavonoids, possibly also with the sterols [2]. There are, however, studies, in which the antilipidemic effect of soy proteins and soy isoflavonoids has not been confirmed. Administration of soymilk (1 l/d) in healthy males caused no anticholesterolemic effect [42]. The same observation was made in healthy menopausal women after administration of soy isoflavonoids (80 mg/d) [55]. Antilipidemic activity of soy lecithin was not observed in another study, wherein hyperlipidemic males were given 20 g soy lecithin/d (in yogurt as the vehicle) for 2 or 4 weeks. It caused no changes in the plasma content of lipoproteins, triacylglycerols and total cholesterol [48].

Partial estrogenic action: The isoflavonoids of soybeans, which soy products also contain in various quantities [45], are weakly estrogenic (phytoestrogens). They exert an extremely low agonistic effect on the reproductive system receptors (uterus, ovaries). They compete, however, with the body-specific estrogens for the estrogen receptor sites and thereby they may possibly inhibit the cell-division promoting effect of the estrogens, e.g. in estrogen-dependent tumor cells in premenopausal women such as those that occur in mammary cancer, among others [61]. This was explained as their contribution in the anti-tumor effect (see above). The low occurrence of climacteric and postmenopausal complaints in East Asian women who consume soy products abundantly is also explained by the partial estrogenic action of the isoflavonoids. Possibly they prevent by feedback the excessive production of gonadotropin pituitary gland hormones [35]. In an ovariectomized rat test model, which should simulate the situation in postmenopausal women, osteoporotic changes could be prevented by soy proteins, but particularly by high doses of the soy isoflavonoids genistein, and even more effectively by daidzein. These constituents

have about the same effect in suppressing bone loss as estrogens. The antiosteoporotic action in humans is still controversially discussed [2, 3, 8, 22, 41, 51].

Cardiovascular protective action: The cardiac- and other blood vessel protective action of soybeans does not depend alone on their possible antilipidemic action. The antiatherogenic acting genistein also inhibits the oxidation of LDL, whose oxidation product taken up by macrophages is a starting point for the genesis of arteriosclerotic vascular changes. Moreover, it disrupts the effect of tyrosine kinase and therefore of the numerous growth factors (e.g. PDGF, FGF), which participate in the formation of pathological vascular changes. Besides that it also exerts antithrombotic action. The partial estrogenic action of the isoflavonoids probably also contributes to the cardiovascular protective effect. Epidemiological studies have shown, that women, who frequently consume soy products, suffer less often from cardiovascular diseases [35, 61]. In rat model studies with experimentally induced myocardial ischemia-reperfusion injury, the cardioprotective action of genistein (1 mg/kg body weight, i.v.) was observed by its lowering of myocardial necrosis [16].

Other actions: Soy oil emulsion doubled the gastric emptying time in patients with dumping syndrome (early gastric emptying after postvagotomy and consequences thereof) [32]. Feeding of raw soybeans in rats led to an increased expression of insulin-mRNA in β-cells. In these animals, compared to animals given a normal diet, only a few β-cells were killed by streptozotocin, so the occurrence of streptozotocin-induced diabetes was diminished [33]. Soyasaponins were shown in vitro to prevent the formation of lipid peroxides caused by the heating of oxygen-perfused corn oil [47].

Toxicology: Based on existing data, there is no acute or chronic toxicity with the use of fermented soy products, soy oil or soy lecithin as a seasoning or therapeutic agent at usual doses. The safety evaluations for genetically engineered soy, issued by an EU-panel, conclude that there are no risks associated with the consumption of these products [4]. The enzyme protein that occurs additionally in genetically engineered soy has no allergenic properties [52].

The phytic acid present in soybeans can reduce the bioavailability of trace elements and phosphate ions and inhibit a few digestive enzymes. It has an anti-nutritional effect similar to the protease inhibitors [19].

Symptoms of food intolerance against products with soy proteins have only been observed very rarely; they are probably caused by the lectins and include inflammation of the gastric mucosa and loss of intestinal villi, accompanied by fever, vomiting, bloody diarrhea and dehydration [1]. In particular, raw or insufficiently cooked, ripe soybeans can lead to these symptoms. Soy flour but not heat-treated soy flour (inactivation of the protease inhibitors and lectins during heating!), fed to rats over a period of 60 weeks, led to the occurrence of pancreas carcinoma [39]. Animals (pigs and rats) which were fed a soybean diet, showed a weight increase of the thyroid gland as well as elevated T_3 and T_4 serum-concentrations and increased iodine uptake. Increased thyroxin elimination in the feces was also observed. There is one case report on the goitrogenic effect of soy diet [60].

The sensitization potential of the soybean protein is small. Cross-reaction with proteins from other legumes is possible. Particularly in baking with the handling of soy flour, asthmatic complaints and rhinitis have been documented. Children with neurodermatitis can also be allergic to soy proteins. Soy lecithin and soy oil can also cause, even though very rarely, allergic reactions due to the presence of soy protein impurities [9, 11, 14, 23, 49].

Culinary use: Soy products are an indispensable food and seasoning in the Far East. But they are also found increasingly in western conventional- and healthy-cooking and used in the manufacture of vegetarian food products.

Products made from ripe soybeans or soybean flour used as seasonings include, among others, soy sauces, miso, natto or meju (see above).

Soy sauces, thin- to viscous liquids, in Asia serve as seasoning for soups, meat- and fish dishes. Mainly dark types are traditionally used in Northern China and lighter types in Japan. Today they are also popular in European and North American cooking.

The long-fermented, dark-brown, viscous Chinese types have a rich, sweetish-spicy taste, that also contain molasses as a sweetener and colorant, and are used as a seasoning and colorant for red stewed chicken, but also of beef- and pork dishes. Mushroom soy sauce is a flavored dark soy sauce made with straw mushrooms. It has a strong aroma and is used the same as dark soy sauce.

The thin, light brown Chinese type that is fermented for a shorter period of time is very salty. It is used mainly for seasoning of soups, seafoods, vegetables and dips. The Japanese light soy sauces are somewhat sweeter and not as salty as the Chinese types. They are used as table seasonings and for the flavoring of meat dishes, soup broths and stews.

Miso, pasty, rarely solid, of various colors (yellow to dark red-brown), tastes acrid and wine-like, is used mainly in Asian cooking for the seasoning of soups, sauces, marinades, dips, meat-, fish-, rice- and vegetable dishes, but also as a bread spread [Ü11, Ü55].

Natto, paste-shape, accented with an ammonia note, is used as a seasoning for cooked rice, meat-, vegetable- and seaweed dishes [Ü55].

Unripe soybeans and sprouts are eaten as vegetables. Soybean sprouts are a good source of ascorbic acid, riboflavin and niacin. During germination the content of lectins decreases, phytic acids and the trypsin inhibitors are broken down [10]. On the contrary, the ripe seeds taste unpleasant (bitter saponins!), are difficult to digest (protease inhibitor!) and can lead to digestive problems (lectins, saponins). They can be eaten after lengthy soaking and cooking [Ü82].

Combines well with: Chillies, and soy sauces.

As a component of spice mixes and preparations: See above (Meju, Miso, Natto, Soy sauce), → Soybean pastes, → Table spice.

Other uses.

Soy oil is used especially in foods, as an ingredient of cooking oils and as a carrier for lipid-soluble active ingredients, e.g. fat-soluble vitamins, and as a raw material for margarine production [Ü24, Ü82].

Soy lecithin serves as a an emulsifier in pharmaceutical technology (for example for the manufacture of fat emulsions for parenteral alimentation), stabilizer for suspensions for the preparation of liposomes, in the cosmetic industry as an emulsifier, in the food industry as an additive for numerous foods (e.g. chocolate, cacao powder, margarine, baked goods), in industry for the manufacture of paints, printing ink, as a component in animal feed, and in form of a spray solution against botanical fungal diseases in agriculture [Ü82].

Soybeans, soy flour, and **soy protein** are used in the food industry for the manufacture of:

Soy sauce (see above),

Soymilk is obtained by boiling the suspension obtained from the ground and moistened soybeans (inactivation of the enzymes and proteinase inhibitors) and enzymatic removal of the bitterness, also produced as a soy protein isolate. Enriched with calcium salts, vitamins, L-carnitine, malt extract and sometimes with iodine (to counteract goitrogenic effects), phosphate and zinc ions (to compensate for the absorption losses caused by the phytates), it serves as a base ingredient for baby food, particularly for infants who are allergic to cow milk, or show galactosemia or lactose intolerance [62].

Dried powdered soymilk, obtained by gentle drying of soymilk, e.g. Soyalac, Mullsoy, Soybee, Proton.

Tofu (soybean curd), precipitate obtained from soymilk upon acidifying and addition of table salt and by almost complete water removal under pressure; it is especially valued as source of protein by vegetarians and added to soups, salads and casseroles as well as a component of pizza toppings and sweet cheesecakes.

Soy cheese (Sufu, Fuyu, Toufuru, Furu, Tosufu, Fusu, Fuyu, Chao, Tahuri, Taokaoan, Tachuyi), obtained by fermentation of Tofu. The main culture used is from *Actinomucor elegans*, rich in salt, as a seasoning or condiment for vegetables or meat.

Meat-like foods or ingredients obtained by extrusion of soy protein concentrate or soy flour and formation of a stringy mass (textured vegetable protein), e.g. as an additive to fast-food products.

Foods made from fermented soybeans, for example

Tempeh (Tempe, Kedelee, Kedele): obtained from sprouted, boiled and fermented soybean (soy tempeh), or other grains, and used as food and seasoning; the main culture are Rhizopus-species, duration of fermentation 24 to 72 hours, for industrial production, commercial yeasts (Ragi, Ragi-Tempeh) are employed; the cake-like product, which is also dried to extend shelf-life, is added to soups or eaten in fried form; tempeh is used as a source of protein (containing 20%), particularly by vegetarians (high vitamin B_{12} content) in the USA and Western Europe.

Meitauza: Dried soycake, covered with fungal mycelium and baked in oil or eaten with vegetables [Ü98].

In the food industry, soy flour or soy lecithin is used, due to its rheological properties, particularly of the proteins, as a stabilizer for emulsions, as well as a water- and fat-binding agents for the manufacture of synthetic fibers, adhesives, for impregnating textiles, and as a foaming agent in fire extinguishers [36, Ü61, Ü82, Ü98].

Extracted soybean meal is used as a concentrated feed for cattle and pigs.

Soy foliage is used as a forage and feed for livestock and is also suitable for silage [Ü82].

Medicinal herb

Herbal drugs: Sojae semen, Soybeans, Oleum Sojae raffinatum, Refined Soyabean oil [Ph Eur], Oleum Sojae hydrogenatum, Hydrogenated soya-bean oil [Ph Eur], Lecithinum ex soja, Soy lecithin [ÖAB].

Indications: In Eastern Asia, soybeans are used for fever, infectious diseases, dropsy, flatulence, and as an invigorating tonic, among other uses, [34], emulsified soy oil is used as a supplement in parenteral alimentation, and soy lecithin, due to its essential fatty acid content, is used for mild forms of hypercholesterolemia, so far as dietetic measures alone are not sufficient for lowering of cholesterol levels (daily dose corresponding to 3.5 g 3-sn-phosphatidylcholine) [6]. In folk medicine, soy lecithin is used as an invigorating tonic.

Chicken with Soy Sauce
(4 to 6 portions)
1 whole chicken (about 2 kg), salt, 300 ml soy sauce, 300 ml dry sherry, 150 g sugar, 3 tablespoons honey, 1 star anise fruit, 1 small piece of tangerine peel.

Rinse the chicken under running tap water, spot dry and salt on the inside. Mix the soy sauce, sherry, sugar, honey, star anise and mandarin peel in a large pot and bring to a boil. Stir the mixture until the sugar has dissolved. Place the chicken in the liquid and bring again to a boil; then, reduce the heat and let the chicken simmer for about 30 minutes; during this process, frequently pour liquid over it. Turn the chicken around and remove it from the pot after 20 minutes; serve on a large serving plate, cold or warm. The cooking liquid can be passed through a sieve and stored in the refrigerator for future reuse [Ü55].

Literature

[1] Ament M.E., Gastroenterol. 62:227–234 (1972).
[2] Anderson J.J. et al., Public Health Nutr. 2(4):489–504 (1999).
[3] Anderson J.J., S.C. Garner, Baillieres Clin. Endocrinol. Metab. 12(4):543–557 (1998).
[4] Anonym, Dtsch. Apoth. Ztg. 136(43): 3811 (1996).
[5] Anonym, Dtsch. Apoth. Ztg. 138(8): 597–600 (1998).
[6] Anonym, BAnz. Nr. 85 vom 05.05.1988.
[7] Anthony M.S. et al., J. Nutr. 126(1):43–50 (1996).
[8] Arjmandi B.H. et al., J. Nutr. 126(1): 161–167 (1996).
[9] Awazuhara H. et al., Clin. Exp. Allergy 28(12):1559–1564 (1998).
[10] Bau H.M. et al., J. Sci. Food Agric. 73(1):1–9 (1996).
[11] Baur X et al., J. Allergy Clin. Immunol. 102(6 Pt 1):984 (1998).
[12] Becker F.F., Carcinogenesis 2:1213–1214 (1981).
[13] Berhow M.A. et al., Mutat. Res. 448(1): 11–22 (2000).
[14] Codina R. et al., J. Allergy Clin. Immunol. 105(3):570–576 (2000).
[15] Coward L. et al., Am. J. Clin. Nutr. 68(6 Suppl): 1486S–1491S (1998).
[16] Deodato B. et al., Br. J. Pharmacol. 128(8):1683–1690 (1999).
[17] Duane W.C., Metabolism 48(4):489–494 (1999).
[18] Franz H. (Ed.): Advances in Lectin Research, VEB Verlag Volk und Gesundheit, Berlin 1988.
[19] Garcia M. et al., Crit. Rev. Food Sci. Nutr. 37(4):361–391 (1997).
[20] Gotoh T. et al., Jap. J. Cancer Res. 89(2):137–142 (1998).
[21] Grant G. et al., Pancreas 20(3):305–312 (2000).
[22] Harrison E. et al., J. Nutr. Sci. Vitaminol. (Tokyo) 44(2):257–268 (1998).
[23] Helm R. et al., Int. Arch. Allergy Immunol. 117(1):29–37 (1998).
[24] Iritani N. et al., J. Nutr. Sci. Vitaminol. 34:309–315 (1988).
[25] Kennedy A.R., Am. J. Clin. Nutr. 68(6):1406S–1412S (1998).
[26] Key T.J. et al., Br. J. Cancer 81(7):1248–1256 (1999).
[27] Kihara K., Nippon Shoyu Kenkyusho Zasshi 22(6):293–296 (1996), ref. CA 126:170556y.
[28] Kim B.N. et al., Hanguk Yongyang Siklyong Hakhoechi 24(2):219–227 (1995), ref. CA 123:284145g.

In folk medicine, anise oil is also taken as a galactagogue for insufficient breast milk production, for menstrual disorders and for potency debility [14].

Similar culinary herbs

Seeds of *Illicium cambodianum* Sarg., native to and cultivated in Vietnam, Laos, Cambodia, and Malaysia, used as a seasoning and for the production of essential oil [Ü61].

Fruits of *Illicium anisatum* L. (Synonym: *I. religiosum* SIEB. et ZUCC., Japanese star anise, holy star anise, shik(k)im(m)i fruit), native to Japan and Korea, cultivated in Japan, contains 1% essential oil, of which the main components are predominantly monoterpenes (cineole, linalool, β-caryophyllene and α-terpinyl acetate) besides small amounts of phenylpropane derivatives (methyleugenol, myristicine, safrole). Due to their content of toxic sesquiterpene dilactones (0.02% anisatin, furthermore neoanisatin), the fruits are used as a seasoning but in very small amounts. Use with caution! [14, Ü61].

Literature

[1] Albert-Puleo M., J. Ethnopharmacol. 2(4):337–344 (1980).

[2] Dirks U., K. Herrmann, Z. Lebensm. Unters. Forsch. 179:12–16 (1984).

[3] Formacek V., K.H. Kubeczka: Essential Oils Analysis by Capillary Gas Chromatography and Carbon–13 NMR Spectroscopy, John Wiley & Sons. Chicester etc., 1982.

[4] Knackstedt J., K. Herrmann, Z. Lebensm. Unters. Forsch. 173:288–290 (1981).

[5] Kommission E beim BfArM., BAnz.-Nr. 122 vom 06.07.1989.

[6] Kubeczka K.H., Dtsch. Apoth. Ztg. 122: 2309 (1982).

[7] Lawrence B.M., Perfum. Flavorist 9:26–28 (1984).

[8] Nakamura T. et al., Chem. Pharm. Bull. 44(10):1908–1914 (1996).

[9] Okuyama E. et al., Chem. Pharm. Bull. 41(9):1607–1601 (1993).

[10] Rudzi E. et al., Contact Dermatitis 2:305 (1976), zit. Ü39.

[11] Schultze W. et al., Dtsch. Apoth. Ztg. 130(21):1194–1201 (1990).

[12] Schulz J.M., K. Herrmann, Z. Lebensm. Unters. Forsch. 171:278–280 (1980).

[13] Seger V. et al., Pharm. Ztg. 132:2747–2748 (1987).

[14] Zänglein A. W. Schultze, Z. Phytother. 10(6):191–202 (1989).

[15] Zänglein A. et al., Dtsch. Apoth. Ztg. 129:2819–2829 (1989).

Literature references identified by Ü can be found in the general listing of books and monographs at the back of this book.

Summer savory

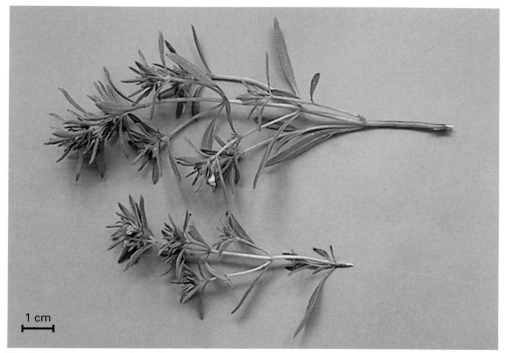

Fig. 1: Summer savory flowering tops

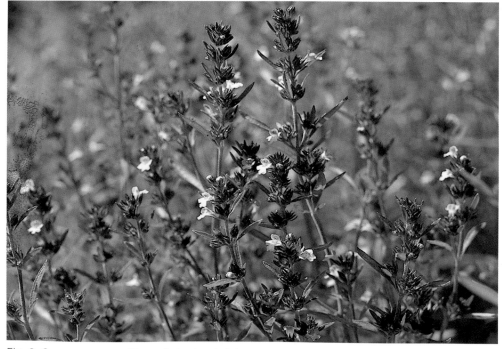

Fig. 2: Summer savory (*Satureja hortensis* L.)

Plant source: *Satureja hortensis* L.

Family: Mint family (Lamiaceae, synonym Labiatae).

Common names: Engl.: summer savory, savory; Fr.: sariette annuelle, savourée, poivrette, sadrée; Ger.: Bohnenkraut, Sommer-Bohnenkraut, Garten-Bohnenkraut, Gartenquendel, Pfefferkraut, Wurstkraut, Weinkraut, Käsekraut, Aalkraut, Saturei, Kölle.

Description: Annual herb, up to 30 cm and more rarely up to 60 cm tall, with an erect, bushy branched stem, softly pubescent, purple pruinose, later becoming woody at the base. Leaves up to 4 cm long and up to 0.5 cm wide, linear-lanceolate, sessile, entire-margined and with ciliated leaf margin. The flowers are arranged in groups of 2 to 5, as false whorls in the upper leaf-axils; the subtending leaves are longer than the flowers, calyx 3 to 4 mm long, softly pubescent with almost even teeth, corolla 4 to 7 mm long, light-violet or white, with red dots in the throat, 4 stamina, superior, diphyllous ovary, divided into 4 chambers, which, in the ripe fruit, separates into about 1 to 1.5 mm large, dark brown nutlets, containing one ovate seed each. Flowering period is from July to October [30, Ü37].

Native origin: Native to the eastern Mediterranean region up to western Iran and Caucasus, and naturalized in western Asia, India, South Africa, and North America.

Main cultivation areas: Throughout Europe (with the exception of northern Europe), Afghanistan, India, Sri Lanka, Java, South Africa, the USA, Argentina, Chile, and Uruguay.

Main exporting countries: Hungary, Czech Republic, Slovakia, Poland, and Bulgaria.

Cultivation: Summer savory prefers light (sandy), loosely packed, humus soils in sunny locations. Seeds are sown directly in the field from the end of April through early May in rows about 30 cm apart (light requirements for germination!). Cultivated varieties include, among others, 'Aromata', 'Budakalaszi', 'Compact', 'Einjähriges Blatt', 'Mestina', 'Pikanta', and 'Saturn' [25, Ü21].

Culinary herb

Commercial forms: Summer savory: the dried, rubbed herb, whole or ground, and also the fresh herb in the vegetable trade, summer savory essential oil.

Production: Summer savory is harvested at the start of the flowering period in July using a cutter loader. After controlled drying, it is mechanically rubbed. When growing for personal use, the young shoots can be clipped off continuously. For drying, the shoots must be cut by hand shortly before or during the flowering period [Ü21, Ü96].

Forms used: The fresh herb, dried sprigs or rubbed herb.

Storage: The fresh herb, stored in a plastic bag, stays fresh for a few days in the refrigerator. It is also possible to store the whole branches in a deep freezer in a freezer bag, or the finely chopped herb can be frozen with water in an ice tray. The dried herb should be stored in a cool place, protected from light and moisture, in airtight porcelain-, glass- or suitable metal containers. The whole dried herb can be stored for a relatively long time. The herb powder loses its aroma quickly.

Description. Whole herb (Fig. 1): Consisting of leaves, stems and flowers; see description of the whole plant.

Powdered herb: In the powdered herb one can find epidermis fragments with wavy cells, with diacytic stomata and with unicellular or bicellular and broad, cone-shaped trichomes, furthermore bi- or tricellular, curved, thick-walled trichomes of the stem with granular surface and terminal cells that are wider than the basal cells (Fig. 3); additionally, 4-celled to multicellular, from a broad base tapered articulate trichomes with smooth, striated or verrucose, robust cell walls, small glandular trichomes with unicellular or bicellular head, as well as lamiaceous, scale-like, glandular hairs with mostly 12 secretory cells, [Ü37].

Odor: Pleasant and spicy, **Taste:** Aromatic and somewhat peppery.

History: Summer savory was already cultivated in Italy during classical antiquity. The 3rd century cookbook "De re coquinaria", which is named after the Roman gourmet Marcus Gavius Apicius (see → Asafetida footnote), describes summer savory as a seasoning for asparagus omelets or truffle salad. Summer savory probably arrived in Germany with the Benedictine Monks in the early Middle Ages. A government decree by Karl the Great, "Capitulare de villis" (authored in about 795 CE, see → Anise footnote), called for its cultivation [26, Ü71].

Constituents and Analysis

DIN- and ISO-Standards: ISO-Standard 7928-1 (Winter savory), ISO-Standard 7928-2 (Summer savory).

Constituents

- Essential oil: 0.3 to 1.5%, in some varieties, e.g. "Aromata", up to 4.2%; the main components are carvacrol (20 to 85%), γ-terpinene (10 to 40%) and p-cymene (5 to 25%), as well as β-caryophyllene, myrcene, α-pinene, α-terpinene and thymol, among others. In the essential oil of Yugoslavian origin, thymol was the main component (about 40%), and in a sample from Moldavia, silvestrene was the principle essential oil constituent [7, 11, 14, 18, 20, 21, 27, 28, Ü31].
- Hydroxycinnamic acid derivatives (known as "labiate tannins"): About 3.4%, particularly rosmarinic acid (0.4 to 2.6%) [6, 10, 12, 23].
- Flavonoids: C-glycosides such as glucuronyl-7-luteolin, glucosyl-7-luteolin and glucuronyl-7-apigenin [2].
- Triterpenes, sterols: β-Sitosterol, ursolic acid, oleanolic acid [1, 19].

Tests for Identity: Sensoric, macroscopic, microscopic, and TLC or GC analyses of the essential oil [28, or following the procedure of the DAC 86, Thymi aetheroleum].

Quantitative assay: Volumetric quantification of the essential oil, according to Ph Eur, with steam-distillation and xylol in the graduated tube. The content of rosmarinic acid can be determined with GC after silylation [23].

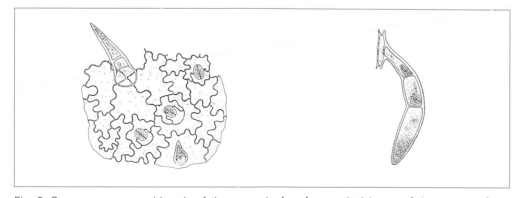

Fig. 3: Summer savory; epidermis of the upper leaf surface and trichome of the stem surface. From Ü29.

Adulterations, Misidentifications and Impurities: Misidentifications are not to be expected since the herb originates from cultivated sources. It is possible that winter savory (see below) is mistaken for summer savory. The former lacks the characteristic features, such as the downwards-pointed trichomes of the stem, among others [Ü37].

Actions and Uses

Actions: Due to its aromatic and slightly pungent taste, summer savory has appetite stimulating and digestion promoting action. The antispasmodic activity of summer savory essential oil has been demonstrated on KCl- and acetylcholine-induced contractions of the isolated ileum of rats. The inhibition of contractions was dose-dependent, and the effect was similar to that of atropine and dicyclomine. Additionally, the essential oil at a dose of 0.1 ml/100 g inhibited castor oil-induced diarrhea in mice [8]. Extracts of summer savory herb and the essential oil have antimicrobial activity [4, 17, 21, 24]. The antiviral action of summer savory extracts, observed in vitro [9, 31], which is predominantly dependent on the rosmarinic acid content, is presumably active only when used topically [31]. The activity of summer savory extracts is due to the content of rosmarinic acid and diphenolic flavonoids acting as hydrogen donators and free radical scavengers with strong antioxidant capacity, therefore the extracts can be used to considerably extend the shelf life of meat products [5, 13, 15].

Toxicology: Based on existing data, there is no acute or chronic toxicity with the regular use of summer savory herb or oil (up to 15 drops/d) as a spice.

Culinary use: Summer savory is used as a food seasoning in the form of a little bundle of sprigs or the rubbed herb placed inside a tea infuser, added to the pot 5 to 10 minutes before completion, depending on the desired strength of seasoning, and then removed from the pot before serving. Due to its strong spice impact, it should be used only sparingly.

Fresh or dried summer savory herb serves as a spice for bean dishes (white and green beans), pea and lentil dishes, soups (e.g. onion soup), salads (chopped fresh leaves added, especially, to cucumber-, bean-, tomato- or potato salads), meat stew dishes (venison, pork, rabbit, lamb), fish dishes (mackerel, pike, trout or carp), fowl dishes (chicken, dove), vegetable dishes (especially kohlrabi, cauliflower, red cabbage, white cabbage and carrots), egg dishes, mushroom dishes, pizzas, ragouts, soufflés, gratins, sauces and marinades. It is also used as a spice in sautéed potatoes, and bacon and potato omelets. A pinch of summer savory gives hash browns (potato fritters) a piquant taste. It is used as a grill spice (shortly before the grilling is finished, lay a sprig directly on the coals), and it is also well suited as a spice for lard [26, Ü55, Ü59, Ü71, Ü74, Ü79, Ü93].

Combines well with: Bay leaf, fennel, garlic, onion, parsley, rosemary, sage, and thyme [Ü55].

As a component of spice mixes and preparations: → Bread spice mix, → Fines Herbes, → Fish spice, → Hamburger meat spice, → Herb vinegar, → Herbes de Provence, → Poultry spice, → Roast spice, → Soup spice, → Table mustard, → Tschubritza → Vegetable spice.

Other uses: Summer savory oil is used in the food industry in the manufacture of spice essences and as an aromatic flavor component of sweets and baked goods [3].

Medicinal herb

Herbal drug: Saturejae herba, Summer savory herb, contains not less than 0.4% essential oil [EB 6].

Indications: Folk medicinal use in the form of tea infusions, taken orally, for digestive disturbances, biliary problems, bronchial disorders, helminths, and menstrual complaints (1.5 g/150 ml), and externally as a rinse for inflammations in the mouth (5 g/100 ml) [Ü37]. As with many herbs that contain essential oil, it was also considered to be an aphrodisiac [26].

Other Satureja-species used as spice herbs

Winter savory (mountain savory, Italian savory, savory, karst savory)**,** *Satureja montana* L., occurs with several subspecies, which are also differentiated by the compositional spectrum of their essential oils. Winter savory is a perennial, hardy, dwarf shrub. Sowing can take place in August (light requirements for germination!). Harvest is possible beginning from the third year. The plant is productive for 5 to 6 years. In the home garden, sprigs can also be harvested in the winter as needed. It is native to southern Europe, and eastwards up to the Ukraine. It is cultivated, especially in Southern- and Central Europe (although rarely in Germany), Central Asia, India, South Africa, and France. It is used similarly as summer savory, although its spice flavor impact is not as strong. The main components of its essential oil are carvacrol (28 to 68%), *p*-cymene (8 to 20%), thymol (0 to 40%) and γ-terpinene (5 to 15%) [16, 18, 29, Ü37]. There are also chemotypes of *S. m.* L. ssp. *montana*, which are dominated by *p*-cymene, *trans*-sabinene hydrate, linalool, borneol, *p*-cymene-8-ol or silvestrene [27]. The essential oil of *S. m.* var. *citriodora* is predominately composed of geraniol (about 66%), estragole (about 10%) and β-caryophyllene (about 10%) [18].

Thyme-leaved savory, Persian Zatar, *Satureja thymbra* L., is native to Sardinia, Crete, Greece, and Spain. The main components of its essential oil are either carvacrol or thymol. In its countries of origin, it is used as a spice for soups and stews, especially with meats [22].

Creeping savory, *Satureja spicigera* (K. KOCH) BOISS., is native to the Caucasus region, and is cultivated in Georgia. The essential oil has a similar composition to that of summer savory.

Potato-Tomato Salad

(For 4 persons)

500 g potatoes (of a hard variety that does not burst during cooking), 8 tablespoons of vegetable oil, 6 tablespoons of broth (instant), 4 tablespoons of vinegar, 500 g salad tomatoes, 1 to 2 bundles of summer savory, 150 g sheep cheese, salt and pepper.

Wash the potatoes and boil them unpeeled. Mix together the oil, broth and vinegar, and season with salt and pepper. Peel the potatoes while still warm, slice them not too thinly into the salad dressing. Let stand at room temperature for 15 minutes. Separate the summer savory leaves from the stem and carefully mix them in. Place the potato and tomato slices in a deep serving dish and sprinkle with crumbled sheep cheese. The remaining salad dressing is seasoned with pepper and salt to taste, and poured evenly over the tomatoes. Serve immediately. Thinly cut ham is an excellent side dish [Ü95].

Literature

[1] Brieskorn C.H. et al., Arch. Pharm. 286: 501–506 (1953).

[2] Darbour N. et al., Pharm. Acta Helv. 8:239–240 (1990).

[3] De Vincenzi M. et al., Fitoterapia 65:49–53 (1994).

[4] Deans S.G., K.P. Svoboda, Horticultural Sci. 64:205–210 (1989).

[5] Gerhardt U., P. Blat, Fleischwirtschaft 64:484–486 (1984).

[6] Gerhardt U., A. Schröter, Fleischwirtschaft 63:1628–1630 (1983).

[7] Gora J. et al., J. Essent. Oil Res, 8(4): 427–428 (1996).

[8] Hajhashemi V. et al., J. Ethnopharmacol. 71(1/2):187–192 (2000).

[9] Herrmann E.C. jr., L.S. Kucera, Proc. Soc. Exp. Biol. Med. 124:874–878 (1995).

[10] Herrmann K., Z. Lebensm. Unters. Forsch. 116:224–228 (1961).

[11] Kustrak D. et al., J. Essent. Oil Res. 8: 7–13 (1996).

[12] Lamaison J.L. et al., Ann. Pharm. Franc. 48:103–108 (1990).

[13] Lamaison J.L. et al., Plant Méd. Phytothér 22:231–234 (1988).

[14] Lawrence B.M., Perfumer Flavorist 13:46–48, 17:51–52 (1992).

[15] Lindberg Madsen H. et al., Z. Lebensm. Unters. Forsch. 203(4):333–338 (1996).

[16] Lokar L.C. et al., Webbia 37:197–206 (1983).

[17] Menphini A. et al., Riv. Ital. EPPOS 4(Spec. Num.):566–571 (1993).

[18] Mikus B. et al., Drogenreport 10(18): 68–73 (1997).

[19] Nicholas H.J., J. Am. Pharm. Assoc. 47:731–735 (1958).

[20] Nikolajev A.G., Y. Andrejeva, Uchenye Zapiski Kshinev Univ. 23:69 (1957), ref. CA 52:14907.

[21] Panizzi L. et al., J. Ethnopharmacol. 39(3):167–170 (1993).

[22] Ravid U., E. Putievsky, Planta Med. 49:248 (1983).

[23] Reschke A., Z. Lebensm. Unters. Forsch. 176:116–119 (1983).

[24] Sattar A.A. et al., Pharmazie 50(1):62–65 (1995).

[25] Schmidt L., Drogenreport 6(9):39–40 (1993).

[26] Scholz H., Natürlich (6):33–37 (1998).

[27] Slavkovska V. et al., J. Essent. Oil Res. 9:629–634 (1997).

[28] Thieme H., Nguyen-Thi-Tam, Pharmazie 27(4):255–265 (1972).

[29] Thieme H., Nguyen-Thi-Tam, Pharmazie 27(5):324–331 (1972).

[30] Weymar H., Buch der Lippenblütengewächse, Neumann Verlag, Radebeul 1961.

[31] Yamasaki K. et al., Biol. Pharm. Bull. 21(8):829–833 (1998).

Literature references identified by Ü can be found in the general listing of books and monographs at the back of this book.

Sweet cicely

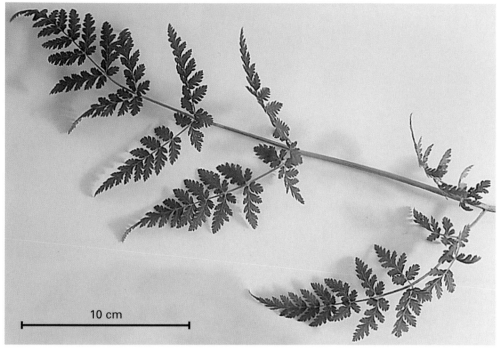

Fig. 1: Sweet cicely leaf

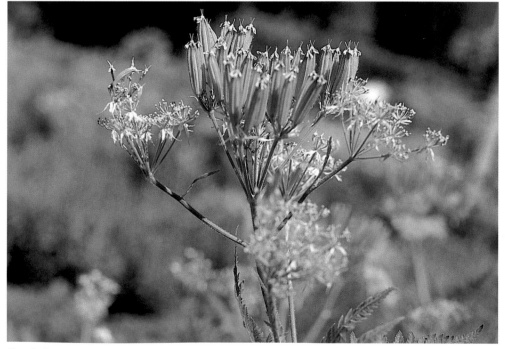

Fig. 2: Sweet cicely (*Myrrhis odorata* (L.) SCOP.)

Plant source: *Myrrhis odorata* (L.) SCOP.

Synonym: *Scandix odorata* L.

Family: Umbelliferous plants (Apiaceae, synonym Umbelliferae).

Common names: Engl.: garden myrrh, Amer. Engl.: sweet cicely; Fr.: cerfeuil musqué, cerfeuil anisé; Ger.: Süßdolde, Myrrhenkerbel, Aniskerbel, Spanischer Kerbel, Englischer Kerbel, Süßkerbel, Wilder Anis.

Description: Perennial plant, up to 1.5 tall. Stem roundish, tubular, branched in the upper part, root carrot-like, very fleshy, white under the upper brown surface. The tender, double or threefold pinnate leaves with pinnately cleft pinnules with oblong-ovoid, dentate lobes, pubescent on the lower side, appear fern-like. The inflorescences are terminal arranged, 6- to 20-radiate compound umbels without bracts and fimbriate involucels. The quinate flowers with white petals are male or bisexual, the male ones have 5 stamina, the bisexual ones have 5 stamina and an inferior 2-chambered ovary with 2 styles. The fruit is a bipartite yellowish to black-brown shiny diachene, up to 2.5 cm long, disintegrating after ripening in 2 closed mericarps, hanging on a bifurcate carpophore. Flowering period is from June to August [9, Ü17, Ü37].

Native origin: Northern Spain, the Pyrenees, the Alps, mountains of the Western Balkans to Albania, in the rest of Europe occurring rarely in vegetations formed by tall perennial herbs.

Source: Only sporadic cultivation, mostly for home use.

Cultivation: The plant prefers nutrient rich, damp, porous soil, half-shaded, but can also tolerate full sun locations. Sowing takes place in April to May or in the autumn. It can also be started in the greenhouse and then planted out in May, 4 to 6 plants/m². It is a perennial crop [Ü2, Ü21, Ü47, Ü67].

Culinary herb

Commercial forms: Not commercially traded.

Production: The fresh leaves can be harvested throughout the entire year. The fruits are harvested immature or ripe, the ripe fruits are dried at 40 °C.

Forms used: Fresh leaves, immature fresh fruits, ripe, dried fruits.

Storage: The fresh leaves can be stored for a few days in plastic bags in the vegetable compartment of the refrigerator, or minced in water and frozen in the ice-tray. Drying is not recommended due to the considerable aroma loss.

Description: For the leaves and fruits, see plant description.

Odor: Anise-like with slight musk-note, **Taste:** Anise-like, licorice-like and sweet.

History: This plant was already used in the Middle Ages as a sugar substitute in fruit dishes.

Constituents and Analysis

Constituents of the fruit
- Essential oil: In unripe fruits about 4%, in ripe fruits about 0.8%, the main component is *trans*-anethole (75 to 85%), and, among others, α- or/and γ-terpineol, elemol and β-bisabolene, [4, 5].
- Fatty oil (12 to 15%).

Constituents of the leaves
- Essential oil: 1 to 1.5%, the main component is *trans*-anethole (75 to 83%), furthermore, among others, methylchavicol (about 2.5%), germacrene D (about 1%), δ-cadinene (about 1%), β-caryophyllene (about 1%), myrcene (about 1%), and according to older sources, α-terpinene (2.4%) and methyleugenol (eugenol methyl ether, 9%) [3, 4, 6–8].
- Flavonoids: Apigenin-7-*O*-β-ᴅ-glucoside, luteolin-7-*O*-β-ᴅ-glucoside [1, 2].

Tests for Identity: No methods cited in the literature.

Quantitative assay: The content of essential oil can be determined volumetrically with steam-distillation, with xylol in the graduated tube, according to the European Pharmacopeia [Ph Eur].

Adulterations, Misidentifications and Impurities: Since the herb originates from cultivated sources, misidentifications are unlikely.

Actions and Uses

Actions: Due to its aromatic aroma and taste, sweet cicely has appetite stimulating and digestion promoting action. On the basis of its high content of anethole, similar to → Anise or → Fennel, it has mildly spasmolytic as well as antibacterial and therefore anti-dyspeptic and carminative action. Moreover it is supposed to have expectorant activity, and possibly also a mild estrogenic effect.

Toxicology: Based on existing data, there is no acute or chronic toxicity with its use as a spice at normal doses. At high doses, an estrogenic effect similar to → Anise and → Fennel is likely due to the anethole content.

Culinary use: Sweet cicely has now, probably unjustly so, fallen into oblivion as a culinary plant.

Chopped fresh leaves can be used as a seasoning of fruit salads and compotes, especially of apricot-, pear-, nectarine-, rhubarb- and gooseberry compote, of green salads, vegetable salads, herb butter, quark, yogurt, cream, rice pudding, root vegetables and pumpkin dishes as well as a flavoring of fruit juices, fruit syrups and fruit punches [Ü2, Ü47, Ü53, Ü74].

Chopped immature fruits serve as a seasoning of salads and cream dishes, ripe fruits as an ingredient of desserts, cakes or sweet cream sauces [Ü2, Ü47, Ü74].

The flowers can be used as a garnish of compote or fruitcakes [Ü47]. The roots can be dug up in the autumn, cooked briefly, and eaten as a vegetable with white sauce or vinaigrette, just like parsnip [Ü17].

Combines well with: Bay, lemon balm, and mint.

Other uses: The essential oil is used in the perfume industry.

Similar culinary herbs: → Anise, → Star anise, → Fennel.

Medicinal herb

Herbal drugs are now obsolete, formerly used was Cerefolii hispanici herba, Myrrh herb, Sweet-scented cicely herb.

Indications: Today the herb is used medicinally only rarely. Formerly it served as a "blood purifying" remedy, an expectorant, and, in the form a smoked dried herb, for alleviating asthmatic difficulties, among other uses.

Fruit juice-wine punch

500 ml orange juice, 250 ml lemon juice, 1 bottle of dry red wine, 2 teaspoons finely minced sweet cicely leaves.

Put all the ingredients in large juice bowl and mix well. Chill in the refrigerator until serving. Fill large drink glasses (250 ml) to the rim with punch and 2 to 3 ice cubes [Ü55].

Literature

[1] Ciskowski W., Herba Pol. 31:13–19 (1985).

[2] Harborne J.B., C.A. Williams, Phytochemistry 11(5):1741–1750 (1972).

[3] Hussain R.A. et al., Econ. Bot. 44:174–182 (1990).

[4] Kubeczka K.H. et al., in K.H. Kubeczka (Hrsg.): Ätherische Öle, Thieme Verlag, Stuttgart 1982, p.158–187.

[5] Kudrzycka-Bieloszabska F.W., W. Sawicka, Acta Pol. Pharm. 27:305–307, 307–310, 313–317 (1970).

[6] Sawicka W., Acta Pol. Pharm. 26:565–568 (1969).

[7] Tkachenko K.G., I.G. Zenkevich, J. Ess. Oil Res. 5:329–331 (1993).

[8] Uusitalo J.S. et al., J. Ess. Oil Res. 11:423–425 (1999).

[9] Weymar H., Buch der Doldengewächse, Neumann Verlag, Radebeul 1959.

Literature references identified by Ü can be found in the general listing of books and monographs at the back of this book.

Sweet marjoram

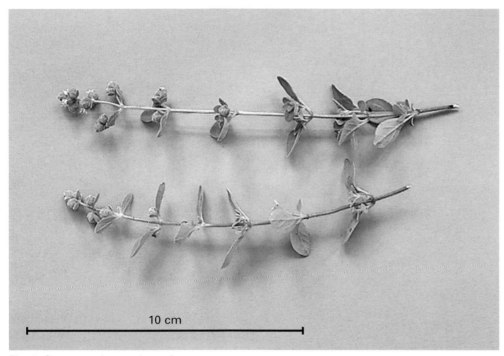

Fig. 1: Sweet marjoram shoot tip

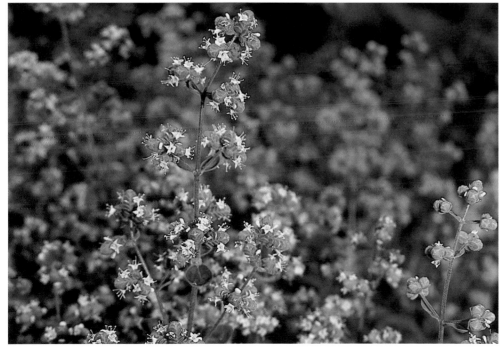

Fig. 2: Sweet marjoram (*Origanum majorana* L.)

Plant source: *Origanum majorana* L.

Synonyms: *Majorana hortensis* MOENCH, *Majorana vulgaris* MILL.

Family: Mint family (Lamiaceae, synonym Labiatae).

Common names: Engl.: sweet marjoram, annual majoram, knotted majoram; Fr.: marjolaine; Ger.: Majoran, Süßer Majoran, Garten-Majoran, Gartendost, Wurstkraut, Mairan, Süßer Majoran.

Description: Annual in Central Europe, perennial in warmer climate regions, stem up to 50 cm in height, erect, quadrangular, with many branches, reddish-brown, more or less softly pubescent. Leaves ovate to elliptical, short petiolate, 0.5 to 2.5 cm long, 0.5 to 1 cm wide, entire-margined, roundish, with dense and matted, gray pubescence on both surfaces, without prominent venation. The flowers are situated in the axils of circular, up to 4 mm wide bracts with capitular arrangement; corolla white to pale pink, about 4 mm long, lips only indistinct, 4 stamina, calyx without teeth, obliquely split, superior ovary, diphyllous, divided into 4 compartments. The fruit separates into 4 single, smooth, nutlets, light to dark brown. Flowering period is from June to September [47, Ü37].

Native origin: Cyprus and southern Turkey, today occurring from the Mediterranean region to Hindustan.

Main cultivation areas: Southern France (Bouches du Rhône, Provence), Germany (especially in the area around Aschersleben), Poland, Czech Republic, Austria, Italy, Hungary, Bulgaria, Greece, Egypt, Tunisia, Morocco, South Africa, northern India, south- and southeastern USA, Mexico, Chile, and Bolivia.

Main suppliers: Egypt followed by Morocco (especially as an exporter of sweet marjoram essential oil), France, Hungary, Romania, Germany (predominantly for domestic use), Czech Republic, and Tunisia.

Cultivation: The plant needs well drained, humus rich, neutral to chalky, slightly warmed up soil. It will tolerate frost down to –7 °C. The plant is self-incompatible, which means it should not be grown for years on the same spot. Seeds can be sown directly outside in May in rows of 25 to 50 cm apart (germination is light dependent!). The cultivation on a small scale can be started indoors at 10 to 15 °C in containers or in a cold frame. Due to its shallow root system, it must be watered as soon as possible when the soil dries out. The preferred cultivar-groups for cultivation in Central Europe are 'Blattmajoran' (French bush marjoram) and, very rarely, bud marjoram (German marjoram). Other widely cultivated varieties include 'Marcelka', 'Miraz' ('Mirage'), 'Max', and 'Francia' [Ü14, Ü21].

Culinary herb

Commercial forms: Sweet marjoram: dried, rubbed herb, essential oil of sweet marjoram, sweet marjoram oleoresin.

Production: Harvest takes place during the budding stage prior to full bloom (July to August) using loader combine harvesters in industrial cultivation. Under optimal conditions a second harvest is possible, and with sprinkler irrigation a third harvest may be possible. The herb must be dried rapidly at 35 to 45 °C, rubbed and sieved. Because it grows so close to the soil and is covered with hairs, the herb must be thoroughly cleaned. For personal use, one can harvest the fresh shoots throughout the entire summer. Only the shoot tips are cut off, after which the plant regenerates soon thereafter [Ü21].

Forms used: The fresh shoot tips and leaves, the dried, rubbed or cut herb, rarely the powdered herb, and the essential oil.

Storage: The fresh leaves or the fresh herb can be stored for a few days refrigerated in plastic bags or, with little water, frozen in the ice-tray. The dried herb is stored in airtight porcelain-, glass- or suitable metal containers. Dried marjoram retains its spicy aroma for 1 to 2 years.

Description. Whole herb: Consisting mostly of the dried leaves and inflorescences which have been scraped off from the stems by rubbing, and, more rarely, of the whole herb; see description of the whole plant.

Powdered herb: Characteristic are the uni- to tri- cellular, often bent trichomes with cuticular warts, and the epidermal cells of the upper leaf surface with distinctly wavy outline, sometimes punctate, with capitate hairs and few diacytic stomata (Fig. 3). Also present are, among others, lamiaceous, glandular scales and large pollen grains, about 35 µm in diameter, with 6 slit-like pores [Ü25, Ü29, EB 6].

Odor: Strongly aromatic, **Taste:** Spicy, somewhat bitter and burning, camphor-like.

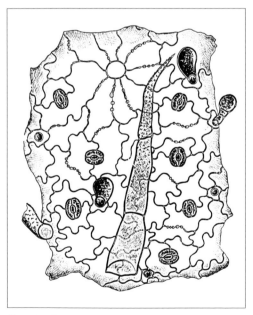

Fig. 3: Sweet marjoram. Epidermis of the upper leaf surface with broken off, articulate trichome.

History: This herb was already cultivated by the ancient Egyptians, 3000 years ago. It is described in Dioscorides' "De materia medica" (around 50 CE). In the cookbook "De re coquinaria", authored by the Roman gourmet Apicius in the 3rd century (see footnote in → Asafetida monograph), sweet marjoram is mentioned as a kitchen seasoning for cooked fish and sauces. In Central Europe it was introduced by Benedictine monks in the 16th century [35, Ü92].

Constituents and Analysis

DIN- and ISO-Standards: ISO-Specification 10620 (Dried sweet marjoram – Specification).

Constituents

- Essential oil: 0.8 to 3% (0.2 to 0.4% in the fresh herb); the main components of the genuine essential oil are *cis*-sabinene hydrate (40 to 80%, during steam distillation mostly transformed to, among other constituents, terpinenol-4, α-terpinene, γ-terpinene and limonene; at pH 8, this conversion can be largely avoided), *cis*-sabinene hydrate acetate (3 to 40%, during steam distillation partially transforming to terpinenol-4, among others) and sabinene (traces to 10%). The components *cis*-sabinene hydrate and terpinenol-4 determine the odor. The composition of the essential oil obtained by steam distillation does not only depend significantly on the chemical race but also on the method of production. The main components of such essential oils are usually terpinenol-4 (20 to 40%), *cis*-sabinene hydrate (7 to 60%), α-terpineol (4 to 8%), γ-terpinene (2 to 12%), α-terpinene (1 to 7%), *p*-cymene (1 to 10%), sabinene (2 to 6%) and *trans*-sabinene hydrate (2 to 6%). There are also marjoram oils with a high proportion of carvacrol (78 to 80%), thymol (up to 75%) or linalool and linalyl acetate (up to 35%) [4, 7, 8, 10, 13, 14, 17, 24, 26, 33–36, 38, 41]. Some of the essential oil compo-

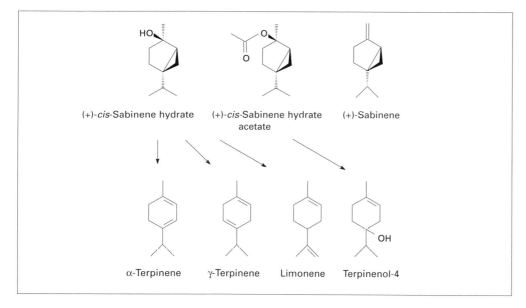

(+)-cis-Sabinene hydrate   (+)-cis-Sabinene hydrate acetate   (+)-Sabinene

α-Terpinene   γ-Terpinene   Limonene   Terpinenol-4

nents occur as glycosides in the intact plant [32].

- Flavonoids: Including, among others, diosmetin, vitexin, orientin, cynaroside, dinalin, thymonin ("majoranin"), vicenin-2, diosmetin-β-glucuronide, luteolin-7-rutinoside and apigenin-7-glucoronide [12, 45].
- Phenol glycosides: Arbutin (0.4 to 1%), methylarbutin, hydroquinone [6, 23, 31, 42].
- Hydroxycinnamic acid derivatives (labiate tannins): About 5%, including, among others, rosmarinic acid (0.1 to 3.3%) and chlorogenic acid [21, 29, 39].
- Bitter substances: Possibly diterpenes.
- Saponins: Murwaoside [48].
- Triterpenes, sterols: Ursolic acid (about 0.5%), oleanolic acid (about 0.2%) and β-sitosterol [9, 30].

Tests for Identity: Sensoric, macroscopic and microscopic analysis as well as TLC of the extract, and TLC or GC of the essential oil [16, 34, 35, 37].

Quantitative assay: The content of essential oil can be determined volumetrically with steam-distillation [Ph Eur]; rosmarinic acid is analyzed quantitatively with GC after silylation [39].

Adulterations, Misidentifications and Impurities are possible, with other thymol-

or carvacrol-containing Origanum species, which occur as weeds in marjoram fields of southern regions. They can be differentiated from genuine marjoram with TLC based on their content of thymol and carvacrol [35].

Actions and Uses

Actions: Due to its aromatic and slightly bitter taste, sweet marjoram has appetite stimulating and digestion promoting effects. Antiviral activity of an aqueous extract of sweet marjoram has been observed in vitro [20], with the effect mainly dependent on the rosmarinic acid content, and probably only effective with topical application. The essential oil of sweet marjoram has antimicrobial action [10, 11].

Toxicology: Based on existing data, there is no acute or chronic toxicity with the normal use of marjoram as a spice. Hydroquinone, contained in the herb only in small amounts (in free form or cleaved from arbutin in the intestinal tract), has shown hepato- and nephrotoxic as well as possibly carcinogenic effects in animal tests when administered in large amounts over longer periods of time [3]. But it does not have the potential for toxic effects in humans with the use of the

herb as a spice. The sensitization potential is not known.

Culinary use: Sweet marjoram is especially popular in France, Italy, and Greece. It is also used to a large extent in Central European cooking. Usually the dried, rubbed herb is used, but the fresh leaves are also an excellent seasoning. Heating sweet marjoram not only causes some of its essential oil to evaporate, but it also changes the aromatic quality (due to decomposition of the cis-sabinene hydrates). Sweet marjoram should therefore be added to the dish only shortly before finishing.

Sweet marjoram is a very intense seasoning so it should be measured carefully. The dried herb serves predominantly as a sausage spice, especially as a spice for cooked sausages such as blood- and liver sausage, but also of Thuringian and Nuremberg frying sausages (bratwurst). One can also season soups with fresh or dried sweet marjoram (e.g. potato soups), piquant puddings, meat dishes (e.g. roasted lamb, -fawn, -venison, -goose, -duck, meat loaf, roasted meats, ragouts, Bavarian liver dumplings, fillings for roasted goose, and meat vol-au-vent), sauces (e.g. gravy, tomato- and salad sauces with vinegar and oil), fish dishes (e.g. Hamburger eel soup, carp), peas and beans dishes, sauerkraut, noodle dishes, eggplant, salads (leaf-, potato- and bean salads), mushrooms, pizzas, quark, omelets, baked potatoes and lard. One can also strew it over mozzarella or other fresh cheeses and on lard bread [Ü7, Ü30, Ü45, Ü55, Ü59, Ü71, Ü74]. It is recommended to sprinkle sweet marjoram over cooked spinach to add flavor [Ü111].

Sweet marjoram macerated in olive oil (add 1 small bunch of dried sweet marjoram to 1 liter olive oil and leave for at least 2 weeks) produces a spicy oil, which can be brushed on meat before putting it on the grill [Ü86].

The essential oil of sweet marjoram is used in the liqueur industry in the production of herbal liqueurs, and in the food industry as a component of spice essences.

Combines well with: Black pepper, garlic, onions, and also (sparingly) with rosemary, sage and thyme.

As a component of spice mixes and preparations: → Barbecue sauce, → Bouquet garni, → Fines herbes, → Fish spice, → Hamburger meat spice, → Herb butter, → Herb mixture for smoking and grilling meats, → Herb oil, → Herb salt, → Herb vinegar, → Herbes de Provence, → Mélange classique, → Parisian pepper, → Pizza spice, → Poultry spice, → Quark spice, → Roast spice, → Salad spice, → Sausage spice, → Table mustard, → Venison spice.

Other uses: The rancidity of fats can be delayed with the addition of 0.1% marjoram [22, 43].

Medicinal herb

Herbal drug: Majoranae herba, Marjoram herb, contains not less than 1% essential oil [EB 6].

Indications: In folk medicine, sweet marjoram is used internally for stomach and intestine problems, among other uses, as a urinary- and diaphoretic remedy, for migraines, nervous headaches, and coughs in the form of tea infusions (1 to 2 teaspoonfuls of dried herb/250 ml water, 1 to 2 cups daily, unsweetened for digestive complaints, sweetened when taken as an expectorant, and in this case sipped slowly as hot as possible). Externally, marjoram ointment [EB 6] is applied for coughs, rhinitis and neuralgia. Due to its hydroquinone content and not sufficiently substantiated efficacy, the German Commission E of the BfArM did not approve its therapeutic use [28].

Other Origanum-species used as culinary herbs

Dittany of Crete (Cretan dittany, hop marjoram), *Origanum dictamnus* L., cultivated in Crete and in England, the main compo-nents of its essential oil are carvacrol, *p*-cymene and γ-terpinene [19, 25, 32, 44]

Greek oregano (false bush oregano), *Origanum vulgare* L. ssp. *viride* (BOISS.) HAYEK (Synonyms: *O. heracleoticum* L., *O. viride* (BOISS.) HALACSY), distributed from Sardinia to the Aegean Sea, the main components of its essential oil are carvacrol (40 to 60%), thymol, (5 to 20%), *p*-cymene (8 to 11%), γ-terpinene (about 15%), and *trans*-sabinene hydrate (about 6%) [1, 2, 27, Ü92]. In contrast, the main components found in the oil of an Iranian race were linalyl acetate (about 20%), β-caryophyllene (about 15%), sabinene (about 13%) and γ-terpinene (about 6%), with carvacrol and thymol occurring only in traces [1]. This

---

Pork filet with marjoram
500 g champignons, 1 bundle of fresh sweet marjoram, 1 onion, 50 g butter or margarine, 600 to 800 g pork filet, salt, freshly ground, black pepper, 175 g crème fraîche or sour cream, 2 tablespoons of whipped cream.

Clean the mushrooms and cut them into thin slices. Wash the marjoram, dab it dry, then finely chop the herb. Peel the onion, finely mince and fry it in a large pan until golden-brown. Add the mushrooms and 2 tablespoons of marjoram, and cook the ingredients for another 5 to 10 minutes. Meanwhile, wash the pork filet, dry the surface with a paper towel and cut the meat into fine slices. Fry the pork on both sides in a separate pan until brown and add it to the cooked mushrooms; season to taste with salt and pepper. Mix the crème fraîche and the whipped cream with the remaining marjoram and add it to the filet. Heat the contents of the pan again, but don't let it boil. Serve with freshly prepared, fried potatoes [Ü91].

---

herb is used as a pizza-, pasta- and tidbits spice as well as for pickling of fish (anchovies) [Ü46].

Cretan oregano (Spanish hops, French marjoram, pot marjoram, ragani), *Origanum onites* L., cultivated in France and Cyprus, a garden plant in England and Germany, the main components of its essential oil are race-specific, carvacrol (67 to 80%) or linalool (90 to 92%), and it can also contain, among others, γ-terpinene, *p*-cymene and borneol. Cretan oregano is used, among other uses, as a pickling spice, e.g. for anchovies, and as a seasoning in potato-, noodle- and meat dishes [2, 8, 40, 46, Ü46, Ü92].

Syrian marjoram (Arabian marjoram, bible hyssop, true za'tar), *Origanum syriacum* L. (Syn. *O. maru* L.), cultivated and used in the Mediterranean region, the main components of its essential oil are carvacrol (80 to 90%) or thymol (about 60%), as well as *p*-cymene (6 to 14%) [2, 5, 15, 18].
→ **Oregano.**

Literature

[1] Afshaypuor S. et al., Planta Med. 63(2): 179–180 (1997).
[2] Akgül A., A. Bayrak, Planta Med. 53:114 (1987).
[3] Anonym, NPT Technical Report on the Toxicology and Carcinogenesis Studies of Hydroquinone (CAS No. 123-31-9) in F344/N Rats and B6C3F1 Mice (Gavage Studies), National Toxicological Programm, NTP TR 366, Publication No. 90–2821, US Department on the Toxicolog. (1989).
[4] Anonym, Drogenreport 11(19):59–63 (1998).
[5] Arnold N. et al., J. Ess. Oil Res. 12: 192–196 (2000).
[6] Assaf M.H. et al., Planta Med. 53(4): 343–346 (1987).
[7] Baser K.H.C. et al., J. Ess. Oil Res. 5:577–579 (1993).
[8] Baser K.H.C. et al., J. Ess. Oil Res. 5:619–623 (1993).
[9] Brieskorn C.H. et al., Arch. Pharm. 285: 290–296 (1952).
[10] Charai M. et al., J. Ess. Oil Res. 8:657–664 (1996).

[11] Deans S.G. et al., Flavour Fragrance 5:187–190 (1990).

[12] Dolci M., S. Tira, Riv. Ital. 62:131–132 (1980).

[13] Fischer N. et al., Flavour and Fragrance 2:55–61 (1987).

[14] Fischer N. et al., J. Agric. Food Chem. 36:996–1003 (1988).

[15] Fleisher A., Z. Fleisher, J. Ess. Oil Res. 3:121–123 (1991).

[16] Franz Ch., M. Auer, Drogenreport 4(6): 31–37 (1999).

[17] Góra J. et al., Riv. Ital. EPPOS (Spec. Num., 15th Journees Internat Huiles Essentielles, 1996):761-766 (1997).

[18] Halim A.F. et al., Int. J. Pharmacogn 29:183–187 (1991).

[19] Harvala C. et al., Planta Med. 53:107–109 (1987).

[20] Hermann E.C. jr., L.S. Kucera, Proc. Soc. Exp. Biol. Med. 124:874–878 (1967).

[21] Herrmann K., Pharmazie 11:433–448 (1956).

[22] Herrmann K., Z. Lebensm. Unters. Forsch. 116:224–228 (1961).

[23] Husain S.Z., R.R. Markham, Phytochemistry 20:1171–1173 (1981).

[24] Junghans W., H. Krüger, Herba Germanica 3(3):78–81 (1995).

[25] Katsiotis S. G.N. Ikonomou, Sci. Pharm. 54:49–52 (1986).

[26] Kirimer N. et al., Khim. Prir. Soedin. (1): 49–54 (1995).

[27] Kokkini S. et al., Phytochemistry 44(5): 883–886 (1997).

[28] Kommission E beim BfArM, BAnz. 226 vom 02.12.92 (1994).

[29] Lamaison J.L. et al., Ann. Pharm. Franc 48:103–108 (1990).

[30] Lossner G., Pharmazie 20:224–228 (1965).

[31] Nguyen H. et al., Ann. Pharm. Fr. 23:297–305 (1965).

[32] Nitz S. et al., Chem. Mikrobiol. Technol. Lebensm. 9:87 (1985).

[33] Nykänen I., Z. Lebensm. Unters. Forsch. 183:172–176 (1986).

[34] Oberdieck R., Deutsche Lebensm. Rdsch. 77:63–74 (1981).

[35] Oberdieck R., Fleischwirtschaft 70: 391–398 (1990).

[36] Oberdieck R., Fleischwirtschaft 63:1–4 (1983).

[37] Pino J.A. et al., J. Ess. Oil Res. 9(4): 479–480 (1997).

[38] Pluhar Z. et al., Olaj, Szappan, Kozmet 45(Spec. Issue): 70–74 (1996), ref. CA 126:242580b.

[39] Reschke A., Z. Lebensm. Unters. Forsch. 176:116–119 (1983).

[40] Ruberto G. et al., Flavour Fragr. 8: 197–200 (1993).

[41] Sarer E. et al., Planta Med. 46:236–239 (1982).

[42] Schreck D., Neuere Methoden zur umfassenden Untersuchung komplexer Naturstoffgemische am Beispiel von Majorana hortensis, Dissertation Marburg 1985.

[43] Shahidi F. et al., J. Food Lipids 2(3):145–153 (1995).

[44] Skrubis B., J. Ethnopharmacol. 1(4): 411–415 (1979).

[45] Voirin B. et al., Phytochemistry 23:2973–2975 (1984).

[46] Vokou D. et al., Econ Bot. 42:407–412 (1988).

[47] Weymar H., Buch der Lippenblütler und Rauhblattgewächse, Neumann Verlag, Radebeul 1961.

[48] Yadava R.N., Adv. Exp. Med. Biol. 405(Saponins used in Food and Agriculture):223–230 (1996), ref. CA 126:290669j.

Literature references identified by Ü can be found in the general listing of books and monographs at the back of this book.

Sweet woodruff

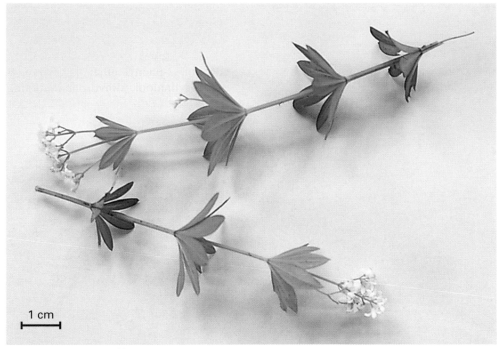

Fig. 1: Sweet woodruff herb

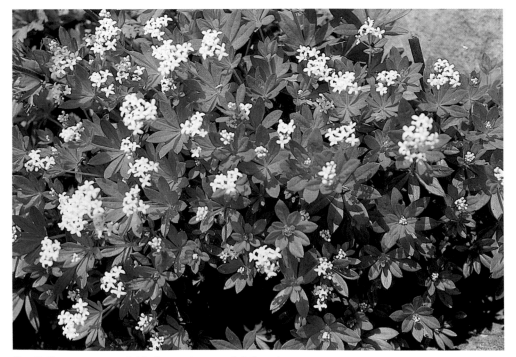

Fig. 2: Sweet woodruff (*Galium odoratum* (L.) Scop.)

Plant source: *Galium odoratum* (L.) Scop.

Synonym: *Asperula odorata* L.

Family: Madder family (Rubiaceae).

Common names: Engl.: sweet woodruff, woodruff asperule; Fr.: aspérule odorante, muguet des bois, petit muguet, reine de bois, hépatique étoilee; Ger.: Waldmeister, Echter Waldmeister, Duftlabkraut, Maikraut.

Description: Perennial plant with thin creeping rootstock, 10 to 30 cm (seldom up to 60 cm) tall. Stem tetragonal, occasionally short-hairy on the nodes. Whorls of 6 to 9 leaves respectively are arranged upon one another on the stem; the leaves are lanceolate, 1.5 to 5 cm long, 6 to 14 mm wide, short-mucronate, flat, entire margined, with fine bristles on the margin and on the costa. The flowers are arranged in a terminal, many-branched cyme, the bracts are small, lanceolate, often almost bristle-like, the flowers are funnel-shaped quadrilobate, the corolla is white, 4 to 6 mm long, the lobes are pubescent on the inner surface. The fruits are almost globose, grayish-green to dark-brown, up to 3 mm in diameter, bearing hook-like bristles [Ü28, Ü42, Ü85].

Native origin: Northern- and Central Europe, southwards to the mountains of Italy, and the Balkan Peninsula, Siberia, and Northern Africa.

Main cultivation areas: In the regions where it naturally occurs (see above) in gardens or in semi-cultivation.

Main exporting countries: There is no meaningful world trade.

Cultivation: Sweet woodruff prefers lime-deficient humus soil in shady positions. It thrives best in semi-cultivation in shady woods or in gardens situated near deciduous trees or bushes. Propagation is carried out by direct drilling in the autumn or January (dark germinator, frost effect is necessary for germination, in the first winter cover with foliage) or with young plants planted in advance, for domestic use it is easiest cultivated by stock division. Growing width 5 to 15 cm. Sweet woodruff spreads its reptant rhizomes very rapidly and is well suited as a ground cover plant under deciduous trees and shrubs [Ü21, Ü41, Ü47].

Culinary herb

Commercial forms: Sweet woodruff: the dried herb.

Production: Sweet woodruff originates mostly from wild- or garden plants. It is harvested shortly before the flowering period with a hand sickle, and in the garden with pruning shears. It is shade-dried in ventilated rooms. For domestic use, the herb can be harvested at any time, but preferably prior to flowering [Ü41].

Forms used: The fresh, and rarely the dried herb.

Storage: The fresh herb can be stored for a few days in plastic bags in the refrigerator. It also can be frozen in freezer bags in the deep freezer. The dried herb must be stored protected from light and moisture in airtight porcelain-, glass-, or suitable metal containers.

Description. Whole herb (Fig. 1): See description of the whole plant.

Cut herb: Characteristic are the fragments of the entire-margined leaves and leaf-tips with a short mucro as well as parts of the angular stem [EB 6].

Powdered herb: Gray-green, characterized by unicellular, short and hooked bristles, occurring on the leaf margin and on the lower leaf surface, as well as by numerous oxalate raphides in the mesophyll of leaf pieces [EB 6].

Odor: The fresh plant is odorless, the dried material smells like coumarin ("hay-like"), **Taste:** Spicy, bitter, somewhat astringent.

History: The use of sweet woodruff for making "May Day Punch" was already mentioned by a Benedictine monk in 854 [Ü42, Ü56].

Constituents and Analysis

Constituents

- Melilotoside: (*o*-Hydroxycinnamic acid glucoside, mostly occurring in *trans*-form, odorless). During drying or processing of the herb with 10 to 50% ethanol, the glucoside is cleaved by β-glucosidase, released upon tissue injury. The formed *o*-coumaric acid (*trans-o*-hydroxycinnamic acid) converts (probably catalyzed by an isomerase) to coumarinic acid (*cis-o*-hydroxycinnamic acid), which, by formation of lactone, transforms to the aroma-determining coumarin. The coumarin content of the fresh herb, using ethanol/water (1:1) as the extraction solvent, is 0.4 to 1.7% (calculated with reference to the dry weight, particularly high contents are reached in spring). The extractable amount of coumarin decreases rapidly upon drying of the herb (volatility of coumarin!) [3, 13, 14].
- Iridoids: About 0.3%, mainly asperuloside (asperulin), furthermore, monotropein, scandoside and desacetylasperulosidic acid [17, 18].
- Essential oil: Very small amount, over 200 volatile substances, including, among others, linalool, borneol, anethole, thujone, menthone, camphor, carvone, β-ionone, benzaldehyde, benzyl alcohol, 2-phenyl ethanol, thymol, 8-hydroxylinalool, dihydroactinidiolide, (*Z*)-hex-3-ene-1-ol and 7,11,15-trimethylhexadecan-2-one (the latter is a suitable marker for identification of woodruff extracts) [20].
- Phenylacrylic acids, phenolcarboxylic acids: Caffeic acid, *p*-coumaric acid, *p*-hydroxybenzoic acid, gallic acid [11].

The anthraquinone derivatives that are typical for Galium-species occur only in the roots [4].

Tests for Identity based on morphological and anatomical characteristics of herb and with TLC [Ü102].

Quantitative assay: The coumarin content is determined with quantitative TLC [13, 14].

Adulterations, Misidentifications and Impurities are possible with other Galium-species, e.g. *G. mollugo* L. or *G. sylvaticum* L., however, they all lack the typical coumarin odor.

o-Coumaric acid   Coumarinic acid   Coumarin

Actions and Uses

Actions: There are no known studies on the therapeutic action of sweet woodruff.

In animal tests (rats, dogs), coumarin in doses of 12.5 to 50 mg/kg body weight accelerates the dehydration of experimentally induced edema. This effect takes place through its antiphlogistic and its capillary stabilizing, therefore antiexudative and lymphokinetic action [7, 19].

The spasmogenic effect of pentetrazol and isonicotinic acid hydrazide in rats and guinea pigs was decreased by coumarin (50 or 100 mg/kg body weight) [22].

The growth of mammary gland tumors in rats was inhibited by coumarin and its metabolite 7-hydroxycoumarin (20 mg/kg body weight) [15]. Because in these cases the coumarin doses applied were very high, it is questionable, as to whether antitumor coumarin activities could be expected with therapeutic doses of sweet woodruff (1 g sweet woodruff corresponds to about 10 mg coumarin).

Toxicology: Based on existing data, there is no acute or chronic toxicity with the occasional use of woodruff as an aromatic additive at normal doses. The use of large amounts of "May Day Punch" can lead to drowsiness and headache [14].

High doses of coumarin, which, however, cannot be attained with the use of sweet woodruff, have acute toxicity. In animal tests at doses of 0.6 to 0.8 g (dog), 5 g (sheep) and 40 g (horse and cattle) per animal, coumarin induced narcosis, reduced reflex- and respiratory functions and led finally to a lethal coma. In humans, 4 g of coumarin may cause nausea, vomiting, headache, dizziness, and general weakness [Ü58].

In chronic administration of high doses of coumarin, a few animals (particularly rodents) developed liver necrosis and liver tumors. The degree of hepatotoxicity is dependent on the dose and the animal species. In rats for example, coumarin is metabolized in the liver mostly to the hepatotoxic coumarin-3,4-epoxide (alkylates DNA and proteins) [12]; in humans and old-world primates, with the intake of very small amounts of coumarin, it is mostly metabolized to the non-toxic 7-hydroxycoumarin (umbelliferone). In humans, it is likely that only very high doses of coumarin or a congenital deficiency of CYP2A6 (enzyme that catalyzes hydroxylation of coumarin to 7-hydroxycoumarin), lead to a relevant epoxidation of the coumarin. Coumarin-3,4-epoxide is metabolized, particularly in the liver, to the non-toxic acetyl-*S*-(3-coumarinyl)cysteine by reaction with reduced glutathione. If the detoxification capacity of the liver is limited, for example in cases of liver damage, liver damage can occur [6, 9].

Culinary use: The fresh and rarely the dried branches or sweet woodruff syrup (see below) are used as flavor ingredients. To add flavoring to liquids, the whole branches are added for 10 to 15 minutes, for sweet woodruff punch in wine, for non-alcoholic May drinks, and jellies, in apple- or grape juice, and for milk drinks in milk, after which time the branches are removed. For one to add sweet woodruff to hot dishes, one must pre-wilt it beforehand in order to make the glycoside cleavage possible. For the production of alcoholic beverages from fresh sweet woodruff herb, the starting concentration of ethanol should be maximum 50% because higher concentrations will denature β-glucosidase.

Sweet woodruff serves as a flavoring of sweet dishes, baked goods, apple-, pear-, strawberry- or melon compote as well as of apple- and grape juice. It is an indispensable component of sweet woodruff pudding and sweet woodruff parfait. It can also be used to improve the taste of marinades and sauces [Ü45, Ü51, 71, Ü90].

It is used as a flavor component of May Day Punches (May drink and May wine) and of lemonades. For May wine, not more than 3 g of fresh herb/liter should be used [14, Ü1].

Sweet woodruff syrup is made with 2 to 3 handfuls of sweet woodruff, 2 liters water, 3 kg sugar, 70 g citric acid, 6 slices of oranges and 3 lemon slices. The water is cooked with sugar and then cooled down to room temperature; the other ingredients are added and macerated for 1 to 2 days, frequently stirred. Afterwards the extract is decanted, poured into clean bottles and sealed [Ü75]. Sweet woodruff syrup is used as a flavoring of desserts, creams, and cakes.

Food law regulations: In the Federal Republic of Germany, the use of coumarin and sweet woodruff for the manufacture of essences is forbidden [2]. An exception is allowed for commercially produced May Day Punches that are made from sweet woodruff herb as long as the maximum amount of coumarin in the drink does not exceed 5 mg/l [1]. Instead of coumarin, 6-methylcoumarin (toncarine, cocodescol, maximum allowable limit 30 mg/kg), which has a coumarin-like odor, can be used [2, 16].

Other uses: Sweet woodruff bundles, which are hung up inside laundry closets, are supposed to repel moths.

Medicinal herb

Herbal drug: Asperulae oderatae herba (Galii odorati herba), Sweet woodruff herb [EB 6].

Indications: In folk medicine, sweet woodruff is used for the prevention and treatment of conditions and diseases of the respiratory tract, the gastrointestinal tract, the liver and gall bladder as well as the kidneys, and the lower urinary tract, furthermore for peripheral blood flow disorders, venous insufficiency and other venous diseases, hemorrhoids, as an anti-inflammatory and vascular widening remedy, moreover as a sedative for sleep disturbances, to promote readiness to fall asleep, as well as for spasms, abdominal pain, skin diseases, as a diaphoretic, roborant for nerves and heart, and also as a "blood purifier" [10]. The average single dose is 1 g [EB 6]. Efficacy for the above listed indications has not been proven. Therefore the therapeutic use of sweet woodruff was not approved by the Commission E of the German BfArM [10].

Similar culinary herbs

Tonka beans (Tonka seeds, elbo), seeds of *Dipteryx odorata* (AUBL.) WILLD. (Synonym: *Coumarouna odorata* AUBL.), rarely from other Dipteryx-species (Fabaceae), native to Northeastern South America (particularly Guyana and Venezuela, to Northeastern Brazil), cultivated in Venezuela, in Trinidad, and on other Caribbean Islands, rarely in tropical Africa (e.g. Nigeria), however it is obtained mainly from collection of wild populations. *Dipteryx odorata* is an up to 25 m high tree that resembles Robinia-species. Post-harvest the seeds are covered with rum (hydrolysis of melilotoside, see above [8]), which after 24 hours is poured off, followed by drying of the seeds. After fermentation they contain 1 to 3%, rarely up to 10% coumarin, coumarin in part is crystallized on the surface of the pruinose-looking seeds. Other identified compounds include, among others, dihydrocoumarin, melilotic acid, methyl melilotate, ethyl melilotate, terpinenol-4, fenchone, camphor, carvone, *p*-cymene, anethole, 1-phenylpropanol, 2-phenol ethanol, 2-phenylethylformiate, pentan-1-ol, hexanal, 2-butanone, 2-nonanone, nonanal and 5-hydroxymethylfurfural [5, 21]. Tonka beans are used for the flavoring of herbal- and bitter liqueurs, bakery products, ice creams, and tobacco as well as in the perfume industry. The use of tonka beans as a food ingredient in Germany is forbidden [Ü89, Ü92, Ü98].

May Day Punch

1 bottle of white wine or dry sparkling wine, 2 oranges (peeled and sliced), 2 sweet woodruff twigs.

Pour the wine into a large jug and add the orange slices with juice as well as the sweet woodruff twigs. Let the mixture stand for 10 minutes, remove the sweet woodruff and serve the punch with ice cubes [Ü74].

Literature

[1] Anonym, BGBl. I:1078 (1983), BGBl. I:256 (1986), BGBl. I:1266 (1986), BGBl. I:1386(1987).

[2] Anonym, BGBl. I:1625–1627 (1981), BGBl. I:601(1983), BGBl. I:897 (1984).

[3] Bourquelot E., H. Hérissey, Compt. Rend. 170:1545–1550 (1920).

[4] Burnett A.R., R.H. Thomson, Phytochemistry 7:1421 (1968), ref. Ü43.

[5] Ehlers D. et al., Z. Lebensm. Unters. Forsch. 201(3):278–282 (1995).

[6] Fentem J.H., J.R. Fry, Xenobiotica 22(3): 357–367 (1992).

[7] Földi-Börcsök E. et al., Arzneim. Forsch. 21:2025–2030 (1971).

[8] Haskins et al., Science 139:496 (1963), ref. Ü60.

[9] Huwer T. et al., Chem. Res. Toxicol. 4: 586–590 (1991).

[10] Kommission E beim BfArM., BAnz. Nr. 193 vom 15.10.87 (1987).

[11] Kooiman P., Acta Bot. Neerl. 18:124–137 (1966).

[12] Lake B.G. et al., Food Chem. Toxicol. 32:723–751 (1994).

[13] Laub E., W. Olszowski, Z. Lebensm. Unters. Forsch. 175:179 (1982).

[14] Laub E., W. Olszowski, R. Woller, Dtsch. Apoth. Ztg. 125:848–850 (1985).

[15] Maucher A., E. von Angerer, J. Cancer Res. Clin. Oncol 120(8):502–504 (1994).

[16] Seidemann J., Drogenreport 9(14):24–27 (1996).

[17] Sticher O., Pharm. Acta Helv. 46:121–128 (1971).

[18] Sticher O., Dtsch. Apoth. Ztg. 111:1795 (1971).

[19] Szabó G., Z. Magyar, Arzneim. Forsch. 27(II):2332–2335 (1977).

[20] Wörner M., P. Schreier, Z. Lebensm. Unters. Forsch. 193:3117–3120 (1991).

[21] Wörner M., P. Schreier, Z. Lebensm. Unters. Forsch. 193:21–25 (1991).

[22] Zoltan Ö, M. Földi, Arzneim. Forsch. 20(11a):1625 (1970).

Literature references identified by Ü can be found in the general listing of books and monographs at the back of this book.

Tamarind

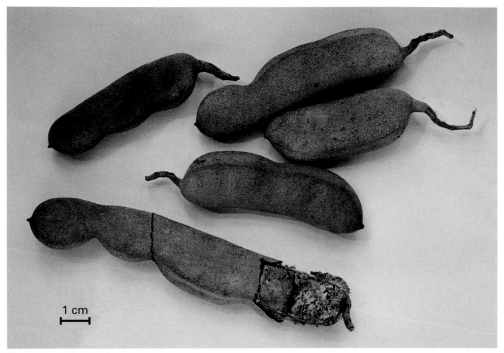

Fig. 1: Tamarind fruits

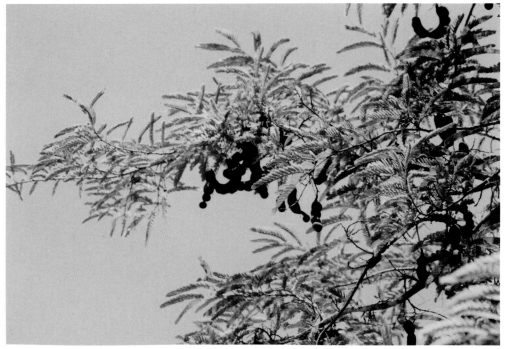

Fig. 2: Tamarind (*Tamarindus indica* L.)

Plant source: *Tamarindus indica* L.

Family: Cassia family (Caesalpiniaceae, with some authors also combining it with Fabaceae and Mimosaceae in the family of leguminous plants, Leguminosae).

Common names: Engl.: tamarind; Fr.: tamarinier, tamarine; Ger.: Tamarinde, Sauerdattel, Indische Dattel, Indische Feige.

Description: Evergreen tree, up to 30 m tall. Leaves are 5 to 12 cm long, paripinnate, pinnules in 10 to 20 pairs, glabrous, with narrow stipules that are caducous. The sweet scented flowers are arranged in terminal racemes. The cup shaped calyx has 4 membranous lobes, the 3 about 1 cm long petals are whitish, later becoming yellowish with red stripes, the 3 stamina are connate; the superior ovary is unilocular. The fruit is a gray-brown to yellowish-brown, up to 20 cm long and 3 cm wide indehiscent pod, often with many constrictions, it contains 3 to 12 seeds, surrounded with parchment-like endocarp. The seeds are roundish, shiny brown, up to 17 mm long. The mesocarp has a mash-like consistency and contains branched vascular bundles. Flowering period is from June to July [Ü60, Ü76].

Native origin: Probably native to tropical Eastern Africa, possibly already reaching India in prehistoric times, naturalized in many subtropical and tropical locations.

Main cultivation areas: Grown in almost all tropical and subtropical countries.

Main exporting countries: India, Pakistan, Myanmar, China, Islands of the West Indies (particularly Barbados), the Philippines, Java, and Spain.

Cultivation: Tamarind prefers dry tropical climates. Propagation is by seeds or cuttings. Tamarind is also planted as a shading avenue tree.

Culinary herb

Commercial forms: Tamarind: dried tamarind fruits, dried tamarind fruit slices, tamarind bricks (made from broken, pressed dried fruits), tamarind pulp (Asem Koening, West Indian or East Indian tamarind pulp, see below), sugarcoated tamarind balls.

Production: The fully ripe pods are harvested from wild growing trees or trees in plantations. To obtain tamarind pulp (Fig. 3), the pericarp is removed and the pulp with vascular bundle fibers and seeds enclosed is kneaded into a paste, with hot sugar syrup poured over and filled into casks (West Indian tamarind pulp) or after diminution of the consistency with hot water the pulp is freed from seeds and vascular bundles by filtering (East Indian tamarind pulp) [Ü92]. The pods are also cut and pressed into bricks or cut into slices and dried.

Forms used: Aqueous extracts of the pods or dilutions of tamarind concentrates.

Storage: The ripe pods are stored in dry form in a ventilated area. Tamarind pulp should be stored in closed containers (nonmetal containers, acids!) or plastic sacks in a cool location.

Description. Whole fruit (Fig. 1): Whole pods (see description of the plant) or black-brown, soft and viscous masses traversed with coarse vascular bundles (Fig. 3), which usually contain numerous seeds, enclosed by the parchment-like endocarp [DAB 6].
Microscopic image: The chloral hydrate slide preparation shows the numerous parenchymatic cells with brown content, as well as small starch grains, up to 18 μm in size, and many crystals. The vascular bundles contain many fibers. In the endo-carp, there is a layer of elongated, toothed stone cells and a layer of closely connected fibers. The testa consists of 1 or 2 rows of palisade sclereids [Ü49, Ü60].

Odor: Sweetish-sour, reminiscent of plum sauce, **Taste:** Strongly sour.

History: Tamarind pulp was already mentioned in the Vedic texts. Around 1270, the import of tamarind pulp from India to Greece has been reported. In the 15th century, it was introduced to the German herbal drug trade. In the 17th century, this tree was brought to the Caribbean and to Mexico by the Spaniards [Ü2, Ü55, Ü92].

Constituents and Analysis

Constituents of the pulp

- Fruit acids: 8 to 24%, D-(+)-tartaric acid (3 to 12%, partially occurring as potassium hydrogentartrate), citric acid, succinic acid, malic acid, lactic acid, formic acid and acetic acid, mostly in free form, but also partially in form of their salts [7].
- Monosaccharides: 20 to 40%, invert-sugar [5].
- Pectin [6].
- Aroma substances: In traces (about 10 mg/kg), in the steam-distillate, 66 components have been identified, main components furfural, 2-acetylfuran, 5-methylfurfural, 5-methyl-2 (3H)furanone (furan derivatives are artifacts which were probably formed during steam distillation by acid-catalyzed dehydration of monosaccharides), ethyl

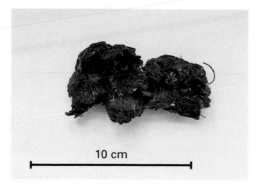

Fig. 3: Tamarind pulp

acetate, *trans*-hex-2-enol, hexanol, isobutanol, phenylacetaldehyde, isopropylvinylether, 2-ethylthiazol, 2-methylthiazol and pyrazine [1, 9, 13, 17, 19]. After extraction with supercritical CO_2, aromadendrene has been found to be the main component (90% of the extract) [13].

Constituents of the seeds
- Proteins: 15 to 20%.
- Ketonic acids: γ-Methyl-α-ketoglutaric acid, γ-methylene-α-ketoglutaric acid [11].
- Mucilage (tamarind mucilage): D-galacto-D-xylo-D-glucanes, the backbone is made up of β-1→4-linked glucose moieties, in the side chains mostly α-1→6 linked D-xylose moieties with partial β-1→2-glycosidic linkage to D-galactose moieties, also, in smaller amounts, L-arabinose and glucuronic acid moieties, M_r about 50 000 da, producing highly viscous solutions with cold water; in presence of highly concentrated saccharose solutions, it gelatinizes without the addition of acid [3, 15, 16, 18, Ü98].
- Fatty oil (about 20%) [Ü60].

Tests for Identity are carried out with macroscopic and microscopic examination as well as by detection of tartaric acid with TLC [12].

Quantitative assay of the water-extractable matter with gravimetric method [DAB 6]. Acid content is determined titrimetrically [DAB 6]; the content of the individual acids can be determined with HPLC [10], as acid esters with GC [10] or as *p*-nitrobenzylester with HPLC [2].

Adulterations, Misidentifications and Impurities have not been reported in recent times. In the past, adulteration of tamarind pulp with prune pulp has been observed.

Actions and Uses

Actions: Due to its spicy acid taste, tamarind pulp is appetite stimulating and digestion promoting.

Because of difficult absorbability of the fruit acids and their salts, tamarind pulp has osmotic laxative action.

Polysaccharide fractions of tamarind fruits have shown in vitro immunostimulant properties [14]. Similar to many other mucilaginous substances (see Actions: → Fenugreek), tamarind mucilage reduces the intestinal absorption of food constituents by elevation of viscosity and retarding the diffusion speed. Thereby it prevents postprandial blood sugar peaks. A hypoglycemic effect was demonstrated in studies with diabetic rats [4].

Toxicology: Based on existing data, there is no acute or chronic toxicity with the use of tamarind pulp as a spice at normal doses. L-(–)-Di-n-butyl malate had in vitro cytotoxic effects on sea urchin eggs [8].

Culinary use: Tamarind pulp (Asem) plays a considerable role in India in the preparation of soft drinks (Asem water, tamarind water), fruit syrups, marmalades, chutneys and relishes; salted, it is served with fish (tamarind fish), and it is also used as a seasoning for lentil- and vegetable dishes (sambhars) or strongly spiced lentil soups (rasams). In Thailand, sour soups are prepared with tamarind pulp. In Jamaica, the fruit is used as a flavoring for rice- and stew dishes as well as for desserts [Ü2, Ü73, Ü98]. Most practical for use in cooking is the commercially available tamarind pulp (tamarind concentrate) with the seeds and pods removed. From the fruit pulp obtained from the pods, from tamarind blocks, tamarind slices or tamarind pulp, an extract is made by soaking in as much warm water as needed to make it pourable. The seeds and remains of the pods are separated from the fruit pulp and the resulting liquid is filtered through a plastic sieve or through gauze (not a metal sieve, acids!). This extract is used as a seasoning. If not used immediately, it should be stored in the refrigerator.

In Central Europe, tamarind pulp serves as a component in the production of chutneys, semi-frozen food items, bakery goods, soft drinks, syrups, marmalades and jellies. However it is also suitable as a sea-soning of sour soups, stews, rice, lentils, seafoods (especially of shrimps), meat- and poultry dishes [Ü53, Ü55, Ü68, Ü91]. In the liqueur industry, tamarind pulp is also used, e.g. as a component of bitter liqueurs (Erzgebirgs-Bitter) [Ü92].

As a component of spice mixes and preparations: → Worcestershire sauce.

Other uses: Tamarind pulp is used in the tobacco industry for the flavoring of chewing and smoking tobacco. The seeds of tamarind are used as a feed for cattle. After roasting or soaking of the seeds, the seed coats are peeled off and then the seeds are eaten boiled or fried, respectively; they are also used to produce flour for baking. Tamarind mucilage is used in the food industry as a gelatinizing and thickening agent as well as a stabilizer, e.g. in ice cream and mayonnaises, or in pharmaceutical technology as a binder for tablets. In the textile industry, it is used as a finish. The fatty oil of the seeds can be used for the manufacture of dyes and varnishes. The sourish smelling young flowers, leaves, unripe fruits and cotyledons are used as a vegetable. The reddish-yellow pigments (anthoxanthins) of the leaves can be used as a dye for wool or silk [Ü61].

Medicinal herb

Herbal drugs: Tamarindorum pulpa cruda, Tamarind pulp, Tamarindorum pulpa depurata, Purified tamarind pulp [DAB 6].

Indications: As a laxative for constipation (dose 10 to 50 g purified tamarind pulp), also used for hepato- and biliary complaints [Ü37].

Furfural   5-Methylfurfural   2-Acetylfuran   Aromadendrene

Literature

[1] Askar A. et al., Dtsch. Lebensm. Rdsch. 83:108–110 (1987).

[2] Badoud R., G. Pratz, J. Chromatogr. 360: 119–136 (1986).

[3] Courtois J.E. et al., Carbohydr. Res. 49: 439–449 (1976).

[4] Ibrahim N.A. et al., Acta Hortic. 390 (Intern. Symp. Medic. Aromat. Plants 1994): 51–57 (1995), ref. CA 126: 222849.

[5] Ishola M.M. et al., J. Sci. Food Agric. 51: 141–143 (1990).

[6] Karawya M.S. et al., Planta Med. (Suppl): 68–75 (1980).

[7] Khurana A.L., C.T. Ho, J. Liq. Chromatogr. 12:419–430 (1989).

[8] Kobayashi A. et al., Z. Naturforsch. C: Biosc. 51(3/4):233–242 (1996).

[9] Lee P.L. et al., J. Agric. Food Chem. 23: 1195–1199 (1975).

[10] Linskens H.F., J.F. Jackson (Eds.): Analysis of Nonalcoholic Beverages, Springer-Verlag Berlin, Heidelberg 1988.

[11] Mukherjee D., M.M. Laloraya, Biochem. Physiol. Pflanz. 166:429–436 (1974).

[12] Rohdewald P. et al.: Apothekengerechte Prüfvorschriften, Dtsch. Apoth. Verlag Stuttgart 1986, 1. Erg. Lfg. 1992.

[13] Sagrero-Nieves L. et al., J. Ess. Oil Res. 6:547–548 (1994).

[14] Sreelekha T.T. et al., Anticancer Drugs 4(2):209–213 (1993).

[15] Srivastava H.C., P.P. Singh, Carbohydr. Res. 4:326–342 (1967).

[16] Taylor I.E.P., E.D.T. Atkins, FEBS Lett. 181:300–302 (1985).

[17] Wong K.C. et al., J. Ess. Oil Res. 10:219–221 (1998).

[18] Youcef A.D. et al., Carbohydr. Res. 61: 169–173 (1978).

[19] Zhang Y.G. et al., J. Ess. Oil Res. 2:197–198 (1990).

Literature references identified by Ü can be found in the general listing of books and monographs at the back of this book.

Tansy

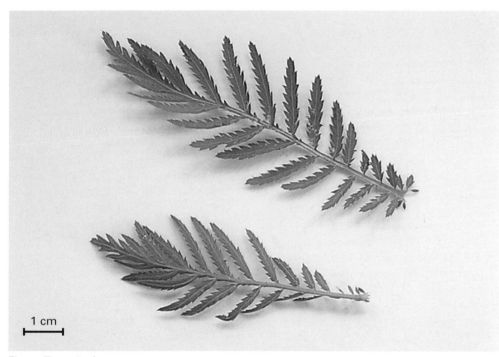

Fig. 1: Tansy leaf

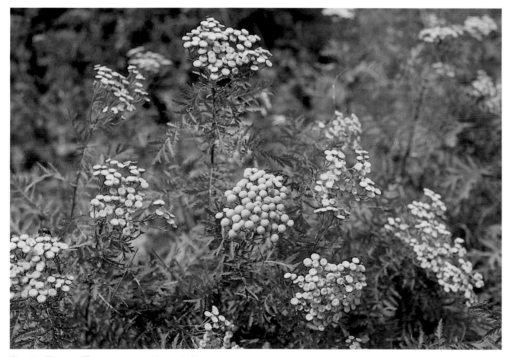

Fig. 2: Tansy (*Tanacetum vulgare* L.)

Plant source: *Tanacetum vulgare* L.

Synonyms: *Chrysanthemum vulgare* (L.) BERNH., *Chrysanthemum tanacetum* KARSCH.

Taxonomic classification: *Tanacetum vulgare* can be divided, depending on the shape of the leaflets, into the varieties *T. v.* f. *typicum* BECK, *T. v.* f. *tenuisectum* BECK and *T. v.* f. *crispum* DC.

Family: Composite plants (Asteraceae, synonym Compositae).

Common names: Engl.: tansy, common tansy, golden-buttons, bitter buttons; Fr.: tanaisie, tanacée, athanase, barbotine, ganelle; Ger: Rainfarn, Wurmkraut, Milchkraut, Frauenkraut, Donnerkraut, Gänserich.

Description: Perennial plant, up to 1.2 m tall. Stalk angulate, branched in the upper part. The leaves are up to 25 cm long and up to 20 cm wide, petiolated in the lower part of the stalk, sessile and amplexicaul in the upper part, initially hairy, contours obovate, single or double pinnatisect, with pinnules with a sharply serrate margin. The 8 to 10 mm wide capitula are arranged in terminal paniculate corymbs, their coat consists of many layers of tegular arranged leaflets, the receptacle is leafless, ligulate flowers are lacking, the tubular flowers are golden-yellow colored. Flowering period is from July to September [44, Ü37].

Native origin: Europe up to the Caucasus, Armenia, Siberia, naturalized in North America.

Main cultivation areas: Rarely cultivated in Europe, for essential oil production it is cultivated in India, and in the USA.

Main exporting countries: No commercial trade of significance.

Cultivation: Tansy prefers nutrient rich, not too dry, humic sandy-, loam- or clay soil. Propagation is carried out through advance planting in trays in the spring. The seedlings are reset at a distance of about 45 cm. Propagation can also be carried out with root runners in the spring or autumn. Tansy spreads rapidly in gardens! Cultivation in tubs is possible. Industrial cultivation rarely occurs due to the low demand. There are a few ornamental varieties (*T. v.* 'Isala Gold', *T. v.* 'Silver Lace') [Ü68].

Culinary herb

Commercial forms: Not in European commerce.

Production: For culinary end use the fresh leaves are taken, for pharmaceutical end use the herb or flowers are harvested during the flowering period.

Forms used: Fresh leaves, and rarely the dried leaves.

Storage: The fresh leaves stay fresh in plastic bags in the refrigerator for a few days. They can also be frozen in freezer bags or chopped and frozen with water in the ice-tray.

Description. Whole leaf (Fig. 1): For the leaf, see description of the plant; microscopical examination reveals the 5- to 7-celled hairs.

Odor: Aromatic, camphor-like, **Taste:** Aromatic, with persistent bitterness.

History: Its cultivation was already made mandatory in the government decree "Capitulare de villis" (authored in about 795, see footnote → Anise) by Karl the Great. Hildegard von Bingen (1110 to 1179) recommended tansy as a spice for confectioneries and baked goods, as well as for meat and sausage dishes. During the Elizabethan era in England, tansy was especially known as a spice for cakes [Ü92].

Constituents and Analysis

Constituents

- Essential oil: 0.5 to 0.9%, in the fresh leaves about 0.2%. There are numerous chemical races. The main components of the essential oil can be, among others, artemisia ketone, bornyl acetate, carvacrol, *trans*-chrysanthenol/chrysanthenyl acetate, 1,8-cineole, camphor, davadone D, dihydrocarvone, germacrene D, linalool, lyratol/lyratyl acetate, α-pinene, piperitone, α- and β-sabinene, β-terpinyl acetate, (+)- or (–)-thujone and umbellulone. Mixed types also occur, which also contain, among others, artemisia alcohol, camphor, chrysanthenol, 1,8-cineole, davadone D, lyratol, lyratyl acetate, myrcene, terpinenol-4 and tricyclene in relatively high concentrations. Also detected were, among other components, borneol, camphene, dihydrocarvone, carveol, chrysanthenone, isobornyl acetate, limonene, *cis*-longipinane-2,7-dione, pinocarvone, sabinaketone and (+)-vulgarone A and B. Chemical races occur within regional limits; they were found to be especially diverse in Hungary (38 races) and Finland (15 races). By hybridization of pure races, mixed types could be produced. In Central Europe, races with a high (+)-thujone content (37 to 96%) of the essential oil are predominant. In Germany, 6 types with mostly (–)-thujone, (+)-thujone or (–)-camphor have been found up to this date. The essential oils from the leaves and flowers have different compositions [3, 5, 8–12, 14, 16, 19, 22, 23, 26, 32, 33, 38–40, Ü37, Ü100].
- Sesquiterpene lactones: Over 20 race-specific constituents, including armefolin, artemorin, chrysanthemin, costunolide epoxide, crispolide, desacetylpyrethrosin, parthenolide, pyrethrosin, reynosin, santamarin, tamirin (desacetylchrysanolide), tanacetin, tanachin (desacetyldihydrochrysanolide), tatri-

din A, tatridin B and vulgarolide, among others. The sesquiterpene lactones are responsible for the bitter taste [4, 35].
- Flavonoids: Apigenin-7-glucoside, luteolin-7-glucoside, luteolin-7-glucuronide, 6-hydroxyluteolin-7-glucoside, acacetin-7-glucobioside, epatilin, cosmosiin, cynaroside, orientin, tilianin, among others, and also methylated analogs, particularly methylether of scutellarein and 6-hydroxyluteolin [1, 25, 27, 45].
- Hydroxycinnamic acid derivatives: Chlorogenic acid, isochlorogenic acid, among others [Ü37].
- Polyines: Ponticaepoxide, artemisiaketone, *trans*-dehydromatricaria ester, di- and terthiophenes (among others, 5-(methyl-prop-1-inyl)-2-thiophene-acrylate and 5-(4-acetoxy-1-butenyl)-2,2′-bithenyl, phototoxic!) [6, 41].
- Triterpenes, sterols: α- and β-amyrine, β-sitosterol and stigmasterol, among others [7, 15].

Tests for Identity: Tansy can be identified with macroscopic and microscopic analysis. The essential oil composition for the distinction of the chemical races can be determined with GC or GC-MS [8, 9, 14, 17, 18].

Quantitative assay: The content of essential oil is determined volumetrically with steam distillation, based on the method of the European Pharmacopoeia, with xylol in the graduated tube [Ph Eur].

Actions and Uses

Actions: Due to its spicy-bitter taste it has appetite stimulating and digestion promoting action.

The chloroform soluble constituents of the dried herb have antiinflammatory effects. In relatively high doses (80 to 160 mg/kg body weight), oral application reduced the extent of Freunds-Adjuvant-induced inflammation of the rat-tail [31]. Local application suppressed the development of TPA (12-*O*-tetradecanoylphorbol-13-acetate)-induced mouse ear edema [37]. The genesis of gastric ulcers in rats, induced through administration of absolute ethanol, was slowed down by oral application of pure parthenolide and of the chloroform extractable active principles of tansy [42].

Tansy oil and its isolated sesquiterpene lactones have an antimicrobial effect [19–21, 24, 33, 36].

Numerous in vitro studies with ascarides, earthworms and leeches prove the anthelmintic action of (thujone-containing?) extracts and essential oils of tansy. Positive therapeutic outcomes after use of tansy as an anthelmintic have also been reported [36]. Tansy or its essential oil act as a repellent for various insects including potato beetles, among others [10].

Toxicology: Based on existing data, there is no acute or chronic toxicity with the occasional use of tansy as a spice in typical doses. However, lethal cases have been observed when tansy extracts were used in high doses as an abortifacient [36].

In addition to the local, irritant effect, following absorption thujone exhibits central excitatory and psychotomimetic effects. Chronic consumption leads to permanent damage of the CNS as well as to disturbances of the liver, kidney and cardiac functions [34, 36, Ü58, Ü100]. Poisonings with tansy, however, have only been observed with therapeutic use of very high doses (possibly using materials with a high thujone content) or with misuse of the drug as an abortifacient. Symptoms included gastroenteritis, convulsions, but also paralysis, cardiac arrhythmia, liver and kidney damage [2, 28, 36, Ü58]. Since the amount used for seasoning is very low, any adverse effects on human health based on the thujone content can be ruled out. Chronic use, however, should be avoided. Tansy herb should not be used during pregnancy.

The sensitization potential of tansy herb is moderate; cases of contact dermatitis have been documented. Cross-reactions with other Asteraceae (e.g. chrysanthemums, motherwort or chamomile) have been observed [30, Ü39]. The essential oil from tansy herb is highly toxic in doses of 7 to 15 g; doses above 15 g are fatal to humans [Ü58, Ü100].

Culinary use: Tansy is used today only in England to a large extent. Due to its bitter, penetrating taste it must be measured carefully. The fine-cut pinnules from 2 to 3 fresh, young leaves are enough for a salad- or meat dish.

Fresh, finely chopped tansy leaves can be used as a seasoning of omelets, meat dishes (e.g. braised meat, lamb), egg dishes, freshwater fish (in the fillings), sausage, mixed drinks, salads, dressings, dips, vinaigrettes, quark, and cream cheese. In England, the powder of dried tansy leaves is used in the same manner as cinnamon, especially at the Easter holiday as a component of cakes, pancakes and puddings, but also of rhubarb- and gooseberry-cream dishes [Ü1, Ü2, Ü17, Ü65, Ü79].

The fresh leaves can be used to smear onto meat before grilling.

In a few countries, Germany among them, tansy is not allowed as an ingredient for the production of flavors and essences for the food industry [Ü55, Ü92].

Combines well with: Marjoram, parsley, and thyme.

Other uses: Dried pansy herb is used in moth bags to keep the insects away from laundry and clothing [Ü2, Ü47].

Medicinal herb

Herbal drugs: Tanaceti flos, Tansy flower, contains minimum 0.8% essential oil [EB 6], Tanaceti herba, Tansy herb, contains minimum 0.25% essential oil [EB 6], Tanaceti aetheroleum, Tansy oil [EB 6].

Indications: The herb, flowers and essential oil of tansy were used prior to the development of synthetic anthelmintic drugs, in the same way as other thujone-containing drugs, e.g. absinthe, predominantly as a vermifuge for treating ascariasis and oxyuriasis. Moreover these drugs were used for treating, among other conditions, indigestion, digestive disorders, dysmenorrhea, gout and rheumatism. In more recent times, it has also been used for migraine and neuralgia. The average single-dose for the leaves is 1 g, for the herb 2 g, for the essential oil 0.1 g [36]. Due to the sensitization potential and the possibly high thujone content, the therapeutic use of tansy is not recommended [28].

Other Tanacetum-species used as culinary herbs

Balsam herb (alecost, costmary, Roman balsam), *Tanacetum balsamita* L. (Synonym: *Chrysanthemum balsamita* (L.) L.), native to Asia Minor, Transcaucasia, and Northern Iran, and naturalized in the Balkan countries, Southern Italy, France, and Spain, today only rarely cultivated, almost exclusively in gardens as an ornamental plant. The main components of its essential oil are L-camphor (72 to 86%, predominantly in the variety *T. b.* var. *balsamita*, without white ray florets), or camphor + thujone [13, 43, 46, 47]. In hexane extracts of the dried plant of Brazilian origin, numerous α,β-unsaturated aldehydes including (*E*)-hept-2-enal, among others, with high antimicrobial activity have been detected [29]. The fresh leaves are used especially in England for the seasoning of soups (e.g. carrot soup), game-, poultry-, mutton- and lentil dishes, in Russia also of sweet dishes and cakes (e.g. plum cakes), and of homemade beer and kvass. The fresh leaves are used as a vegetable [Ü74, Ü45, Ü92].

Literature

[1]   Adikhoedzhaeva K.B. et al., Farmatsiya (Moskau) 27:24–28 (1978).
[2]   Antonov N., G. Iotob, Nevro. Psichiat. Neurochirurg 23:281 (1984).
[3]   Appendino G. et al., Phytochemistry 23: 2545–2551 (1984).
[4]   Appendino G. et al., Phytochemistry 21: 1099–1102 (1982).
[5]   Bankowski C., Z. Chabudzinski, Acta Pol. Pharm. 31(6):755–757 (1974).

[6] Bohlmann F. et al., Chem. Ber. 97: 1179–1192 (1964).

[7] Chandler R.F. et al., Lipids 17(2): 102–106 (1982).

[8] Charles R. et al., J. Ess. Oil Res. 11: 406–408 (1999).

[9] Collin G.J. et al., J. Ess. Oil Res. 5:629–638 (1993).

[10] De Pooter H.L. et al., J. Ess. Oil Res. 1:9–13 (1989).

[11] Forsen K., M. von Schantz, Arch. Pharmaz. 304:944–952 (1971).

[12] Gallino M., Planta Med. 54:182 (1988).

[13] Göckeritz D., Pharmazie 23:515–518 (1968).

[14] Hendriks H. et al., J. Ess. Oil Res. 2:155–162 (1990).

[15] Hendriks H., R. Bos, Planta Med. 56: 540 (1990).

[16] Hendriks H., R. Bos, Woerdenbag, Z. Phytother. 14(6):333–336 (1993).

[17] Héthelyi E. et al., Biomed. Envir. Mass Spectrom. 14:627–632 (1987), ref. in Ü37.

[18] Héthelyi E. et al., Herba Hung. 27: 89–105 (1988).

[19] Héthelyi E. et al., Phytochemistry 20: 1847–1850 (1981).

[20] Héthelyi E. et al., Herba Hung. 30:82–90 (1991).

[21] Héthelyi E. et al., Herba Hung. 28: 99–115 (1989).

[22] Hethelyi E(va) et al., Olaj, Szappan, Kozmet. 45(3):109–114 (1996), ref. in CA: 125:163460p.

[23] Holopainen M. et al., Planta Med. 53: 284–287 (1987).

[24] Holopainen M. et al., Planta Med. 55:102 (1989).

[25] Ivancheva S., M. Behar, Fitoterapia 66(4):373 (1995), ref. CA 124:025548b.

[26] Keskitalo M. et al., Biochem. Syst. Ecol 29(3):267–285 (2001).

[27] Khovorost P.P. et al., Med. Prom. S.S.S.R. 20(2):19–21 (1966).

[28] Kommission E beim BfArM., BAnz-Nr. 122 vom 06.07.1988.

[29] Kubo A., Kubo I., J. Nat. Prod. 58(10): 1565–1569 (1995).

[30] Mark K.A. et al., Arch. Dermatol. 135(1):67–70 (1999).

[31] Mordujevich-Buschiazzo P. et al., Fitoterapia 67:319–322 (1996).

[32] Nano G.M. et al., Planta Med. 35: 270–274 (1979).

[33] Neszmelyi G.W.A. et al., J. Ess. Oil Res. 4:243–250 (1992).

[34] Rice K.C., R.S. Wilson, J. Med. Chem. 19:1054 (1976).

[35] Sanz J.F., J.A. Marco, J. Nat. Prod. 54: 591–596 (1991).

[36] Schenck G., W.H. Hein, Pharmazie 4: 520–521 (1949), siehe auch 2:524 (1947) und 3:284 (1948).

[37] Schinella G.R. et al., J. Pharm. Pharmacol. 50(9):1069–1074 (1998).

[38] Stahl E., D. Scheu, Arch. Pharmaz. 300: 456–458 (1967).

[39] Stahl E., D. Scheu, Naturwissenschaften 52:394 (1965).

[40] Stahl E., G. Schmitt, Arch. Pharm. 298: 385–391 (1964).

[41] Tosi B. et al., Phytother. Res. 5:59–62 (1991).

[42] Tournier H. et al., J. Pharm. Pharmacol. 51(2):215–219 (1999).

[43] Voigt R.F. et al., J. Am. Pharm. Assoc. 27:643 (1938).

[44] Weymar H., Buch der Korbblütler, Neumann Verlag, Radebeul 1957.

[45] Williams C.A. et al., Phytochemistry 51(3):417–423 (1999), Erratum in Phytochemistry 52(6): 1181–1182.

[46] Wolbis M., Acta Pol. Pharm. 36:707–714 (1979).

[47] Wolbis M., Acta Pol. Pharm. 38:705–710 (1981).

Literature references identified by Ü can be found in the general listing of books and monographs at the back of this book.

Tarragon

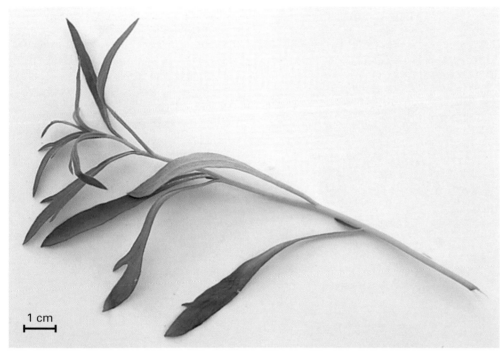

Fig. 1: Tarragon leaf

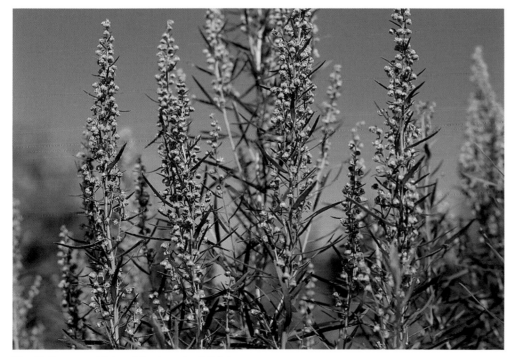

Fig. 2: Tarragon (*Artemisia dracunculus* L.)

Plant source: *Artemisia dracunculus* L.

Family: Composite plants (Asteraceae, synonym Compositae).

Common names: Engl.: tarragon, estragon, dragon sagewort; Fr.: estragon, dragon, herbe dragonne; Ger: Estragon, Bertram, Drachantkraut, Dragon, Dragonbeifuß, Dragunwermut, Eierkraut, Esdragon, Escadronkraut, Kaisersalat, Schlangenkraut.

Description: Perennial herb, stem up to 1.5 m high, branched, bushy, glabrous, root beet-like, creeping. Leaves sessile, lanceolate to linear, the lower ones triple-forked at the tips, entire margined, 3 to 8 cm long and 0.3 to 1 cm wide. The anthodia are arranged in loose, racemose panicles, nodding, nearly spherical, 2 to 3 mm wide, outer involucral leaves oblong elliptic, mostly green, the inner ones are ovate, with a wide, skin-like margin; the base of the receptacle is glabrous, with only tubular florets. Corolla whitish-green, then brownish-red; marginal florets female, the ones in the middle only with stamens. Flowering period is from July to October [22, Ü37].

Native origin: Southern- and Eastern Russian Federation, Afghanistan, Mongolia, Western North America, and also introduced via cultivation in Central Europe, North America (from Colorado to Texas), and Northern Mexico.

Main cultivation areas: Southern France, Italy, Germany (Bavaria and Saxony-Anhalt), Republics of the former Yugoslavia, the Netherlands, Russian Federation, Egypt, USA, Brazil, Argentina, India, and Indonesia.

Main exporting countries: France, Germany, Southern Europe, and the Russian Federation.

Cultivation: Tarragon prefers fresh, humus soil in warm, sunny or half-shaded locations and a good water supply. After 3 to 4 years in the same location, a cultivation pause is necessary. Growing tarragon in the vicinity of parsley should be avoided. Propagation of Russian tarragon takes place through direct seeding in April, and French tarragon must be propagated due to its sterility, with approximately 5 cm long head cuttings which take root in summer under foil, or by root cuttings planted in May or in the late autumn. The plants should be spaced about 30 × 40 cm. For personal use, 1 to 2 plants are sufficient. It is possible to cultivate tarragon in buckets if stored during winter in a frost-free and dry location. Cultivated regional varieties include 'Russian (or Siberian) tarragon' (*A. d.* f. *redowskii* hort., also known as *A. dracunculoides*; fertile, undemanding, frost tolerant), 'Aromatic (or French or German) tarragon' (*A. d.* f. *dracunculus*; sterile, vegetative propagation only, prefers nutrient-rich soil and warm locations, frost-sensitive), and the Hungarian variety 'Zöldzamat' (Type: aromatic tarragon) [Ü21, Ü96].

Culinary herb

Commercial forms: Tarragon: dried leaves, dried herb, the fresh bundled or cut, deep-frozen herb (in the vegetable trade), herb tops, and the essential oil of tarragon.

Production: Tarragon can be harvested at the time of bud formation in the first year at the end of August, and in the second year in June and September. For personal use, fresh leaves or shoot tips can be clipped off regularly [Ü21].

Forms used: Fresh or dried leaves, and the fresh shoot tips.

Storage: The fresh leaves and shoot tips stay fresh wrapped in plastic and stored in the refrigerator for a few days. They can also be chopped and frozen with water in the ice tray or kept in oil or vinegar. The dried herb is stored in well-sealed glass-, porcelain- or suitable metal containers, protected from light, heat and moisture. During drying and storage, tarragon loses its aroma quickly.

Description. Whole herb (Fig. 1): See description of the plant.

Odor: Aromatic, **Taste:** French tarragon: anise-like, spicy, mildly bitter, weakly burning. Russian tarragon: distinctly bitter, chervil-like.

History: Tarragon has a long history of use as a medicinal- and culinary herb in Central Asia and Siberia. In the 13th century, it was brought to Europe by the crusaders [Ü86, Ü92].

Constituents and Analysis

DIN- and ISO-Standards: ISO-Standard 7926 (Dried tarragon).

Constituents

- Essential oil:
  French tarragon: 0.25 to 3.1%, the main components are estragole (methylchavicol, 58 to 80%, with anise-like odor), *trans*-β-ocimene (5 to 22%), *cis*-β-ocimene (5 to 14%), anethole (up to 10%), and in herb material of some provenances also γ-terpinene (up to 17%); other constituents include limonene (up to 4%), sabinene, eugenol, elemicin, myrcene and α-pinene.
  Russian tarragon: 0.1 to 2.1%, mainly sabinene (30 to 48%), methyl eugenol (eugenol methyl ether, 9 to 29%), elemicin (5 to 28%), isoelemicin (prop-2-enyl-analogue of elemicin, 11 to 19%) as well as *trans*- and *cis*-β-ocimene (4 to 12%), nerolidol and spathulenol, among others [2, 3, 7, 15–18, 20].
- Glucosides of eugenol, 8-hydroxygeraniol, vomifoliol and (*Z*)-hexene-3-enol [7].

- Hydroxycinnamic acid derivates: *p*-Hydroxyphenylethyl-*O*-β-D-glucoside-6′-caffeat [7].
- Lignans [7].
- Polyines: Capillarin, hepta-4,6-diyn-1,3-diol and its 1-*O*-β-D-glucoside, among others [5–7].
- Flavonoids: Glycosides of quercetin, patuletin, pinocembrin, naringenin, hesperitin, eriodyctiol, annagenin (annagenin-8-*O*-L-rhamnoside = estragonoside) and the lipophilic 3′-dihydroxy-7,4′-dimethoxyflavone (a strong fish poison) [1, 7–9, 21, Ü43].
- Hydroxycoumarins: Herniarin, scopoletin, scoparone [14, 19, Ü94].
- Isocoumarins: Artemidin, artemidal, artemidinol, among others [6, 10].
- Cyclitols: Pinit (0.5 to 0.9%) [13].

Tests for Identity: Macroscopic and microscopic analysis of the herb or TLC of the essential oil [16].

Quantitative assay: Following the volumetric steam distillation method of the Ph Eur with xylol in the graduated tube.

Adulterations, Misidentifications and Impurities: None known.

Actions and Uses

Actions: Due to its aromatic, slightly pungent and mildly bitter taste it is appetite stimulating and digestion promoting. Tarragon essential oil has shown antimicrobial action [11]. Other pharmacological studies on the activity of tarragon and tarragon essential oil are not known.

Toxicology: Based on existing data, there is no acute or chronic toxicity with the normal use of tarragon as a spice. Estragole, which occurs in high concentrations in French tarragon, had hepatocarcinogenic effects in animal tests (rats, mice) [4, 12, see also: → Fennel]. The use of estragole in foods is not permitted in EU countries. Due to low essential oil levels in the herb, negative effects on human health are not to be expected. In the USA, it is classified as a food additive permitted for direct addition to food for human consumption (§172.515), however in California estragole has been added to the list of chemicals known to the State to cause cancer, and may not be added to foods.

Culinary use: Tarragon is an indispensable spice in not only French cooking but also in Armenian cooking. It is also very popular in the USA. French tarragon has a spicier taste than Russian tarragon, the latter is recommended less. Due to its intense taste, tarragon is used only sparingly. Its aroma intensifies with cooking. Dried tarragon must be used in larger quantities due to the rapid loss of the aroma during drying and storage.

The fresh leaves or shoot tips, and less often the dried herb, serve as a spice for salads (especially tomato-, eggplant-, and zucchini salads, but also for green salads, fish-, meat- and potato salads, and even fruit salads), mixed pickles, cucumber-, pumpkin-, and tomato conserves, sauces (sauce béarnaise, sauce hollandaise, ravigotte sauce, gribiche sauce, tartar sauce, mustard sauce), marinades, meat- and fish soups, meat dishes (e.g. sauerbraten, mutton, veal), poultry dishes (e.g. poultry ragouts, poulet à l'estragon), ground meats, fish dishes (e.g. eel, trout), shrimp, crabs, lobster, scallops, vegetables (carrots, tomatoes), mushrooms, potato salads, eggs in aspic, omelets, quark, soft cheeses and canapés, as well as for the production of tarragon butter, tarragon vinegar and tarragon cooking mustard [Ü13, Ü23, Ü30, Ü55, Ü65, Ü74, Ü79, Ü81].

Combines well with: Chervil, chives, parsley, pepper, rosemary, shallots, and thyme. The aroma of tarragon easily masks that of other spices, therefore in spice combinations it should be used sparingly.

As a component of spice mixes and preparations: → Bouquet garni, → Pickling spice, → Fines Herbes, → Frankfurter green sauce, → Hamburger meat spice, →

Herb butter, → Herb oil, → Herb vinegar, → Mixed pickles spice, → Parisian pepper, → Roast spice, → Sauce spice, → Table mustard, → Venison spice.

Other uses: The essential oil is used in the liqueur and perfume industries.

Other Artemisia species used as culinary spices: → Mugwort.

Medicinal herb

Herbal drug: Dracunculi herba, Tarragon herb.

Cold Tarragon-Cucumber Soup
(Serves 6)
1 cucumber (about 500 g), 1 shallot, 1/2 l cold broth, 1 to 2 teaspoons of fresh tarragon, 1 teaspoon (tarragon)-mustard, 1 teaspoon (tarragon)-vinegar, 200 g crème fraîche, 2 tablespoons olive oil, table salt, 100 g crab meat, 2 teaspoons graded (organic) lemon peels and tarragon leaves to garnish.

Wash the cucumber, keep a few slices for garnishing; peel the rest and cut the cucumber longitudinally, remove the seeds and dice it into small cubes. Peel the shallot and dice. Remove the fat from the broth, chop the tarragon and mix it with the cucumber pieces, shallot, broth, tarragon, mustard, vinegar and crème fraîche, and olive oil, then puree with a mixer, add salt to taste and place the dish in refrigerator. Mix again quickly before serving and garnish with cucumber slices, crabmeat, lemon peels and tarragon leaves [Ü95].

Literature

[1] Balza F., G.H.N. Towers, Phytochemistry 23:2333–2337 (1984).
[2] De Vincenzi M. et al., Fitoterapia 71(6):725–729 (2000).
[3] Deans S.G, K.P. Svoboda, J. Hortic. Sci. 63:503–508 (1988).
[4] Drinkwater N.R. et al., J. Nat. Cancer Inst. 57:1323–1331 (1976).
[5] Greger H., Phytochemistry 18:1319 (1979).
[6] Greger H. et al., Phytochemistry 16:795 (1977).
[7] Jakupovic J. et al., Planta Med. 57: 450–453 (1992).
[8] Kurkin V.A. et al., Rastit Resur 32(1–2):88–92 (1996).
[9] Kurkin V.A. et al., Chem. Nat. Compd. (Transl. of Khim Prir Soedin):33(1): 46–49 (1997), ref. CA 127:356966h.
[10] Mallabaev A., GP. Sidyakin, Khim Prir Soedin 811 (1976).
[11] Mehrotra S. et al., Fitoterapia 64:65–68 (1993).
[12] Miller E.C. et al., Cancer Res. 43: 1124–1134 (1983).
[13] Plouvier V., Compt. Rend. 243:1913 (1956), zit. in Ü43.
[14] Steinegger E., A. Brantschen, Sci. Pharm. 27:184 (1959).
[15] Tateo F. et al., J. Ess. Oil Res. 1:111–118 (1989).
[16] Thieme H., Nguyen-Thi-Tam Pharmazie 27(4):255–265 (1972).
[17] Thieme H., Nguyen-Thi-Tam, Pharmazie 27(5):324–331 (1972).
[18] Tomitaka Y. et al., Tokyo Nogyo Daikagu Nogaku Shuho 41(4):229–238 (1997), ref. CA 127:031580j.
[19] Tunmann P., E. Mann, Z. Lebensm. Unters. Forsch. 138:146–150 (1968).
[20] Venskutonis R. et al., Spec. Publ.-R. Soc. Chem. 197 (Flavour Science):46–51 (1996).
[21] Vienne M. et al., Biochem. Syst. Ecol 17:373–374 (1989).
[22] Weymar II., Buch der Korbblütler, Neumann Verlag, Radebeul 1957.

Literature references identified by Ü can be found in the general listing of books and monographs at the back of this book.

Thyme

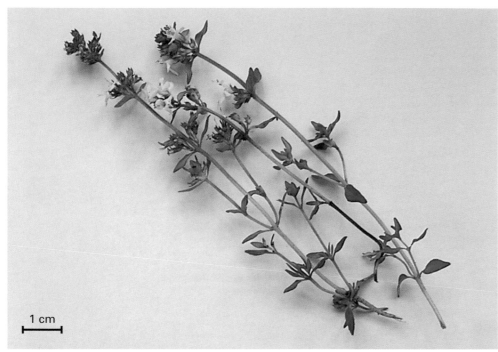

Fig. 1: Thyme branch

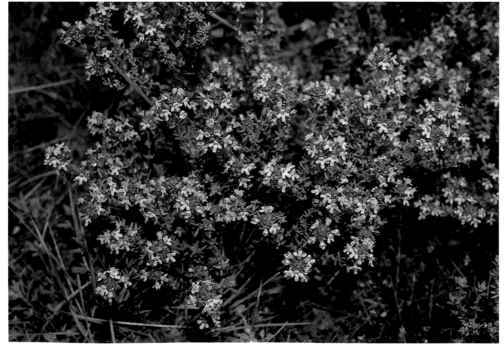

Fig. 2: Thyme (*Thymus vulgaris* L.)

Plant source: *Thymus vulgaris* L.

Taxonomic classification: The species is morphologically quite variable. Agreement on subdivisions into subspecies and/or varieties however does not exist.

Family: Mint family (Lamiaceae, synonym Labiatae).

Common names: Engl.: thyme, common thyme, garden thyme; Fr.: farigoule, frigoule; Ger.: Thymian, Echter Thymian, Garten-Thymian, Römischer Thymian, Kuttelkraut.

Description: Dwarf shrub, up to 40 cm tall. Stalk with many branches, in the lower part lignified. Leaves 3 to 12 mm long, 0.5 to 3 mm wide, small elliptic, with entire, revolute margin, short-stalked or sessile, on the lower surface, densely pubescent, with numerous glandular trichomes situated in punctiform depressions, on the upper surface in most cases glabrous. 3 to 6 flowers respectively, are arranged in false whorls; the two lipped calyx is 3 to 4 mm long; the two lipped pale violet, seldom white corolla has a bell-shaped tube, with 4 stamina; the superior ovary is divided in 4 chambers. The fruit is composed of four one-seeded nutlets [75, Ü37, Ü106].

Native origin: Western Mediterranean Europe to Southern Italy.

Main cultivation areas: Europe, particularly Spain, France, Greece, Portugal, Italy, Czech Republic, Hungary, Poland, Germany (Saxony-Anhalt, Thuringia), Russian Federation (especially in the Ukraine), Morocco, USA, some of the Islands of the Antilles, India, Indonesia (Java), Argentina, Eastern- and Southern Africa.

Main exporting countries: Spain, Poland, Hungary, furthermore Morocco, Austria, Italy, Albania, Russian Federation, Bulgaria, Romania, Portugal, France, England, Germany, and North America.

Cultivation: Thyme occurs in natural settings in light, calcareous soil, but also thrives in very argillaceous, but not too damp soils. It needs locations in full sun and tolerates draught relatively well. It will develop the best aroma when grown in poor soils. Covering in winter is recommended in locations with a high risk of frost. However it often does not endure very cold winters. Propagation is carried out by direct drilling (light germinator!) in mid-April, rarely in August, in row widths of about 20 to 30 cm. Starting the plants under glass in mid-March and planting outside by the end of May is possible. Due to the heterogeneity of the seed materials, propagation by stock divisions or cuttings is recommended, usually in the spring. Thyme fits well in stone garden and also grows well in flowerpots. Productivity of 4 to 6 years is possible. Varieties that are cultivated include, among others, 'Deutscher Winter', 'Sloneczko', 'Krajovy', 'Aroma', 'Lemonal' and 'Mixta', 'Varico'. French summer thyme is not sufficiently winter hardy in Central Europe. It can only be grown there as an annual crop [61, Ü21].

Culinary herb

Commercial forms: Thyme: the stripped, dried foliage leaves and flowers, whole or ground, essential oil of thyme and thyme oleoresin.

Production: In the first growing year, it is cut shortly before full bloom (up until the end of September), after the second growing year harvest takes place in June and early September, with a cutter bar mower, a rebuilt combine harvester or green forage harvester about 10 cm above the soil. After drying at 35 to 40 °C, it is machine rubbed and sieved. For domestic use, the fresh leaves and branches can be continuously harvested. For the production of

dried herb used by industry, some of the supply is still also collected in the wild [Ü21].

Forms used: The dried, rubbed herb, rarely the fresh herb, and thyme essential oil.

Storage: The fresh leaves or the tips of the shoots can be kept fresh in plastic bags in the refrigerator for a few days. They can also be frozen in freezer bags or with water in the ice-tray. Thyme can also be dried without significant aroma loss. Dried thyme supposedly has a 3-times stronger spice flavor than the fresh herb(?). The dried herb has a relatively good shelf life if kept cool, protected from moisture and light in air-tight porcelain-, glass- or suitable metal containers. The loss of essential oil in the first 15 months of post-harvest storage is only 0.075 ml/100 g [20].

Description. Whole herb: Fresh thyme branches (Fig. 1), rubbed dried thyme consisting of leaves and flowers, and sometimes also containing finely pubescent, blue-violet pruinose or brownish stem pieces, see description of the plant.

Powdered herb: The powder contains, besides the leaf fragments, the wavy-sinuate epidermis cells with diacytic stomata and pointed (so called "canine-tooth") trichomes with fine oxalate crystals, numerous 2- to 3-celled trichomes, known as "geniculate" trichomes with warty cuticula (Fig. 3), furthermore, labiate glandular scales with 12 secretory cells, a few upright articulate trichomes of the calyx and corolla, glandular trichomes with globular head, pollen grains with a diameter of 35 µm and 6 slit-like germination pores [Ph Eur].

Odor: Strongly aromatic, **Taste:** Aromatic, mostly reminiscent of thymol, somewhat bitter.

History: Thyme was already known as a kitchen spice in antiquity but it is unclear which thyme species was indeed used. Dioscorides (2nd half of 1st century) and Hippocrates (460–370 BCE) mentioned it in their writings. The Romans brought it to

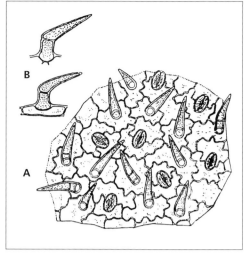

Fig. 3: Thyme. **A** Epidermis of the lower leaf surface with so-called "canine-tooth" trichomes, **B** Geniculate trichomes of the leaf nerves. From Ü29.

England. It was probably introduced to Central Europe in the early Middle Ages by the Benedictine monks, as many other medicinal and spice plants were [Ü91].

Constituents and Analysis

DIN- and ISO-Standards. ISO Standard 6754 (Thyme).

Constituents

Essential oil: 1.5% to 4% (in French summer thyme up to 6.5%). Due to the occurrence of numerous chemical races, the main components vary considerably. The dominant components are thymol or carvacrol (up to 85%, respectively), p-cymene (up to 45%), linalool, α-terpineol, camphor, thymol (up to 65%) + carvacrol (5 to 10%), thymol (about 35%) + γ-terpinene (about 18%) + p-cymene (about 18%), geraniol and geranyl acetate (together up to 90%), linalool + linalyl acetate (together up to 95%), α-terpineol + α-terpinyl acetate (together 96%), trans-sabinene hydrate (up to 56%) + terpinenol-4 (up to 43%), 1,8-cineole + camphor or 1,8-cineole + trans-thujanol + terpinenol-4 [2, 15, 16, 23, 27, 56, 64, Ph Eur]. In the essential thyme oils of commerce, thymol dominates (30 to 50%) besides other significant components such as *p*-cymene (15 to 20%), γ-terpinene (5 to 10%) and carvacrol (1 to 5%); also present are, among others, thymol methyl ether, carvacrol methyl ether, (–)-borneol, camphor, limonene, linalool, β-myrcene, β-pinene, *cis*-sabinene hydrate, α-terpinene and terpinenol-4 [10, 23, 39, 48, 54, 64, 69, 71].

The European Pharmacopeia has the following requirements for thyme oil: 36 to 55% thymol, 15 to 28% *p*-cymene, 5 to 10% γ-terpinene, 4 to 6.5% linalool, 1 to 4% carvacrol, and 0.2 to 2.5% terpinenol-4 [Ph Eur].

- Flavonoids: Free flavones, e.g. apigenin, 6-hydroxyluteolin, luteolin, flavanonols, e.g. taxifolin, flavanones, e.g. naringenin, numerous methoxylated flavones, such as cirsilineol, 8-methoxycirsilineol, cirsimaritin, eriodyctiol, genkwanin, sakuranetin, salvigenin, sideritoflavone, thymonin and thymusin, among others, as well as flavone glycosides, including apigenin-7-glucoside, luteolin-7-glucoside and vicenin-2 [1, 3, 8, 30, 70].
- Hydroxycinnamic acid derivatives (so called Labiate tannins): About 4%, particularly rosmarinic acid (about 0.8 to 2.6%) [26, 36, 37, 41, 59].
- Acetophenone derivatives: 4-Hydroxyacetophenone and its glycosides, esterified with benzoic acid [74].
- Triterpenes: Ursolic acid (1.9%), oleanolic acid (0.6%) [11].

Tests for Identity can be carried with sensoric, macroscopic and microscopic analysis or TLC of the herb extract [63, Ü77, Ü102, Ph Eur] as well as TLC [Ph Eur], GC [Ph Eur] or GC/MS [15] of the essential oil respectively.

Quantitative assay of the essential oil with volumetric analysis after steam distillation without xylol in the graduated tube [Ph Eur]. The phenol content of the essential oil is determined colorimetrically by liquid/liquid extraction of the orange-red reaction product of the phenols with ami-nopyrazolone (4-aminoantipyrin) using dichloromethane (Emerson Reaction). The content of the individual components is determined with GC [Ph Eur]. The rosmarinic acid content is measured with HPLC [26] or after silylation with GC [59].

Adulterations, Misidentifications and Impurities: Since the material of pharmacopoeial quality can also be obtained from *Thymus zygis*, such an admixture should be expected in the herb for culinary use. *Th. zygis*, Spanish thyme, has no geniculate trichomes but instead, it shows 1- to 3-celled, short, and sometimes upright or bent hairs of the lower leaf surface, with warty surface; in contrast to garden thyme, it shows about 1 mm long ciliate trichomes of the leaf base.

Actions and Uses

Actions: Due to its spicy taste, thyme causes a reflex stimulation of the secretion of saliva, gastric juices and biliary fluids and therefore has appetite stimulating and digestion promoting action.

Dilutions of the thyme fluidextracts, isolated flavonoids from the dried herb, thyme essential oil, thymol and carvacrol are able to counteract against spasms induced by $BaCl_2$, carbachol, noradrenaline, histamine or $PGF_{2\alpha}$ in vitro in isolated guinea pig ileum and trachea [12-14, 47, 51, 73].

In older research, the secretolytic and secretomotor action of thyme oil and thymol were reported [22, 24, 25, 40, 72]. Studies investigating the stimulation of ciliary function of frog mucosa has led to contradictory results [21, 76].

Addition of thyme oil in the feed of rats lessened age-related regression of antioxidative capacity of the liver, heart and brain. Age-related changes in fatty acid composition can also be stopped [77, 78]. Thymol (1 to 10 mg/kg body weight) acted as a calcium channel blocker and lowered blood pressure in rats [4].

Thyme extract and thyme oil have strong antimicrobial action [6, 7, 17, 19, 29, 31, 32, 42, 44, 55, for an overview see Lit. 51, Ü37]. The growth of *Helicobacter pylori* was also inhibited [67]. Some bacteria and fungi are however resistant to the growth inhibition influence of thyme powder [60, 79]. The antiviral action of thyme extracts observed in vitro [35], which mainly depends on the rosmarinic acid content, is probably only relevant for topical application.

Dilutions of thyme oil (1 : 2000) killed ascarids [5].

Extracts of thyme inhibit the tendency to rancidity of fats and fatty meat products due to the antioxidative effects of rosmarinic acid, the essential oil, the flavonoids and other components [18, 28, 62, 68].

Toxicology: Based on existing data, there is no acute or chronic toxicity with the normal use of thyme and thyme oil (up to 20 drops/day) [51].

The application of large amounts of thyme extracts to mice (corresponding to 0.9 g of the dried herb/animal, about 45 g/kg body weight) over 90 d, led to an elevated liver weight, among others (hepatotoxicity?). 30% of the male and 10% of the female mice died [58].

The sensitization potential of thyme herb is small. A few cases of allergic reactions have been observed however. Cross-reactivity occurs with a few other Labiatae [9, Ü39]. Thyme oil did not cause any sensitization [52].

Culinary use: Thyme is an indispensable spice in French, Spanish, Mexican, and Latin American cooking. There it is used preferably for stews, soups and sauces. The Italians season pizzas and lasagna with thyme. The English add thyme in fillings, jugged hare and beef stews, and even sweet dishes. In the USA, the American "national soup" clam chowder is seasoned with thyme.

Fresh thyme is used chopped. For dried thyme, which should have a more intense seasoning strength than fresh thyme, either the whole branches are used, which can be cooked with one time, and then the stem is removed before serving (the leaves usually fall off) or the dried rubbed or ground herb can be sprinkled before cooking over roast- and grill- meat or added to pot dishes, best inside of a metal tea ball. Due to its intense seasoning strength, thyme should be measured carefully.

Fresh, chopped thyme leaves, rubbed, dried or ground thyme or fresh or dried branches are used as seasonings of soups (e.g. of potato-, pea-, lentil-, bean-, tomato- or vegetable soups), meat dishes (mainly with fatty meats of lamb, mutton, pork or duck, of kidneys, liver and liver noodles), of fillings for roast pork and roast poultry, tortellini and ravioli, of fish dishes (especially trout), vegetable dishes (e.g. of eggplant, paprika or zucchini), mushroom-, noodle- or egg dishes (e.g. of scrambled eggs and herb omelets), of boiled potatoes, salads (e.g. finely chopped leaves are used for tomato-, potato-, bean salads, red beet salad, lemon thyme is used for fruit salads, see below), sauces (especially tomato-based and wine sauces) and marinades (e.g. for pork and venison). Thyme is also used as a flavoring for sheep- and goat cheese, quark, and even yogurt, as well as herb vinegar. It is also used as a component of sausage spice mixes, especially for cooked sausages (blood sausage and liverwurst). Combined with dill, it serves as a pickling spice for cucumbers and tomatoes [Ü1, Ü2, Ü13, Ü17, Ü30, Ü55, Ü59, Ü79, Ü80, Ü86, Ü91, Ü92, Ü111].

Ground thyme can be used for preventing rancidity of fatty meat [62].

Combines well with: Basil, bay, dill, garlic, lavender, marjoram, olives, onions, oregano, parsley, rosemary, sage, and summer savory.

As a component of spice mixes and preparations: → Barbecue sauce, → Bouquet garni, → Cajun spice, → Cocktail sauce, → Fines herbes, → Grill spice, → Gravy spice, → Hamburger meat spice, → Herb butter, → Herb oil, → Herb salt, → Herb vinegar, → Herbes de Provence, → Meat spice, → Mélange classique, → Parisian pepper, → Pizza spice, → Poultry spice, → Roast spice, → Sausage spice, → Table mustard, → Vegetable spice, → Venison spice, → Zahtar.

Other uses: Thyme oil is used in the liqueur industry (Abtei, Alpenkräuter, Benedictiner, Kartäuser, Stonsdorfer) and as a perfume of soaps and bath products as well as an ingredient of Eau de Cologne, oral hygiene products, deodorants and hair lotions [Ü24].

Medicinal herb

Herbal drugs: Thymi herba, Thyme herb, contains minimum 12 ml/kg essential oil of which a minimum of 40% is thymol and carvacrol [Ph Eur], Thymi aetheroleum, Thyme oil [Ph Eur]. Both drugs may also be obtained from *Thymus zygis* L. [Ph Eur].

Indications: Internally in the form of tea infusions (1 to 2 g/150 ml, several times daily), fluidextracts (1 to 2 g, 1- to 3 times daily), rarely dry extracts (loss of essential oil during processing!) or other preparations for the symptomatic treatment of bronchitis and pertussis as well as other catarrhs of the upper respiratory tract [34, 51]. Thyme oil is applied externally in the form of baths (minimum 0.004 g/l, bath temperature 35 to 38 °C, duration of bath 10 to 20 minutes) for supportive therapy of acute or chronic diseases of the respiratory tract and for dermatosis with pruritus [33].

In folk medicine, thyme is used in the form of baths (500 g dried herb/4 l water, extract added to the full bath, with the usual restrictions for bath applications) or in the form of cataplasms with 5% infusion for supportive therapy of acute and chronic diseases of the upper respiratory tract, and for pruritus. The tea infusion (1 to 2 g/cup, several times daily) is also used for digestive problems, such as colic, flatulence, diarrhea in children, for combating against feverish colds, and as a gargle for inflammations of the pharynx [51, Ü37]. Thyme oil is used in the form of a 10% embrocation for treatment of rheumatic complaints and of neuralgia. Internally it is used for acute bronchitis (4 to 5 drops on sugar, 3- to 5 times daily) [51, Ü37].

Other Thyme-species used as culinary herbs

Lemon thyme, *Thymus × citriodorus* (PERS.) SCHREB. ex SCHWEIGG. et KOERTE (hybrid of *Th. pulegioides* L. × *Th. vulgaris* L., also occurs spontaneously in growing areas of garden thyme). Sometimes strains of → *Th. pulegioides* (see below) that also have a lemon-like odor are also described as lemon thyme. Lemon thyme is a perennial, as a hybrid it can only be vegetatively propagated and requires covering in strong frost. Varieties cultivated in Spain, Southern Italy, and Switzerland, include, among others, 'Fragantissimus' and 'Aureus'. The main components of the essential oil are geraniol (60 to 75%) and citral (8 to 15%) [49, 50, 66]. Fresh lemon thyme is used especially as a seasoning of salads, fruit desserts and cream sauces, but also as a seasoning of fish dishes, seafoods, chicken or roast veal [Ü61, Ü74].

Caraway-thyme, *Thymus herba-barona* LOISEL., native to Sardinia, the main components of its essential oil are carvone + dihydrocarvone, carvone + limonene, thymol, carvacrol or thymol + carvacrol [Ü43]. It is suitable as a seasoning of meat, poultry, carrots, parsnips, and cheese dishes [Ü74].

Russian steppe-thyme, *Thymus pallasianus* H. BRAUN, native to the southern parts of the Russian Federation, particularly suited as a seasoning of dessert sauces [Ü55].

Common thyme (large thyme, wild thyme), *Thymus pulegioides* L. (aggregate species, numerous subspecies, varieties and chemical races), widely distributed throughout Central Europe, and cultivated in numerous crop forms. The main components of its essential oil can be thymol, carvacrol, fenchone, linalool, linalyl acetate, citral, citral + geraniol (lemon thyme), linalool + *p*-cymene, geraniol + linalool, thymol + β-caryophyllene + carvacrol or carvacrol + γ-terpinene + β-caryophyllene [38, 45, 46, 64, 65]. Common thyme is used the same as garden thyme [Ü74].

Japanese thyme, *Thymus quinque-costatus* Celak., native to Northeastern China, Korea, and Japan, cultivated in Japan, the main component of its essential oil is thymol. It is used especially as a seasoning of soups and meat dishes [64, Ü61].

Wild thyme (wild creeping thyme, mother-of-thyme), *Thymus serpyllum* L. emend. MILL. (Aggregate species with numerous varieties or subspecies), native to temperate Eurasia, cultivated in the Ukraine, in the Balkan countries, in Morocco, and in Spain, due to its low essential oil content it is less aromatic than garden thyme. The main components of its essential oil are very diverse including, among others, predominantly thymol, carvacrol, linalool + linalyl acetate, 1,8-cineole + myrcene, 1,8-cineole + -camphor or myrcene + 1,8-cineole + linalool, in commercially traded oils mainly carvacrol (20 to 45%), *p*-cymene (5 to 15%), γ-terpinene (5 to 15%) and thymol (1 to 10%), as odoriferous compounds also citral and citronellal (*Th. s.* var. *citriodorus*). Wild thyme is used especially in the Mediterranean countries as a seasoning of some meat dishes, fish- and poultry farces, soups, dark sauces, uncooked salads and fried potatoes [43, 48, 50, 53, 64, Ü92].

Spanish thyme (south of France thyme), *Thymus zygis* L., native to Spain, Portugal, and Southern France, cultivated and wild collected in Spain, in Central Europe it is not winter hardy. There are numerous varieties and chemical races. The main components of its essential oil are therefore quite variable, including, among others, predominantly thymol, carvacrol, linalool, geranyl acetate, α-terpinyl acetate, thymol + carvacrol, thymol + *p*-cymene, carvacrol + *p*-cymene, linalool + 1,8-cineole, 1,8-cineole + thymol, 1,8-cineole + linalool + thymol, geraniol + geranyl acetate, linalool + thymol, α-terpinyl acetate + myrcenol + terpinenol-4, or myrcenol + terpinenol-4 + *trans*-thujanol [2, 57, 64]. Spanish thyme is used in the same manner as garden thyme, especially for seasoning of Spanish thyme soup "Tonill" [Ü92].

Thyme grog

1 twig of thyme, fresh or dried, 60 ml Rum Havana Club (42%), a shot of hot water, peel of one lemon (organic) cut in form of a spiral, 1 teaspoon brown sugar.

Heat up the rum (don't boil!) and pour the liquid into a heat-resistant glass (mulled wine glass). Add a shot of hot water as well as the thyme, the lemon peel spiral and sugar. Mix and let the liquid stand for a short while [Ü57].

Literature

[1] Adzet T. et al., Planta Med. Suppl. 1980: 52–55 (1980).

[2] Adzet T. et al., Biochem. Syst. Ecol. 5: 269–272 (1977).

[3] Adzet T. et al., J. Ethnopharmacol. 24: 147–154 (1988).

[4] Aftab K. et al., Phytomedicine 2(1):35–40 (1995).

[5] Akacic B., J. Petricic, Pharmazie 11:628–632 (1956).

[6] Aktug S.E., M. Karapinar, Int. J. Food Microbiol. 3:349–354 (1986).

[7] Aureli P. et al., J. Food Prot. 55:344–348 (1992).

[8] Bauer F. et al., Chem. Mikrobiol. Technol. Lebensm. 11:181–187 (1988).

[9] Benito M. et al., Ann. Allergy Asthma Immunol. 76(5):416–418 (1996).

[10] Bestmann H.J. et al., Z. Lebensm. Unters. Forsch. 180:491–493 (1985).

[11] Brieskorn C.H. et al., Arch. Pharm. 286:501–506 (1953).

[12] Broucke van den C.O., Fitoterapia 54: 171–174 (1983).

[13] Broucke van den C.O., J.A. Lemli, Pharm. Weekbl. Sci. 5:9–14 (1983).

[14] Broucke van den C.O., J.A. Lemli, Planta Med. 41:129–13 (1981).

[15] Daferra DJ. et al., J. Agric. Food Chem. 48(6):2576–2581 (2000).

[16] Delpit B. et al., Riv. Ital. EPPOS 7(Spec. Num.):403–408 (1996), ref. CA 125:081836b.

[17] Dorman H.J., S.G. Deans, J. Appl. Microbiol. 88(2):308–316 (2000).

[18] Economou K.D. et al., J. Am. Oil Chemist's Soc. 68:109–113 (1991).

[19] Farag R.S. et al., Fette, Seifen, Anstrichm. 88:69–72 (1986).

[20] Fehr D., G. Stenzhorn, Pharm. Ztg. 124: 2342–2349 (1979).

[21] Freytag A., Pflügers Arch. 231:346–348 (1933).

[22] Freytag A., Pflügers Arch. 232:346 (1933).

[23] Góra J. et al., Riv. Ital. EPPOS (Spec. Num., 15th Journees Internat. Huiles Essentielles, (1996):761–766 (1997), ref. CA: 128:016268r.

[24] Gordonoff T., F. Janett, Z. Exper. Med. 79:486 (1931), zit. bei Lit. 12 (s.o.).

[25] Gordonoff T., H. Merz, Klin. Wschr. 10:928 (1931), zit. bei Lit. 12 (s.o.).

[26] Gracza L, P. Ruff, Arch. Pharmaz. 317: 339–345 (1984).

[27] Granger R., J. Passet, Phytochemistry 12: 1683–1691 (1973).

[28] Haraguchi H. et al., Planta Med. 62(3): 217–221 (1996).

[29] Huhtanen C.N., J. Food Prot. 43:195–196, 200–202 (1980).

[30] Husain S.Z, K.R. Markham, Phytochemistry 20:1171–1173 (1981).

[31] Ismaiel A., M.D. Pierson, J. Food Sci. 55:1676–1678 (1990).

[32] Janssen A.M. et al., Pharm. Weekbl. 10: 277–280 (1988).

[33] Kommission B8 beim BfArM., BAnz. 115 vom 26.06.1990.

[34] Kommission E beim BfArM., BAnz. 228 vom 05.12.84, Berichtigung BAnz. vom 13.03.1990 und 02.12.

[35] Kucera L.S., E.C. Herrmann, Proc. Soc. Exp. Biol. Med. 124:865–869 (1967).

[36] Lamaison J.L. et al., Ann. Pharm. Franc. 48:103–108 (1990).

[37] Lamaison J.L. et al., Ann. Pharm. Franc. 46:103–108 (1990).

[38] Länger R. et al., Sci. Pharm. 63:325 (1995).

[39] Lawrence B.M., Perfum. Flavor 20(3):67–68, 70, 72 (1995).

[40] List P.H. et al., Dtsch. Apoth. Ztg. 40: 1392 (1964), zit. bei Lit. 12 (s.o.).

[41] Litvinenko V.I. et al., Planta Med. 27: 372–380 (1975).

[42] Llewellyn G.C. et al., J. Assoc. Off. Anal. Chem. 64:955–960 (1981).

[43] Loziene K. et al., Planta Med. 64(8):772–773 (1998).

[44] Marino M. et al., J. Food Prot. 62(9):1017–1023 (1999).

[45] Mártonfi P., J. Ess. Oil Res. 4:173–179 (1992).

[46] Mastelic J. et al., Planta Med. 58(7):A679 (1992).

[47] Meister A. et al., Planta Med. 65(6):512–516 (1999).

[48] Messerschmidt W., Planta Med. 13:56–72 (1965).

[49] Mikus B. et al., Drogenreport 10(18):68–73 (1997).

[50] Mikus B., I. Zobel, Drogenreport 9(15): 10–15 (1996).

[51] Mills S. et al. (Eds.): Principles and Practice of Phytotherapie, Churchill Livingstone, Edinburgh 2000.

[52] Opdyke D.L.J., Food Cosmet. Toxicol. 12:1003–1004 (1974).

[53] Oszagyan M. et al., J. Ess. Oil Res. 8(3):333–335 (1996).

[54] Oszagyán M. et al., Flavour Fragrance J. 11:157–165 (1996).

[55] Patakova D., M. Chládek, Pharmazie 29: 140–143 (1974).

[56] Pino J.A., J. Ess. Oil Res. 9:609–610 (1997).

[57] Proenca da Cunha A., L. Salgueiro, J. Ess. Oil Res. 3:409–412 (1991).

[58] Qureshi S. et al., Fitoterapia 62:319–323 (1991).

[59] Reschke A., Z. Lebensm. Unters. Forsch. 176:116–119 (1983).

[60] Salmeron J. et al., J. Food Prot. 53: 697–700 (1990).

[61] Schmidt L, Drogenreport 6(9):39–40 (1993).

[62] Shahidi F. et al., J. Food Lipids 2(3):145–153 (1995).

[63] Stahl E. (Hrsg.): Chromatographische und mikroskopische Analyse von Drogen, Fischer Verlag Stuttgart, New York 1978.

[64] Stahl-Biskup E., J. Ess. Oil Res. 3:61–82 (1991).

[65] Stahl-Biskup E., Planta Med. 52:233–235 (1986).

[66] Stahl-Biskup E. et al., Flavour Fragrance J. 10(3):225–229 (1995).

[67] Tabak M. et al., J. Appl. Bacteriol. 80(6):667–672 (1996).

[68] Takacsova M. et al., Nahrung 39(3):241–243 (1995).

[69] Vampa G. et al., Plantes Med. Phytothér. 22:195 (1988).

[70] Van den Broucke C.O. et al., Phytochemistry 21:2581–2583 (1982).

[71] Venskutonis R. et al., Flavour Fragrance J:11(2):123–128 (1996).

[72] Vollmer H., Klin Wschr. 11:590, zit. bei Lit. 12 (s.o.) (1932).

[73] Wagner H. et al., Planta Med. 52:184–187 (1986).

[74] Wang M. et al., J. Agric. Food Chem. 47(5):1911–1914 (1999).

[75] Weymar H: Buch der Lippenblütler und Raublattgewächse, Neumann Verlag, Radebeul 1961.

[76] Yong Bong Han et al., Arch. Pharm. Res. 7:53–56 (1984).

[77] Youdim K.A., S.G. Deans, Mech. Ageing Dev. 109(3):163–175 (1999).

[78] Youdim K.A., S.G. Deans, Br. J. Nutr. 83(1):87–93 (2000).

[79] Zaika L.L. et al., J. Food Sci. 48: 1455–1459 (1983).

Literature references identified by Ü can be found in the general listing of books and monographs at the back of this book.

Turmeric

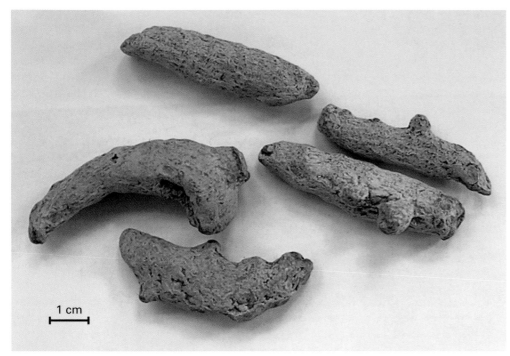

Fig. 1: Turmeric rhizome

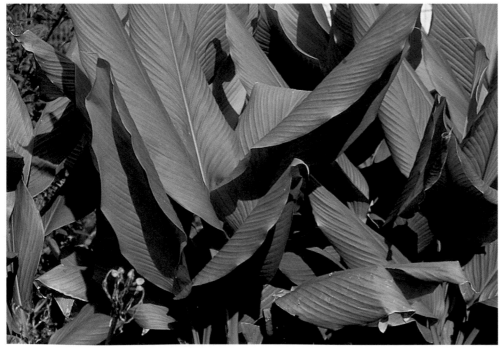

Fig. 2: Turmeric (*Curcuma domestica* VAL.)

Plant source: *Curcuma domestica* VAL.

Synonym: *Curcuma longa* auct. plur. non L.

Taxonomic classification: The validity of the epitheta domestica and longa is again and again disputed according to the priority rules because it is unclear, whether the plant, described first by Linné 1753 as *Curcuma longa* is identical with *Curcuma domestica* described 1918 by Valeton.

Family: Ginger family (Zingiberaceae).

Common names: Engl.: turmeric, Indian saffron, long rooted curcuma; Fr.: curcuma, Terre-mérite; Ger.: Kurkuma, Gelbwurz, Gelbwurzel, Indischer Safran, Safranwurzel, Langer Gelbwurzelstock, Tumerik, Gelber Ingwer.

Description: Rhizomatous perennial. The main rhizome is tuberous with numerous rootlets, which are partially thickened at the end to form elliptical tubers; the secondary rhizomes are finger-shaped. All rhizomes bear reduced leaves, which appear as annular scars after they have died off. The leaves are basal, up to 1.2 m long with ovate-lanceolate lamina and almost parallel venation, narrowing to a sheath-like petiole. The inflorescences are cone-shaped spikes, situated on about 15 to 20 cm long peduncles, which are enclosed by sheath-like petioles; the large 5 to 6 cm long, pale-green bracts that are fused to form pocket-like leaf aggregates, as well as white or often pink-colored bracteoles. The few flowers, yellowish white or yellow, appear in small pauciflorous coils in the axils of the bracts; they have a tube-like, three-lobed outer perigone (calyx) and large funnel-like, three-lobed inner perigone (corolla). Each flower only contains one fertile stamen;

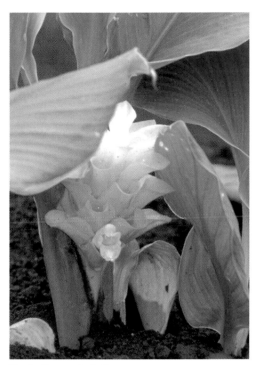
Fig 3: Turmeric inflorescence

the other two stamens from the inner ring are corolla-like, fused to a yellow, circular lip, and the lateral staminodes of the outer ring are yellow, petal-like and oblong-ovoid. The inferior ovary is filaceous with a two-lipped stigma. The fruit capsule is spherical and membranous [Ü37, Ü76].

Native origin: Probably native to India in the region of Bihar at altitudes of about 1800 to 2000 m.

Main cultivation areas: Tropical Asia, especially India, and furthermore Pakistan, Cambodia, Thailand, Sri Lanka, Indonesia, Southern China, Taiwan, Japan, the Philippines, Madagascar, and Réunion, as well as in the Caribbean, especially Jamaica and Haiti, and in southern parts of the Russian Federation.

Main exporting countries: India (Madras-, Bengal-, and Alleppey turmeric), with smaller amounts exported by China, Thailand, Indonesia (Java), and Haiti.

Cultivation: Turmeric cultivation requires a tropical, frost-free climate with relatively consistent temperatures and consistent humidity. Propagation is carried out vegetatively using pieces of the main rhizome. The young plants are mounded up. The inflorescences are removed. After about 8 to 10 months, the aerial parts wither after which the rhizome harvest takes place [Ü56].

Culinary herb

Commercial forms: Turmeric: Curcumae rotundae rhizome, the tuberous, oval- to pear shaped, dried main rhizomes ("bulbs"), Curcumae longae rhizoma, the finger shaped, dried secondary rhizomes ("fingers"), turmeric "slits", and turmeric powder. Furthermore, the commercial forms are often named according to their origin, e.g. Curcumae longae rhizoma Haiti and Curcumae longae rhizoma Madras. A few Asian countries also export the fresh rhizome. Alleppey- and Madras-turmeric are considered to be good quality and West Indian turmeric has a lower value. Lipid- and water-soluble turmeric oleoresins are also commercially traded (containing 30 to 40% curcumin).

Production: After being dug up, the rhizomes are separated from the roots and washed. Then the secondary rhizomes (the fingers) are separated from the primary rhizomes (the bulbs). They are then cured by boiling in water for 5 to 45 minutes, and more rarely they only have boiled water poured over them (perhaps in order to prevent sprouting during the drying process). The cork layer is then extensively peeled off. The cooking process gelatinizes the starch, allows the pigment to release from the secretory cells and to penetrate the entire tissue causing more uniform coloration. Finally they are dried for 5 to 10 days on bamboo mats or on drying racks [Ü90].

Forms used: The fresh rhizome, the dried rhizome (briefly cooked with cork layer peeled off), powder from processed rhizomes, turmeric essential oil and turmeric oleoresin, obtained by extraction with 75% ethanol.

Storage: Turmeric powder should only be stored for a short time in airtight glass- or porcelain containers protected from light and heat. Taste and aroma loss occur relatively quickly while the dye strength remains constant for an almost unlimited time.

Description. Whole rhizome (Fig. 1): Consisting of secondary and tuberously thickened main rhizomes. The pieces of the yellowish brown or gray-brown rhizome branches, orange-colored in the cross section, are 2 to 5 cm long, finger-shaped, cylindrical or somewhat compressed, straight or bent and up to 1.8 cm thick. The pieces of the main rhizome are ovoid, up to 5 cm long and 3 cm thick. All pieces are almost horn-like hard, show wrinkled surfaces and uniformly yellow-orange cross sections [DAC].

Powdered rhizome: The yellow to brown-yellow powder shows, in the water slide preparation, large, yellow, gelatinized starch aggregates. Also present are a few single, ungelatinized, colorless, eccentric and flattened starch grains, 15 to 30 µm long. The chloral hydrate slide preparation, yellow-colored due to curcuminoids, reveals the multi-layered cork fragments (Fig. 4) and polygonal epidermis cells with somewhat curved outer walls, which occasionally contain small, tetrahedral calcium oxalate crystals. The remains of thick-walled, mostly broken off, pointed and cylindrical, unicellular trichomes can also be present. The cells of the endodermis are corky, not thickened and starch-free. The large-celled parenchyma is thin-walled. Between the parenchyma cells, one can find numerous smaller, orange-yellow secretory cells. Occasionally, pieces of reticulate and scalariform vessels can also be found. Sclerenchymatic fibers are absent [DAC, Ü49].

Taste: Mildly spicy, faintly burning, slightly bitter, ginger-like, **Odor:** Strong and aromatic, spicy.

History: Turmeric has been used as a spice and particularly for dyeing textiles and as a

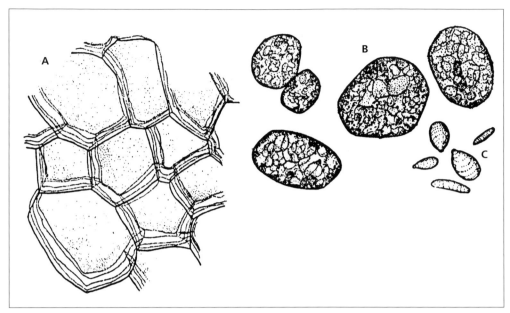

Fig 4: Turmeric. **A** Cork cells (top view), **B** Gelatinized starch aggregates, **C** Individual starch granules. From Ü49

medicine for 3000 years. First, its use was limited to India and Indochina. At the end of the 1st century, turmeric was introduced as "yellow ginger" to Greece by Arab traders and later reached Central Europe. Since the 7th century, the plant has also been cultivated in China. Around 1200, turmeric was brought to Africa and later also to the Caribbean. In Germany, turmeric is claimed to be known since 1150, when it was named "Indian saffron" to replace the much more expensive genuine saffron as a dye for foods [Ü89, Ü92].

Constituents and Analysis

DIN- and ISO-Standards: ISO-Standard 5562 (Turmeric, whole or ground (powdered) – Specification), ISO-Standard 5566 (Turmeric: Determination of coloring power – Spectrophotometric method).

Constituents
- Essential oil: 2 to 7%; the main components are sesquiterpene ketones (about 65%), particularly turmerone (α-turmerone. 30 to 70%), *ar*-turmerone (17 to 26%) and curlone (β-turmerone, 14 to 18%), as well as, among others,

germacrone, germacrone-4,5-epoxide, germacrone-13-al, 4-hydroxybisabola-2,10-diene-3-one and dehydrozingerone, as well as other sesquiterpenes, particularly zingiberene (up to 25%); furthermore, β-sesquiphellandrene, β-curcumene, *ar*-curcumene (α-curcumene), β-bisabolene, curcumenol, procurcumadiol and β-caryophyllene, among others. Turmeric from most origins contains only small amounts of monoterpenes, e.g. linalool (in a batch from Malaysia about 15%), Δ^3-carene, α-terpinene, γ-terpinene, terpinolene, cineol, α-phellandrene, sabinene and borneol [16, 17, 19, 22, 30, 36, 40, 52, 55, Ü43].
- 1,7-Diaryl-heptane derivatives:
– Curcuminoids (1,7-diaryl-hepta-1,5-diene-3,5-diones, dicinnamoylmethane derivatives): 3 to 6%; yellow to red-orange, not steam-distillable pigments, hardly soluble in water, easily soluble in ether, ethyl acetate and fatty oils, thermostable, light sensitive. The main component is curcumin (diferuloylmethane) in addition to monodesmethoxycurcumin (*p*-coumaroylferuloylmethane), bisdesmethoxycurcumin (di-*p*-coumaroylmethane) and feruloylcaffeoyl-

methane; the proportions of the different curcuminoids are race-specific.
– Dihydrocurcuminoids (1,7-diaryl-hepta-1-ene-3,5-dione) and
– 1,7-Bis-(4-hydroxyphenyl)-1,4,6-hepta-triene-3-one [17, 23, 58, Ü43].
- 1,5-Diaryl-pentane derivatives: 1,5-Diaryl-penta-1,4-diene-one, biogenetically related to curcuminoids [35].
- Diterpene aldehyde: Labda-8(17)12-diene-15,16-dial [49].
- Turmerin, a peptide with reported antioxidant activity [56].
- Starch: 30 to 40%.
- Monosaccharides: Glucose, fructose, arabinose.
- Water soluble polysaccharides with immune-stimulating activity: Ukonan A (a complex, acidic arabinogalactan).

Tests for Identity: Organoleptic, macroscopic and microscopic examination, as well as TLC analysis for establishing identity [Ü102, Ü106]; the constituents can be assayed with GC, GC-MS [36, 52] or HPLC [19], respectively.

Quantitative assay: The content of curcuminoids can be determined photometrically based on the intensely red rubrocurcumin-complex, which develops after turmeric powder is heated with boric- and oxalic acid, dissolved in acetic acid; the absorption is measured at 530 nm [DAC]. The quantitative determination of the curcuminoid mixture is carried out with HPLC [57], and the content of essential oil is measured volumetrically with steam-distillation and xylene in the graduated tube [DAC].

Adulterations, Misidentifications and Impurities: Turmeric from Indonesian and Chinese origins is sometimes confused with *Curcuma xanthorrhiza* ROXB. (Javanese turmeric). In Chinese materials, misidentifications with rhizomes of *Curcuma aromatica* SALISB. (Wild turmeric) or *C. zedoaria* (CHRISTM.) ROSCOE (zedoary) have also been encountered. The differentiation is possible by the detection of camphene and camphor with TLC of a hexane extract [45]; these two markers are absent

Turmerone (α-Turmerone)

ar-Turmerone

Curlone

Zingiberene

Curcumin: (R₁=R₂=OCH₃)

Monodesmethoxycurcumin (R₁= OCH₃, R₂=H)
Bisdesmethoxycurcumin (R₁= R₂=H)
Feruloylcaffeoylmethane (R₁= OCH₃, R₂=OH)

from *C. domestica* [45]. More conclusive is the GC-analysis of the essential oil (see above). Sometimes, the powder was "beautified" with lead chromate; in these cases, the lead content reached 410 to 3700 ppm [51].

Actions and Uses

Actions: Due to its mild aromatic odor and slightly pungent taste, turmeric has a reflex action, through mild, direct stimulation of the stomach, the secretion of gastric juices and the flow of bile are stimulated, thereby promoting digestion [18, 23, 24]. The application of curcuminoids through a duodenal tube, bypassing the mouth and stomach, as well as by parenteral application also stimulated the production of bile fluids and increased cholekinesis [17, 25, 37, 53, 54]. Feeding curcumin to rats (0.5% in feed) over an 8-week period increased the activity of pancreas lipase, pancreas amylase, trypsin and chymotrypsin. Curcumin fed to mice (0.5% in feed) caused an increase in the excretion of bile and the breakdown of gallstones (80% with 10 weeks) [21].

Turmeric has **antimutagenic**, **anticarcinogenic** and **antitumor** action [37]. In animal experiments, curcumin and other curcuminoids, mostly in concentrations of 1 to 2% in feed or drinking water, inhibited not only carcinogenesis that was induced by the cocarcinogen 12-O-tetradecanoyl phorbol-13-acetate (TPA) and carcino gens (e.g. 2-acetamidofluorene, benzo[a] pyrene, 4-nitrochinoline-1-oxide, *N*-nitrosomethylbenzylamine, azoxymethane, *N*-ethyl-*N*′-nitro-*N*-nitrosoguanidine, 7,12-dimethylbenz[a]anthracene), but also inhibited tumor progression. Genesis of uterus-, skin-, duodenal-, intestinal-, esophageal-, and stomach tumors has been prevented as well as papillomas. The mechanism of action probably involves, among other mechanisms, the induction of detoxifying enzymes in the liver (e.g. glutathione-S-transferase) and suppression of carcinogen adduction to DNA, and of the production of oncogenes (p-21(ras), p53) as well as of cell division promoting factors (AP-1, cyclin E, p34(cdc2), NF-κB), and through induction of apoptosis (programmed cell death) of tumor cells. Curcumin also inhibits the growth of estrogen-dependent tumors by way of a blockade of the estrogen receptors [4, 13, 14, 20, 26, 27, 33, 34, 42, 44, 59, 60]. The tumor protective effect of turmeric may also be caused through its ability to prevent the formation of carcinogenic nitrosamines (e.g. nitrosomethyl carbamide) in foods (especially through reaction of the secondary amines in meat with the added nitrite) and in the stomach [37].

Turmeric has **antioxidative** and through it **cytoprotective** and **antiphlogistic** action [6, 37, Ü83]. Due to the ability of curcuminoids to inactivate oxygen radicals, it protects unsaturated fatty acids from autoxidation [Ü83]. Turmeric protects cells in vivo from oxidative stress. Tetrahydrocurcuminoids, which are formed in the liver as biotransformation products, have stronger antioxidative effects than the curcuminoids themselves and are especially good at protecting cell membranes from oxidative attacks.

The antihepatotoxic effect has been demonstrated in animal tests [10, 15, 29]. For example, the addition of turmeric to feed given to rats before or during the application of hepatotoxic carbon tetrachloride, reduced the serum levels of such liver damage indicators as aspartate-aminotransferase, alanine-aminotransferase, and alkaline phosphatase. Without application of turmeric there was 2 to 3 fold increase in all parameters [15]. By investigation of isolated liver cells, the curcuminoids have been identified as the antioxidative active constituents [28]. In rats, administration of high doses of curcumin (200 or 600 mg/kg body weight, orally) effectively suppressed diethylnitrosamine (DEN)-induced liver inflammation and liver hyperplasia, which commonly precede liver tumor genesis [10].

The neuroprotective effect of curcumin (applied orally) has been demonstrated in rats in which ethanol-induced brain damage was attempted. Curcumin led to a drop in lipid peroxidation and to an increase in the glutathione level in the brain [46].

In ex vivo studies it has been shown that in rats that received curcumin (75 mg/kg body weight in corn oil), their lenses in vitro were much more resistant to 4-hydroxy-*trans*-non-2-enal-induced cataract formation than were lenses from control animals [7]. Patients suffering from chronic anterior uveitis (inflammation of anterior part of the eye) given high doses of curcumin (375 mg, t.i.d.) improved within a few weeks [32].

In animal tests, turmeric extracts and curcumin have limited the skin inflammation triggered by TPA (12-*O*-tetradecanoyl phorbol-13-acetate) and edemas triggered by arachidonic acid [20, 37, Ü83]. Administration of curcumin (120 mg/day) to patients suffering from rheumatoid arthritis caused considerable improvement in symptoms [37]. Possibly this antiphlogistic effect is due to the inhibition of cyclooxygenase and of 5- and 12-lipoxygenase, observed in vitro, caused by the antioxidative action of turmeric [1, 8, 17, 37, Ü37].

Upon exposure to light in the presence of oxygen, curcumin catalyzes the formation of reactive oxygen species and thus demonstrates bactericidal and cytotoxic effects. Its application as a photosensitizing agent in the phototherapy of psoriasis and infections was proposed [11, 37].

In animal experiments, turmeric has shown antiarteriosclerotic action through its **antihyperlipidemic**, **antioxidative**, **antithrombotic** and **fibrin level lowering** effects [37]. The antihyperlipidemic action of turmeric extracts or curcuminoids has been demonstrated repeatedly [37, Ü37]. In mice, the feeding of curcumin (4 mg/kg body weight per day) over a four-week period led to a decrease of the peroxides concentration in blood plasma and in the liver [38]. In rabbits that were fed an atherogenic diet in addition to turmeric extract (1.7 mg/kg body weight per day) for 7 weeks, there was, compared to the control group, a lower susceptibility of LDL for oxidative changes as well as lowered blood levels of cholesterol, phospholipids and triacylglycerols [48]. In ex-vivo animal tests, curcumin or turmeric extracts were shown to inhibit blood platelet aggregation induced by ADP, collagen, arachidonate and adrenaline, an effect that is probably dependent on reduced thromboxane production [37, 41]. Aqueous-ethanolic extracts of turmeric have been shown to lower abnormally elevated plasma fibrinogenic values in humans [47]. Furthermore, turmeric extracts have **antibacterial** and **fungistatic** action [37]. The effects occur especially in light (phototoxicity!) [12]. The antibacterial effect of turmeric is dependent on the curcumin

and the essential oil, and the fungistatic effect is due only to the essential oil and labda-8(17)-12-dien-15,16-dial. Curcumin has shown no effect against dermatophytes and yeast [5, 49]. It does have, however, antiprotozoic action, as shown against *Plasmodium falciparum* (IC_{50} for curcumin 3.5 µg/ml) and *Leishmania major* (IC_{50} 7.6 µg/ml) [50]. Turmeric extracts have also shown insect repellent and insecticidal properties [2, 3, 40, 49].

Toxicology: No acute or chronic toxicity was ascertained even with administration of high doses in animal tests. Only with application of very high doses of the oleoresin (296 and 1551 mg/kg body weight), pathological changes, e.g. of the bladder and kidney, were observed [37].

As with most spices, the stimulation of gastric juice secretion can cause hyperacidity-induced gastric complaints (e.g. stomach ulcers) if unusually high amounts are consumed for an extended period of time. Due to their cholagogic effect, turmeric extracts have the potential to trigger biliary colic in predisposed individuals with gallstones. It is therefore advisable that patients suffering from gallstones talk to a physician before using turmeric therapeutically [31]. With the admixture of very high amounts of turmeric (over 10%) to animal feed, hair loss was observed. The sensitization potential of turmeric is very low [37].

Culinary use: Turmeric is an indispensable spice in rice dishes of India and Indonesia, where it is also used in meat-, fish- and vegetable curries. Because of the close connections of India with England in the past it is understandable that turmeric has gained popularity in Europe, especially in English cooking. In England, turmeric plays a role mainly in traditional kedgeree (Hindi: khichri; rice dish with fish, peas, onions, eggs and butter) and in piccalilli (various vegetables cooked with a mixture of vinegar, mustard, garlic, turmeric and other spices and served with cold meat). Turmeric is also added to bean- and lentil dishes. Turmeric has been in use for a long time in central eastern and northern

Africa, where it is used as a component of sofrito sauces, which are used to spice fish- and chicken dishes. Couscous also contains turmeric. In Morocco, turmeric is an essential component of la-kama mix. In American cooking, turmeric is used when making mayonnaise, cream sauces, bread spreads and fish salads. It is also used in the preparation of egg dishes, e.g. of the American breakfast yellow scrambled eggs. In Central Europe, turmeric was, up until recently, almost exclusively known as a component of curry powders. With the introduction of Asian cooking, it is now used more frequently as a single spice.

In the west, turmeric powder is always used, but in the countries where turmeric grows the grated fresh rhizome is also used. It should be measured carefully however. For 1 kg of rice dish, one level teaspoon of turmeric is all that is necessary, and it should be added at 3 to 5 minutes prior to the end of cooking time.

Turmeric can serve to improve taste and color of poultry ragouts, boiling fowl, fish, seafoods and vegetables (especially of baked cauliflower). It can also be added to sauces (especially sauces for crabs, lobster, mussels and escargot), mustard sauces, egg dishes (e.g. scrambled eggs, omelets), chutneys, relishes, bread spreads, fish salads as well as bean- and lentil dishes. It is used mainly for its coloring effect as a component of rice dishes, couscous, potatoes, mayonnaise and pickled vegetables. As a substitute for saffron in sweet dishes, e.g. cakes, it is not suitable due to its pungent taste.

Turmeric essential oil is used to improve or round out the taste of stomach bitters. Turmeric oleoresin is used in the food industry as a spice in sauces, soups and instant meals [Ü1, Ü2, Ü55, Ü56, Ü59, Ü89, Ü90, Ü93].

Combines well with: Chillies, garlic, ginger, onions, paprika, star anise, and naturally with all of the spices used in → Curry powder.

As a component of spice mixes and preparations: → Arabian spice mix, → Bomboe, → Curry powder, → La kama, → Sambhar powder, → Sarawak spice mix, → Table mustard, → Tandoori, → Tika paste, → Worcestershire sauce.

Other uses: The essential oil from turmeric is occasionally used in the perfume industry. By soaking the starch in water, the bitterness is removed and the obtained product (known as Bombay-arrowroot, Malabar-arrowroot or East-Indian arrowroot) is used as a food ingredient in its country of origin and also internationally, as a raw material for the manufacture of dietetics, infant formulas and confectioneries. Turmeric extracts were often employed as a dye for cotton, silk, leather or wood, among others. Ground turmeric is used to repel pests feeding on stored foods, e.g. as an admixture to stored rice or wheat. Curcumin is an approved food colorant (E 100) for butter, margarine, cheese and medicines; it is also a reagent for the detection of borates [Ü89].

Medicinal herb

Herbal drugs: Curcumae longae rhizoma, Turmeric rhizome, contains not less then 2.5% dicinnamoyl methane derivatives and not less than 2.5% essential oil [DAC].

Indications: Turmeric is used for digestive problems in the form of powder, tea infusions and aqueous-ethanolic extracts. Dry extracts may be less effective than powder and/or liquid dosage forms due to the contribution of the essential oil to the efficacy. The daily dosage is 1.5 to 3.0 g dried turmeric or equivalent quantities of preparations [31]. It should be taken 2 to 3 times daily between meals.
Furthermore, the following indications are based on positive outcomes in clinical testing: arthritis (curcumin) and osteoarthritis [37]. Local application of turmeric essential oil (1 : 80 dilution) caused dermatomycosis to disappear within one week [5].

Turmeric is traditionally used for skin diseases. In India, it is also used for treating fever, vomiting of pregnancy, liver diseases and externally for conjunctivitis, skin infections and eczema. In China, the turmeric rhizome is used as a stimulant with analgesic properties for chest- and abdominal pain, jaundice, amenorrhea, and also as a post-partum anodyne, and styptic [37].

Similar culinary spices

Zedoary, *Curcuma zedoaria* (BERG.) ROSCOE, is native to northeastern India and cultivated in India, China, Madagascar, and Sri Lanka. Its rhizome is conical, grayish-brown to pale red in the cross section. The commercial forms are usually its slices. Its essential oil contains, among other compounds, 1,8-cineole, α- and β-caryophyllene, α- and β-caryophyllene epoxide, β-eudesmol and zerumbone. Extracts of the rhizome or its essential oil serve as aromatic components in the production of bitter liqueurs (Boonekamp, Stonsdorfer). Small amounts of the rhizome are used, similarly to the buds and leaves of the plant, as a cooking spice, especially as a component of curry powder [43, Ü61].

Wild turmeric, *C. aromatica* SALISB., is native to and cultivated in India. The main components of the essential oil obtained from the rhizome are camphor (26 to 32%), curzerenone (about 11%), germacrone (about 11%), 1,8-cineole (6 to 10%), turmerone (α-turmerone, about 7%) and *ar*-turmerone (about 6%). The curcuminoids content corresponds to that of *C. domestica*. The rhizome is only rarely used, in the Russian Federation among other countries, as a spice or colorant [9, 58, Ü61, Ü92].

Javanese turmeric (Indonesian: temu lawak), *C. xanthorrhiza* (BERGIUS) ROSCOE, is native to Indonesia and is cultivated in Malaysia, Thailand, the Philippines and Java. Even though its aroma and flavor can hardly be differentiated from turmeric, it is only rarely used as a spice and almost exclusively as a medicinal herb for dyspeptic complaints, among other conditions. It contains 3 to 12% essential oil (according to Ph Eur not less than 5%) of which the main components are xanthorrhizol (about 45%), and zingiberene (about 10%) as well as 0.8 to 2.0% curcuminoids [17, 22, Ü61].

Temu pauh, *C. mangga* VAL. et VAN ZIJP, is cultivated in Java and Malaysia. The main components of its essential oil are myrcene (about 80%) and β-pinene (about 10%). Its rhizome tips and young shoots have significance as spices only locally in Java [22, Ü61, Ü93].
Zander, Dictionary of plant names, 17. Ed., 2002 [Ü22] unites *C. mangga* and *C. xanthorrhiza* under *C. zedoaria* (?).
See also → Ginger; similar culinary spices: Mango ginger.

Turmeric-potatoes with green and yellow peppers
800 g potatoes, 500 g green and yellow peppers, 500 g onions, 4 tablespoons vegetable oil, 1 1/2 teaspoons turmeric, 1/2 teaspoon salt, black pepper (freshly ground).

Wash the evenly sized potatoes and boil them unpeeled. Let them cool and dice them along with the peppers and onions. Heat the oil in a frying pan and add the turmeric with the diced vegetables. After frying the ingredients for a few minutes, add 1 to 2 tablespoons of water. Reduce the temperature and let the vegetables simmer for 10 min while stirring occasionally. Season to taste with salt and ground pepper [Ü91].

Literature

[1] Ammon H.P. et al., J. Ethnopharmacol. 38(2/3):113–119 (1993).

[2] Ammon H.P.T. et al., Planta Med. 58:226 (1992).

[3] Ammon H.P.T., M.A. Wahl, Planta Med. 57:1–7 (1991).

[4] Anto R.J. et al., Mutat. Res. 370(2): 127–131 (1996).

[5] Apisariyakul A. et al., J. Ethnopharmacol. 49(3):163–169 (1995).

[6] Asai A. et al., Biosc. Biotechnol. Biochem. 63(12):2118–2122 (1999).

[7] Awasthi S. et al., Am. J. Clin. Nutr. 64(5):761–766 (1996).

[8] Bonté F. et al., Planta Med. 63(3): 265–266 (1997).

[9] Bordoloi A.K. et al., J. Ess. Oil Res. 11:537–540 (1999).

[10] Chuang S. et al., Food Chem. Toxicol. 38(11):991–995 (2000).

[11] Dahl T.A. et al., Photochem. Photobiol. 59(3):290–294 (1994).

[12] Dahl Th.A. et al., Arch. Microbiol. 151: 163–185 (1989).

[13] Deshpande Sh. et al., Cancer Lett. (Shannon, Irel.) 123(1):35–40 (1998), ref. CA 128:175859a.

[14] Deshpande Sh.S. et al., Cancer Lett. (Shannon, Irel.): 118(1):79–85, ref. CA 127: 272388h (1997).

[15] Deshpande U.R. et al., Indian J. Exp. Biol. 36(6):573–577 (1998).

[16] Gopalan B. et al., J. Agric. Food Chem. 48(6):2189–2192 (2000).

[17] Hänsel W., Z. Phytother. 18(5):297–306 (1997).

[18] Harnischfeger G., H. Stolze, notabene medici 12: 562 (1982).

[19] Hiserodt R. et al., J. Chromatogr. A 740(1):51–63 (1996).

[20] Huang M.T. et al., J. Cell Biochem. Suppl. 27:26–34 (1997).

[21] Hussain M.S. et al., Indian J. Med. Res. 96:288–291 (1992).

[22] Jantan bin I. et al., J. Ess. Oil Res. 11:719–723 (1999).

[23] Jentzsch K. et al., Sci. Pharm. 36:251 (1968).

[24] Kalk H., K. Nissen, Dtsch. Med. Wochenschr. 58:1718 (1932).

[25] Kalk H., K. Nissen, Dtsch. Med. Wschr. 57:1613–1615 (1931).

[26] Kawamori T. et al., Cancer Res. 59(3): 597–601 (1999).

[27] Khar A. et al., FEBS Lett. 445(1):165–168 (1999).

[28] Kiso Y. et al., Planta Med. 49:185–187 (1983).

[29] Kiso Y. et al., Shoyakugaku Zasshi 36:238 (1982).

[30] Kojima H. et al., Planta Med. 64(4):380–381 (1998).

[31] Kommission E beim BfArM., BAnz-Nr. 223 vom 30.11.85, Berichtigung vom 01.09.90.

[32] Lal B. et al., Phytother. Res. 13(4):318–322 (1999).

[33] Limtrakul P. et al., Cancer Lett. 116(2): 197–20 (1997).

[34] Manoharan Sh. et al., J. Clin. Biochem. Nutr. 21(2):141–149 (1995).

[35] Masuda T. et al., Phytochemistry 32: 1557–1560 (1993).

[36] Mc Carron A. et al., Flavour Fragrance 10:355–357 (1995).

[37] Mills S. et al. (Eds.): Principles and Practice of Phytotherapie, Churchill Livingstone, Edinburgh 2000.

[38] Miquel J. et al., Age (Chester, Pa.): 18(4):171–174 (1995).

[39] Nagabhushan M. et al., Mutat. Res. 202(1):163–169 (1988).

[40] Ohshiro M. et al., Phytochemistry 29: 2201–2205 (1990).

[41] Olajide O.A., Phytother. Res. 13(3):231–232 (1999).

[42] Paek S.H. et al., Arch. Pharmacol. Res. 19(2):91–94, ref. CA 125: 000555j (1996).

[43] Phan M.G. et al., Hoa. Hoc. Cong. Nghiep. Hoa. Chat. 1997(4):9–11, 26 (1997), ref. CA 128:280838r.

[44] Piper J.T. et al., Int. J. Biochem. Cell Biol. 30(4):445–456 (1998).

[45] Raghuveer K.G., V.S. Govindarajan, J. Assoc. Off. Anal. Chem. 62:1333–1337 (1979).

[46] Rajakrishnan V. et al., Phytother. Res. 13(7):571–574 (1999).

[47] Ramirez Bosca A. et al., Mech. Ageing Dev. 114(3):207–210 (2000).

[48] Ramirez-Tortosa M.C. et al., Atherosclerosis 147(2):371–378 (1999).

[49] Roth G.N. et al., J. Nat. Prod. 61(4):542–545 (1998).

[50] Rasmussen H.B. et al., Planta Med. 396–398 (2000).

[51] Sayed A.M. et al., J. Chem. Soc. Pakistan 9:387–390 (1987).

[52] Sharma R.K. et al., J. Ess. Oil Res. 9(5):589–592 (1997).

[53] Siegers C. et al., Planta Med., 45th Ann. Congr. Soc. Med. Plant Res. (Abstracts) I0 (1997).

[54] Siegers C.P. et al., Pharm. Pharmacol. Lett. 7(2/3):87–89 (1997).

[55] Srinivasan K.R., J. Pharm. Pharmacol. 5:448 (1953).

[56] Srinveas L. et al., Arch. Biochem. Biophys 292:617–623 (1992).

[57] Tonnesen H.H., J. Karlsen, Z. Lebensm. Unters. Forsch. 182:215–218 (1986).

[58] Tonnesse H.H. et al., Z. Lebensm. Unters. Forsch. 194:570–571 (1992).

[59] Ushida J. et al., Jpn. J. Cancer Res. 91(9):893–888 (2000).

[60] Van Dau N. et al., Phytomedicine 5(1): 29–34 (1998).

Literature references identified by Ü can be found in the general listing of books and monographs at the back of this book.

Vanilla

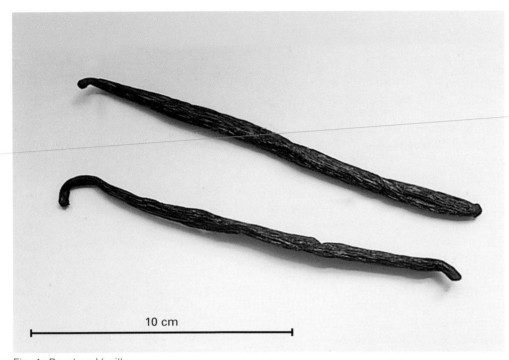

Fig. 1: Bourbon-Vanilla

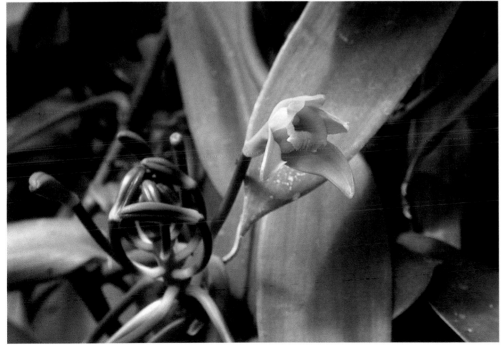

Fig. 2: Vanilla (*Vanilla planifolia* ANDR.)

10 cm

Plant source: *Vanilla planifolia* ANDR.

Synonym: *Vanilla fragrans* (SALISB.) AMES.

Family: Orchid family (Orchidaceae).

Common names: Engl.: vanilla, common vanilla, Bourbon vanilla; Fr.: vanille, vainilles, vanille de Mexique; Ger.: Vanille, Echte Vanille, Gemeine Vanille, Mexikanische Vanille.

Description: Perennial evergreen climber, with green unlignified, 2 to 3 cm wide stem. The leaves are petiolated, oval, succulent, up to 15 cm long, up to 7 cm wide, yellowish- to dark-green. The stem bears adhesive rootlets opposite to the leaves, which enables the plant to climb up to 20 m high to the treetops of primeval forest. The adhesive rootlets are accompanied with hanging aerial roots, being finely hairy on their thickened ends, and short-stalked racemes with up to 15 flowers. The flowers have 6 whitish-green perigone leaves, one of them enlarged (labellum), the gynostegium (little column, formed of stamen and stigma) arillate embracing; the stigma is separated from the stamen by a small shield (rostellum); the content of the anther forms a so-called pollinarium (pollen mass with stipellus and adhesive disc); the inferior ovary is composed of 3 carpels, the margins of them project as biangular placentas to the interior of the capsule. The ripe yellow, one-celled capsules (no pods!) open with two longitudinal splittings. The fruit pulp contains numerous very small seeds [6, Ü82, Ü89].

Native origin: Southeastern Mexico to northern South America (Bolivia, Paraguay, Northern Argentina), and the Antilles.

Main cultivation areas: Madagascar, the Comoros, Indonesia, and Réunion, furthermore, among others, Mexico (exported almost exclusively to the USA and Canada), Guatemala, Nossi-Bé, Costa Rica, Tonga, Seychelles, Mauritius, Uganda, and India.

Main exporting countries: Madagascar, Indonesia, the Comoros, Tonga, and Réunion, furthermore, among others, Mexico, Costa Rica, French-Polynesia, Uganda, and a few of the Pacific Islands.

Cultivation: Vanilla grows between 25° north and 25° south latitude with average temperatures of 23 to 29 °C without daily or annual fluctuations, and 1000 to 3000 mm rainfall, preferably evenly distributed throughout the year, protected from too much direct solar radiation by shade trees, in deep, humus-rich soil. Propagation is carried out exclusively by cuttings, which are about 1.5 m long, and tied to a trellis, trestle or to living trees. The very small seeds only germinate in symbiosis with certain mycorrhizal fungus. In order to facilitate plant care, the vines should be regularly pruned back to a height of about 2 m. Outside of their native region the flowers must be artificially pollinated, because of the absence of insect species that are necessary for the pollination (especially bees from the Meliponinae subfamily). Therefore, the flowers, which are only fertilizable for about 8 hours, are slit open with a needle or a bamboo splinter, the rostellum is lifted up or removed and the pollen mass is pressed with the fingers onto the stigma. Only some of the flowers are fertilized in order to prevent too many fruits on one stalk. After about 4 weeks, short- or poorly growing fruits are removed. Harvest maturity occurs 6 to 8 months after fertilization. The plants reach the optimal yield in the 5th year and remain productive rarely longer than 12 years [11, Ü82, Ü83, Ü89].

Culinary herb

Commercial forms: Vanilla beans: **Mexican vanilla** (qualities: superior, good, fair, ordinary, origin Mexico and Central America), **Bourbon-vanilla** (Ceylon-vanilla, qualities: extra fine, fine, medium-fine, fendue, origin Madagascar, Comoros and Réunion), **Indonesian vanilla** (Javanese vanilla, similar to Bourbon vanilla, but has a harder outer shell). First quality vanilla is composed of fine, thick, fatty oil looking pods of a chocolate brown color and delicate aroma; the succulent fruits without defects do not break upon bending. The pods of lower quality vanilla are relatively thin and/or they have cracks and scars. Also commercially traded are **Vanilla powder**, **Vanilla extract** (extracted with 50% ethanol, USA-Standard 10 g (= 7.5 g dry weight)/100 ml, single fold), **Vanilla oleoresin** (obtained by evaporation of the menstrum of solvent-extracted beans), **Vanilla sugar** (made by mixing a minimum of 5% finely rubbed vanilla with raw sugar, the addition of vanillin is considered adulteration) and **Vanillin sugar** (made from a combination of vanillin, 1 to 2%, or ethyl vanillin with raw sugar) [Ü89, Ü92, Ü98].

Production: The odorless fruits are plucked when the green color begins to turn to yellow. In order to release the aromatic components from the glycosides, the cells must be destroyed, without inactivating the enzymes (by solar influence, hot water or dry heat), thereby the glycosidase comes into contact with the glycosides through destruction of the cell structures. Through hot temperatures and high moisture content, the glycoside cleavage is then advanced (sweating process). With this process, moreover, the diphenols contained in the fruits convert into blackish-brown polyphenols by polyphenol oxidase. In Mexico, the fruits are spread out on trays in the sun for a few hours post harvest, midday they are covered with woolen cloth and in the evenings they are wrapped in the cloth, put into closed boxes in order to "sweat". This process, depending on the state of the fruits, is repeated for 8 days up to a month (dry method). Subsequently, the moisture content is reduced to 20 to 30% by careful drying (volatile aroma components!).

In the cultivation areas around the Indian Ocean, the harvested fruits are placed in baskets and plunged into hot water (65 °C) in kettles. The dried off fruits are then put into closed chests. Subsequently, they are placed between cloths for several days until midday when they are laid out in the sun (wet method). Then they are dried in ventilated rooms.

Finally a one- to several-month "aging" (conditioning) process is carried out in tin cans lined with wax paper, in which the full aroma develops through oxidation- and hydrolysis- processes, and often white vanillin crystals occur on the surface of the fruits (frosted vanilla, Eng.: frosted = Fr.: givré = Ger.: Raureif) [Ü82, Ü83, Ü89].

Forms used: Whole or ground fruits, vanilla extracts, and vanilla sugar.

Storage: Protected from light and moisture, in a cool place, stored in airtight porcelain- or glass containers, vanilla pods keep their aroma for several years. Extracts are best stored in the refrigerator.

Description. Whole fruit (Fig. 1): Vanilla pods are 14 to 20 cm long and at most 1 cm wide (Bourbon-vanilla: 14 to 18 cm long, 3 to 8 mm wide; Mexican vanilla: 16 to 20 cm long, 4 to 8 mm wide), narrowed on both ends, more or less flattened, with long furrows, flexible, shiny black-brown and sometimes covered with white vanillin crystals (only in Bourbon-vanilla). At the thin, usually hook-like end, there is a scar of the fruit stalk, and at the pointed end, there is a scar from the fallen off flower parts. The inner part of the single-celled fruit shows the numerous globose, up to 0.3 mm thick, black-brown, shiny seeds, located in a black fruit pulp with a pleasantly fragrant odor [21, EB 6].

Powdered fruit: The black brown powder reveals the prominent seeds, up to 300 μm in size, as well as fragments thereof with polygonal, brown stone cells. Also present are, among others, shreds of the epidermis with flat, thick-walled, dotted cells with yellowish cuticula, single crystals of oxalate, small stomata and the hypoderm

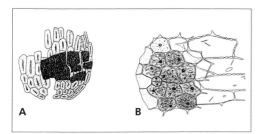

Fig. 3: Vanilla. **A** Fragments of the testa, **B** Epidermis of the epicarp (roundish cells with dark content) and elongated cells of the hypoderm. From Ü29.

beneath with elongated and also dotted cell walls with oxalate needles (Fig. 3), thin-walled parenchyma of the fruit pulp with fine vascular bundles and long, narrow cells, which contain mucous-embedded bundles of calcium oxalate raphides. Upon microsublimation, the powder yields an oily sublimate from which vanillin crystals separate, taking on a red color with phloroglucin solution and hydrochloric acid [Ü29, EB 6].

Odor: Flowery, vanillin-like, **Taste:** Very spicy, agreeable, vanillin-like.

History: Vanilla was already used in Mexico for a long time before the discovery of the Americas by Columbus (1492). The Aztecs grew this plant and used it for the flavoring of foods and beverages (particularly chocolate). At the beginning of the 16th century, the first vanilla pods were brought to Europe by the Spaniards. At the start of the 17th century, vanilla established itself as an aroma component for chocolate in European courts. In 1819, the Dutch brought vanilla stock to Java. Only after the introduction of artificial pollination, the production of vanilla pods became possible outside of Mexico. From green house cultures in France, the first plant stocks were established on the Isle de Bourbon (now Réunion) [11, 21, 25, Ü83, Ü89, Ü97].

Constituents and Analysis

DIN- and ISO-Standards. ISO-Standard 3493 (Vanilla-Vocabulary), ISO-Standard 5565, parts 1 and 2 (Vanilla, specification, classification into 4 commercial forms, test methods in Annex A and Annex B).

Constituents

- Benzaldehyde derivatives: The main odorous component is vanillin: about 1.5 to 4.0% (high levels in Bourbon-vanilla), in a few cultivars up to 10% [5], in the intact unripe fruit, occurring as vanilloside (vanillin-β-glucoside, gluco-vanillin) and released when fermented; also present in the intact fruit in form of their p-hydroxybenzaldehyde-β-glucosides are protocatechuic aldehyde and anisaldehyde [2, 9, 20, 22, Ü43].

- Benzyl alcohol derivatives: Vanillylalcohol, in the intact fruit present as vanilloside (vanillylalcohol-4-β-glucoside), p-hydroxybenzylalcohol, p-hydroxybenzylmethylether (contributing to the aroma), anise alcohol, and benzyl benzoate (General Section, Fig. 9) [2, 22, Ü8, Ü43].

- Benzoic acid derivatives: p-Hydroxybenzoic acid, vanillinic acid, in the intact fruit occurring as p-hydroxybenzoic acid-β-glucoside or vanillinic-β-glucoside, respectively, anisic- and protocatechuic acid [2, 9, 22, Ü43].

- Esters: Numerous esters, including esters of salicylic acid, e.g. ethylsalicylate, pentyl salicylate, isoamyl salicylate and hexyl salicylate, among others, as well as esters of acetic acid, e.g. fenchyl acetate, menthyl acetate and α-terpinyl acetate and also hexylbutanoate and anisylformiate [32].

- Furan derivative: Furfural, 5-hydroxymethylfurfural and 2,5-dimethylfuran (possibly formed from the monosaccharides by acid-catalyzed dehydration during production) [?, 29, 22].

- (+)-trans-α-Ionone (contributing to the aroma) [Ü8].

- Vitispiranes (cis/trans isomers of 2,10,10-trimethyl-6-methylene-1-oxaspiro-(4,5)dec-7-enes, contributing to the aroma) [26].

- Mucilage.

- Monosaccharides, oligosaccharides: Glucose, fructose (together about 15 to 20%) and saccharose (35%) [Ü60].

- Fatty oil [21].

- Waxes: Epicuticular wax with high content of long-chained 2,4-dicarbonyl compounds, particularly hepta-cos-18(Z)-ene-2,4-dione (nervonoylacetone) [23].

- Residual moisture: 24 to 35%.

Vanilloside   Vanillin   Protocatechuic aldehyde   p-Hydroxybenzaldehyde

Vanillyl alcohol   p-Hydroxybenzyl alcohol   Anise alcohol   Piperonal

trans-α-Ionone   Vitispirane

Tests for Identity: Based on morphological and anatomical characteristics as well as with TLC [22, 28, Ü38, ISO-Standard 5565, Annex A], GC [21], GC/MS [27], LC [1, 3, 8, 9, 12, 15, 29, 30], GC-IRMS or NMR (for a differentiation of natural vanillin from synthetic based on the isotope index: content of ^{2}H as well ^{13}C) [18, 19, 24].

Quantitative assay of vanillin and other constituents of vanilla in the fermented beans, in vanilla extracts and preparations with HPLC [1, 3, 8, 9, 12, 14–16, 29–31] or UV-spectroscopy [ISO-method 5565-1982/Annex B]

Adulterations, Misidentifications and Impurities: Adulterations are rare. Mentioned are musk-like smelling, up to 14 cm long fruits of the Tahiti-vanilla, the up to 12 cm long but 1.5 to 3 cm wide "vanillons", split fruits (obtained by harvesting of the ripe beans) as well as spent fruits, already partially extracted [EB 6].

Actions and Uses

Actions: Due to its aromatic taste, vanilla is appetite stimulating and digestion promoting. Vanillin has good antioxidative properties, also in products with low water content [4].

Toxicology: Based on existing data, there is no acute or chronic toxicity with the use of vanilla at normal doses.

In female workers with frequent exposure to vanilla beans during packaging, skin reactions (allergies, see below) as well as increased menstrual bleeding have been reported [Ü58].

The sensitization potential of vanilla is moderate [Ü39]. Contact allergies ("vanillism") occur particularly in people who harvest or package vanilla beans. After the intake of vanilla-containing foods, for example vanilla ice cream, urticaria and swelling of the face have been observed in allergic individuals. Lip balm containing vanilla has also caused allergic reactions [10]. In 9 out of 10 children with neurodermatitis, vanilla (50 mg) or vanillin (12.5 mg) caused eczema, and in one child Quinke's edema. After elimination of the flavoring from the food, the conditions improved in 6 of the 11 children [17].

Culinary use: Vanilla is used especially in the USA and to a lesser extent in Western Europe. The main consumers are the food industry (bakery goods, confectionaries, beverages, sweet sauces, yogurt, fermented milk, cream cheese, ice cream), the chocolate industry, the beverage industry (eggnog, coffee liqueurs, cacao liqueurs, crème de cacao, Galliano, cordial Medoc, Swedish punch) and the perfume industry. To some extent, industrial use of vanilla has been replaced by the significantly less expensive semi-synthetic vanillin, which however has a less fine aroma.

For the production of desserts or ice creams, the vanilla pods are crushed with a knife and immersed in about 1/2 l warm milk or cream. After cooling, the pods are removed, washed off, and dried again. They can be used more than once.

Due to its fine aroma, vanilla is preferred for the seasoning of cold dishes. In all dishes wherein the spice will be heated, vanillin-sugar will suffice, because in the cooking- or baking-process the components that besides vanillin determine the aroma of vanilla are mostly lost from the heating.

Sugar can be flavored by preserving with dried vanilla pods, with the fruit pulp removed, for a few weeks in a tightly closed jar. The vanilla pods can be used repeatedly. The fruit pulp can be used for production of ice creams. Vanilla sugar can be prepared by grinding the vanilla pods with sugar in a mixer.

Vanilla pods, vanilla extracts or vanilla sugar are used as seasonings of sweet dishes (e.g. of vanilla pudding, vanilla sauce, quark, yogurt, sweet soups), sweet drinks (cacao), chocolates, ice creams, cold bowls, milk products, confectionaries, pastries (e.g. vanilla pretzels, vanilla rolls, vanilla streusel cakes), fruit desserts (e.g. rhubarb, pear, apricot, plum), punch and liqueurs [Ü2, Ü13, Ü30, Ü51, Ü59, Ü92, Ü95]. Vanilla is also suitable for poultry- and veal dishes [Ü13].

Vanilla is sometimes also used for the flavoring of coffee or tea. Some tea lovers place a piece of vanilla pod in the tea caddy, in order to enhance the aroma of the tea [Ü59].

In very small amounts, vanilla is also used as a seasoning of sausage products such as blood sausage and liverwurst, veal or lobster [Ü30, Ü55, Ü108].

Combines well with: Cinnamon, clove, and ginger.

As a component of spice mixes and preparations: → Egg spice, → Gingerbread spice, → Pastry spice.

Other uses: Vanilla is also used as a tobacco flavoring [21].

Medicinal herb

Herbal drug: Vanillae fructus, Vanilla, Vanilla fruit [EB 6, Ph Helv V].

Indications: Vanilla can be used, usually in the form of vanilla tincture, as an aromaticum (daily dose corresponding to 0.5 g dried fruit [EB 6]). In folk medicine it also serves as an aphrodisiac and as a remedy for dysmenorrhea [Ü60]. Today vanilla is used mainly as a flavoring component of galenical preparations.

Similar culinary herbs

Tahiti vanilla, fermented, dried fruits of *Vanilla tahitensis* J.W. Moore, native to Tahiti, Society Islands, and Hawaii, cultivated on islands of Polynesia, exported mainly to France, and the USA. The curviform pods are about 14 to 20 cm long, up to 2.5 cm wide, reddish to blackish, triangular and have a musk-like odor. The main aromatic components are anise alcohol, vanillin and *p*-hydroxybenzaldehyde, furthermore anisaldehyde, anisic acid, *p*-hydroxybenzoic acid and vanillic acid have been identified [7, 9]. Tahiti vanilla is used the same as vanilla [Ü30, Ü61, Ü92, Ü98].

West Indian vanilla (pompon, Ger.: Vanillon, Pompona-Vanille, Pompon-Vanille, Vanille aus Guadeloupe, Große Vanille, Westindische Vanille), fermented, dried fruits of *Vanilla pompona* SCHIEDE (Synonym: *Vanilla grandiflora* LINDL.), native to southern Mexico, Nicaragua, Panama, and northern South America, cultivated in the Lesser Antilles (Martinique, Guadeloupe, Dominica). The fruits are 1.5 to 3 cm thick and up to 12 cm long. The main constituents are vanillin and anise alcohol, and furthermore p-hydroxybenzaldehyde p- and m-anisaldehyde, p-hydroxybenzoic acid, vanillic acid and anisic acid have been detected. West Indian vanilla is used the same as vanilla, but has little importance as a spice, serving instead mainly for the manufacture of perfumes and for flavoring of tobacco products [Ü61, Ü98].

Chocolate macaroons

75 g of chocolate, 125 g sugar, 150 g ground almonds, 1/2 vanilla bean, 3/4 teaspoon ground cinnamon, 2 egg whites.

Melt the chocolate in a bowl over a hot water bath. Take the bowl off the heat and add the remaining ingredients while mixing until a soft batter is obtained. Line the oven tin with parchment paper, mold the dough into small balls and place them on top of the tin.
Flatten the dough balls slightly using a knife. Bake them in a preheated oven at 100 °C for 12 to 15 minutes until they feel solid to the touch. After reaching room temperature, the paper lining is peeled off (if the macaroons stick to the paper, wipe the lower side with a wet cloth) [Ü73].

Fruits of *Vanilla abundiflora* J.J. SMITH, native to and cultivated in Indonesia, and used the same as vanilla [Ü61].

Fruits of *Vanilla gardneri* ROLF, native to and cultivated in Brazil, and used the same as vanilla [Ü61].

Literature

[1] Archer A.W., J. Chromatogr. 462: 461–466 (1989).

[2] Bohnsack H. et al., Riechst. Aromen Körperpflegemittel 21:125 -128, 163–166 (1971), 15:284–287, 321–324, 407–410 (1965), 16: 512–514 (1966), 17:133–136 (1967).

[3] Brodelius P.E., Phytochem. Anal. 5:27–31 (1994).

[4] Burry J. et al., J. Sci. Food Agric. 48:49–56 (1989).

[5] Cambornac M., Riv. Ital. EPPOS 7 (Spec. Num.):478–480 (1996), ref. CA 125: 053512z.

[6] Dressler R.L., Die Orchideen, Biologie und Systematik der Orchidaceae, Eugen Ulmer Verlag, Stuttgart 1987.

[7] Ehlers D. et al., Z. Lebensm. Unters. Forsch. 199:38–42 (1994).

[8] Ehlers D. et al., GIT Fachz. Lab. 39:765–768 (1995).

[9] Ehlers D., M. Pfister, J. Ess. Oil Res. 9:427–431 (1997).

[10] Ferguson J.E., M.H. Beck, Contact Dermatitis 33(5):352 (1995).

[11] Havkin-Frenkel D., R. Dorn, ACS Symp. Ser. 1997, 660 (Spices):29–40 (1997), ref. CA 126:292519j.

[12] Hermann A., M. Stocki, J. Chromatogr. 246:313–315 (1982).

[13] Hjorth N., Acta Derm. Venerol. 41, Suppl 46:1–216 (1961).

[14] Jagerdeo E. et al., J. Assoc. Off. Anal. Chem. 83(1):237–240 (2000).

[15] Kahan S., J. Assoc. Off. Anal. Chem. 72:614–618 (1989).

[16] Kahan Set al., J. Assoc. Off. Anal. Chem. Int. 80(3):564–570 (1997).

[17] Kanny G. et al., Aller. Immunol. 26(6): 204–206 (1994).

[18] Kaunzinger A. et al., J. Agric. Food Chem. 45(5):1752–1757 (1997).

[19] Lamprecht G. et al., J. Agric. Food Chem. 42:1722–1727 (1994).

[20] Negishi O., T. Ozawa, J. Chromatogr. A. 756(1+2):129–136 (1997).

[21] Oberdieck R., Dtsch. Lebensm. Rundsch. 94(2):53–59 (1998).

[22] Poole S.K. et al., J. Planar Chromatogr-Mod TLC 8(4):257–268 (1995).

[23] Ramaroson-Raonizafinimanana B. et al., J. Agric. Food Chem. 48(10):4739–4743 (2000).

[24] Renaud G.S. et al., J. Agric. Food Chem. 45:859–866 (1997).

[25] Scholz H., Natürlich 18(11):37–45 (1998).

[26] Schulte-Elte K.H. et al., Helv. Chim. Acta 61:1125 (1978), ref. Ü43.

[27] Sostaric T. et al., J. Agric. Food Chem. 48(12):5802–5807 (2000).

[28] Stahl E. (Hrsg.): Chromatographische und mikroskopische Analyse von Drogen, Fischer Verlag Stuttgart, New York 1978.

[29] Taylor S., Flavour Fragrance J. 8:281–287 (1993).

[30] Thompson R.D., T.J. Hoffmann, J. Chromatogr. 438:369–382 (1988).

[31] Voisine R. et al., J. Agric. Food Chem. 43(10):2658–2661 (1995).

[32] Werkhoff P. et al., Food Sci. Technol. (London) 30(4):429–431 (1997).mistry 21:2581–2583 (1982).

Literature references identified by Ü can be found in the general listing of books and monographs at the back of this book.

Watercress

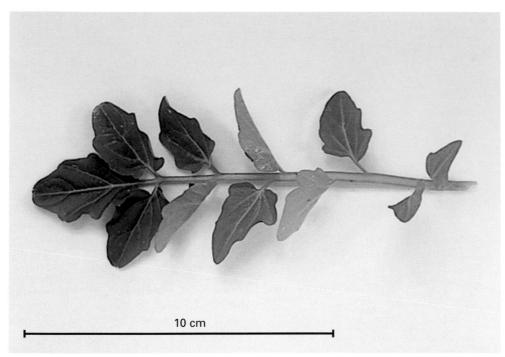

Fig. 1: Watercress leaf

(scale bar: 10 cm)

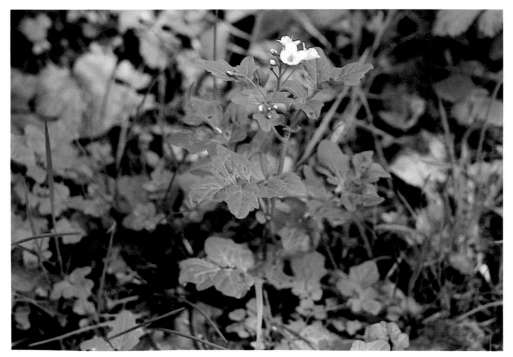

Fig. 2: Watercress (*Nasturtium officinale* R. Brown)

Plant source: *Nasturtium officinale* R. Brown.

Synonym: *Rorippa nasturtium-aquaticum* (L.) Hayek.

Family: Mustard family (Brassicaceae, synonym Cruciferae)

Common names: Engl.: watercress; Fr.: cresson de fontaine; Ger.: Brunnenkresse, Gemeine Brunnenkresse, Bachkresse, Wasserkresse, Wassersenf, Wiesenkren.

Description: Perennial plant, stem creeping in the lower part, with rootlets and stolons, ascending in the upper part, 25 to 70 cm long, hollow, angular and furrowed, almost glabrous. The leaves are dark-green throughout the winter, the lower of which are trifoliate with broad-elliptic, entire-margined or sinuous-crenate side leaves and roundish and broad-cordate larger, terminal leaf; the upper ones are imparipinnate, divided into 6 to 18 lyrate leaflets. The terminal and axillary inflorescences are racemose, umbel-like compressed; the flowers have 4 sepals, 4 petals, which are white, later on becoming purple and indistinctly unguiculate, 2 short and 4 long stamina with yellow anthers and with a small, green and knotty honey leaf on each side of the two smaller stamina. The ovary is superior, and the fruit is a husk, 13 to 18 mm long, over 2 mm wide and 1.8 to 2.5 mm thick. The seeds are flat, ovoid, about 1 mm long and coarsely reticulate. The shape of the underwater plant parts varies depending on the depth of immersion. Flowering period is from June to October [23, Ü37].

Native origin: Probably native to southeastern Europe, now distributed worldwide, occurring circumpolar in the northern hemisphere, but also in the mountains of the tropics, and elsewhere in the southern hemisphere.

Main cultivation areas: Because it is a highly labor intensive crop, it is cultivated only on a small-scale in Central- and Western Europe (especially in Germany, e.g. near Erfurt, in France, the south of England, and the Netherlands), Hawaii, China, and to a lesser extent also in tropical areas of eastern Africa, and southeastern Asia.

Main exporting countries: Rarely France. Most of the supply is traded locally.

Cultivation: Watercress prefers humus, nutrient-rich soil and shaded to half-shaded, cool locations. Seeds can be sown from May to July in watertight pots that are not completely filled with soil. The soil must be kept continually very moist. After germination, thin out the plants to about 7 cm apart and fill the pots with water so that only the tips of the starts rise above the water. There must always be about 1 cm of water covering the soil. The water should be changed repeatedly. [Ü96].

Culinary herb

Commercial forms: Watercress herb: fresh plants in bundles, stored in water or packed in plastic bags.

Production: The flowering tops are harvested when the plants reach 6 to 8 cm in height. An additional harvest in the autumn is possible. Collection in its natural habitat (along running water rich in oxygen) is not advisable due to river pollution.

Forms used: Flowering aerial parts of young plants.

Storage: Immediate use is preferred. The fresh herb can be stored in water at 0 to 5 °C or in a plastic bag for 1 week.

Description. Whole herb (Fig. 1): Fresh shoots of the young plant; see description of the whole plant.

Odor: Absent; pungent if rubbed, **Taste:** Pungent and burning.

History: Watercress was already known in antiquity as a medicinal and wild edible plant. Cultivation was first carried out in the 18th century, particularly around Erfurt, Germany ("Dreibrunnengebiet"). Since the beginning of the 19th century, it has been cultivated also in France and England [Ü61].

Constituents and Analysis

Constituents

- Glucosinolates: About 1% (calculated with reference to the fresh young leaves), with the main component gluconasturtiin (phenylethyl glucosinolate); upon tissue damage, the glucosinolates undergo enzymatic hydrolysis and convert to mustard oils (isothiocyanates) and small amounts of nitrile (see Fig. 12 on page 12). Gluconasturtiin is primarily converted to 2-phenylethyl mustard oil (2-phenylethyl-isothiocyanate, volatile, with a pungent odor) and small amounts of 3-phenyl-propionitrile; also present are glucotropaeoline (converting to benzyl mustard oil = benzylisothiocyanate), 7-methylsulfinylheptyl glucosinolate (converting to 7-methylsulfinylheptyl-isothiocyanate) and 8-methylsulfinyloctyl glucosinolate (converting to 8-methylsulfinyloctyl isothiocyanate) [12, 14, 20].
- Flavonoids: Rhamnazin and rhamnetin-3-O-sophoroside, among others [5].
- Vitamin C: About 50 to 80 mg/100 g (calculated with reference to the fresh herb) [10, Ü98].

Tests for Identity: Based on sensoric and macroscopic examinations. TLC [19, 21], HPLC and RP-HPLC analyses are suitable for the determination of the glucosinolate or desulfoglucosinolate constituents [1, 9, 13, 15, 24].

Quantitative assay: The glucosinolates can be determined with RP-HPLC or as desulfoglucosinolates with HPLC or GLC [1, 13, see also → Sarepta mustard].

Adulterations, Misidentifications and Impurities: It is possible to mistake the similarly bitter-tasting large bitter-cress (*Cardamine amara* L.) for watercress. In contrast to watercress, this herb has a pithy stem, the lower pinnate leaves have more than 3 leaflets, and the anthers have a violet color [Ü37]. Possible misidentification with fool's watercress (*Apium nodiflorum* (L.) LAG., Apiaceae), which is supposedly toxic, has also been described [Ü54]; this herb can be distinguished from watercress by the occurrence of large leaf sheaths.

Actions and Uses

Actions: Due to its pungent taste, it has appetite stimulating and digestion promoting action. After consuming 56 g of watercress with each meal over a period of three

2-Phenylethyl-isothiocyanate

3-Phenyl-propionitrile

7-Methylsulfinylheptyl-isothiocyanate

8-Methylsulfinyloctyl-isothiocyanate

days, 11 smokers showed an increase in the concentration of detoxification products from carcinogenic nitroso compounds in the urine. It was postulated that mustard oils, in this case phenylethyl-isothiocyanate, but particularly 7-methylsulfinylheptyl-isothiocyanate and 8-methylsulfinylheptyl-isothiocyanate, prevented the metabolic activation of carcinogenic nitroso-compounds (e.g. 4-(methylnitrosamino)-1-(3-pyridyl-1-butanone) by inhibition of Phase I Enzymes, and through the induction of Phase II Enzymes (e.g. quinone-reductase, UDP-glucuronosyltransferase), promoted the detoxification and excretion of carcinogens, consequently preventing tumor genesis [6, 7, 8, 16]. For the inhibition of oxidative changes of xenobiotics, after the consumption of watercress a decrease in the levels of oxidative metabolites, e.g. of acetaminophen, in the urine, occurred [2].

Toxicology: Based on existing data on healthy individuals, there is no acute or chronic toxicity with the regular use of watercress in salads or as an addition to salads. People with preexisting kidney disease can experience kidney pain and painful micturition. After the intake of large amounts of watercress by healthy individuals, nausea, heart palpitations and gastrointestinal complaints, including colic, among others, have been reported [11, 17, Ü58]. Allergic reactions have also been observed [3, 4, 22].

The inhibition of iodine accumulation in the thyroid gland caused by rhodanides (present as breakdown products in all glucosinolate-containing plants) and thus the occurrence of goiter, only occurs with long-term use of very high doses that cannot be reached during normal consumption of watercress [Ü100].

Culinary use: The fresh flowering tops are coarsely chopped and used as an addition to salads (leaf-, cucumber-, tomato- or potato salads), and with quark, or mixed with fresh cheese or butter as a bread topping. Finely chopped or pureed, it is also used as a spice for sauces (especially with sour cream), soups (e.g. of cream soups), vegetables (e.g. finocchio or Florentine fennel, leek, wild parsnip, blanched celery, parsley roots), omelets, scrambled eggs and stew dishes, as well as mixed with butter as a spice for meat and fish [18, Ü45, Ü54, Ü55, Ü71].

The flowering tops are steamed, like spinach, and eaten as a vegetable [18].

The seeds are used similarly as brown mustard [Ü45].

Medicinal herb

Herbal drug: Nasturtii herba, Watercress herb [EB 6], dried or fresh, aerial parts, collected during the flowering period.

Indications: For catarrh of the upper respiratory tract (daily dose: 20 to 30 g fresh herb or 60 to 150 g freshly pressed plant juice). Due to its irritant effect, it is contraindicated in gastric and intestinal ulcers, inflammatory diseases of the kidneys, and for children less than four years of age [11]. It is also used as a cholagogue and stomachic.

Similar culinary herbs

Brown watercress, *Nasturtium × sterile* (Airy Shaw) Oefelein (hybrid of *N. officinale* L. × *N. microphyllum* Boenningh., triploid, sterile), is cultivated on a small scale, especially in the UK, and is more frost-resistant than watercress [Ü98].
→ **Garden Cress.**

Literature

[1] Björnquist B., A. Hase, J. Chromatogr. 435:501–507 (1988).
[2] Chen L. et al., Clin. Pharmacol. Ther. 60(6):651–660 (1996).
[3] Derrick E., C. Darley, Br. J. Dermatol. 136(2):290–291 (1997).
[4] Diamond S.P. et al., Dermatol. Clin. 8:77–80 (1990).
[5] Goda Y. et al., Biol. Pharm. Bull. 22(12): 1319–1326 (1999).
[6] Hecht S.S, J. Nutr. 129(3):768S–774S (1999).
[7] Hecht S.S et al., Cancer Epidemiol. Biomarkers Prev. 4(8):877–884 (1995).
[8] Hecht S.S et al., Cancer Epidemiol. Biomarkers Prev. 8(10):907–913 (1999).
[9] Helboe P. et al., J. Chromatogr. 197: 199–205 (1980).
[10] Jones E., R.E. Hughes, Phytochemistry 22: 2493–2499 (1983).
[11] Kommission E beim BfArM, BAnz-Nr. 22a vom 01.02.90.
[12] MacLeod A.J., R. Islam, J. Sci. Food Agric. 26:1545–1550 (1975).
[13] Minchington I. et al., J. Chromatogr. 247:141–148 (1982).
[14] Newmann R.M. et al., J. Chem. Ecol. 16:245–259 (1990).
[15] Olsen O., H. Sorensen, Phytochemistry 18:1547–1552 (1979).
[16] Rose P. et al., Karzinogenesis 21(11): 1983–1988 (2000).
[17] Schilcher H., Dtsch. Apoth. Ztg. 124: 2430–2435 (1984).
[18] Scholz H., Natürlich 18(3):46–51 (1998).
[19] Schultz O.E., W. Wagner, Z. Naturforsch. 11b:73–78 (1956).
[20] Spinks E.A. et al., Fette, Seifen, Anstrichm. 86:228 (1984).
[21] Wagner H., L. Hörhammer, Arzneim. Forsch. 15:453–457 (1956).
[22] Wetzig, T. et al., Contact Dermatitis 42(2):110 (2000).
[23] Weymar, H.: Buch der Kreuzblütler, Neumann Verlag, Leipzig-Radebeul 1988.
[24] Zrybko C. et al., J. Chromatogr. A 767 (1/2):43–52 (1997).

Literature references identified by Ü can be found in the general listing of books and monographs at the back of this book.

West Indian lemongrass

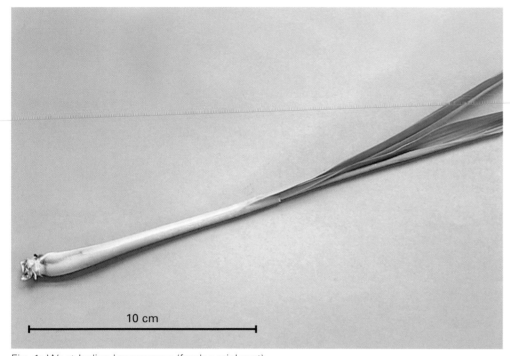

Fig. 1: West Indian lemongrass (fresh aerial part)

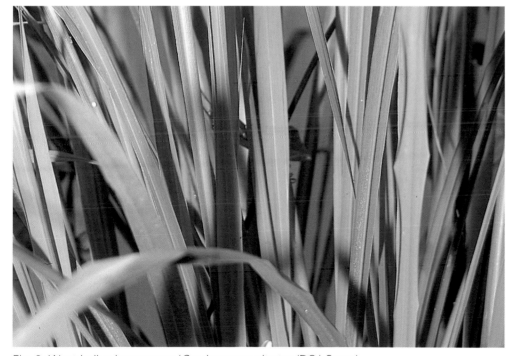

Fig. 2: West Indian lemongrass (*Cymbopogon citratus* (DC.) Stapf.)

Plant source: *Cymbopogon citratus* (DC.) Stapf.

Synonym: *Andropogon citratus* DC.

Taxonomic classification: Clones have been developed through crossbreeding and selection, which makes assignment to a single species uncertain, particularly because the plant blooms only exceedingly rarely.

Family: Sweet grass (Poaceae, synonym Gramineae).

Common names: Engl.: West Indian lemongrass, lemongrass, fever grass, citron grass, sereh; Fr.: verveine des Indes; Ger.: Lemongras, Zitronengras, Indisches Zitronengras, Westindisches Zitronengras, Serehgras, Takrai.

Description: Perennial grass plant with an up to 1.5 m tall stalk, smooth, glabrous. Leaves with lineal leaf-blade with pointed end, up to 90 cm long and up to 3 to 5 cm wide, glabrous on both sides, leaf sheath with circular cross section, paper-like ligula, less than 1 mm long. At the lower end, the plant is somewhat bulbous. Flowers are very rare; spurious spikes 30 cm long, sessile spikelets 6 mm long [Ü37].

Native origin: Probably native to eastern India, and Indonesia, it is only known as a cultivated plant.

Main cultivation areas: Cultivated worldwide in the tropics, but especially in southern Asia (India, Vietnam Sri Lanka, Java), but also in Australia, Brazil, Africa (western African countries as well as Egypt, and Kenya), the USA (Florida), Central America (Guatemala), and South America.

Main exporting countries: Malaysia, Vietnam, Guatemala, and Egypt, among others. Additionally, lemongrass essential oil is exported from Zambia, Guatemala, Brazil, and China.

Cultivation: Lemongrass is not winter hardy and therefore can only be cultivated in tropical regions. Propagation is done by rhizome division. Growing lemongrass in pots or pails with a sandy soil mix is possible without a problem, but the plant must overwinter at temperatures above 10 °C. The fresh plant with roots removed is sold commercially and forms new roots rapidly after being placed in water.

Culinary herb

Commercial forms: Lemongrass: the lower, 10 to 25 cm long parts of the herb, fresh or dried, whole or pulverized (often also commercially traded under the common names from the countries of origin: Serai, Sereh, and Tabrai), lemongrass oil (West Indian lemongrass oil, distilled from the fresh plant).

Production: The first harvest is possible 4 to 6 weeks after planting, and further harvests are possible following every 3 to 4 months.

Forms used: Fresh plant, dried plant, whole or pulverized, essential oil.

Storage: The fresh plant parts can be stored wrapped in plastic in the refrigerator for 2 to 3 weeks or in the freezer for 2 to 3 months. Drying is not recommended (due to aroma loss). Commercial lemongrass powder can be stored in well-closed screw-top glass jars, protected from light and heat. Lemongrass oil should be stored in completely filled and appropriately sized, airtight containers, protected from light and heat.

Description. Whole herb (Fig. 1): Commercially traded are the lower parts of the plant, which are 10 to 25 cm long; see description of the whole plant.

Powdered herb: Characteristic are the leaf fragments with the epidermis of the lower surface, consisting of elongated cells with stout, punctate and wavy walls, and typical for Poaceae, the stomata with dumbbell-shaped guard-cells and numerous cylindrical trichomes (50 μm long, 30 μm wide); the parenchyma contains yellowish brown oil cavities (about 60 μm in diameter) and the epidermal cells of the upper leaf surface consisting of elongated, thin-walled, somewhat sinuous cells. Fragments of the leaf margin show the serrate-like hairs along the margin [30].

Odor: Lemon-like, **Taste:** Lemon-like.

History: The use of aromatic grasses was already reported by Dioscorides (2nd half of the 1st century) and Pliny the Elder (23-79 CE). Only later, after 1820, the commercial distillation of Cymbopogon species, and their introduction to global trade started [9].

Constituents and Analysis

Constituents

- Essential oil: 0.2 to 0.5%, the main components are citral (65 to 86%, with about equal amounts of neral and geranial), myrcene (traces to 20%), limonene (3 to 16%), camphene (traces to 10%) and geraniol (2 to 10%); furthermore, geranyl acetate, linalool, nerol, citronellal and 2-methylhept-5-ene-2-one [3, 4, 6, 14, 17, 34, Ü83]. In a cultivar from Ethiopia, the main components were found to be geraniol (about 40%), citral (about 14%), borneol (5%) and α-oxobisabolene (12%, sesquiterpene ketone) [8]. In materials from Bhutan, up to 6% piperitone was detected [27].
- Flavonoids: Luteolin, 6-C-glucosylluteolin [10].
- Triterpenes, sterols: β-Sitosterol, cymbopogonol, a fucosterol glucoside [11,12].

Tests for Identity: Organoleptic, macroscopic and microscopic examination, as well as TLC analysis [Ü101].

Quantitative assay: The essential oil content can be determined with steam-distillation, according to Ph Eur, with xylol in the graduated tube. Citral is assayed quantitatively using a titrimetric method [Ph Eur, → Lemon oil, see → Lemon monograph] or TLC-densitometry [26], and citronellal, citronellol and geraniol contents are determined by GC [33] or GC/MS [29].

Adulterations, Misidentifications and Impurities have been observed, particularly with essential oils from other Cymbopogon-species (see below). They can be recognized by GC-analysis.

Actions and Uses

Actions: Due to its aromatic taste, lemongrass has appetite stimulating and digestion promoting effects.

Administration of a tea infusion made from fresh lemongrass in rats let to a dose-dependent analgesic effect. The infusion alleviated pain that was induced by injections of carrageenan or prostaglandin E_2. β-Myrcene was isolated from the tea via activity-guided-fractionation as the main active constituent [19]. A similar effect was observed in mice following application of lemongrass oil (50 to 200 mg/kg body weight, orally), which strongly inhibited acetic acid-induced writhing of the animals [35].

No changes in blood parameters (e.g. transaminase-, LDH-, cholesterol-, and triacyl glycerol levels, among others) were observed after ingestion of lemongrass tea in healthy subjects. Sedative and anxiolytic effects have also not been confirmed [15]. In animal tests (mice, rats), the oral application of lemongrass tea infusion or isolated citral (200 mg/kg body weight) was shown to have no hypothermic or sedative effects [2]. Lemongrass has shown merely mild diuretic and antiphlogistic activity [1].

Application of ethanolic extracts of lemongrass (0.5 or 5 g/kg body weight, orally) in rats, beginning one week prior to the application of azoxymethane (subcutaneous, 2 injections at one week apart), significantly inhibited DNA adduct formation (6-O-methylguanine, 7-N-methylguanine) in both the colonic mucosa and the muscular layer but not in the liver, and over a 12 week treatment period it prevented aberrant crypt foci (ACF) formation in the rat colon and thereby tumor genesis [31].

Lemongrass oil and its main component citral have shown good antimicrobial action [12, 16, 23-25].

Toxicology: Based on existing data, there is no chronic or acute toxicity with the regular use of lemongrass as a flavoring [7]. With ingestion of high doses of lemongrass tea infusions, drowsiness, polyuria and diarrhea have been observed [15]. Animal tests in rats and their offspring (in utero exposure) showed no signs of chronic toxicity (4 or 8 ml infusion of a 6.7% solution/kg body weight for 2 months) [29].

Citral and citronellal have sensitization potential. Skin inflammations and vesicular exanthema have occurred in workers who frequently come into contact with lemongrass oil [13, Ü39].

Culinary use: Lemongrass is used mainly in Thai and Vietnamese, but also in Indian and Indonesian cooking. Combined with coconuts it is used in the preparation of Malaysian fish dishes.

The lower, whitish, approximately 10 cm long, bulbously widened ends of the grass are used, similar to leeks. The outer, fibrous leaves are removed, then squeezed, chopped or finely cut. Lemongrass, prepared in this way, is added to the dish after cooking is completed, but sometimes it is, however, also cooked with the meal. The dried lemongrass or powder thereof must be soaked in hot water before use.

Lemongrass serves as a spice of steamed fish or chicken (lemongrass is placed in the steam water), hot chicken ragout, of soups (e.g. mussel soup), stews, roast dishes, wok dishes, sea foods, beef or pork, broccoli, cabbage, eggplant, salads, mushrooms and marinades [Ü2, Ü51, Ü55, Ü74, Ü95].

Combines well with: Basil, cilantro (in wok dishes), chillies, garlic, paprika, and shallots.

As a component of spice mixes and preparations: → Bomboe sajoer lodeh.

Other uses: The young, inner leaves are cooked and eaten as a vegetable [Ü61]. Lemongrass oil is used to scent cleaning products, air fresheners, deodorants and liquid soaps [27]. In the food industry, it is used as a flavoring for confectionaries and lemonades [17]. Some insect repellents also contain lemongrass oil as an active ingredient [7]. Furthermore, it serves as a raw material for the isolation of citral, which, among other uses, is used for partial synthesis of vitamin A and ionons [28].

Medicinal herb

Herbal drug: Cymbopogonis citrati aetheroleum, Lemongrass oil (West Indian lemongrass oil).

Indications: The therapeutic use of Cymbopogon-species and their essential oils were evaluated and not approved by Germany's Commission E of the BfArM due to insufficiently substantiated efficacy [13]. In Indian folk medicine, lemongrass is taken internally in the form of tea infusions (single dose 2 g, daily dose 6 g) for loss of appetite and gastrointestinal complaints; in Brazilian folk medicine, it is used for nervous restlessness and feverish colds and in Cuba for high blood pressure. Lemongrass oil is taken internally (dose: 3 to 5 drops on sugar) for cramp-like gastrointestinal pains, and in India, also for diarrhea combined with vomiting. Externally, it serves as a hyperemic remedy for the treatment of rheumatic pains, lumbago and sprains, diluted at minimum 1:1 ratio with a neutral fatty oil, or it is used in the form of baths. Evidence of efficacy for the aforementioned conditions is not available [Ü37]. The essential oils of West Indian lemongrass or East Indian lemongrass (see below) are used as substitutes for Melissa oil, and sometimes are described as "Indian Melissa Oil."

Similar spices

East Indian lemongrass (Cochin lemongrass), *Cymbopogon flexuosus* (NEES ex STEUD.) STAPF, native to tropical and subtropical Asia, is cultivated in India, Southeastern Asia, Equatorial Africa, and the Caribbean, and supplies Malabar oil (East Indian lemongrass oil, Cochin lemongrass oil), of which the main component is citral (75 to 80%). In some Indian chemical races, the main component is isointermedeol (sesquiterpene alcohol). Other races have been described with oil that is dominated by geraniol (30 to 50%), (+)-citronellol (about 25%) or geranyl acetate, and some that contain up to 20% methyleugenol (eugenol methylether). It is used the same as West Indian lemongrass, especially in Thai, Indian, Vietnamese and Indonesian cooking, as a spice in salads, clear fish- or chicken soups, roasted dishes and seafoods [7, 20, 32, Ü13, Ü43].

Selected Cymbopogon-species used primarily for the production of essential oil

Ceylon citronella, *Cymbopogon nardus* (L.) RENDLE, native to India, cultivated in Southeastern Asia, especially in Sri Lanka as well as in Central- and Eastern Africa, supplies Ceylon citronella oil (lenabuta oil), of which the main components are geraniol (17 to 39%), citronellal (5 to 16%), camphene and limonene (10 to 15%) [33].

Java citronella, *Cymbopogon winterianus* JOWITT, native to Sri Lanka, cultivated throughout almost all of the tropics, especially in Taiwan, Java, China, and Guatemala, supplies Java citronella oil, of which the main components are citronellal (32 to 50%), geraniol (12 to 25%) and citronellol (9 to 15%), geranyl acetate (3 to 8%) and citronellyl acetate (2 to 4%) [3, 29, 33].

Inchigras, *Cymbopogon travancorensis* BOR., native to and cultivated in southern

India, supplies inchigras oil, of which the main components are borneol (15-30%) and camphene (about 20%) [Ü42].

Palmarosa (rhosha grass), *Cymbopogon martinii* (ROXB.) WATSON var. *motia* auct., p.p., native to India, cultivated in India, Brazil, Madagascar, Zimbabwe, South Africa, and Indonesia, supplies palmarosa oil (rosha grass oil, East Indian geranium oil), of which the main components are geraniol (72 to 94%), geranyl acetate (4 to 17%) and linalool (2 to 3%), in addition to, among other, pyrazine derivatives [5, 18].

Gingergrass, *Cymbopogon martinii* (ROXB.) WATSON var. *sofia* GUPTA, cultivated in India, supplies gingergrass oil, of which the main components are perillalcohol (*p*-mentha-1,8-diene-3-ol, possibly an artifact, about 45%), and some races also contain geraniol. Gingergrass oil is of lower quality than palmarosa oil. [21, Ü43].
These oils are used mainly as perfume components of cosmetics and soaps, but are also used medicinally.

Literature

[1] Carbajal D. et al., J. Ethnopharmacol. 25(1):103–107 (1989).

[2] Carlini E.A. et al., J. Ethnopharmacol. 17(1):37–64 (1986).

[3] Chagonda L.S. et al., J. Ess. Oil Res. 12:478–480 (2000).

[4] Chisowa E.H. et al., Flav. Fragr. 13:29–30 (1998).

[5] Collin P., Forum Aromather. Aromapflege 14/98: 17–18 (1998).

[6] De Silva M.G., Mfg. Chemist. 30: 415–416, ref. CA: 363d (1959).

[7] De Smet P.A.G.M. et al. (Eds.), in: Adverse Effects of Herbal Drugs, Springer Verlag Berlin, Heidelberg, New York 1992, Bd. 1, p. 115–124.

[8] Demissew S., J. Ess. Oil Res. 5:465–479 (1993).

[9] Dürbeck K., Forum Aromather. Aromapflege 18/98 (1998).

[10] Gunasingh E.A. et al., Indian J. Pharm. Sci. 43:115 (1981), ref. CA: 96:139659x.

[11] Hanson S.W. et al., Phytochemistry 15: 1074–1075 (1976).

[12] Kishore N. et al., Mycoses 36(5/6):211–215 (1993).

[13] Kommission E beim BfArM, BAnz-Nr. 22a vom 01.02.1990.

[14] Leclerque P.A., J. Ess. Oil Res. 12:14–18 (2000).

[15] Leite J.R. et al., J. Ethnopharmacol. 17: 75–83 (1986).

[16] Lemos T.L. et al., Phytother. Res. 4(2): 82–84 (1990).

[17] Leung A.Y., in: Encyclopedia of common natural ingredients used in food, drugs and cosmetics, John Wiley & Sons, Cichester, Brisbane, Toronto 1980, p. 37 (1980).

[18] Locksley H.D. et al., Planta Med. 45:20–22 (1982).

[19] Lorenzetti B.B. et al., J. Ethnopharmacol. 34(1):43 (1991).

[20] Nath S.C. et al., J. Ess. Oil Res. 6:85–87 (1994).

[21] Naves Y.R., A.Y. Grampoloff, Bull. Soc. Chim. Franc. 1960:37 (1960).

[22] Olaniyi A.A. et al., Planta Med. 28:187–189 (1975).

[23] Onavunmi G.O. et al., J. Ethnopharmacol. 12(3):279–286 (1984).

[24] Pattnaik S. et al., Cytobios. 97(386):153–159 (1999).

[25] Ramadan F.M. et al., Chem. Microbiol. Technol. Lebensm. 1:96–102 (1972).

[26] Rossini C. et al., J. Planar. Chromatogr. Modern TLC 4:259 (1991).

[27] Schmidt E., Forum Aromather. Arompflege 14/98:3–5 (1998).

[28] Schultze W. et al., Dtsch. Apoth. Ztg. 135(7):557–577 (1995).

[29] Souza Formigomi M.L. et al., J. Ethnopharmacol. 17(1):65–74 (1986).

[30] Strauss D., Dtsch. Lebensm. Rdsch. 65: 176–177 (1969).

[31] Suaeyun R. et al., Carcinogenesis 18(5): 949–955 (1997).

[32] Thappa R.K. et al., Phytochemistry 18: 671 (1979).

[33] Thieme H. et al., Zbl. Pharm. 119(9):953–956 (1980).

[34] Torres Rosalinda C., A.G. Ragadio, Philipp. J. Sci. 125(2):147–156 (1996), ref. CA 126: 334188h.

[35] Viana G.S. et al., J. Ethnopharmacol. 70(3):323–327 (2000).

Literature references identified by Ü can be found in the general listing of books and monographs at the back of this book.

White mustard

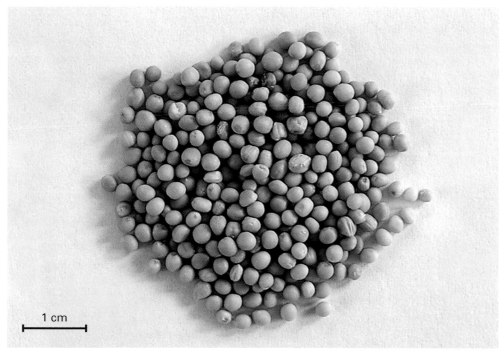

1 cm

Fig. 1: White mustard seed

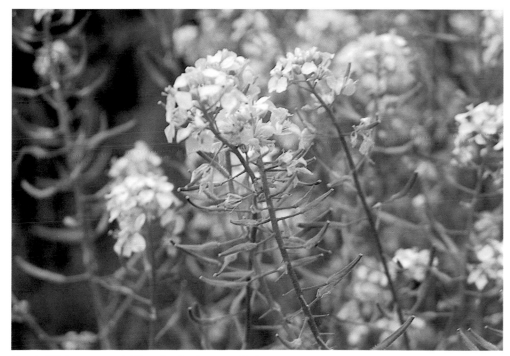

Fig. 2: White mustard (*Sinapis alba* L. ssp. *alba*)

Plant source: *Sinapis alba* L. ssp. *alba*.

Synonyms: *Brassica hirta* MOENCH, *Eruca alba* NOUL.

Taxonomic classification: The species *Sinapis alba* can be subdivided into the subspecies *S. a.* ssp. *alba* and *S. a.* ssp. *dissecta* (LAG.) BONNIER. Only *S. a.* ssp. *alba* is cultivated as a culinary- and medicinal plant.

Family: Mustard family (Brassicaceae, synonym Cruciferae).

Common names: Engl.: white mustard, yellow mustard; Fr.: moutarde blanche, herbe au beurre; Ger.: Weißer Senf, Echter Senf, Englischer Senf, Gelber Senf, Gelb-Senf, Gewürz-Senf, Garten-Senf, Mostard-korn.

Description: Annual plant, up to 1 m tall, stem with backward bent stiff hairs on the lower part, ramified in the upper part. The stalked, hirsute leaves are lyrate-pinnatifid to lyrate-pinnatipartite, with a large terminal lobe. The typical cruciform flowers are arranged in corymbs, have 4 horizontally spreading sepals, 4 bright-yellow unguiculate petals, 2 short and 4 longer stamina. The superior ovary develops to rostrate, hispid, 1 to 2 cm long (seldom 5 cm) long, 3 to 7 mm wide pod with 3 to 8 seeds. The seeds are yellow or sand-brown, nearly globular, pitted, with diameters of 1.8 to 2.5 mm. The subspecies is very variable (e.g. with varying leaf shapes, hairiness, color of seeds). Flowering period is from June to July [35, Ü37].

Native origin: Mediterranean region, Anterior Asia up to the Caucasus and to the Crimea, and introduced in many regions of Europe, Eastern Asia, and the Americas.

Main cultivation areas: Canada, Denmark, France, Hungary, Republics of the Russian Federation, England, Northern regions of the USA, as well as in, among others, the Balkan countries, Holland, Poland, Sweden, Switzerland, Czech Republic, Argentina, Chile, and Australia.

Main exporting countries: Canada, Hungary, Holland, and France.

Cultivation: The plant prefers humic, calcareous soil with sufficient water supply in sunny to half-shaded locations. Repeated cultivation in the same location or after growing other mustard family plants is to be avoided. Propagation is done through direct sowing in the early spring (in-between row width of about 20 cm, sowing depth 1 to 2 cm). The plants also thrive in pots in the autumn and winter. For the production of mustard seeds, suitable varieties include, among others, 'Budakalaszi sarga', 'Borowska', 'Carla', 'Condor', 'Kastor', 'Litember', 'Mansholt', 'Maxi', 'Metex', 'Mirly', 'Mustang', 'Nakielska', 'Santa Fe', 'Signal', 'Tilney', 'Trico', 'Ultra', 'Valiant' and 'Zlata' [6, Ü21]. Mustard sprouts can be obtained by placing the mustard seeds on damp cloth or cotton wool. If the substrate is kept constantly damp, the seedlings can be harvested after about 2 weeks, if they are about 5 cm long [Ü55].

Culinary herb

Commercial forms: Yellow mustard: ripe, dried seeds, mustard flour (mustard seed powder, for avoidance of the tendency to become rancid thereby causing a negative influence on taste, the fatty oil is usually removed).

Production: The harvest takes place with a combine harvester after the stems and leaves die off, and when the seeds rattle in the pods [Ü21].

Forms used: Ripe, whole or ground seeds, young leaves, flowers, and sprouts.

Storage: The seeds are stored as cool as possible, in well-closed containers, protected from light and moisture. They have a several year shelf life.

Description. Whole seed (Fig. 1): For the seeds or leaves, respectively, see description of the plant.

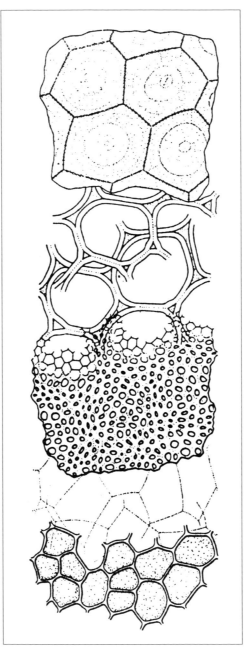

Fig. 3: White mustard. Testa, top view. Epidermis, from top to bottom, large cells, palisade cells, colorless "pigment cells", aleuron grains. From Ü29.

Powdered seed: Microscopic examination of the yellowish powder reveals the epidermis fragments of the testa with almost rectangular, transparent mucilage cells which are rounded at the top with concentric striations. Situated below are the 2 to 3 rows of thin-walled, collenchymatically thickened larger cells and a palisade layer with colorless, thick-walled cells with narrow lumen, followed by a layer of small, indistinctly visible cells, which, in contrast to the cells of black mustard, are not pigmented. The endosperm, fused to the testa, consists of a layer of thick-walled cells containing aleuron grains (Fig. 3). The fragments of the embryo are rich in fatty oil and aleuron grains. Starch must be absent. [DAC].

Odor: Odorless, **Taste:** The seeds first taste mildly sweetish then pungent and burning; cotyledons, leaves and flowers taste pungent.

History: There is archeological evidence from Iraq indicating the use of white mustard in ancient Sumer. In ancient Rome and Greece, mustard played an important role as a spice. In the 1st century, the Romans produced the first recipe for → Table mustard. Since the early Middle Ages, white mustard has also been cultivated in Central Europe [6, Ü59, Ü97].

Constituents and Analysis

DIN- and ISO-Standards. DIN Standard 10204 (Mustard seed, technical delivery conditions), DIN Standard 10225 (Determination of *p*-hydroxybenzylisothiocyanate, photometric method for mustard seed), ISO Standard 1237 (Mustard seed), DIN Standard 10221-2 (Determination of water content and volatile components, oven-drying method for mustard seed and saffron).

Constituents of the seeds
▪ Glucosinolates: The main components are sinalbin (2.5 to 5%). Upon tissue injury, the glucosinolates come into contact with the enzyme myrosinase, which

is located in the so-called myrosine cells; thereby mustard oils (alkyl- or alkarylisothiocyanates) are formed (Fig. 12, → General Section). From sinalbin, the non-volatile, pungent tasting *p*-hydroxybenzylisothiocyanate (*p*-hydroxybenzyl mustard oil) forms. The seeds also contain smaller amounts of gluconapin and progoitrin [9, 11, 23].

- Phenylpropane derivatives: Sinapin (1.2 to 2%, possibly an artifact from the isolation procedure), 4-hydroxybenzoyl-choline [11].
- Fatty oil: 20 to 45%, the main fatty acid is erucic acid (depending on the cultivar, 2 to 60%), oleic acid (18 to 33%), linolic acid (8 to 20%) and linolenic acid [6, 19].
- Protein: About 25 to 40% [6].
- Mucilage: About 25% [3].
- Triterpenes, sterols: β-Sitosterol, campesterol, brassicasterol, 24-ethylidene-cholesterol [1, 8].

Constituents of the leaf and sprouts

- Glucosinolates: In the leaves sinalbin (about 0.2%, upon tissue injury, transforming into the pungent tasting *p*-hydroxybenzylisothiocyanate), furthermore, glucoputranjivin, glucobrassicanapin, glucotropäolin, sinigrin and ω-methylthioalkylglucosinolate, in the sprouts, however, only a small amount of sinalbin but particularly glucobrassicin and methoxyglucobrassicin [2, 4, 12]. Upon infection, the plant produces the phytoalexins sinalexin, sinalbin A and sinalbin B (indole derivatives with 2,3-condensed sulfur- and nitrogen-containing 5- or 6-ring) [15].
- Sterols: β-Sitosterol, campesterol [8].

Tests for Identity: The identity of white mustard seeds can be determined with sensoric examination, macroscopic and micro-scopic analysis, as well as with TLC of the glucosinolates [11, 21, DAC] or the mustard oils after fermentation [10, 21].

Quantitative assay: The determination of the glucosinolate content is carried out indirectly by quantifying the isothiocyanates after fermentative cleavage. Alkalization with NaOH, transforms the formed *p*-hydroxybenzylisothiocyanate to sodium thiocyanate, which is determined colorimetrically as red iron(III)thiocyanate [9, 16, DIN-Standard 10225], iodometrically [17] or acidimetrically, after reaction with piperidine [18]. The direct quantification of the glucosinolates is also possible, for example with RP-HPLC [23] or in form of the desulfoglucosinolates by HPLC or GLC [7]

Adulterations, Misidentifications and Impurities: Seeds from other cruciferous plants are possible adulterants. Differentiation is possible based on size and color or composition of the testa as well as by differences in the glucosinolate spectrum.

Actions and Uses

Actions: Due to its pungent taste, it is appetite stimulating and digestion promoting. Extracts of the ground, fermented seeds have skin irritant action and therefore induce hyperemia and enhance peripheral blood flow [13, 18]. They also have good antibacterial properties [5]. In murine hepatic cell lines, sinalbin and some breakdown products of glucosinolates induced the activity of the enzyme quinone reductase, which can block the action of a few carcinogens [20].

Toxicology: Based on existing data, there is no acute or chronic toxicity with the use of the seeds, or of the leaves, flowers or sprouts as a salad or salad ingredient at normal doses. Intake of larger amounts of the seed powder (e.g. for stimulating digestion or regulating defecation) should, however, be avoided due to possible irritation and damage to the gastrointestinal mucosa. The development of antibodies against Sin a I, a low molecular albumin from mustard seeds, was observed in many clinical trial volunteers. Therefore, allergic reactions to mustard seeds are possible [14].

Culinary use: In order to not prevent the enzymatic release of the flavor-determining mustard oils, the mustard seed must not be heated over 55 °C in the preparation of meals (denaturing of myrosinase!).

Mustard flour, stirred with cold or luke-warm(!) water and left to stand for 15 minutes, is used, for example, as a seasoning of sauces for salads, fish, meat and egg dishes, soups and stews. In mayonnaises, mustard flour serves also as a pseudo-emulsifier due to its mucilage content.

The whole seeds are used as a seasoning of mixed pickles, such as mustard cucumbers, pumpkin, red beets, onions or mixed pickles. They also serve as an ingredient for sauerkraut, fish marinades, roasted meat, and sausage products (e.g. large frankfurters, bratwurst or salami), light sauces for fish, eggs or vegetables [Ü1, Ü30, Ü46, Ü92].

The young leaves can be added in small quantities to salads (up to 30%) or chopped and added to stew dishes (after cooking!). They also serve as a seasoning of sausage-, quark- and egg dishes or as a bread topping. They are eaten as a salad especially in Southern- and Eastern Asia. The flowers are also used as a food ingredient [Ü63, Ü95].

Mustard sprouts are used in the same way as those of → Garden cress, as a salad ingredient as well as garnish or sandwich spread [Ü55].

Combines well with: Dill, ginger, lemon, onions, and pepper.

Sinalbin   →   *p*-Hydroxybenzyl mustard oil

As a component of spice mixes and preparations: → Barbecue sauce, → Curry powder, → Fish spice, → Frankfurter green sauce, → Sambhar powder, → Table mustard.

Similar culinary herbs: → Sarepta mustard.

Medicinal herb

Herbal drug: Erucae semen, White mustard seed [DAC].

Indications: In the form of cataplasms made from powdered mustard seeds for catarrhs of the respiratory tract and for segmental therapy of chronic joint diseases and soft tissue rheumatism. For these conditions 4 tablespoonfuls of powdered mustard seeds are stirred immediately before use in lukewarm (enzymes!) water until making a paste. The cataplasm is left on the skin for 10 to 15 minutes (for children 5 to 10 minutes). Due to the possible absorption of mustard oils, it should not be applied to persons with renal diseases and children under 6 years of age. Because there is a risk of skin- and nerve- damage with long-term use, the duration of use should not exceed 2 weeks [13].

Literature

[1] Appelquist L.A.D. et al., Phytochemistry 20:207–210 (1971).
[2] Bergmann F., Z. Pflanzenphysiol. 62:362–375(1970).
[3] Ciu W. et al., Food Chem. 46:169–176 (1993).
[4] Cole R., Phytochemistry 15:759–762 (1976).
[5] Crasselt E., Arch. Pharm. 283:275–280 (1950).
[6] Hackl G., Arznei- und Gewürzpflanzen 1(2):48–54 (1996).
[7] Hrncirik K. et al., Z. Lebensm. Untersuch. Forsch. A. 206:103–107 (1997).
[8] Ingram D.S. et al., Phytochemistry 7:1241–1245 (1968).
[9] Josefsson E., J. Sci. Food Agric. 21:94 (1970), zit. Ü37.
[10] Karig F., J. Chromatogr. 106:477–480 (1975).
[11] Kerber E. et al., Angew. Bot. 55(5/6):457–467 (1981).
[12] Kjaer A., K. Rubinstein, Acta Chem. Scand. 4:1276 (1953), zit. Ü37.
[13] Kommission E beim BfArM., BAnz.-Nr. 22a vom 01.02.90.
[14] Menendez-Arias L. et al., Eur. J. Biochem. 177(1):159–166 (1988).
[15] Pedras M.S., I.L. Zaharia, Phytochemistry 55(3):213–216 (2000).
[16] Raghavan B. et al., Microchimica Acta (6):818–822 (1972).
[17] Raghavan B. et al., J. Sci. Food Agric. 22:523–525 (1971).
[18] Shankaranarayana M.L. et al., Agric. Biol. Chem. 35:959–961 (1971).
[19] Sietz F.G., Fette Seifen Anstrichm. 74:72–80 (1972).
[20] Tawfiq N. et al., Carcinogenesis 16(5):1191–1194 (1995).
[21] Wagner H. et al., Arzneim. Forsch. 15:453–457 (1965).
[22] Weymar H., Buch der Kreuzblütler, Neumann Verlag, Leipzig-Radebeul 1988.
[23] Zrybko C. et al., J. Chromatogr. A 767(1/2):43–52 (1997).

Literature references identified by Ü can be found in the general listing of books and monographs at the back of this book.

Spice mixtures

Spice mixtures and other seasoning ingredients

(Bibliographical data denoted with an arrow (→) refer to literature with recipes for preparation of the special spice mixture)

A.1. Sauce: A sweet-piquant seasoning sauce that contains garlic, onions, oranges, undeclared herbs and spices, and serves as a table condiment for steaks and grilled meat or fish, also as a seasoning of marinades for chicken and beef [Ü55].

Adshika paste: A seasoning blend, used in Grusinia (Caucasia region), composed of a mixture of spices, which upon the adding of vinegar and salt turns into a paste, it serves as a seasoning of meat-, vegetable-, and rice dishes [Ü92].

Almond biscuit spice: Contains cardamom, cinnamon, clove, coriander, and mace, among others [Ü30].

Apple cake spice: 4 parts cinnamon, 1 part ground clove, 1/2 part ground nutmeg [Ü2].

Arabian spice mix: Contains caraway, cardamom, clove, pepper, and turmeric, it is used in Arab countries as a seasoning of soups and meat dishes [Ü92].

Baharat: A seasoning blend made from cardamom, clove, coriander, cumin, nutmeg, and pepper, sometimes also cinnamon and chillies, it is used especially in the Gulf States as a seasoning of meat, fish, legumes, rice- and potato dishes [Ü30, → Ü73].

Barbecue spices: Are rubbed onto the meat before grilling, they usually contain black pepper, celery fruits, chillies, clove, garlic, marjoram, mustard, paprika, thyme, table salt and brown sugar [→ Ü73].

Berbere: An Ethiopian variety of → Garam masala.

Beurre Maître d'hôtel: → Parsley butter.

Bologna spice mix (Hamburger spice mix): Contains allspice, anise, caraway, coriander, dill, mace, nutmeg, onions, paprika, and white pepper, it is used as a seasoning of meat dishes [Ü92].

Bomboe (Boemboe): An Indonesian spice blend, which is made fresh just before use, it contains predominantly garlic, onions and paprika. **Bomboe nasi goreng** contains paprika, turmeric, lesser galangal, garlic and onions, and is used in Indonesia for regional specialty dishes, e.g. Nasi goreng, a rice dish, **Bomboe sajoer lodeh** contains additional cumin, lemongrass and pepper and serves as a seasoning of meat [Ü30, Ü92].

Bouquet garni: A bunch bundled together with a string or a in a muslin sack, an herb bouquet used as a seasoning of soups, stews, cooked fish or sauces, in the classic form composed of one bay leaf, a small thyme stalk and 2 stalks of parsley or chervil, which are added at the end of the cooking process and then removed when cooking is finished. Any of the following herbs can also be added according to the type of meal and personal taste: basil, celery, chives, clove, leeks, marjoram, mints, rosemary, sage, summer savory or tarragon, [Ü30, Ü47, → Ü91].

Bread spice: Suitable for seasoning of bread it contains, among others, anise, coriander, caraway and onions, but spice mixtures made from summer savory, fennel and sage are also used, 10 g/kg is added [Ü30].

Café de Paris spice mix: Contains → Curry powder, chives, garlic, onions, parsley, pepper, rosemary, sodium glutamate and herb salt. A rich spice mixture used as a seasoning of herb butter, marinades for steaks, grilled plates, commercially traded in a paste form [Ü92].

Cake spice: → Pastry spice.

Cajun spice: A North American spice mixture that contains black pepper, chillies, cumin, garlic, onions, oregano, paprika, thyme, and salt, it is rubbed over the meat or fish before roasting or used as a seasoning of stews or rice dishes [→Ü73].

Celery salt: Contains 85 to 90% salt and 10 to 15% ground celery fruits, leaves and tubers [Ü30].

Char masala: A typical spice mixture of Afghanistan that contains black cardamom, cinnamon, clove and cumin, it is used as a seasoning of rice dishes [Ü92].

Chat masala: A typical seasoning of Northern India made from ajowan or dill fruits, asafetida, black pepper, chillies, cumin, ginger, mango, mint, pomegranate seeds, and salt, it is used as a seasoning of soups, vegetable- and fish dishes, vegetable salads, but also used on fruit [Ü73].

Chemen: A spice mixture used in Turkey and Armenia that contains powdered fenugreek, garlic and pepper, that is served on a dried meat called patuma [Ü73].

Chili con carne seasoning: A spice mixture composed of chillies, caraway, coriander, garlic and oregano, it is used as a seasoning of the Mexican dish chili con carne, but also of other meat dishes as well as tomato dishes [Ü92, Ü98].

Chili powder: A dark red powder, prepared from ground, dried chillies (usually ancho-chillies), allspice, clove, cumin, garlic powder, onion powder, oregano, and salt, it is used mostly as a seasoning of chili con carne, but also of fish- and vegetable soups, marinades and dressings. It is also suitable for egg dishes, goulash and tartar [→ Ü2, Ü13, Ü55].

Chili sauce: Contains chillies, vinegar and sugar, flavored with cinnamon, ginger, and onions, it is offered in the flavor types "sweet" and "hot", used as an ingredient in other seasoning sauces, but also as a seasoning of fish- and vegetables conserves and mixed pickles [Ü92, Ü98].

China spice: → Five-spice-mix.

Citrus comminuted: A mixture of ground lemon peels, lemon juice and lemon oil, used in the food industry as a flavoring [Ü92].

Cocktail sauce: In addition to vegetable oil, egg yolk and vinegar as seasonings it contains, among others, chillies or white pepper, bay leaf, dill, parsley and thyme, it serves as a seasoning of fish dishes and egg dishes [Ü92].

Cumberland sauce: A seasoning sauce that originally contained meat broth, red wine, orange peels and spices, but today commercially produced Cumberland sauce usually contains meat extract, orange- or lemon juice, currant- or apple jelly, mustard flour, olive oil and dessert wine, it serves as a seasoning of venison dishes, poultry and pasties [Ü92, Ü98].

Curry powder: Developed in India, a quite variable, more or less pungent spice mixture made from 10 to 15 (sometimes up to 35) individual spices. In India it serves as a seasoning of curry (kari), a dish made from meat, fish and vegetables. Curry powder contains, among others, turmeric, mainly for the color it provides, and other spices such as ajowan, allspice, anise, black pepper, caraway, cardamom, chillies, Chinese cinnamon, clove, coriander, cumin, curry herb, fennel, fenugreek seeds, ginger, lesser galangal, mace, mustard, nutmeg, paprika, and white pepper, rarely also asafetida, sometimes also salt and other ingredients such as legume flour, starch and/or dextrose. The proportion of salt amounts to maximum 5%, and the other ingredients maximum 10%. Commercially available curry powder is offered in different flavor types including, among others, mildly aromatic Madras curry powder and spicy-hot Bengali curry powder. It is used as a seasoning of roast- lamb or veal, poultry,

fish dishes, stews with legumes, cauliflower dishes, soups (e.g. fish soup), sauces, rice- and noodle dishes, egg dishes, butter and salads, among others. The full aroma of curry powder is unfolded when stewed in fat [Ü13, → Ü30, Ü33, Ü40, → Ü73, Ü89, Ü90, DIN-Standard 10203, ISO-Standard 2253].

Delicatessen spices: Spice mixtures that are used for the seasoning of dressings, meat salads, mayonnaises and seasoning sauces, among others. Their composition is customized according to the intended use [→ Ü30].

Dukkah: An Egyptian spice mixture that contains coriander, cumin, filberts, pepper, sesame, and salt, it serves as a spice for bread dipped in oil [Ü93].

Egg spice: For sweet dishes like egg pancakes it contains cinnamon and vanilla, and for salty dishes like scrambled eggs or fried eggs it contains basil, chervil, chives, mace, paprika, and pepper, among others [Ü30].

English pudding spice: One part each of powdered allspice, cinnamon bark, clove, coriander fruits, mace and nutmeg.

Fines herbes: A mixture prepared according to French recipes composed of freshly chopped or dried rubbed herbs: chervil, chives, parsley, tarragon, others can also be added including basil, hyssop, lavender, marjoram, rosemary, sage, salad burnet, summer savory, and thyme. It is added to roasts, stews, salads, quark, soups, sauces and omelets [Ü30].

Fish spice: Serves as a base seasoning composed of, among others, allspice, basil, black pepper, caraway, cardamom, clove, coriander, dill, garlic, ginger, juniper berries, lemon balm, lovage, marjoram, onions, paprika, parsley, peppermint, rosemary, sage, summer savory, white mustard and white pepper. Fish spice is usually used not ground. Variations depend on the type of fish and the preparation [→ Ü30].

Five-spice-mix (China spice): A cocoa-colored spice mixture that contains 1 part Japanese pepper, 1 part star anise, 1/2 part cinnamon, 1/2 part clove and 1 1/4 parts fennel, sometimes supple-

mented with cardamom or ginger. It serves as a seasoning of fish, meat, meat and liver pastes, grilled lobster or shrimp, bouillon or soup broth [Ü30, Ü33, → Ü73, → Ü93, Ü90].

Frankfurter green sauce: Contains mainly borage, chervil, chives, dill, garden cress, garden sorrel, lemon balm, mustard, parsley, salad burnet, and tarragon. It is mostly used for egg, fish- and meat dishes, but is also suitable for potatoes boiled in their jacket [Ü30, → Ü86].

Garam masala (= warm mixture): A North Indian, quite variable seasoning mix, that in the base mix usually contains cumin (about 27%), coriander (about 17%), black pepper (about 14%), cardamom (about 14%), clove (about 10%), mace (about 10%), cinnamon (about 5%), and bay leaf (about 1.5%). The mixture is often prepared from roasted spices and is usually added at the end of the cooking process or sprinkled over the finished dish [Ü30]. This spice mix is used for the seasoning of rice, vegetable dishes (e.g. cauliflower), fish, grilled fish and lamb. For certain fish dishes, the uncut spices are also used [→ Ü2, Ü33, → Ü73, Ü90].

Gingerbread spice: The main components are anise, cinnamon, clove, cardamom, mace, allspice and coriander, occasionally also orange peels, ginger, nutmeg and vanilla [→ Ü30].

Gomasio: A Japanese seasoning salt that contains 3 parts roasted black sesame seeds, which are ground fine with 1 part salt, used especially for the seasoning of rice dishes, raw vegetables and uncooked vegetarian salads [→ Ü2].

Green masala: → Masala.

Gremolata: An Italian spice mixture composed of freshly chopped parsley, grated lemon peel and finely chopped garlic cloves, sprinkled over the classic Milanese meat dish ossobuco just prior to serving, it can also be used as a seasoning for pasta or risotto [Ü51].

Grill spice (shish kebab spice, shashlik spice): Contains, among others, allspice, caraway, chillies or paprika, coriander, garlic, mace, nutmeg, pepper, rosemary, and thyme, it serves as a seasoning of grilled meats or sausages, but also of poultry, ground chuck, marinades and pizzas [→ Ü2, Ü30, → Ü91, Ü92].

Hamburger meat spice (minced meat seasoning): Usually contains garlic, marjoram, onions, paprika, pepper, sage, summer savory, tarragon, thyme and sometimes also salt [Ü92].

Hamburger spice mix: → Bologna spice mix.

Harissa: A typical seasoning paste of Tunisia prepared from dried chillies, caraway, coriander, garlic, mint, salt and olive oil. It is added in marinades before grilling chicken, lamb or fish, also suitable for Northern African dishes like couscous [Ü55, → Ü73].

Herb butter: Made by allowing butter to become soft at room temperature and then mixing up the butter with fresh, well washed, dried off herbs (1 table-spoonful of about 125 g butter) using a hand blender and chill for 3 hours. Individual herbs can be used, e.g. parsley or garlic, or herb mixtures, e.g. of marjoram, rosemary, and thyme. Herb butter has a shelf life of about one month in the refrigerator. It is suitable not only as a bread spread, but also as an addition to vegetable, poultry, fish or grilled and roasted meat [Ü1]. For the preparation of herb butter with dried spices one can use borage, celery, chervil, chives, dill, parsley, salad burnet, and tarragon, among others [Ü30, → Ü64].

Herb cubes: A very convenient form of preservation of dried, comminuted herbs is the embedding in anhydrous vegetable fat, e.g. in the form of so-called herb cubes. Due to its high viscosity, the fat slows down the diffusion of the essential oils through the surface thereby preventing evaporation as well as penetration of oxygen into the deeper fat layers. Due to their antioxidative, radical scavenging activity, the herbs do their part to prevent the fat from rapidly becoming rancid. Herb cubes, usually containing also salt, are added after cooking, to season sauces, soups and stews.

Herb oil: Fresh herbs (e.g. basil, marjoram, oregano, tarragon, and thyme) are rubbed into a paste and mixed with slightly warmed oil. Sieve it after storage for a duration of about 2 weeks in the refrigerator. Furthermore the herb oil must be stored cool, because this type of preparation does not kill the microorganisms. It is suitable for the seasoning of salads, sauces, marinades and soups as well as for brushing onto meat and fish before grilling. About 10 g of mixed herbs are added per 250 ml oil [→ Ü64, Ü67].

Herb salt: Contains 80 to 90% table salt (usually iodized) or sea salt and about 15% dried herbs including, among others, basil, celery, dill, marjoram, onions, parsley, rosemary, and thyme, → Celery salt [Ü30].

Herb vinegar: A nonperishable, easily homemade seasoning preparation. 50 to 100 g of fresh, washed, then dried off herbs are rubbed into a paste; 1 liter of 5%, heated vinegar is poured over 2 to 3 tablespoons of bruised spices or 10 crushed garlic cloves and is left to macerate in a warm place for 3 to 6 weeks, afterwards decanted and filtered. Well suited for the preparation of herb vinegars, individually or mixed, are basil, bay, dill, fennel, garden nasturtium (adds color!), lemon balm, lovage, marjoram, mint, rosemary, sage, southernwood, summer savory, tarragon, and thyme. Herb vinegars are suitable for the seasoning of stews, marinades and sauces [Ü1, → Ü30, → Ü64, Ü67].

Herbes de Provence: May contain anise, basil, hyssop, lavender, marjoram, oregano, rosemary, sage, summer savory, and thyme, used especially for savory tasting dishes, e.g. of lamb, potato-, vegetable- and tomato dishes. The herbs should always be cooked with the dish [Ü30, Ü54].

Herbs for grilling and smoking: A spice mixture for grilling that is sprinkled over the charcoal embers, it may contain, among others, fennel, marjoram, rosemary and spruce needles [Ü92].

Hoisin-sauce: A viscous, reddish-brown sauce made from red bean paste, seasoned with → Five-spice-mix and chillies [Ü51].

Honey cake spice: → Gingerbread spice.

HP-sauce (HP = House of Parliaments): A pungent seasoning sauce produced in England made from malt vinegar, molasses, fruits and undeclared spices, used as a seasoning of minced meat added before cooking or after grilling, of soups, stews and gravies [Ü55].

Ketchup: A salty seasoning sauce common in Eastern Asia, arrived in Central Europe via England, generally composed of tomato puree, salt, vinegar and onions, frequently paprika is also added, offered in numerous flavor variations, most often as → Tomato ketchup [Ü92].

La kama: A Moroccan spice mixture composed of black pepper, cinnamon, ginger, nutmeg, and turmeric, it serves as a soup- and stew seasoning [Ü93].

Lemon pepper: A classic Italian paste-like seasoning mixture made from grated lemon peels, ground black pepper, garlic, raw sugar, dextrin, salt, citric acid and olive oil, it is used as a seasoning of fish, roasted, baked or grilled sea foods as well as of salads, together with grated Parmesan cheese used as a pasta sauce [Ü92].

Masala: An Indian seasoning mix either in the form of a spice powder composed of bay leaf, cardamom, cinnamon, mace, and nutmeg, heated together with ghee (a clarified butter-like product), or in the form of a spice paste (green masala) made from freshly peeled ginger, garlic (or onions), fresh pitted chillies and fresh cilantro leaves, pounded with water until it becomes a thick paste, it is used as a seasoning of fish or chicken [→ Ü2, Ü55, → Ü73, Ü92].

Meat spice: The most frequently used component is pepper, in addition to, for cooked pork, bay leaf, celery, clove, garlic, mace, and parsley, for cooked beef, bay leaf, horseradish, lovage, onions, and parsley, for roasted meat, among others, basil, bay leaf, celery, → Herbes de Provence, juniper berries, rosemary, thyme, and a mixture made from capers, caraway, → Curry powder, green pepper, onions, paprika, and pepper is used for the seasoning of tartar

[Ü30, → Ü91]. See also → Hamburger meat spice.

Meju: → Soybean.

Mélange classique: A seasoning blend made from bay leaves, chillies, clove, coriander, marjoram, nutmeg, rosemary, thyme, and white pepper [→ Ü73].

Mignonette pepper: A mixture of coarsely ground or minced black pepper, used especially in France as a table spice, mainly for seasoning already prepared, pan-fried or grilled meat [Ü13].

Miso: → Soybean.

Mixed pickles spice: Usually contains allspice, bay leaf, capers, chillies, dill, and tarragon [Ü30, → Ü73].

Mostert, Mostrich: → Table mustard.

Mulled wine spice (Punch spice): Contains cardamom, cinnamon, clove, nutmeg, star anise, dried lemon- or orange peels and citric acid, among others [→ Ü2].

Multi-colored pepper: Composed of about the same proportions of green, white and black pepper as well as pink pepper [Ü92], and sometimes allspice is also added.

Mustard: → Table mustard.

Nam prik: A paste-like Thai seasoning mix made with, among others, chillies, garlic, shallot, shrimp, and sugar, it serves as a seasoning of vegetables, rice, and fish [→ Ü73].

Natto: → Soybean.

Nonaya-spice: A Malaysian or Chinese spice mixture that contains 2 parts chilli powder, 2 parts garlic powder, 2 parts onion powder, 1 part lemongrass powder and 1 part sugar [Ü2].

Panch phoron (= 5 seeds): An East Indian 5-spice-mix made from 2 3/4 parts fennel, 2 parts cumin, 1 3/4 parts brown mustard, 1 to 2 parts cumin, and 1 part fenugreek seeds, mainly used as a seasoning of dishes made from legumes or vegetables (tomatoes, eggplant), but also as an addition for roasting of fish and meat [→ Ü73, Ü93].

Parisian pepper: A seasoning blend made from bay leaves, black pepper, chillies, coriander, marjoram, nutmeg, paprika, rosemary, sage, tarragon, and thyme, sometimes a flavor enhancer and salt are also added, it serves as a seasoning of meat, especially venison, grilled dishes and marinades [Ü49].

Parsley butter (Beurre Maître d'hôtel): 120 g foamy whipped butter is mixed with 2 to 3 tablespoons of finely chopped parsley and 1 tablespoon lemon juice as well as salt and pepper to taste, suitable for grilled steak or roasted fish [Ü47].

Pastry spice: Contains anise, cardamom, clove, coriander, ginger, saffron, and vanilla, among others [Ü30].

Pepper bouquet: A French seasoning blend made from ground black pepper as well as red and green paprika, it is used as a seasoning of cheese and meat dishes [Ü92].

Pepper sauce (Devil's sauce): A commercially produced very hot seasoning sauce composed of cayenne pepper, salt, vinegar and other spices, it is used as a seasoning of meat- and fish dishes and egg dishes [Ü92].

Persillade: A French seasoning mix composed of finely chopped parsley leaves and garlic, roasted shortly and, added to the meal before serving, it is used as a seasoning of soups, stews, vegetables, grilled lamb, beefsteak, roasted fish or chicken [Ü55, Ü92].

Pesto (In France 'pistou', in Russia 'pestu'): An Italian pasty, green seasoning sauce made by pureeing 200 g finely cut, lightly roasted pine nuts, 200 g ramsons leaves, and 100 ml olive oil in the mixer, then adding 50 g grated Parmesan- or Pecorino-cheese; it can be stored for several weeks in the refrigerator in a sealed jar. Garlic (2 cloves) and basil (25 g fresh leaves) can be used instead of ramsons leaves. It is suitable as a seasoning of sauces, soups, pasta, spaghetti, risotto, vegetable dishes as well as gnocchi- and homemade noodles [Ü80, → Ü92].

Pickling spice: Used for pickling cucumbers, gherkins, pickled gherkins, herbed gherkins and mixed pickles, it usually contains allspice, bay leaf, celery, chillies, clove, coriander, dill, ginger, horseradish, juniper berries, mugwort, nutmeg, paprika, pearl onion, pepper, tarragon, and white mustard. Pickling spice is dispersed in a warm mixture of vinegar and water, which is poured hot over the items to be pickled or marinated [→ Ü2, Ü13, → Ü30, Ü92].

Pizza spice: The main component is oregano, and it may also contain garlic, marjoram, paprika, pepper, rosemary, and thyme [Ü30].

Plum jam spice: Contains cinnamon and clove or cardamom, coriander, clove, ginger, and mace [Ü30].

Poultry spice: Is dominated by marjoram, sage, and thyme, but may also contain, among others, anise, basil, cardamom, celery, coriander, dill, ginger, nutmeg, onions, paprika, pepper, and summer savory [Ü30].

Punch spice: → Mulled wine spice.

Quark spice: Contains caraway, celery, chives, → Curry powder, dill, garlic, green pepper, marjoram, onions, paprika, and parsley, among others [Ü30].

Quatre épices (= 4 spices): A French seasoning mixture composed of allspice, cinnamon, clove, and nutmeg, it is used in the preparation of sausage and for the seasoning of stews as well as braised meat [Ü30, → Ü73]. According to other sources the mixture contains clove, ginger, nutmeg, and white pepper. The Tunisian variety is made from cinnamon, dried rosebuds, paprika, and pepper [Ü13].

Ras el hanout: A North African seasoning mixture that is quite variable in its composition, and may contain, among others, allspice, anise, bay, black cumin, black pepper, cardamom, chaste tree fruit, Chinese cinnamon, cinnamon, clove, cubeb, fennel, ginger, grains-of-paradise, iris rhizome, lavender, lesser galangal, long pepper, mace, rowanberry, saffron, Spanish fly (sic!), thyme, and turmeric, the mixture is ground right before use and it is used especially in Morocco as a seasoning of game-, rice-, mutton dishes and couscous [→ Ü73].

Ravigotte: A sauce made from mixed and chopped herbs such as parsley and tarragon.

Roast spice: May contain, among others, allspice, basil, lovage, marjoram, mugwort, paprika, parsley, pepper, sage, southernwood, summer savory, tarragon, and thyme. It is used as a seasoning of sauces and ragouts, added after infusing and cooked together in the sauce [Ü30].

Salad spice: Suitable as a seasoning of leaf salads, especially borage, celery, chervil, dill, marjoram, parsley, and/or salad burnet [Ü30].

Salsa (the Spanish word for sauce): Normally understood to be a tomato-based seasoning sauce, seasoned with cilantro leaves, chillies, and onions [Ü51].

Salsa comum: An old Italian seasoning mixture that contains black pepper, cinnamon, clove, coriander, ginger, and sometimes also saffron, it is used as a seasoning of rice- and noodle dishes [92].

Sambal (Samballan): A typical Indonesian and Indian paste-like seasoning mixture that contains as its base components mostly ground chillies, salt and brown sugar (**Sambal oelek**) and other ingredients, e.g. **Sambal assem** with the addition of comminuted shrimps, **Sambal manis** with the addition of nutmeg, **Sambal nasi goreng** with the addition of onions, **Sambal trassi** with crab paste. **Sambal badjak** has a complex composition besides chillies it contains, among others, clove, coriander, garlic, lesser galangal, onion, pepper, and shrimps [→ Ü2, Ü80, Ü95].

Sambhar powder: A South Indian seasoning mixture made from asafetida, black pepper, chillies, coriander, cumin, fenugreek seeds, mustard, turmeric, peas and mung beans, it is used as a seasoning of peas and beans [→ Ü73, Ü92].

Sarawak spice mix: Made from ajowan, dried barberry fruits and turmeric, it serves as a seasoning of pilaws in the Southern parts of the Russian Federation [Ü92].

Sauce spices: As a seasoning of Hollandaise sauce, parsley, pepper, onions, and lemon peels, of Béarnaise sauce nutmeg, onions, pepper, tarragon, and lemon peels and for brown sauces allspice, bay leaves, garlic, lovage, onions, pepper, and thyme [Ü30].

Sausage spices: The composition of the seasonings vary depending on the type of sausage. Mixed spices for cooked sausages contain, among others, clove, coriander, ginger, nutmeg, paprika, and pepper, mixes for liverwurst contain first of all marjoram, further allspice, cardamom, cinnamon, ginger, mace, pepper, and thyme, mixes for blood sausage contain allspice, black pepper, clove, ginger, and marjoram, uncooked sausages are often seasoned only with pepper, but they may also contain cardamom, coriander, mace, nutmeg, and paprika [→ Ü30, Ü92].

Scappis spice mix: An old Italian seasoning mixture that contains cinnamon, clove, ginger, nutmeg, saffron, and brown sugar [→ Ü73], it serves as a seasoning of bakery goods and confectionaries as well as sweet dishes [Ü92].

Seven-spice: → Shichimi tograrashi.

Seven-seas-spice: An Indonesian and Malaysian seasoning mixture composed of cardamom, cayenne pepper, celery fruits and cinnamon, clove, coriander, and cumin, [Ü93].

Seven-pepper-spice: → Shichimi tograrashi.

Shichimi tograrashi (Schichmi tograrashi, seven-spice, seven-pepper-spice): A Japanese seasoning mixture that contains mostly black and white sesame seeds, Japanese pepper, chillies, poppy seeds, seaweed (nori) and dried tangerine peels, it serves as a seasoning of meat-, vegetable-, rice- and noodle dishes [→ Ü73, Ü92].

Shish kebab spice: → Grill spice.

Sichuan spice: A Chinese seasoning composed of 1 part Japanese pepper and 1 part salt [Ü2].

Stollen spices: Contain predominantly cinnamon, clove, ginger, and lesser galangal, as well as, among others, cardamom, mace, and nutmeg [→ Ü30].

Soup greens: Made up of fresh plant parts, mostly composed of carrots, celery root, leeks, and parsley (root and/or leaves), and commercially sold in bundles, used for the seasoning of stew dishes. The leafy material (leek, parsley) is an indicator for the freshness [Ü98].

Soup spices: Contain mainly basil, cardamom, chervil, chillies, → Curry powder, dill, garlic, lovage, nutmeg, paprika, pepper, and summer savory [Ü30].

Soy sauce: → Soybean.

Soybean pastes: Made from crushed yellow or brown soybeans, soy sauce, garlic, salt and sugar [Ü2].

Sukiyaki sauce: A seasoning made from soy sauce, sugar and rice wine [Ü51].

Tabasco sauce (Tabasco): A very hot, North American condiment, prepared by mixing hot chillies (Tabasco chillies) with salt, aged for about 3 years in oak casks, afterwards brandy vinegar is added and the mixture is filtered through a sieve. The sauce is used only in drops (!), e.g. as a seasoning of tomato juice, Bloody-Mary cocktails, jambalayas, pizzas, scrambled eggs and veal fricassee. A mild form is the green Tabasco-jalapeno-sauce, which is made from the milder jalapeno chillies [→ Ü73].

Tabil: A Tunisian seasoning mixture that contains caraway, chillies, coriander, and garlic [Ü73].

Table mustard (Mostrich, Mostert): Prepared from ground, sometimes also peeled and de-oiled seeds of Sarepta mustard, brown mustard and/or white mustard, vinegar, fruit must, wine, salt, sugar and spices including, among others, allspice, caraway, cardamom, cinnamon, clove, coriander, dill, horseradish, lovage, marjoram, nutmeg, pepper, summer savory, tarragon, thyme, and turmeric (adds color!). Special varieties include, among others, **Bavarian mustard** (Munich mustard, Sweet mustard, White sausage mustard, rich in herbs, very mild), **Bordeaux-mustard** (French specialty mustard, Tarragon mustard, dark-brown, coarse-grained, the herbal component is composed mainly of tarragon, along with sugar and vinegar, mild, sweet-sour), **Dijon mustard** (French specialty mustard, pale yellow, because the mustard seeds are peeled, contains the must of unripe grapes, vinegar, salt and spices, fruity, various classes of pungency, with extended storage becomes bitter, stored in the refrigerator after opening), **Champagne mustard** (A French specialty mustard, contains wine from champagne, mild), **Düsseldorf mustard** (Düsseldorfer Löwensenf, a German speciality, extra hot), **Moutarde au poivre vert** (French specialty mustard, contains green pepper, medium-hot), **Mostarda di frutta** (Italian specialty mustard composed of mustard seeds, honey and white wine), **English mustard** (Coleman brand, powdered form, made from the powder of white mustard and Sarepta mustard, sometimes with the addition of turmeric as a colorant component, it must be stirred with water and left to stand for about 15 minutes), and **American mustard** (light yellow, made from white mustard, sugar and wine or vinegar, mild, quite watery).

Table mustard serves as a seasoning of meat, e.g. spread onto roulade or meat prior to roasting, of meatballs, for production of mustard sauces, e.g. for cooked eggs, of Roquefort sauce, cream sauces, salad dressings, sauces for fish, dressings, vinaigrettes, marinades, mayonnaises, as a seasoning for the table, e.g. of cooked sausages, pickled pig knuckles, cold brats and sandwiches. Due to the volatility of the aromatic components, mustard should be added to taste just before serving the meal [Ü2, → Ü30, Ü59, Ü70, Ü90, for history Ü2].

- **Table spice:** A protein hydrolyzate in liquid, pasty or powder form, obtained from animal- and/or plant protein (including, among others, blood meal, meat meal, casein, yeast, wheat gluten, soybean meal, ground nut meal, cotton seed) by heating with hydrochloric acid in an autoclave followed by neutralizing with sodium carbonate, it is used as a component of vegetable-, herb- or mushroom extracts including, among others, Weizenin-spice, Bino-spice, Erwa-spice, Wawi-spice, Knorr-spice, Maggi-spice, as a seasoning and flavor enhancer [Ü92, Ü98]
- **Tahini paste:** A gray-brown, thick paste made from finely ground sesame seeds, it serves as a seasoning of noodle-, veg-etable- and rice dishes, but also of fruit plates and as a basis for salad dressings, it is eaten together with garlic and lemon as 'meze' with bread [Ü2].
- **Tai-ping China:** A Chinese spice mixture composed of the powder from chillies, → Curry powder, garlic, onions, paprika, glucose, salt and flavor enhancers, it is used as a seasoning of grilled dishes, steaks, pan-fried meats, rice- and egg dishes [Ü92].
- **Tandoori** (Tadoori): An Indian spice mixture for stews prepared in a fired clay oven (tandoor), mainly composed of cayenne pepper, coriander, cumin, garlic, ginger, and turmeric, applicable for the seasoning of rice, vegetables, poultry, fish and meat, and well suited for marinades [Ü33].
- **Tartar sauce:** A mayonnaise-like seasoning sauce that contains capers, parsley and onions, as well as, among others, pickled fruits, olives, lemon juice, suitable for seasoning of sea foods [Ü30].
- **Teriyaki sauce:** Prepared from soy sauce, wine, vinegar, sugar and spices, it is used for marinades and grilled dishes [Ü51].
- **Tika paste:** An Indian spice mixture composed of 1 part chilli powder, 1 part chopped garlic, 2 parts chopped ginger, 2 parts turmeric powder, 1 part ground pepper, and 4 parts, fresh, chopped cilantro leaves [Ü2].
- **Tofu spice:** Contains yeast extract, fennel, oregano, sesame seeds, tomatoes, wheat meal and tofu powder, used as a table spice for fried → Tofu [Ü92].
- **Tomato ketchup:** The base components are tomato puree (about 40%), vinegar, salt, starch and sugar, as a seasoning it may also contain: allspice, celery, cinnamon, clove, garlic, ginger, nutmeg, onions, and pepper. **Tomato chutney** has a similar composition, but it is more hotly seasoned. Both mixtures are used as a seasoning of briefly fried or grilled meat and fish, of cooked sausages, pizza, French fries, rice and pasta dishes [→ Ü30, Ü92, Ü98].
- **Tridschataka:** An Indian seasoning that contains ginger and black pepper, among other spices, used as a seasoning of rice dishes [Ü30].
- **Tschubritza:** A Hungarian spice mixture that contains fenugreek seeds, paprika, summer savory, roasted corn meal, and salt, used the same as → Curry powder [Ü45].
- **Vegetable spices:** For seasoning of cauliflower and broccoli, the herbs used include, among others, mace, nutmeg, parsley, and/or pepper, for beans and lentils, among others, summer savory, thyme and/or pepper, for cabbage dishes, allspice, caraway, celery, nutmeg, paprika, and/or thyme, for sauerkraut, among others, allspice, bay leaf, celery, clove, juniper berries, nutmeg, and/or onions, for mashed potatoes, caraway, chives, dill, nutmeg, onions, paprika, and/or parsley, for spinach, basil, mace, onions and/or pepper [Ü30].
- **Venison spice:** Contains allspice, bay leaves, juniper berries, pepper, and/or thyme, among others, and depending on the type of game it may also contain clove, garlic, marjoram, paprika, rosemary sage or tarragon [Ü30].
- **Vinegar spice:** Used for the production of → Seasoned vinegar with spices.
- **Worcestershire sauce:** Prepared in England according to an originally Indian recipe with vinegar, sherry, brandy, soy sauce, salt, sugar, caramel, pig's liver, shallots, tamarind sauce, malt vinegar, anchovies and incompletely declared spices, of which allspice and turmeric are components, but the exact composition is proprietary, it is used as a table spice to season sauces, soups, fish- and meat dishes [Ü55].
- **Zahtar:** A spice mixture made from Sicilian sumac, roasted sesame seeds and dried, ground thyme, it is used in Northern Africa, Turkey and Jordan as a seasoning of meat dumplings and vegetables [→ Ü74].
- **Zhug:** A pasty Yemeni spice mixture that contains cardamom, chillies, coriander, garlic, paprika, and lemon juice.

Literature references identified by Ü can be found in the general listing of books and monographs at the back of this book.

Indexes

Index of books and monographs used as general references

Ü1 Anonym, Kräuter und Gewürze. Die feine Kunst der richtigen Anwendung, Unipart-Verlag Stuttgart 1996 (Lizenzausgabe von Peter Halfar Media GmbH & Co Holding KG, Remseck 1996)

Ü2 Anonym, Kräuter und Gewürze. Ein illustrierter Führer über einheimische und exotische Gewürze, Kräuter und natürliche Aromen, Unipart-Verlag, Stuttgart 1995 (Lizenzausgabe von A. Nicholas Enterprise Book, London)

Ü3 Anonym, Kochen mit Kräutern & Gewürzen, Naumann & Göbel Verlagsgesellschaft mbH, Köln, 1990

Ü4 Anonym, Das große Lexikon der Lebensmittel, Südwest Verlag GmbH, München, 1998 (Lizenzausgabe von Les Editions Québec/Ameriqué, Montreal)

Ü5 Anonym, Enzyklopädie der Haus- und Gartenpflanzen, 8. Bde, Bechtermünz Verlag im Weltbild Verlag GmbH, Augsburg, 1996

Ü6 Anonym, Chinesische Küche, Unipart-Verlag GmbH, Remseck 1994 (Lizenzausgabe von Hilit Publishing Co. Ltd, Taipei)

Ü7 Baumgart J, Mikrobiologische Untersuchung von Lebensmitteln, Behr's Verlag, Hamburg 1993

Ü8 Belitz HD, Grosch W, Lehrbuch der Lebensmittelchemie, 4. Aufl., Springer Verlag, Berlin, Heidelberg, New York 1992

Ü9 Boldt KJ, Needon Ch, Gewürzbüchlein, Buch Verlag für die Frau GmbH, Leipzig 1997

Ü10 Bown D, DuMont's große Kräuterenzyklopädie, DuMont Buchverlag, Köln 1998

Ü11 Bowring J, Price J, Das große Buch der asiatischen Küche, Könemann Verlagsgesellschaft, Köln 1998 (Lizenzausgabe von Murdoch Books, North Sydney)

Ü12 Braun R, Standardzulassungen für Fertigarzneimittel. Ringbuch, Fortsetzungswerk, Govi-Verlag, Pharmazeutischer Verlag, Deutscher Apotheker-Verlag, Stuttgart 1986

Ü13 Bültjer U, Falken Lexikon der Gewürze, Falken Verlag, Niederhausen/Ts. 1998

Ü14 Bundessortenamt BSA, Beschreibende Sortenliste 1996, Heil- und Gewürz-pflanzen, Landbuchverlagsgesellschaft, Hannover 1996

Ü15 Bundessortenamt BSA, Beschreibende Sortenliste 1995, Wurzelgemüse, Zwiebelgemüse, Kohlgemüse, Landbuchverlagsgesellschaft-, Hannover 1995

Ü16 Bundessortenamt BSA, Beschreibende Sortenliste 1996, Fruchtgemüse, Blattgemüse, Landbuchverlagsgesellschaft, Hannover 1996

Ü17 Callery E, Das große Buch der Kräuter, Anbau, Verarbeitung und Verwendung von 50 beliebten Kräutern, Könemann Verlagsgesellschaft mbH, Köln 1997 (Lizenzausgabe von Quintet Publishing Limited, London)

Ü18 Carter G, Das Garten-Praxisbuch Kräuter, Bertelmanns Club GmbH, Rheda-Wiedenbrück 1997 (Lizenzausgabe von Ryland Peters & Small, London)

Ü19 Clevely, A, Richmond K, Dumont's grosses Kräuterbuch, Dumonts Buchverlag, Köln 1994 (Lizenzausgabe von Anness Publishing Limited, London)

Ü20 Craze R, Gewürze, das Handbuch für Genießer, Benedikt Taschen Verlag, Köln 1999 (Lizenzausgabe von Quintet Publishing Limited)

Ü21 Dachler M, Pelzmann H, Arznei- und Gewürzpflanzen, Anbau, Ernte, Aufbereitung, Österreichischer Agrarverlag, Klosterneuburg 1999

Ü22 Erhard et al. (Hrsg.), Zander Handwörterbuch der Pflanzennamen, 17. Aufl., Ulmer Verlag, Stuttgart, 2002

Ü23 Ettl A, Ideenreich kochen, Kräuter & Gewürze, Sirius, Künzelsau, keine Jahresangabe

Ü24 Fey H, Otte I, Wörterbuch der Kosmetik, 4. Aufl., Wissenschaftliche Verlagsgesellschaft mbH, Stuttgart 1997

Ü25 Fischer R, Praktikum der Pharmakognosie, Springer Verlag, Wien 1952

Ü26 Franke G, Nutzpflanzen der Tropen und Subtropen, 3 Bde, 2. Aufl, Hirzel Verlag, Leipzig 1975

Ü27 Frohne D, Pfänder HJ, Giftpflanzen. Ein Handbuch für Apotheker, Ärzte, Toxikologen und Biologen, 4. Aufl, Wissenschaftliche Verlagsgesellschaft mbH, Stuttgart 1997

Ü28 Garcke A, Illustrierte Flora, 23. Aufl., Verlag Paul Parey, Berlin, Hamburg 1997

Ü29 Gassner G, Mikroskopische Untersuchung pflanzlicher Nahrungs- und Genussmittel, Fischer Verlag, Jena 1931

Ü30 Gerhardt U, Gewürze in der Lebensmittelindustrie: Eigenschaften – Technologien – Verwendung, 2. Aufl., B. Behr's Verlag, Hamburg 1994

Ü31 Gildemeister E, Hoffmann F, Hrsg.: Treibs W, Bournot W, Die ätherischen Öle, Bde 4 bis 7, Akademie-Verlag, Berlin, 1956–1961

Ü32 Greiner K et al., Der große Ratgeber Garten, Balkon- und Kübelpflanzen, ADAC Verlag GmbH, München 1995

Ü33 Grosser W, Mein Kräutergarten, Trautwein Garten-Edition, Compact Verlag, München 2000

Ü34 Habersbrunner F, Aroma-Drinks, köstliche Mixgetränke mit ätherischen Ölen, Joy-Verlag, Sulzberg 1994

Ü35 Hahn H, Michaelsen I, Mikroskopische Diagnostik pflanzlicher Nahrungs-, Genuß- und Futtermittel einschließlich Gewürze, Springer Verlag, Berlin, Heidelberg, New York, 1996

Ü36 Hall G, Siewek F, Gerhardt U, Handbuch der Aromen und Gewürze, B. Behr's Verlag, Hamburg, 1999

Ü37 Hänsel R et al.(Hrsg.), Hagers Handbuch der pharmazeutischen Praxis, Drogen, Bde. 4 bis 6, Folgegbde. 2 und 3, Springer Verlag, Berlin, Heidelberg, New York (1992–1998)

Ü38 Hänsel R, Sticher O, Steinegger E, Pharmakognosie, Phytopharmazie, Springer-Verlag, Berlin, Heidelberg, New York 1999

Ü39 Hausen BM, Nothdurft H, Allergiepflanzen-Pflanzenallergene, Handbuch und Atlas der allergie-induzierenden Wild- und Kulturpflanzen. Kontaktallergene, ecomed, Landsberg, München 1988

Ü40 Hauser H (redaktioneller Bearbeiter), Deutsches Lebensmittelbuch, Leitsätze, Bundesanzeiger Verlagsgesellschaft, Köln 2000

Ü41 Heeger EF, Handbuch des Arznei- und Gewürzpflanzenanbaus, Drogengewinnung, Deutscher Bauernverlag, Berlin 1965

Ü42 Hegi G, Illustrierte Flora von Mittel-Europa, 1. Aufl., 1909–1931, 2. Aufl. 1936, 3. Aufl. 1966 begonnen, Carl Hauser Verlag, München 1909

Ü43 Hegnauer R, Chemotaxonomie der Pflanzen, Bde. 1–11, Birkhäuser Verlag, Basel, Stuttgart, 1962–2001

Ü44 Hiller K, Melzig MF, Lexikon der Arzneipflanzen, 2 Bde., Spektrum Akademischer Verlag, Heidelberg, Berlin 1999

Ü45 Hlava B, Lánská D, Küchenkräuter, Karl Müller-Verlag, Erlangen 1995

Ü46 Hohenberger E, Gewürze und Küchenkräuter aus dem eigenen Garten, Naturbuch-Verlag, Augsburg 1999

Ü47 Holt G, Kräuter – In Garten und Küche – Für Gesundheit und Schönheit – Als Duft und Dekoration, Kaleidoskop Buch im Christian Verlag, München 1997

Ü48 Jackson BP, Snowdon DW, Atlas of Microscopy of Medicinal Plants, Culinary Herbs and Spices, Belhaven Press, A Division of Pinter Publisher, London 1990

Ü49 Karsten G et al., Lehrbuch der Pharmakognosie, 9. Aufl, VEB Gustav Fischer Verlag, Jena 1962

Ü50 Karsten G, Weber U, Lehrbuch der Pharmakognosie für Hochschulen, 7. Aufl., Verlag von Gustav Fischer, Jena 1949

Ü51 Kellermann M, Kräuter, Gewürze. Die kleine Schule, Verlag Zabert Sandmann GmbH, München 1999

Ü52 Kettenring M, Aromaküche im Rhythmus der Jahreszeiten, AT-Verlag, Aarau 1997

Ü53 Koch S, Bassermann-Handbuch Gewürze und Kräuter, Bassermann'sche Verlagsbuchhandlung, Niederhausen/Ts. 1996

Ü54 Lafer, J, Johann Lafer kocht mit Kräutern und Gewürzen, Falken-Verlag, Niederhausen/Ts. 1997

Ü55 Lambert Ortiz E, Gewürze, Kräuter und Essenzen, Christian Verlag, München 1993 (Lizenzausgabe von Dorling Kindersley Ltd., London)

Ü56 Laux HE et al., Gewürzpflanzen anbauen, ernten, verwenden, Franckh-Kosmos, Stuttgart 1993

Ü57 Lechthaler E, Kräuterdrinks mit und ohne Alkohol, Walter Hädecke Verlag, Weil der Stadt 1995

Ü58 Lewin L, Gifte und Vergiftungen – Lehrbuch der Toxikologie, 6. Aufl., Nachdruck der Originalausgabe von 1929 Karl F Haug Verlag, Heidelberg 1992

Ü59 Linde G, Linde E, Von Anis bis Zimt. Kleine Gewürzfibel, Verlag für die Frau, Leipzig 1972

Ü60 List PH et al. (Hrsg.), Hagers Handbuch der Pharmazeutischen Praxis, 4. Aufl., Bde I bis VIII, Springer-Verlag, Berlin, Heidelberg, New York 1967–1980

Ü61 Mansfeld R, Verzeichnis landwirtschaftlicher und gärtnerischer Kulturpflanzen (ohne Zierpflanzen), Bde. 1–4, 2. Aufl. herausgegeben von J. Schulze-Motel, Akademie-Verlag, Berlin 1986

Ü62 Matissek R, Wittkowski R, High Performance Liquid Chromatography in Food Control and Research, Behr's Verlag, Hamburg 1992

Ü63 Mayr C, Gewürzfibel, Bechtermünz Verlag im Weltbild Verlag GmbH Augsburg 1996 (Lizenzausgabe von Athesia Verlagsanstalt Ges.mbH, Bozen)

Ü64 McHoy P, Westland P, Die Kräuterbibel, Könemann Verlagsgesellschaft, Köln 1998 (Lizenzausgabe von Quarto Publishing plc, London)

Ü65 McLeod M, Handbook of Herbs, Growing, Cooking, Health, etc., Elliot Right Way Books, Brighton 1976

Ü66 McVicar J, Der große Kräuterführer, Karl Müller Verlag, Erlangen 1997 (Lizenzausgabe von Kyle Cathie Ltd., London)

Ü67 Michalak PS, Kräuter, leicht anbauen und gesund genießen, Bechtermünz Verlag im Weltbild Verlag GmbH, Augsburg 1998 (Lizenzausgabe von Weldon Owen Pty Ltd.)

Ü68 Morris S, Mackley L, Das kulinarische Handbuch der Gewürze, Christian Verlag, München 1999 (Lizenzausgabe von Anness Publishing Ltd., London)

Ü69 Müller G, Grundlagen der Lebensmittelmikrobiologie, VEB Fachbuchverlag, Leipzig 1989

Ü70 Nerger J, Alles mit Kräutern. Würzen. Heilen. Genießen. Weltbild Buchverlag, Augsburg 1998

Ü71 Neuhold M, Gewürze aus dem eigenen Garten: Anbau, Ernte, Verwendung, Leopold Stocker Verlag, Graz 1998

Ü72 Neumann R et al., Sensorische Lebensmitteluntersuchung, Fachbuchverlag, Leipzig 1991

Ü73 Norman J, Das grosse Buch der Gewürze, Verlag Das Beste, Stuttgart, Zürich, Wien 1996 (Lizenzausgabe von Dorling Kindersley Ltd., London)

Ü74 Norman J, Klassische Kräuterküche, AT Verlag, Aarau/Schweiz 1998 (Lizenzausgabe von Dorling Kinersley Ltd., London)

Ü75 Obermair/Schneider, Haltbar machen – Gemüse – Kräuter – Pilze, Leopold Stocker Verlag, Graz, Stuttgart 1997

Ü76 Pabst G (Hrsg.), Köhler's Medizinalpflanzenatlas, Gera-Untermhaus, 1887–1898, Reprintausgabe, Bechtermünz-Verlag im Weltbild Verlag, Augsburg 1997

Ü77 Pachaly P, DC-Atlas, Wissenschaftliche Verlagsgesellschaft mbH, Stuttgart 1991

Ü78 Pahlow M, Gewürze – Genuß und Arznei, 2. Aufl Apotheker-Verlag, Stuttgart 1995

Ü79 Painter G, A Herb Cookbook, Hodder and Stoughton, Auckland 1983

Ü80 Pini U, Das Gourmethandbuch, Könemann Verlagsgesellschaft, Köln 2000

Ü81 Pochljobkin WW, Alles über Gewürze, Arten – Eigenschaften – Verwendung, Verlag MIR Moskau, VEB Fachbuchverlag, Leipzig 1977

Ü82 Rehm S, Espig G, Die Kulturpflanzen der Tropen und Subtropen, Verlag Eugen Ulmer, Stuttgart 1996

Ü83 Risch SJ, Ho ChT, Spices – Flavor Chemistry and Antioxidant Properties, ACS Symposium Series 660, American Chemical Society, Washington, DC 1997

Ü84 Roth L et al., Giftpflanzen-Pflanzengifte, Nikol Verlagsgesellschaft mbH & Co. KG, Hamburg 1994

Ü85 Rothmaler W, Exkursionsflora, Band 4: Kritischer Band, Volk und Wissen Volkseigener Verlag, Berlin 1988

Ü86 Rüegg, K, Feißt, WO, Großmutters Kräuterküche, Müller Rüschlikon Verlags AG, Cham 1997

Ü87 Saller R, Feiereis H (Hrsg.), Erweiterte Schulmedizin, Bd. 1, Beiträge zur Phytotherapie, Hans Marseille Verlag GmbH, München 1993

Ü88 Schinharl C, Italien. Die neue große Schule, Bechtermünz Verlag im Weltbild Verlag GmbH, Augsburg 2000

Ü89 Schröder R, Kaffee, Tee und Kardamom. Tropische Genußmittel und Gewürze. Geschichte, Verbreitung, Anbau, Ernte, Aufbereitung, Ulmer-Verlag, Stuttgart 1991

Ü90 Schubeck A, Alfons Schubecks feine Gewürz- und Kräuterküche, Verlag Zabert Sandmann GmbH, München 1999

Ü91 Schwinghammer H, Ehrenreich P, Heilgewürze und Kräuter, Weltbild Buchverlag, Augsburg 1999

Ü92 Seidemann J, Würzmittel-Lexikon, B. Behr's Verlag, Hamburg 1997

Ü93 Siewek F, Exotische Gewürze, Birkhäuser Verlag, Basel 1990

Ü94 Staesche K, Gewürze, in Handbuch der Lebensmittelchemie, Bd. VI, Springer-Verlag, Berlin, Heidelberg, New York, 1970, S.426–610

Ü95 Stegmann A (Redaktion), Kochen mit Kräutern und Gewürzen, Naumann und Göbel Verlagsgesellschaft, Köln, keine Jahresangabe

Ü96 Stein B, Stein S, Der große Ratgeber Garten: Gemüse und Kräuter, ADAC Verlag GmbH München 1995, Bd. 2

Ü97 Swahn JÖ, Gewürzkunde. Über Ursprung, Geschichte und Verwendung von Gewürzen in aller Welt, Orbis Verlag 1991 (Lizenzausgabe des AB Nordbok, Götheburg)

Ü98 Täufel A et. al. (Hrsg.), Lebensmittellexikon, Behr's Verlag, Hamburg 1993, Nachdruck 1998

Ü99 Teuscher E, Biogene Arzneimittel, 5. Aufl., Wissenschaftliche Verlagsgesellschaft mbH, Stuttgart 1997

Ü100 Teuscher E, Lindequist U, Biogene Gifte, Biologie, Chemie, Pharmakologie, 2. Aufl., Fischer Verlag, Stuttgart 1994

Ü101 Wagner H et al., Drogenanalyse. Dünnschichtchromatographische Analyse von Arzneidrogen, Springer-Verlag, Berlin, Heidelberg, New York 1983

Ü102 Wagner H, Bladt S, Plant Drug Analysis – A Thin Layer Chromatography Atlas, sec. Ed , Springer-Verlag, Berlin, Heidelberg, New York 1995

Ü103 Wagner H, Wiesenauer M, Phytotherapie – Phytopharmaka und pflanzliche Homöopathika, Gustav Fischer Verlag, Stuttgart, Jena, New York 1995

Ü104 Werner M, Kochen mit ätherischen Ölen, Verlag Gräfe und Unzer, München 1995

Ü105 Werner M, Ätherische Öle. Duftende Heilpflanzen-Essenzen zum Helfen und Heilen, Pflegen und Wohlfühlen, zum Würzen und Aromatisieren, Gräfe und Unzer GmbH, München 1999

Ü106 Wichtl M (Hrsg.), Teedrogen und Phytopharmaka, 3. Aufl., Wissenschaftliche Verlagsgesellschaft, Stuttgart. 1997

Ü107 Wilson A, Feine Kräuterküche, Könemann Verlagsgesellschaft mbH, Köln 1997 (Lizenzausgabe von Murdoch Books, North Sydney)

Ü108 Wilson A, Richtig gut kochen mit Kräutern und Gewürzen, Könemann Verlagsgesellschaft, Köln 1998 (Lizenzausgabe von Murdoch Books, North Sydney)

Ü109 Winnington U, Kleines Würzbuch für Kinder, Der Kinderbuchverlag, Berlin 1987

Ü110 Wittkowski R, Matissek R, Capillary Gas Chromatography in Food Control and Research, Behr's Verlag, Hamburg 1992

Ü111 Zittlau, J, Die besten Rezepte aus der Gewürzküche, Südwest-Verlag GmbH & Co. KG, München 1997.

Subject Index

Monograph titles as well as the extended chapters in the general section are shown in **bold face**.

Scientific botanical names are shown in *italics*.

Terms marked with an asterisk * refer to formulas (chemical structure diagrams).

The Latin and English names for the medicinally used herbal drugs are rendered just as they appear in the corresponding pharmacopoeial monographs.

The Subject Index includes only those chemical constituents that contribute to odor, taste and color (e.g. components of essential oils, pungent compounds, bitter substances, coloring matters), as well as to pharmacological or toxicological action.

Secondary entries of constituent groups are only made under primary entries, e.g. specific herbs, if further data on the components of these groups can be found on the indicated page(s).

A

A.1. Sauce   430
Aalkraut   372
Abrahamsstrauch   296
Abrotani herba   359
Abrotone   357
Absinthin   245*, 245
Acafraosamen   69
Acetaldehyde   175
Acetic acid   278, 389
Acetoin   278
Acetoxy-1,8-cineole   223
1′-Acetoxychavicol   223
Acetoxychavicol acetate   222*, 222
4-[(4′-O-Acetyl-α–rhamnosyloxy)ben-zyl]isothiocyanate   200
2-Acetyl-1-pyrroline   344
Acetyleugenol   10*, 138, 139f.
2-Acetylfuran   389, 390*
Acetylintermedine   89
Acetyllycopsamine   89
Acetylpyrazine   344
Ach(i)ote   67
Achiote tree   67
Achiotti semen   69
Acid amides of Piper-species   10
α-Acids   193f.
β-Acids   193f.
δ-Acids   193
Iso-α-Acids   193
Ackerminze   240
Acridone alkaloids   313f.
Acrodiclidium puchury-major   252
Adaptation   15
Adenosine   175
Adhumulone   193, 193*
Adjowan   51
Adlupulone   193, 193*
Adshika paste   430
Aetheroleum Aurantii floris   129
– Carvi   98
– Juniperi   208
Aframomum angustifolium   103
– *daniellii*   103
– *korarima*   103
– *meleguta*   189
– *exscapum*   190

Agastache foeniculum   65
– *mexicana*   216
– *rugosa*   65
Agathophyllum aromaticum   252
Ague tree   337
Ail   173
– blanc   173
– des bois   303
– des ours   303
– fistuleux   340
– stérile   348
Ají   281
Ajipfeffer   281
Ajmud   53
Ajoene   175, 304, 304*
(E)-Ajoene   11*
Ajoenes   175, 175*
Ajowain   51
– seed   51
Ajowainkümmel   51
Ajowan   51
–, essential oil   52
– fruits   51
– oil   52
– oleoresin   52
Ajowankümmel   51
Alcea rosea   322
Aligatorpfeffer   189
Alkamides   293, 295
Alkanna tinctoria   322
– *tuberculata*   322
Alkanna red   322
Alkanna root   322
Alkannin   322
Alkene-thiosulfinate   175*
Alk(en)yl-alkane   175*
Alk(en)yl-alkane/alkenethiosulfinate   10*
Alk(en)ylsulfenic acids   10*
n-Alkylphenols   299
Alliaceous oils   115f., 175, 211, 263, 265, 304, 349
–, Definition   7
–, Structure   7
Allicin   11*, 175, 304
Alligator pepper   189
Alligatorpfeffer   189
Allii ascalonici bulbus   350

– cepae bulbus   265
– sativi aetheroleum   179
– sativi bulbi pulvis   179
– sativi bulbus recens   179
– ursini bulbus   305
– ursini herba   305
Alliin   176f., 304, 304*
(+)-Alliin   11*
Alliins   10*, 115f., 175, 211, 263, 304, 341, 349
Allium ampeloprasum   210
– – var. *porrum*   210
– *angolense*   350
– *angulosum*   116
– *ascalonicum*   348
– *bakeri*   116
– *cepa* var. *aggregatum*   348
– – var. *ascalonicum*   348
– – var. *cepa*   261
– – var. *viviparum*   350
– *cernuum*   266
– *chinense*   116f.
– *fistulosum*   350, 416
– *giganteum*   266
– *grayi*   266
– *kurrat*   116
– *longicuspis*   179
– *macrostemon*   179
    obliquum   179
– *porrum* var. *porrum*   210
– – var. *sectivum*   265
– × *proliferum*   350
– *ramosum*   116
– *sativum*   173
– – var. *ophioscordum*   173
– – var. *pekinense*   173
– *schoenoprasum*   114
– – var. *schoenoprasum*   114
– – var. *sibiricum*   114
– – × *Allium sativum*   116
– *scorodoprasum*   116
– *senescens*   116
– *stipitatum*   265
– *suvorovii*   266
– *tuberosum*   116f.
– *ursinum*   303
Allium-fistulosum whole plant   342
Allium-porrum whole plant   212

Allium-schoenoprasum leaves   116
Allspice   54
–, Brazil   57
–, crown   56
–, essential oil   55
–, flavonoids   56
–, Mexican   57
– oil   55, 56
– oleoresin   55
–, Spanish   57
–, tannins   56
Allylalcohol   212
4-Allylanisol   121
S-Allylcysteine   178
S-Allyl-L-cysteine sulfoxide   116, 175, 304*, 341
1-Allyl-2,4-dimethoxybenzene   9*, 112
Allylisothiocyanate   198, 198*, 334
Allylmercaptan   175
Allyl-methane-thiosulfinate   116f., 304, 304*
Allyl-prop-1-enethiosulfinate   211
Allyl-prop-2-enethiosulfinate   175, 304, 304*
Allyl mustard oil   198, 200, 334f.
Almond biscuit spice   430
Aloysia citriodora   218
– *triphylla*   218
Aloysiae citriodorae aetheroleum   220
Aloysie   218
Alpine wormwood   246
Alpinia galanga   223
– *malaccensis*   221
– *officinarum*   221
– *speciosa*   223
Alpinol   222
Althaein   322
Amabiline   89
Amatisa   281
Amber fenugreek   162
Ammei, Ägyptischer   51
Ammi de l'Inde   51
Amomi fructus   56
Amomum aromaticum   103
– *cardamomum*   100, 103
– *compactum*   103
– *globosum*   103
– *kepulaga*   103

Photo Credits

Herbal drug photographs:

Prof. Dr. E. Teuscher,   All (89)
Triebes

Plant photographs:

A. Bärtels,   *Cinnamomum verum*
Waake   *Sassafras albidum*

Dr. M. Börnchen,   *Crocus sativus*
Drensteinfurt

Th. Brendler,   *Pimenta dioica*
Berlin

Dr. W. Buff,   *Alpinia officinarum*
Biberach/Riß

B. Ernst,   *Bixa orellana*
Basel   *Curcuma domestica*
                 Elettaria cardamomum
                 Piper nigrum
                 Zingiber officinale

H. E. Laux,   *Angelica archangelica*
Biberach/Riß   *Allium cepa* var *ascalonicum*
                   Allium porrum (2)
                   Allium schoenoprasum
                   Allium ursinum
                   Aloysia triphylla
                   Anethum graveolens
                   Anthriscus cerefolium
                   Apium graveolens (2)
                   Artemisia vulgaris
                   Borago officinalis
                   Capsicum annuum
                   Citrus medica
                   Coriandrum sativum
                   Cuminum cyminum
                   Ferula assa-foetida
                   Juniperus communis (2)
                   Laurus nobilis
                   Lepidium sativum
                   Mentha × *piperita*
                   Ocimum basilicum
                   Origanum vulgare
                   Petroselinum crispum, flat-leaf

Pimpinella anisum
Sanguisorba minor
Satureja hortensis
Tanacetum vulgare
Thymus vulgaris

Prof. Dr. P. Schönfelder,
Ingrid Schönfelder,
Pentling

Capparis spinosa
Citrus aurantium
Citrus limon
Mentha pulegium
Myristica fragrans (2)
Nigella sativa
Olea europaea (2)
Rhus corariu
Schinus terebinthifolius
Sesamum indicum

Doz. Dr. Th. Schöpke,
Salzgitter-Ringelheim

Cymbopogon citratus
Vanilla planifolia

Prof. Dr. E. Teuscher,

Allium cepa
Allium fistulosum
Allium sativum
Armoracia rusticana
Artemisia abrotanum
Artemisia dracunculus
Brassica juncea
Carum carvi
Foeniculum vulgare
Galium odoratum
Glycine max
Humulus lupulus
Hyssopus officinalis
Levisticum officinale
Melissa officinalis
Mentha spicata
Monarda didyma
Myrrhis odorata
Nasturtium officinale
Origanum majorana
Petroselinum crispum, curled
Ruta graveolens
Salvia officinalis
Sinapis alba
Trachyspermum ammi
Trigonella foenum-graecum
Tropaeolum majus

Prof. Dr. M. Wichtl, Mödling

Syzygium aromaticum

Dr. E. Yamasaki,
Hiroshima

Illicium verum
Tamarindus indica
Zanthoxylum piperitum